NEUROSCIENCE – DEALING WITH FRONTIERS

Edited by **Carlos M. Contreras**

Neuroscience – Dealing with Frontiers
Edited by Carlos M. Contreras

Published by InTech
Janeza Trdine 9, 51000 Rijeka, Croatia

Publishing Process Manager Silvia Vlase

Technical Editor Teodora Smiljanic

Cover Designer InTech Design Team

Additional hard copies can be obtained from orders@intechopen.com

Neuroscience – Dealing with Frontiers, Edited by Carlos M. Contreras
p. cm.
ISBN 978-953-51-0207-6

For EU product safety concerns:
IN TECH d.o.o., Prolaz Marije Krucifikse Kozulić 3, 51000 Rijeka, Croatia,
info@intechopen.com or visit our website at intechopen.com.

Meet the editor

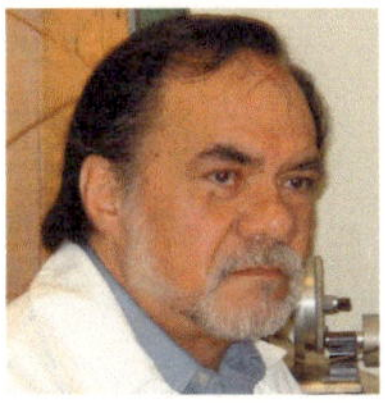

Dr Carlos M. Contreras is a Senior Researcher at the Biomedical Research Institute, National Autonomous University of Mexico (UNAM), Titular Professor of Experimental Clinical Medicine and Pharmacology at the Universidad Veracruzana, and member of the National Researchers System in México. Dr Contreras is a Medical Doctor and Doctor of Sciences at UNAM where he has taught Physiological Psychology for the past three decades. His first studies at the Neurology and Neurosurgery Institute in México involved the pharmacology of sleep, epilepsy, and drug dependence. He later received training in Biological Psychiatry in Mexico and Experimental Psychology at the University of Wisconsin, Madison, USA. During the past 30 years, he has been studying and continuously publishing his results on the neurophysiology, neurochemistry, and ethology of affective disorders and anxiety and more recently the neurobiology of mother-infant linkage processes.

Contents

Preface

Scientific advances are products of the intellectual human effort and a creative activity directed at obtaining knowledge. From the legacy of Ionian culture more than 2000 years ago, with the exception of a long period of interruption that ended with the Renaissance, knowledge based on experimental approaches accumulated such that the ability of humans to store and understand all of the information they receive is almost impossible. The divisions of the sciences thus emerge as exact sciences that comprise social sciences, humanities, and many other disciplines. Is there such a thing as an inexact science? Maybe. But perhaps it is not science. The neurosciences are no exception, denoted by the plural use of the word. Why not conceive neuronal science and behavioral science as a whole? Any division is artificial because functional and even pathological events occur simultaneously in organisms that have evolved with the development of a nervous system. Organisms, in turn, are simultaneously influenced by environmental, social, and cultural phenomena. Therefore, when the aim is to understand the functional processes of the nervous system, attempting to integrate knowledge from several points of view is necessary, eliminating some of the artificial frontiers constructed in the first half of the 20th century and incorporating as many sources of knowledge as possible into the science of the nervous system and behavior. There in one main goal: to understand the natural laws of nervous system function. We cannot invent these laws. They already exist, but we want to identify their rules of operation. The first scientists called themselves "Physiologists." They purported to know how things and the universe work. The authors of the chapters in this book can also be considered physiologists. From different points of view, they attempt to understand the operation of the nervous system under conditions of both health and illness.

The diverse topics contained in this book are grouped by several aspects, from the phenomena that underlie neuronal communication and signaling to how the first affective linkages are established between mammals. In the chapters that deal with homeostatic processes, inflammation is a central topic. Inflammation has long been considered a restorative process that follows trauma, but pain may also be considered an inseparable partner of inflammation that serves as a danger signal. Alcoholism is the most frequently abused, legal drug. To date, its physiopathology is only partially understood. Lastly, around the second half of the 20th century, medical students learned little about chronic degenerative illnesses and the processes that underlie learning and memory. Certainly, human longevity has increased, increasing the prevalence of previously scarce illnesses that affect memory. Unsurprising is the incidence of people who suffer from Parkinson's disease and Alzheimer's disease, illnesses that typically affect individuals in their sixth decade of life. Today, octogenarians are common. The reasonable goal of humans is to live as many healthy years as possible, with the functional cognitive capacity and autonomy to leave this world without becoming a nuisance and endure as little suffering as possible. The venerable old man and woman in antiquity often became a considerable charge for their family when they became ill. It is better to become grandfathers and grandmothers who recount stories, provide advice and orientation, and generously share their experiences every day. But such a life is only possible if one is healthy.

Common denominators of the chapters in this book are the ancient concept of physiology and natural selection. All species possess some form of organization of the nervous system, from coelenterates to mammals, and they have inhabited this planet for thousands or even millions of years. But the natural laws that permit adaptation and survival are only partially known. All of the chapters in this book make contributions in this sense. As scientists, we search for the rules that govern the natural strategies that allow individuals and the species to survive from the viewpoint of the science of the nervous system, unencumbered by frontiers.

Dr. Carlos M. Contreras
Biomedical Research Institute,
National Autonomous University of Mexico,
at Unit Xalapa, Neuroethology Institute,
University of Veracruz,
Mexico

1

Adrenaline and Noradrenaline: Partners and Actors in the Same Play

Vera Marisa Costa[1], Félix Carvalho[1],
Maria Lourdes Bastos[1], Rui Albuquerque Carvalho[2],
Márcia Carvalho[1,3] and Fernando Remião[1]
[1]*REQUIMTE - Toxicology Laboratory, Department of Biologic Sciences, Pharmacy Faculty, University of Porto,*
[2]*Neurosciences Center of Coimbra, Department of Biochemistry, Faculty of Sciences and Technology, University of Coimbra,*
[3]*CEBIMED, Faculty of Health Sciences, University Fernando Pessoa,*
Portugal

1. Introduction

1.1 An overview on the role of catecholamines: Basic physiology and pharmacology

Tremendous advances in the knowledge of catecholamines occurred in the last century, namely the discovery of their chemical structure, the notion of adrenoceptors by Ahlquist or the characterization of (at least in part) their transduction pathways. General concepts related to catecholamines, namely their synthesis, storage, reuptake, release, action termination, the adrenergic receptors, and their transduction pathways will be approached in this chapter. Additionally, the levels of catecholamines and metabolites found in human plasma and urine will be briefly addressed. Special focus will be given to adrenaline (ADR) and noradrenaline (NA) since they are the main actors of the human adaptation to the environment. ADR and NA are responsible for the cross talk between the sympathetic nervous system (and central nervous system) and adrenal medulla.

2. Historic introduction and background

In 1856, Vulpian applied a solution of ferric chloride to slices of adrenal glands and noticed that the medulla stained green while the cortex did not. He also observed that the same reaction occurred in samples of venous blood leaving the adrenal, but not in the arterial blood entering the gland. To account for these observations, Vulpian assumed that the medulla synthesized a substance that was released into the circulation (Vulpian, 1856). In 1895, Oliver and Schäfer demonstrated the first pharmacological action of catecholamines when they showed that the administration of extracts of adrenal gland led to the rise of arterial blood pressure (Oliver and Schäfer, 1895).

In 1897, Abel and Crawford obtained a compound that they called "epinephrin" (Abel and Crawford, 1897). The mono-benzoyl derivative isolated was however less active than the crude extracts, so the quest for the bioactive compound continued. In 1901, Takamine, an industrial chemist, isolated the active principle, then named "adrenalin" (Takamine, 1902) (Figure 1). Takamine's notation was adopted by the Europeans but not by North American researchers, thus resulting in the different nomenclature of both sides of the Atlantic Ocean.

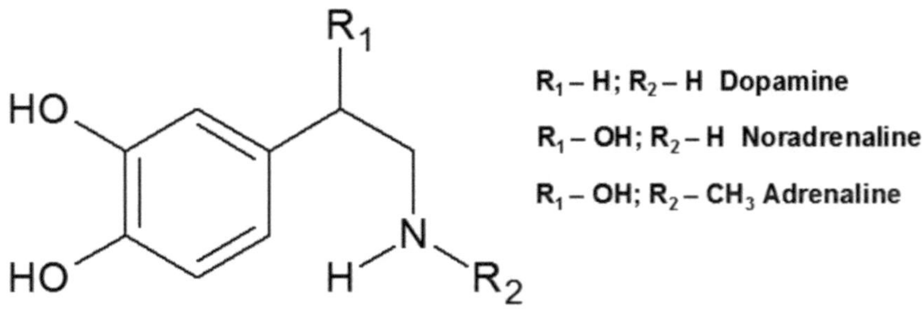

Fig. 1. Chemical structures of biogenic catecholamines.

Catecholamines soon became the centre of one of the most endurable and passionate scientific discussions, with tremendous breakthroughs that crossed the twentieth century. When reporting to catecholamines, under the general heading are NA (also known as norepinephrine), the principal transmitter of sympathetic postganglionic fibres and certain tracts of the central nervous system; dopamine, a known transmitter of the mammalian nigrostriatal, mesocortical, and mesolimbic neuronal pathways; and ADR (also known as epinephrine), the major hormone of the adrenal medulla. Collectively, these three amines are called biogenic catecholamines (Westfall and Westfall, 2006) and are involved in the regulation of motor coordination, learning and memory, sleep-wake cycle regulation, as well as in endocrine and visceral functions (Wevers et al., 1999).

3. Structure and main location of catecholamine-releasing sites

NA, ADR, and dopamine are known as catecholamines, as they contain a catechol moiety, an amine side-chain and they are all derived from the amino acid tyrosine (Westfall and Westfall, 2006, Baynes and Dominiczak, 2007, Rang et al., 2007) (Figure 1). Catecholamines share with 5-hydroxytryptamine (5-HT; serotonin) the amino side chain and altogether are known as biogenic amines. Similar compounds, like isoproterenol (previously isoprenaline), a synthetic derivative of NA, are catecholamines but not biogenic amines (Rang et al., 2007).

Although many before postulated it, von Euler was the first to show that NA was the main neurotransmitter in the sympathetic nervous system (von Euler, 1946). Sympathetic nerves arise from the spinal cord and run to the ganglia situated close to it; from those ganglia the postganglionic noradrenergic nerves run to the target tissues. Stimulation of the sympathetic nerves is inseparable from the "fight or flight" response, which results in the secretion of corticosteroids by the adrenal cortex and the release of ADR and NA by the adrenal medulla and sympathetic nerves (Wang et al., 1999, Baynes and Dominiczak, 2007). Together with ADR and corticosteroids, NA helps to coordinate different body part responses for adaptation to a stressful situation. The main function of NA is to orchestrate the response of the body to stress culminating in increased heart rate and blood pressure, and enhanced energy mobilization and neural reflexes (Wang et al., 1999, Westfall and Westfall, 2006).

NA is a neurotransmitter found in the peripheral and central nervous system, where it regulates a numerous assortment of physiological processes that include mood, arousal, learning and memory, blood flow, and metabolism (Axelrod and Kopin, 1969, Xu et al., 2000, Nolte, 2009). As a central nervous system neurotransmitter, NA is synthesized primarily in the brainstem *nuclei locus ceruleus* and *subceruleus*, which project rostrally to virtually every region of the midbrain and forebrain, dorsoventrally to the cerebellum, and caudally to lumbar segments of the spinal cord (Wang et al., 1999, Westfall and Westfall, 2006, Nolte, 2009). Additionally, the A1, C1, A2, C2, C3, A4, A5, and A7 noradrenergic cell groups also provide projections into the brain. Noradrenergic projections are identified in virtually every region of the midbrain, forebrain and cerebellum (Nolte, 2009). In the peripheral nervous system, NA is synthesized and released from sympathetic neurons connected to a wide variety of endocrine organs and other tissues (Axelrod and Kopin, 1969, Wang et al., 1999, Nolte, 2009). This extensive projection pattern throughout the neuroaxis defines NA as a general regulator of neurotransmission. NA is directly involved in mood stabilization, sleep regulation, aggression and in the general degree of alertness and arousal. NA is also involved in the central control over the endocrine and autonomic nervous systems (Wang et al., 1999, Westfall and Westfall, 2006, Nolte, 2009).

Although generally treated only as an endocrine hormone, ADR also acts as a neurotransmitter released in central and peripheral adrenergic neurons (Loewi, 1936, Jarrott, 1970, Fuller, 1982). Indeed, Loewi demonstrated the presence of an "acceleranstoff" released from sympathetic neurons that innervated the heart of frogs (Loewi, 1921), later found to be ADR (Loewi, 1936, Azuma et al., 1965, Norberg and McIsaac, 1967). The presence of ADR in the mammalian central nervous system was recognized both in biochemical and neuroanatomical studies (Lew et al., 1977, Pendleton et al., 1978, Moore and Bloom, 1979, Armstrong et al., 1982, Goodchild et al., 1984). The existence and function of only ADR-synthesizing neurons are not without controversy (Mefford, 1987). The confirmation of specific neurons in the central nervous system that contain ADR occurred after the development of sensitive enzymatic assays and immunocytochemical staining techniques for phenylethanolamine N-methyltransferase (PNMT), the enzyme responsible for the synthesis of ADR (Axelrod, 1962, Lew et al., 1977, Pendleton et al., 1978). Subsequently, neuroanatomical studies using antibodies against PNMT showed the presence of ADR-synthesizing neurons in the C1, C2, and C3 cell groups of the *medulla oblongata* and the *nucleus tractus solitarii* in multiple species (Goodchild et al., 1984, Carlton et al., 1987, Carlton et al., 1991), including humans (Burke et al., 1986, Halliday et al., 1988, Kitahama et al., 1988). Many other studies have shown the existence of adrenergic neurons in the medullar reticular formation that make restricted connections to a few pontine and diencephalic *nuclei*, eventually coursing as far rostrally as the paraventricular nucleus of the dorsal midline thalamus (Armstrong et al., 1982, Chamba and Renaud, 1983, Goodchild et al., 1984, Ross et al., 1984b, Stolk et al., 1984, Bloom, 2006). It is recognized nowadays that ADR synthesizing neurons are involved in cardiovascular homeostasis in both physiological and pathophysiological conditions (Moore and Bloom, 1979, Goodchild et al., 1984, Reis et al., 1984, Ross et al., 1984a, Johansson et al., 1997).

In adults, ADR accounts for approximately 80% of adrenal medulla catecholamine content, with NA making up most of the remaining (von Euler, 1972). Although the adrenal gland and neurons are the most prominent sites of PNMT expression in the adult mammal, this enzyme has also been detected in the retina (Hadjiconstantinou et al., 1983, Foster et al., 1985, Park et al., 1986), spleen (Pendleton et al., 1978), lungs (Pendleton et al., 1978, Kennedy et al., 1990), and heart (Axelrod, 1962, Pendleton et al., 1978, Culman et al., 1987, Torda et al., 1987, Kennedy and Ziegler, 1991). ADR triggers coordinated metabolic and physiological processes in response to stress (Westfall and Westfall, 2006). ADR is more active than NA in the heart and lungs, it causes redirection of blood from the skin to skeletal muscle and it has important stimulatory effects in the glycogen metabolism of the liver (Westfall and Westfall, 2006, Baynes and Dominiczak, 2007, Rang et al., 2007).

Dopamine (3,4-dihydroxyphenylethylamine) is the immediate metabolic precursor of NA and ADR (Figure 2). Although dopamine originally was regarded only as a precursor of

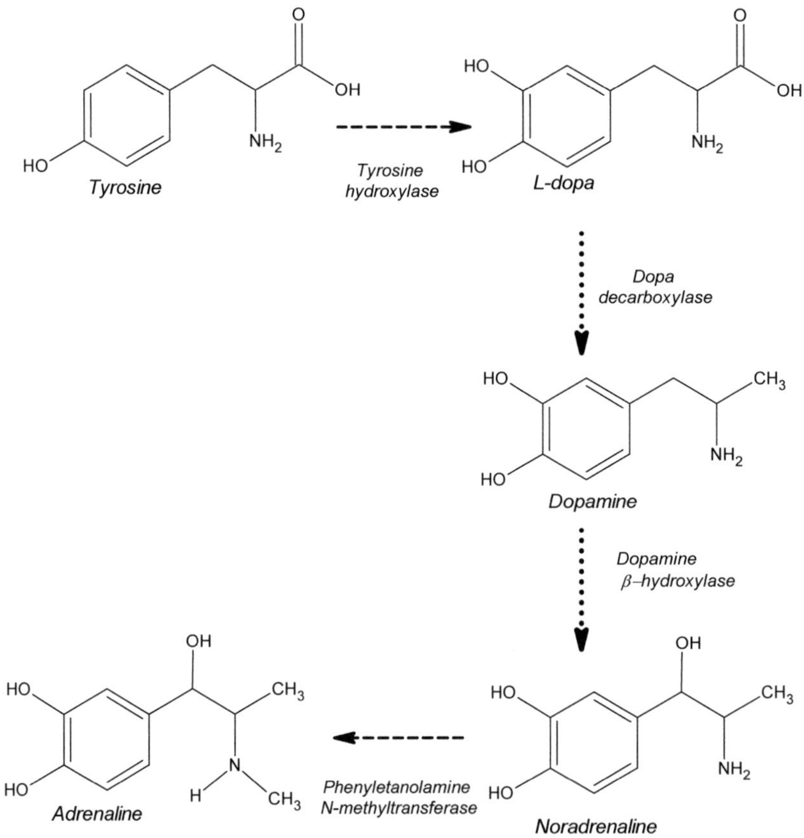

Fig. 2. The synthesis of catecholamines. Tyrosine hydroxylase hydroxylates tyrosine and forms L-3,4-dihydroxyphenylalanine (L-dopa). L-dopa is decarboxylated to form dopamine through the catalysis of dopa decarboxylase. Dopamine β-hydroxylase β-hydroxylates dopamine to yield noradrenaline. Noradrenaline is N-methylated by phenylethanolamine N-methyltransferase to form adrenaline in adrenergic neurons and other adrenaline producing cells.

NA, studies on distinct central nervous system regions revealed that the distribution of dopamine and NA neurons is markedly different (Bloom, 2006). More than half of the central nervous system catecholamine content is dopamine and extremely large amounts are found in the basal ganglia (especially the *caudate nucleus*), the *nucleus accumbens*, the olfactory tubercle, the central nucleus of the amygdala, the median eminence, and restricted fields of the frontal cortex (Bloom, 2006). Of the wide variety of connections, the greatest attention has been given to the long projections between the major dopamine-containing nuclei located at the substantia nigra and ventral tegmentum and their targets in the striatum. In addition, two important central dopaminergic systems are functionally located outside the blood-brain barrier: in the chemoceptor trigger zone and in the anterior pituitary. In the periphery, dopamine is synthesized in epithelial cells of the proximal tubules and it is thought to exert local diuretic and natriuretic effects in the kidneys (Esler et al., 1990, Bloom, 2006). Likewise, dopamine receptors are found in the proximal gastrointestinal tract where their activation delays gastric emptying. Dopaminergic receptors are also present in renal, mesenteric, coronary and intracerebral arteries (Bloom, 2006). At the cellular level, the actions of dopamine depend on the expression of the different receptor subtypes and the contingent actions of other transmitters to the same target neurons (Bloom, 2006). This catecholamine will not be deeply addressed in the present work, except in specific circumstances where it can be of relevance to the theme.

4. Synthesis of catecholamines

The mechanisms of catecholamine synthesis, storage, release, and binding have been mainly studied in sympathetically innervated organs and in the adrenal medulla (Westfall and Westfall, 2006).

The steps that occur in the synthesis of dopamine, NA, and ADR are shown in Figure 2. In the cytoplasm, tyrosine is sequentially 3-hydroxylated by tyrosine hydroxylase to form L-3,4-dihydroxyphenylalanine, which is then decarboxylated to form dopamine by L-3,4-dihydroxyphenylalanine decarboxylase (also known as aromatic L-amino acid decarboxylase) (Axelrod, 1962). Dopamine β-hydroxylase β-hydroxylates dopamine to yield NA, which is N-methylated by PNMT to form ADR, in adrenergic neurons and other ADR producing cells (Rang et al., 2007). The enzymes involved in this synthesis have been identified, cloned, and characterized (Nagatsu, 1991).

In adrenergic neurons, the enzymes that participate in NA formation are synthesized in the cell bodies of neurons and are then transported along the axon to the terminals. In the course of NA synthesis, both the hydroxylation of tyrosine to L-3,4-dihydroxyphenylalanine and the decarboxylation of L-3,4-dihydroxyphenylalanine to dopamine take place in the cytoplasm. About half of the dopamine formed in the cytoplasm is then actively transported into the dopamine β-hydroxylase-containing storage vesicles, where it is converted to NA. The remainder escapes active transport to the vesicles and is deaminated to 3,4-dihydroxyphenylacetic acid and subsequently *O*-methylated to homovanillic acid (HVA) (Westfall and Westfall, 2006). In ADR-producing cells, the NA formed in the vesicles leaves them and it is methylated in the cytoplasm by PNMT to yield ADR. ADR then re-enters the vesicles, where it is stored and concentrated for subsequent release (Masson et al., 1999, Westfall and Westfall, 2006).

The hydroxylation of tyrosine by tyrosine hydroxylase is generally regarded as the rate-limiting step in the biosynthesis of catecholamines (Zigmond et al., 1989). This enzyme is activated after stimulation of sympathetic nerves or adrenal medulla and is tightly regulated. In fact, tyrosine hydroxylase is substrate for protein kinase A (PKA), protein kinase C (PKC) and calcium/calmodulin-dependent protein kinase II (CaMKII). The kinase-catalysed phosphorylation results in the increase of tyrosine hydroxylase activity (Zigmond et al., 1989, Daubner et al., 1992). This is an important acute mechanism to increase the synthesis of catecholamines in response to elevated nerve stimulation. Likewise, tyrosine hydroxylase activity is subject to a feedback inhibition by catechol compounds, which allosterically modulate the activity of the enzyme (Kumer and Vrana, 1996). On the other hand, the expression of tyrosine hydroxylase can be increased at multiple levels, including transcription, ribonucleic acid (RNA) processing, regulation of RNA stability, translation, and enzyme stability (Kumer and Vrana, 1996).

Tyrosine hydroxylase deficiency has been reported in humans and is characterized by generalized rigidity, hypokinesia, among other symptoms. Low cerebrospinal fluid levels of NA and dopamine metabolites, like HVA and 3-methoxy-4-hydroxy-phenylethylene glycol are observed in humans with tyrosine hydroxylase deficiency (Wevers et al., 1999, Carson and Robertson, 2002). The tyrosine hydroxylase knockout is unviable in mice as they die in the embryonic stage, presumably because catecholamine loss results in altered cardiac function (Zhou et al., 1995). Interestingly, residual levels of dopamine are present in these embryonic mice, suggesting that tyrosinase may be an alternate way to form catecholamines. However, the amount of tyrosinase-derived catecholamines is clearly not sufficient for the survival of the animals (Carson and Robertson, 2002).

Dopamine β-hydroxylase deficiency in humans is characterized by orthostatic hypotension, ptosis of the eyelids, retrograde ejaculation, and elevated plasma levels of dopamine (Westfall and Westfall, 2006). In the case of dopamine β-hydroxylase-deficient mice, there is about 90% embryonic mortality (Carson and Robertson, 2002).

At rest, the basal cardiovascular function in PNMT knockout mice showed little change. In fact, ADR was found indispensable for normal blood pressure and cardiac filling responses to stress but it was not required in tachycardia during stress or in normal cardiovascular function at rest (Bao et al., 2007, Sun et al., 2008). Furthermore, glucocorticoids levels are very important in the expression of PMNT and thus in the rate of ADR synthesis. Glucocorticoids are very relevant in the size of the stores of ADR available for release in the brain (Moore and Phillipson, 1975b, a), adrenal medulla (Kelner and Pollard, 1985, Stachowiak et al., 1988, Wan and Livett, 1989, Ross et al., 1990, Betito et al., 1992, Wong et al., 1992), heart (Kennedy and Ziegler, 1991, Krizanova et al., 2001, Kvetnansky et al., 2004) or lungs (Kennedy et al., 1993). The activities of both tyrosine hydroxylase and dopamine β-hydroxylase are also increased in the adrenal medulla under the influence of glucocorticoids (Carroll et al., 1991). Thus, any stress that persists sufficiently to evoke an enhanced secretion of corticotrophin mobilizes the appropriate hormones of both the adrenal cortex (predominantly cortisol in humans) and adrenal medulla.

5. Intracellular storage of catecholamines

Neurotransmission depends mainly on the regulated release of chemical transmitter molecules. That release requires the packing of these substances into the specialized secretory vesicles of neurons and neuroendocrine cells. The neuronal content of catecholamines is confined to vesicles, while in adrenal medulla, catecholamines are stored in chromaffin granules. These vesicles contain extremely high concentrations of catecholamines (approximately 21% dry weight), ascorbic acid, and adenosine-5'-triphosphate (ATP), as well as chromogranins, dopamine β-hydroxylase, and peptides, including enkephalin and neuropeptide Y. Two types of storage vesicles are actually found in sympathetic nerve terminals: large dense-core vesicles equivalent to the chromaffin granules and small dense-core vesicles containing NA, ATP, and membrane-bound dopamine β-hydroxylase (Bloom, 2006). The enhanced activity of the sympathetic nervous system is accompanied by increase of both dopamine β-hydroxylase and chromogranins in circulation, thus supporting the argument that the process of release, following the adrenergic nerve stimulation, involves exocytosis (Westfall and Westfall, 2006).

The storage process decreases the intraneuronal metabolism of the transmitters and their leak out of the cell. This allows to control the concentration gradient across the plasma membrane and to prevent possible toxic effects that could occur when the cytoplasmic concentration of catecholamines exceeds critical levels (Schuldiner, 1994, Masson et al., 1999). The storage process is mediated by specific vesicular transporters (Schuldiner et al., 1978, Erickson et al., 1992, Schuldiner, 1994, Masson et al., 1999). In mammals, there are two closely related vesicular monoamine transporter (VMAT) isoforms that are named VMAT-1 and VMAT-2. VMAT-1 is primarily present in endocrine and paracrine cells, while VMAT-2 is the predominant monoamine transporter in the nervous system (Masson et al., 1999). VMAT-2 is mainly expressed in dense core vesicles of axon terminals (Figure 3) (Nirenberg et al., 1997).

Monoamine vesicular transporters are relatively promiscuous when concerning to their substrates. They transport dopamine, NA, ADR, and 5-HT but they differ in substrate preference and affinity. Several vesicular transport complementary deoxyribonucleic acid (cDNA) have been cloned; these complementary DNAs reveal open reading frames predictive of proteins with 12 transmembrane domains (Masson et al., 1999). Reserpine inhibits the monoamine vesicular transport and ultimately leads to the depletion of catecholamines inside the nerve endings (von Euler, 1972, Masson et al., 1999).

The vesicular transport is driven by pH and potential gradients which are established by ATP-dependent proton pumps. The ATP-driven H^+ pump, on one hand, acidifies the vesicular lumen (ΔpH) and, on the other hand, generates a potential gradient (ΔΨ)(Schuldiner et al., 1978, Johnson and Scarpa, 1979). For every molecule taken in, two internal H^+ ions are extruded by VMAT-2 by an antiport process (Masson et al., 1999). Therefore, the intravesicular concentration of monoamines depends upon ΔΨ and ΔpH (Njus et al., 1986, Rottenberg, 1986, Johnson, 1988, Schuldiner, 1994, Masson et al., 1999). In addition, the monoamine uptake is modulated by vesicle-associated heterotrimeric guanine nucleotide binding regulatory proteins (G proteins), $G_{\alpha o2}$ and $G_{\alpha q}$ (Ahnert-Hilger et al., 1998, Holtje et al., 2000, Holtje et al., 2003). G proteins control transmitter storage: the

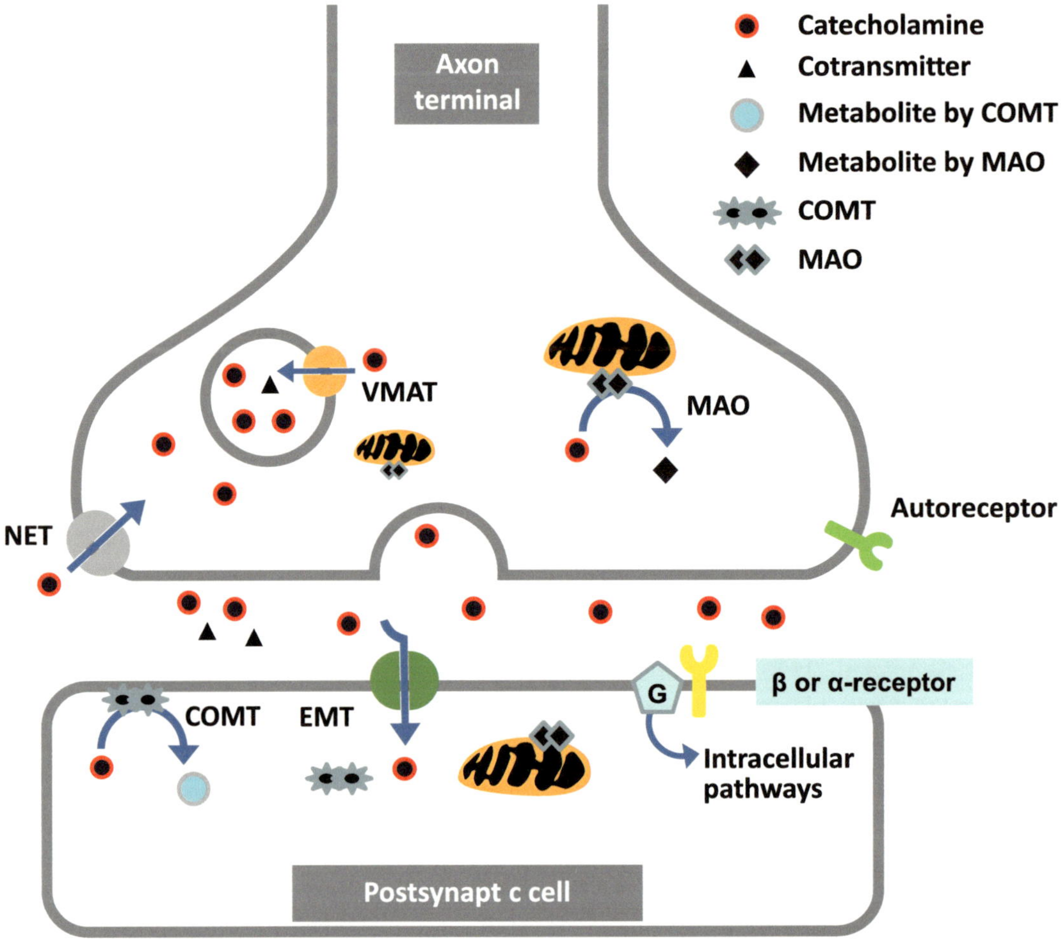

Fig. 3. Catecholamines in axon terminals. The axon terminal has neurotransmitter storage vesicles with catecholamines and cotransmitters. The vesicular monoamine transporter (VMAT) is responsible for the transport of catecholamines to the storage vesicles, maintaining their cytosolic concentration low. After catecholamine release to the synaptic cleft, catecholamines are reuptaken to the presynaptic terminal by noradrenaline transporter (NET), and/or taken to extraneuronal cells by the extraneuronal transporters. The most important extraneuronal transporter for catecholamines is extraneuronal monoamine transporter (EMT). Catecholamines are metabolized by intracellular enzymes. Monoamine oxidase (MAO) is located in the outer membrane of mitochondria in neurons and in extraneuronal cells. Catechol-*O*-methyl transferase (COMT) is located at extraneuronal cells. Both enzymes (COMT and MAO) are the main responsible for the metabolism of catecholamines. The enzymatic process leads to the formation of several metabolites. To exert their actions, the catecholamines and other neurotransmitters in the synaptic cleft bind to different pre- and postsynaptic receptors. Such binding leads to alterations in the postsynaptic cell and activation of intracellular pathways through G proteins. In presynaptic neurons, catecholamines bind to autoreceptors and activate feed-back responses that change their own release.

monoamines stored inside the vesicles represent the upstream signal that mediates the inhibition to further uptake through G proteins. In fact, biogenic amines, with the exception of ADR, lead to G protein-mediated inhibition; VMATs have a receptor-like area in their first luminal loop that senses the intravesicular concentration of monoamines (Brunk et al., 2006).

6. Release of catecholamines

Depolarization of the axonal terminal triggers the release of catecholamines into the cleft. The content of the vesicles, including enzymes, neurotransmitters, and hormones, is discharged to the exterior through a process termed exocytosis (Figure 3). Triggered exocytosis is the most common cellular mechanism for the release of polar molecules and it involves several mechanisms that include vesicle docking, priming, and fusion. It can be regulated or constitutive. In synaptic transmission, a synchronized mechanism provides the cells with a way for precisely timed release of molecules into the extracellular space (Pocock and Richards, 2006). The full sequence of steps by which the nerve impulse affects the release of transmitters from sympathetic neurons is not yet fully understood.

In the adrenal medulla, the triggering event to exocytosis is the release of acetylcholine by the preganglionic fibres; that acetylcholine binds to nicotinic receptors on chromaffin cells which produce a localized depolarization. In most types of cells, regulated exocytosis is triggered by the increase in cytosolic free calcium (Ca^{2+}) (Meir et al., 1999, Pocock and Richards, 2006). This cytosolic Ca^{2+} enters the cells from the extracellular medium, through the voltage-gated Ca^{2+} channels. The voltage-gated Ca^{2+} channels open following depolarization of the plasma membrane, making the Ca^{2+} able to diffuse into the cell down its electrochemical gradient. Ca^{2+} is also mobilized from intracellular stores (mainly the endoplasmic reticulum). As result, the intracellular free Ca^{2+} increases and it triggers the fusion of secretory vesicles with the plasma membrane. Ca^{2+}-triggered secretion involves the interaction of highly conserved molecular scaffolding proteins and leads to the docking of the vesicles (Aunis, 1998, Meir et al., 1999). As fusion continues, a pore is formed and it connects the extracellular space with the interior of the vesicle thus providing a pathway for vesicle content to diffuse into the extracellular space (Pocock and Richards, 2006) (Figure 3).

Other aspects concerning modulation of catecholamine transmission or secretion will be better addressed in a subsequent section where adrenoceptors and their role in augmenting or diminishing the synaptic release will be focused.

7. Neuronal transporters involved in catecholamine reuptake

Synaptic transmission involves the regulated release of transmitters into the synaptic cleft, where they interact with receptors that subsequently transduce the information. The removal of catecholamines from the cleft usually occurs by uptake either back to the presynaptic terminal or into the postsynaptic cell (Iversen et al., 1967, Axelrod and Kopin, 1969). A number of high-affinity transporters have been identified, namely for dopamine, NA, 5-HT, and several aminoacid transmitters (Masson et al., 1999). These transporters are members of an extensive family that share common structural motifs, particularly the putative 12-transmembrane helices (Bönisch and Brüss, 2006). The transporters show a similar configuration of intracellular and extracellular loops or related regions that contain phosphorylation and glycosylation sites and intracellular located amino- and carboxyl-terminal residues (Eisenhofer, 2001). Dopamine is cleared by dopamine transporter whilst NA and ADR are cleared by NA transporter (NET) (Figure 3) (Trendelenburg, 1988, Apparsundaram et al., 1997, Eisenhofer, 2001). These plasma membrane transporters have higher substrate specificity than vesicular transporters and may be viewed as targets ("receptors") for several drugs such as cocaine (NET) or fluoxetine (5-HT transporter) (Bönisch and Brüss, 2006, Capela et al., 2008), but also MDMA (both) (Capela et al., 2009). Dopamine transporter and NET exhibit overlapping, yet distinct, substrate selectivity, translocation efficiency, and antagonist sensitivity (Buck and Amara, 1994, Giros et al., 1994, Pifl et al., 1996, Bönisch and Brüss, 2006). Other than the corresponding neurons, NET is also present in adrenal medulla, liver, and placenta, whereas dopamine transporter is present in the stomach, pancreas, and kidneys (Eisenhofer, 2001).

The neuronal NA uptake system was first reported in the spleen and heart (Axelrod et al., 1959, Axelrod et al., 1961). The availability of radiolabelled catecholamines enabled Axelrod and co-workers to examine the fate of these amines after their intravenous administration to laboratory animals (Axelrod et al., 1959, Axelrod et al., 1961). They observed a selective accumulation of radiolabelled ADR and NA in sympathetically innervated organs, which was dependent on intact sympathetic nerve terminals and it was inhibited by cocaine (Axelrod et al., 1959, Axelrod et al., 1961). It was shown that this accumulation occurred through the activity of NET.

The activity of neurotransmitter transporters, like NET and dopamine transporter, is dependent on intracellular sodium ion (Na^+) and chloride ion (Cl^-) concentrations. The Na^+-gradient (extracellular concentration of Na^+ is higher) across the plasma membrane is the main driving force, dictating the direction of the transport of neurotransmitters and co-substrate ions (in these case Na^+). The normal direction is inwards (Masson et al., 1999, Sonders et al., 2005, Bönisch and Brüss, 2006). The negative intracellular membrane potential also contributes for the above mentioned driving force and it is mainly created by the potassium ion (K^+) gradient (Bönisch and Brüss, 2006).

Transport of NA by NET is saturated and it is characterized by a half-saturation constant or Michaelis constant (Km) of about 0.8 μM; ADR is transported by NET with a Km of 2.8 μM in a maximum velocity two times lower than the transport of NA (Apparsundaram et al., 1997, Bönisch and Brüss, 2006). NET has a high affinity for NA and a somewhat lower affinity for ADR, while isoproterenol is not a substrate for this system (Eisenhofer, 2001, Bönisch and Brüss, 2006). The common structural requirement for uptake by NET is the presence of an ionisable nitrogen not incorporated in the aromatic ring system (Eisenhofer, 2001).

In amphibians, an ADR specific transporter has been identified, with characteristics distinct from those of dopamine transporter or NET (Apparsundaram et al., 1997). In mammals, the presence of an ADR specific transporter was not yet clarified, however *in situ* hybridization studies indicate the absence of both dopamine transporter and NET messenger ribonucleic acid (mRNA) in ADR-synthesizing neurons in the brainstem of adult rats (Lorang et al., 1994). Thus, as ADR is also cleared at these sites, these terminals might have a distinct catecholamine transporter from dopamine transporter or NET; as an alternative, ADR may act as an endocrine regulator that does not require rapid reuptake in those neurons (Lorang et al., 1994, Apparsundaram et al., 1997).

The importance of neuronal catecholamine transporters in maintaining vesicular levels of catecholamines is well illustrated in mutant mice lacking NET. NET is a high-affinity system, relatively selective for NA, with a low maximum rate of uptake, and it is important in maintaining releasable stores of NA (Bönisch and Brüss, 2006). The knockout NET mice showed depletion of NA intraneuronal stores, lack of inhibition of neuronal amine synthesis, protracted clearance, and elevated NA extracellular levels (Wang et al., 1999). Interestingly, in cyclic voltammetry experiments with the knockout NET mice, the rate of NA clearance was decreased by only six fold when compared to the rate of wild-type animals (Xu et al., 2000). The knockout NET mice behave like wild-type animals treated with antidepressant drugs and are hyperresponsive to locomotor stimulation with psychostimulants (Xu et al., 2000).

In summary, the neuronal reuptake process aims to assure constant and high levels of neurotransmitters in the releasing neuron and low concentrations in the cleft (Eisenhofer, 2001, Bönisch and Brüss, 2006). It works as an integrated part of the neurotransmitter recycling process, since in addition to their *de novo* synthesis, the stores of monoamines in the terminal portions of the neural fibres are also replenished by their active transport back to the terminals. Moreover, the reuptake system contributes to the degradation of catecholamines since the metabolizing enzymes are found intracellularly (Westfall and Westfall, 2006). Furthermore, the reuptake of catecholamines maintains the concentration gradient within the neuronal vesicles. Two distinct neuron carrier-mediated transport systems are involved: one across the axoplasmic membrane from the extracellular fluid to the cytoplasm, NET or dopamine transporter, and the other from the cytoplasm into the storage vesicles, the VMAT-2 (Bloom, 2006). The removal of catecholamines from the cytoplasm into the storage system by VMAT-2 acts as an amplification step for the overall uptake process developed by NET or dopamine transporter (Schuldiner, 1994, Sonders et al., 2005). In a broader sense, catecholamine transporters function as part of an integrated system where catecholamine synthesis, release, uptake, and metabolism are regulated in a coordinated fashion (Eisenhofer, 2001). Therefore, neuronal catecholamine transporters function not only as part of metabolizing systems, but perhaps more importantly, as part of the recycling system, operating in series with VMAT-2 to maintain catecholamine neuronal stores (Eisenhofer, 2001) (Figure 3).

8. Catecholamine extraneuronal transporters

Catecholamines are also taken up by extraneuronal transporters. A low affinity, high capacity uptake for NA and ADR in the isolated perfused rat heart was found by Iversen (Iversen, 1963, 1965b,a). Iversen observed that radiolabelled [^{3}H]-NA in the isolated heart entered into at least two intracellular pools with distinct rate constants. In fact, [^{3}H]-NA entered one pool approximately seven-times faster when compared to the other pool (Iversen, 1963). In 1967, Malmfors demonstrated, by fluorescence microscopy, that the myocytes were responsible for an uptake process (Malmfors, 1967). After these discoveries, the neuronal NA uptake system was designated as "uptake-1" and the extraneuronal transport system as "uptake-2" (Iversen, 1965b). The extraneuronal uptake of catecholamines is mediated by organic cation transporters (OCTs), that include the classic corticosterone-sensitive extraneuronal monoamine transporter and traditionally named "uptake-2" that nowadays is called OCT3 (Eisenhofer, 2001, Schömig et al., 2006). Other members of this family are: OCT1 and OCT2.

All three OCTs can transport catecholamines in addition to a wide variety of other organic acids, including 5-HT, histamine, choline, spermine, guanidine, and creatinine (Eisenhofer, 2001). The affinity of extraneuronal monoamine transporter for NA is rather low (Km > 0.5 mM), which is compensated by its high capacity (high turnover number). The transport efficiency of OCT1 and OCT2 for dopamine, NA, ADR, and 5-HT is usually low (Schömig et al., 2006).

OCTs share common features. A single positive charge is required to be an OCT substrate, while uncharged, doubly charged or negatively charged substances are not transported by OCTs (Schömig et al., 2006). A decrease in extracellular pH and the depolarization of the cytoplasmatic membrane will reduce the OCT activity. The OCT mediated transport is independent of Na^+ and Cl^- gradients and all three OCTs are transporters, not just channels, as shown by trans-stimulation experiments. OCT1, OCT2 or extraneuronal monoamine transporter may mediate electrogenic uniport of a substrate or electroneutral exchange of two substrates (antiport). The OCTs are relatively resistant to the inhibitors of the neuronal transporters such as desipramine (Eisenhofer et al., 1991, Schömig et al., 2006), but are inhibited by steroids, such as corticosterone, and the *O*-methylated metabolites of catecholamines, like normetanephrine and metanephrine (Eisenhofer, 2001, Costa et al., 2009a, Nissinen and Männistö, 2010). Other compounds, like GF120918, were shown to inhibit extraneuronal monoamine transporter at low concentrations in isolated rat cardiomyocytes (Costa et al., 2009a).

Extraneuronal monoamine transporter (OCT3) is expressed in many but not all tissues. The expression varies greatly between organs and during organ development (e.g. in placenta). Consistently, high expression has been reported for placenta and heart (Eisenhofer, 2001). Other reports indicate high extraneuronal monoamine transporter expression in the area postrema (Haag et al., 2004, Vialou et al., 2004) and very low in the kidneys (Eisenhofer, 2001). Interestingly, extraneuronal monoamine transporter expression has been also suggested to occur in neurons (Kristufek et al., 2002, Shang et al., 2003).

For NA, the uptake by NET is more relevant for signal termination than extraneuronal uptake. It has been estimated that the sympathetic nerves remove approximately 87% of released NA by NET, while 5% is removed by extraneuronal monoamine transporter. The remainder 8% is diffused into the circulation (Eisenhofer, 2001). This data, however, does not necessarily reflect the relative importance of the two processes. The proximity of the neuronal transporters to the location of catecholamine release (when compared to extraneuronal transporters) implies that the transmitter removed by extraneuronal transport has a higher duration and wider range of action. Extraneuronal uptake, therefore, may be particularly important for the removal of neuronal released catecholamines in tissues where high concentrations of adrenergic receptors exist (Eisenhofer, 2001). The clearance of circulating catecholamines is primarily mediated by non neuronal mechanisms, with liver and kidney accounting for over 60% (Eisenhofer, 2001, Westfall and Westfall, 2006). As stated above, most NA released by sympathetic nerves is removed by neuronal reuptake, which is in contrast with that of ADR. ADR when secreted directly into the bloodstream from the adrenal medulla is predominantly inactivated by extraneuronal uptake and metabolism. ADR has lower affinity for neuronal uptake than NA and consequently the neuronal process contributes approximately 50% less for its elimination when compared with NA (Iversen, 1965a). In contrast, ADR is removed by extraneuronal uptake 2-3 times more efficiently than NA (Iversen, 1965b, Eisenhofer et al., 1992b).

In short, when compared to NET, extraneuronal monoamine transporter exhibits lower affinity (i.e. higher Km) for catecholamines, favours ADR and isoproterenol over NA or dopamine, and shows a higher maximum rate for catecholamine uptake (i.e. higher maximum velocity) (Iversen, 1965a, b, Eisenhofer et al., 1992b, Eisenhofer, 2001, Schömig et al., 2006). Extraneuronal monoamine transporter is not Na^+-dependent and displays a completely different profile of pharmacological inhibition (Schömig et al., 2006, Westfall and Westfall, 2006). Thus, in contrast to the importance of NET in the clearance of neuronal released catecholamines, clearance of circulating catecholamines is predominantly made by non-neuronal mechanisms (Eisenhofer, 2001).

9. Metabolism and action termination

The pharmacological actions of NA and ADR are terminated by: (i) reuptake into nerve terminals by NET; (ii) uptake at extraneuronal sites by extraneuronal monoamine transporter, OCT1, or OCT2; and (iii) metabolic transformation. Catecholamines undergo a complex metabolic fate, mediated by several enzymes, including aldehyde reductase, aldose reductase, aldehyde dehydrogenase, alcohol dehydrogenase, catechol-*O*-methyltransferase (COMT), dopamine β-hydroxylase, monoamine oxidase (MAO) type A and B, monoamine-preferring phenolsulfotransferase, and PNMT (Dooley, 1998, Goldstein et al., 2003). *In vivo*, two of the most important enzymes responsible for the metabolic transformation of catecholamines are MAO and COMT (Westfall and Westfall, 2006).

9.1 Monoaminoxidase metabolism

MAO was first described as tyramine oxidase by Mary Hare-Bernheim in 1928, since it catalyses the oxidative deamination of tyramine. This enzyme was found to oxidize several monoamines, including catecholamines, i.e. dopamine, NA, and ADR, and also 5-HT. MAO [amine: oxygen oxidoreductase (deaminating)] catalyses the following reaction:

$$RCH_2NH_2 + H_2O + O_2 \rightarrow RCHO + NH_3 + H_2O_2$$

MAO acts on primary amines and also on some secondary and tertiary amines (Nagatsu, 1991). It is located in the outer membrane of mitochondria (Schnaitman et al., 1967) both in neuronal and extraneuronal cells (Trendelenburg, 1988) (Figure 3). It is a flavo-protein, with flavin adenine dinucleotide as cofactor (Kearney et al., 1971). Two forms of MAO exist, i.e. MAO-A and MAO-B (Johnston, 1968). In humans, MAO-A is abundant in the brain, liver, and in the syncytiotrophoblast layer of term placenta, whereas liver, lungs, platelets, lymphocytes, osteocytes that surround the blood vessels, and the intestine are rich in MAO-B (Abell and Kwan, 2001, Nagatsu, 2004). In the human brain, MAO-A is located in the catecholamine-containing regions, with the highest levels being found in *locus ceruleus*. MAO-B is prominent in the dorsal *raphe nuclei*, which are known to have serotonergic neurons. MAO-B is also present in the posterior hypothalamus and in glial cells (Abell and Kwan, 2001, Nagatsu, 2004).

5-HT, NA, and ADR are preferential substrates for MAO-A, and clorgyline and Ro 41-1049 are MAO-A inhibitors (Johnston, 1968, Kitaichi et al., 2010); MAO-B prefers β-phenylethylamine as a substrate and it is inhibited by deprenyl and lazabemide (Knoll et al., 1978, Kitaichi et al., 2010). Dopamine, tyramine, and tryptamine are oxidized with equal affinity by MAO-A and MAO-B (Glover et al., 1977). Pargyline inhibits both MAO-A and

MAO-B (Blaha et al., 1996, Carvalho et al., 2001, Carmo et al., 2003, Duarte et al., 2004). MAO-A appears to be the main enzyme in the metabolism of 5-HT and NA, while the location of MAO-B, abundant in serotonergic neurons, remains under debate (Abell and Kwan, 2001).

In the brain of MAO-A-deficient mouse pups, NA levels increased up to two-fold, while a small increase in dopamine levels was observed. Borderline mental retardation and abnormal behavioural are observed in humans with selective MAO-A deficiency. Severe mental retardation in patients with combined MAO-A/MAO-B deficiency and Norrie disease are also observed (Lenders et al., 1996). Human males from a Dutch family with a complete deletion of the *mao-a* gene in the X chromosome were reported to show abnormal aggressive behaviour (Brunner et al., 1993), as observed in adult mice (Cases et al., 1995). MAO-A-deficient adult male mice show enhanced aggressive behaviour and enhanced emotional learning, probably due to elevated levels of 5-HT in the brain in the pup stage (Cases et al., 1995, Kim et al., 1997). Furthermore, MAO-A knockout mice exhibited a dramatic reduction of defensive and fear-related behaviours in the presence of predator-related cues, such as predator urine or an anaesthetized rat (Godar et al., 2010).

All regions of the brain of MAO-B-deficient mouse pups showed increased levels of β-phenylethylamine (Lenders et al., 1996), especially in striatum and prefrontal cortex (Bortolato et al., 2009). The MAO-B knockout mice show behavioural disinhibition and decrease anxiety-like responses partially through a regional increase in β-phenylethylamine levels (Bortolato et al., 2009). In contrast to the borderline mental retardation and abnormal behavioural phenotype in subjects with selective MAO-A deficiency and the severe mental retardation in patients with combined MAO-A/MAO-B deficiency and Norrie disease, the MAO-B-deficient human subjects neither exhibited abnormal behaviour nor mental retardation except increased reactivity to stress (Grimsby et al., 1997). The subjects with the *mao-b* gene deletion have complete absence of platelet MAO-B activity and have increased brain levels and urinary excretion of β-phenylethylamine (Lenders et al., 1996). In fact, the inhibition of MAO-B indicates that this form of MAO has a lower contribution to the metabolism of endogenous catecholamines and of their *O*-methylated metabolites (Eisenhofer and Finberg, 1994).

9.2 Catechol-*O*-methyl transferase metabolism

Another important catecholamine-metabolizing enzyme (COMT) was first described and purified by Axelrod (Axelrod, 1958, Axelrod and Tomchick, 1958) (Figure 3). One single gene for COMT codes for both soluble COMT and membrane-bound COMT. That gene has different transcription starting sites. COMT is an intracellular enzyme, the most abundant form being the soluble COMT with a minor fraction as membrane bound COMT (Mannisto and Kaakkola, 1999). COMT catalyses the transfer of the methyl group of *S*-adenosyl-L-methionine to one of the hydroxyl groups in the catechol in the presence of magnesium ion (Mg^{2+}) (Mannisto and Kaakkola, 1999). COMT is widely distributed throughout the body. High levels of COMT are found in the liver, proximal tubular epithelial cells of the kidneys, and other extraneuronal cells, namely adrenomedullary chromaffin cells (Eisenhofer et al., 1998, Mannisto and Kaakkola, 1999). However, little or no COMT is found in sympathetic neurons. In the presynaptic terminals of the brain, no significant COMT is detected, but it is reported in some postsynaptic neurons and glial cells. The physiological substrates of

COMT include L-3,4-dihydroxyphenylalanine, all three endogenous catecholamines (dopamine, NA, and ADR), their hydroxylated metabolites, catecholestrogens, ascorbic acid, and dihydroxyindolic intermediates of melanin (Mannisto and Kaakkola, 1999, Nissinen and Männistö, 2010).

In COMT knockout mice, minor behaviour changes were detected and the neurochemistry of catecholamines in the brain is virtually unaltered (Gogos et al., 1998). Mutant mice showed sexually dimorphic and region-specific changes of dopamine levels, notably in the frontal cortex. Mutant male mice have almost a three-fold increase of dopamine levels in the frontal cortex, while no changes were observed in the striatum or hypothalamus. In mutant female mice no alterations in dopamine levels were observed when compared to the wild type (Gogos et al., 1998). Despite the complete lack of *comt* gene in homozygous mice, residual HVA levels were detectable in several brain areas, revealing a possible and still unidentified methylation pathway in the brain (Gogos et al., 1998). Female knockout mice showed impaired emotional reactivity, while heterozygous males were more aggressive (Gogos et al., 1998). The work by Gogos and colleagues suggested that the importance of COMT in the emotional and social behaviour has probably been undervalued and the complete lack of COMT can be partially compensated, at least in mice (Gogos et al., 1998).

9.2.1 The cross-talk between catecholamine catabolic enzymes and transporters

Of relevance, the main mechanism that reduces the life span of catecholamines in the extracellular space is their uptake by active transport and not their enzymatic metabolism. It has been shown that NET inhibitors (e.g., cocaine, imipramine, and desipramine) potentiate the effects of the neurotransmitters, while inhibitors of MAO and COMT have relatively little immediate effect (Gonçalves et al., 1989, Eisenhofer, 1994, Eisenhofer and Finberg, 1994, Friedgen et al., 1994, Blaha et al., 1996, Friedgen et al., 1996). Early studies in isolated tissues showed that the inhibition of MAO or COMT could limit the ability of neuronal and extraneuronal uptake to clear extracellular catecholamines (Furchgott and Garcia, 1968, Belfrage et al., 1977). More recent *in vivo* studies however indicate that inhibition of one enzyme under normal physiological conditions has little effect on the overall catecholamine clearance and on their extracellular or circulating levels (Eisenhofer, 1994, Eisenhofer and Finberg, 1994, Friedgen et al., 1994, Blaha et al., 1996, Friedgen et al., 1996). Only when MAO and COMT are both inhibited or subjected to saturating concentrations of substrate, the clearance of catecholamines is significantly impaired (Eisenhofer, 1994, Friedgen et al., 1996). To confirm the redundancy of metabolizing systems, in MAO-A-deficient humans or rats a marked decrease in deaminated catecholamine metabolites and a concomitant marked elevation of *O*-methylated amine metabolites occur (Eisenhofer and Finberg, 1994, Lenders et al., 1996). These neurochemical changes are only slightly exaggerated in patients with combined lack of MAO-A and MAO-B (Lenders et al., 1996).

The activity of metabolizing enzymes can influence the catecholamine net transport and the extracellular levels of catecholamines. Moreover, the metabolizing enzymes are always required for the irreversible chemical alteration of catecholamines following neuronal or extraneuronal uptake. Nevertheless, Trendelenburg stated that understanding the interactions and the functions of the active transport and metabolizing processes is very relevant as they function as "pump and leak systems with enzyme(s) inside" (Trendelenburg, 1988, 1990).

An integrated vision explains the results found *in vivo*. In fact, the presence of only one catecholamine-metabolizing enzyme, MAO, in neuronal systems would lead to the assumption that inhibition of this enzyme would impair the catecholamine's neuronal uptake by changing the concentration gradient. However, the additional presence of VMAT-2 maintains the axoplasmic catecholamine levels low. Furthermore, VMAT-2 has higher affinity for NA than MAO, which implies that over 70% of the recaptured NA through NET is sequestered into storage vesicles before being metabolized (Bloom, 2006). Therefore, under normal physiological conditions, the inhibition of MAO has little effect (Graefe and Trendelenburg, 1970, Graefe and Henseling, 1983). Rather than impairing the catecholamine uptake, short-term inhibition of intraneuronal MAO leads to higher retention of recaptured transmitter by VMAT-2 and, thus, an apparent increase in the net uptake of the transmitter (Furchgott and Garcia, 1968). In the long term, if vesicular storage capacity is overwhelmed, inhibition or saturation of intraneuronal MAO can lead to a decrease in neurotransmitter's uptake (Trendelenburg et al., 1972).

9.3 The metabolites of catecholamines

Complex and dynamic processes are involved in the metabolism of catecholamines, either intracellularly or even after their release into the extracellular fluid. In both neuronal and extraneuronal metabolizing systems, the inactivation of catecholamines occurs in a coordinated fashion, with uptake being followed by metabolism (Graefe and Henseling, 1983). Most of the metabolism of catecholamines takes place in the same cells where they are produced, even before their exocytotic release (Figure 4). Dihydroxyphenylglycol (DHPG, 3,4-dihydroxyphenylethylene glycol) constitutes the main NA metabolite before NA release or reuptake. DHPG is also a deaminated metabolite of ADR (Eisenhofer and Finberg, 1994, Goldstein et al., 2003). DHPG is formed from NA in the cytoplasm of sympathetic nerves by sequential deamination of NA by MAO to form dihydroxyphenylglycoaldehyde. This aldehyde is reduced by aldehyde reductase or aldose reductase to form DHPG or it is oxidized by aldehyde dehydrogenase to form 3,4-dihydroxymandelic acid. DHPG diffuses rapidly across the membrane of the cell into the extracellular fluid and into extraneuronal cells. In the extraneuronal cells, DHPG is metabolized by COMT to form 3-methoxy-4-hydroxy-phenylethylene glycol, or it overflows into the bloodstream (Eisenhofer and Finberg, 1994, Goldstein et al., 2003). Also, the decrease in plasma concentrations of endogenous DHPG and 3,4-dihydroxyphenylacetic acid after inhibition of MAO-A, but not MAO-B, corroborates that NA is a better substrate for the A isoform (Eisenhofer and Finberg, 1994).

COMT has a substantial importance in the metabolism of the deaminated metabolites of NA and dopamine, as corroborated by the increase of plasma levels of 3,4-dihydroxyphenylacetic acid and DHPG after COMT inhibition (Eisenhofer and Finberg, 1994). Alternatively, COMT can catalyse the *O*-methylation of NA to normetanephrine, of ADR to metanephrine, of L-3,4-dihydroxyphenylalanine to 3-methoxytyrosine, and of dopamine mainly to 3-methoxytyramine (Eisenhofer and Finberg, 1994, Goldstein et al., 2003).

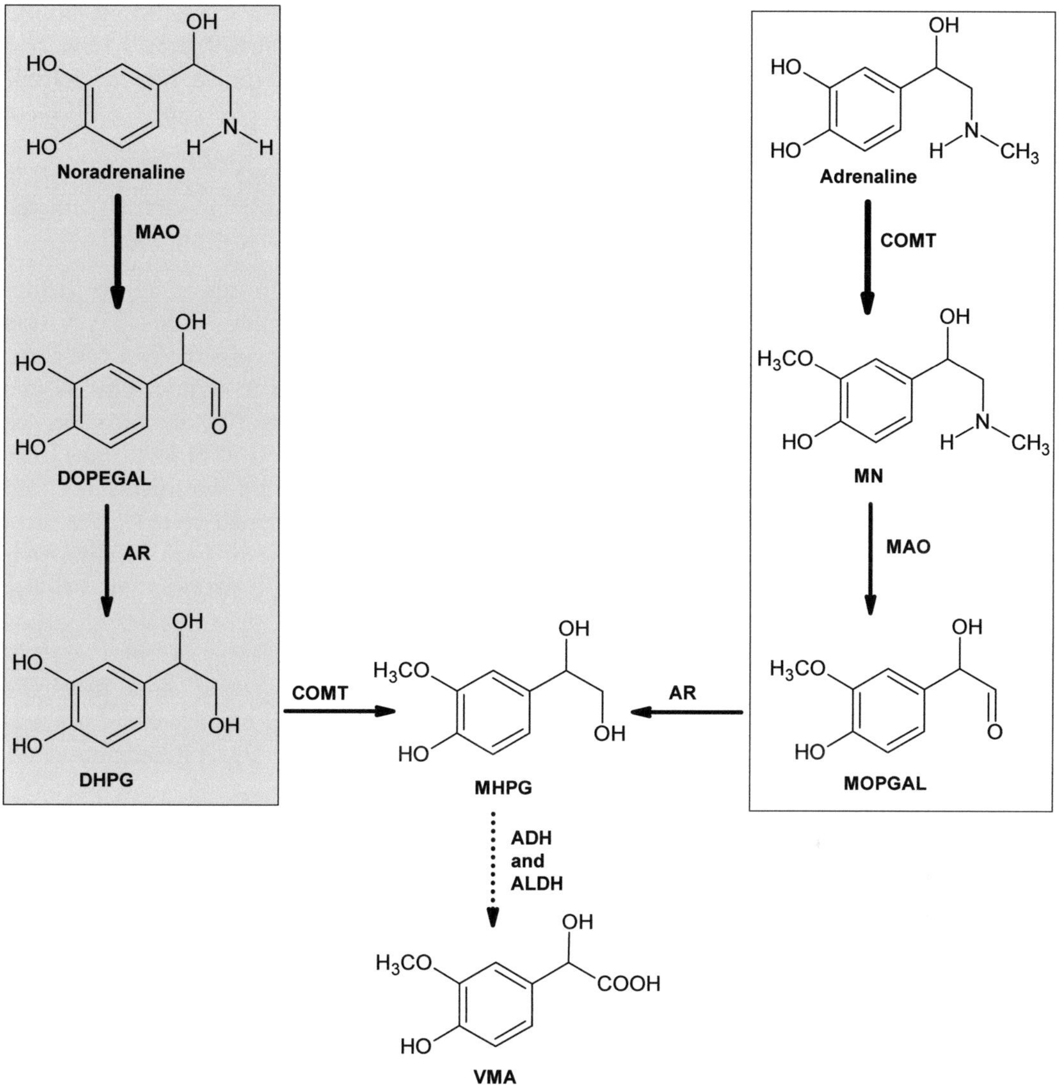

Fig. 4. Representative pathway of the most common metabolic pathways of adrenaline (ADR) and noradrenaline (NA). ADR is synthesized from NA through phenylethanolamine N-methyltransferase (PNMT) catalysis. NA is metabolized preferably by monoamine oxidase (MAO) to dihydroxyphenylglycoaldehyde (DOPEGAL) that is reduced by aldehyde reductase (AR) to form dihydroxyphenylglycol (DHPG). ADR is preferably metabolized by catechol-*O*-methyltransferase (COMT) resulting in metanephrine (MN). MN can be further metabolized by MAO to 3-methoxy-4-hydroxyphenyl-glycoaldehyde (MOPGAL) and by aldehyde reductase (AR) to form 3-methoxy-4-hydroxy-phenylethylene glycol (MHPG). MHPG is further metabolized and can be transformed to vanillylmandelic acid (VMA) by alcohol dehydrogenase (ADH) and aldehyde dehydrogenase (ALDH). VMA is the main catecholamine metabolite in urine (adapted from reference Goldstein et al., 2003).

In adrenal chromaffin cells, as they contain both MAO and COMT, the deamination and *O*-methylation coexist. The COMT present in chromaffin cells is mainly membrane bound COMT while soluble COMT is found in the majority of other tissues (namely liver and kidneys). Membrane bound COMT has a higher affinity for catecholamines than the soluble COMT (Roth, 1992). As a result, in adrenal chromaffin cells, leakage of NA and ADR from storage granules leads to substantial intracellular production of the *O*-methylated metabolites, normetanephrine and metanephrine. In humans, about 93% of circulating metanephrine and between 25% to 40% of circulating normetanephrine result from the catecholamines metabolized within adrenal chromaffin cells (Eisenhofer et al., 2004).

In most cells, the *O*-methylated compounds that contain amine groups undergo further metabolic alterations by MAO. Deamination of 3-methoxytyramine yields HVA and deamination of normetanephrine and metanephrine yields 3-methoxy-4-hydroxy-phenylethylene glycol. 3-Methoxy-4-hydroxy-phenylethylene glycol in human plasma is a very important metabolite with multiple sources, including (i) deamination of normetanephrine after its cellular uptake; (ii) *O*-methylation of DHPG after its uptake from the circulation; and (iii) *O*-methylation of DHPG after its uptake from the interstitial fluid but before its entrance into the circulation. Of the previously mentioned sources, the most relevant is the last (Eisenhofer and Finberg, 1994). The fate of circulating 3-methoxy-4-hydroxy-phenylethylene glycol is complex and includes sulfation, glucuronidation, urinary excretion, and specially conversion to methoxy-4-hydroxymandelic acid [generally, called vanillylmandelic acid (VMA)] through the hepatic sequential oxidation of circulating 3-methoxy-4-hydroxy-phenylethylene glycol by alcohol dehydrogenase and aldehyde dehydrogenase (Goldstein et al., 2003). In fact, the major product of urinary excretion and also an important plasma metabolite of adrenergic catecholamines is VMA (Goldstein et al., 2003) (Figure 4).

The formation of normetanephrine occurs after NA extraneuronal uptake and metabolism. Due to the importance of the reuptake and intraneuronal deamination of endogenously released NA, plasma levels of normetanephrine are lower than those of DHPG, despite the similar plasma clearance of these two compounds. The rate of extra adrenal production of normetanephrine, although low, still provides a unique marker of NA extraneuronal metabolism. Accordingly, during MAO-A inhibition, normetanephrine and metanephrine levels increase as COMT becomes more relevant in the metabolism of NA (Eisenhofer and Finberg, 1994).

As stated, adrenomedullary chromaffin cells contain both MAO and COMT and, in agreement with the different affinities between extraneuronal and neuronal uptake, ADR is less metabolized by MAO than NA, but it is a better substrate for COMT (Paiva and Guimarães, 1978, Eisenhofer and Finberg, 1994). Because of these differences, extraneuronal uptake and *O*-methylation clear more circulating ADR than NA (Axelrod et al., 1959, Eisenhofer, 2001, Goldstein et al., 2003) and metanephrine is the major metabolite of ADR (Axelrod et al., 1959, Goldstein et al., 2003).

In cells that contain monoamine-preferring phenolsulfotransferase, the non-acid metabolites, methoxytyramine, normetanephrine, metanephrine, and 3-methoxy-4-hydroxy-phenylethylene glycol undergo extensive sulphate-conjugation. The urinary metabolites, resulting from monoamine-preferring phenolsulfotransferase metabolization are usually 3-

methoxy-4-hydroxy-phenylethylene glycol-SO_4, normetanephrine-SO_4, and metanephrine-SO_4 (Eisenhofer et al., 2004).

Glucuronides of methoxytyramine, normetanephrine, metanephrine, and 3-methoxy-4-hydroxy-phenylethylene glycol are also formed and they may be excreted in the bile. When these glucuronides enter into the circulation, they are eliminated in the urine (Eisenhofer et al., 2004).

Of relevance, the oxidative deamination of catecholamines by MAO leads to another relevant product, hydrogen peroxide (H_2O_2) which subsequently may be converted into the highly reactive hydroxyl radical (HO•) (Valko et al., 2007), that may cause oxidative stress-related damage (Carvalho et al., 2001, Duarte et al., 2004, Vaarmann et al., 2010, Costa et al., 2011).

9.3.1 Levels of catecholamines and their metabolites in the plasma and urine

Catecholamines enter the plasma mainly after their leakage from the synaptic cleft to the circulation or after the secretion of catecholamines by the adrenal medulla (Esler et al., 1990, Goldstein et al., 2003). The bulk of NA in the plasma results mainly from sympathetic overflow, while the majority of plasma ADR is formed by adrenal medulla secretion (Esler et al., 1990, Goldstein et al., 2003). The metabolites of NA and ADR also spill into the plasma after intraneuronal metabolism (namely oxidative deamination by MAO) or extraneuronal metabolism (preferentially COMT-methylation), since the majority of the metabolism occurs even before the catecholamines reach the circulation (Goldstein et al., 2003). The most abundant human plasma metabolites are VMA, 3-methoxy-4-hydroxy-phenylethylene glycol and its sulphate metabolite (Goldstein et al., 2003). The main human plasma catechols are the three catecholamines, their precursor, L-3,4-dihydroxyphenylalanine, and their deaminated metabolites, 3,4-dihydroxyphenylacetic acid from dopamine, and DHPG from NA (Goldstein et al., 2003) (Figure 4).

In humans, the sympathetic nerves of kidneys and skeletal muscles are the major sources of plasma NA, each contributing with approximately 25% of the total (Esler et al., 1984a, Esler et al., 1984b). The sympathetic innervations of the human heart, skin, gastrointestinal tract, lungs, and liver are responsible for a minor percentage of total plasma NA, but equally important (Esler et al., 1984a, Esler et al., 1984b, Goldstein et al., 1988, Esler and Kaye, 2000).

The rate of NA entrance into the arterial plasma ("total body spillover") can be measured and in healthy people averages 0.3 to 0.5 µg/min (Goldstein et al., 2003). Key players in the rate of NA spillover include the rate of NA release, and consequently nerve firing velocity and density, but also regional blood flow, capillary permeability, neuronal NA uptake, and NA metabolism (Esler et al., 1990). These key aspects have to be taken into account when interpreting NA overflow as an index of sympathetic activity. In fact, when comparing the levels of NA release into interstitial fluid to circulation with NA spillover, the NA release into interstitial fluid in kidneys averages 3 times, in skeletal muscle 12 times, and in the heart over 20 times the NA spillover, due to the efficient local neuronal reuptake of NA. (Goldstein et al., 2003).

The majority of plasma ADR in physiological conditions results from the stimulation of adrenal medulla (Goldstein et al., 2003); it is assumed that ADR overflow from adrenergic nerves is not very relevant (Esler et al., 1990). The only exception is the heart, which at very high stimulation rates can contribute significantly for ADR spillover into the plasma (Peronnet et al., 1988, Johansson et al., 1997).

Plasma levels of ADR in healthy volunteers at rest are as low as 30 pM, while NA reaches 1 nM (Wheatley et al., 1985, Goldstein et al., 2003). Spillover of ADR to arterial plasma in healthy resting humans is typically 30-100 pg/mL, while it can reach 200-600 ng/mL for NA (Esler et al., 1990). Any alteration in the metabolism of catecholamines or disruption of their transport mechanisms might lead to abnormal high concentrations of these substances (Lameris et al., 2000). Elevated levels of circulating and interstitial catecholamines are found in arrhythmias, myocardial necrosis (Lameris et al., 2000, Behonick et al., 2001), heart failure, (Esler and Kaye, 2000), myocardial ischemia (Lameris et al., 2000, Akiyama and Yamazaki, 2001, Killingsworth et al., 2004, Kuroko et al., 2007), exercise (Kjaer, 1998), pheochromocytoma (Gerlo and Sevens, 1994), hypoglycaemia, haemorrhagic hypotension, circulatory collapse, distress (Goldstein et al., 2003), and cirrhosis (Esler et al., 1990). The administration of amphetamines can also lead to peaks of plasmatic levels of biogenic catecholamines. In fact, after high doses of *d*-amphetamine in rats, levels of plasmatic ADR and NA reached 146 nM and 418 nM, respectively (Carvalho et al., 1997).

The levels of urinary and plasma catecholamine or metabolites can also indicate a higher sympathetic overflow or metabolism impairment (Esler et al., 1990, Brunner et al., 1993, Lenders et al., 1996, Behonick et al., 2001, Goldstein, 2003). In fact, the measurement of DHPG gives important information of NA sympathetic nerve neuronal uptake and turnover (Esler et al., 1990, Goldstein et al., 2003). The DHPG values reflect the sum of vesicular leakage, NA deamination (which is mainly neuronal) and reuptake (Eisenhofer et al., 1992a, Goldstein et al., 2003). DHPG plasma levels can reach 4.7 nM in healthy volunteers (Goldstein et al., 2003).

Formation of normetanephrine in the body occurs after extraneuronal uptake and metabolism of NA in the sympathetic terminals, as well as from the *O*-methylation of NA within the adrenal medulla by COMT. Because of the high importance of reuptake and intraneuronal deamination of NA, plasma levels of normetanephrine (~0.3 nM) are significantly lower than those of DHPG (Goldstein et al., 2003).

O-Methylation is the main metabolic pathway of ADR in man (Labrosse et al., 1958). Metanephrine constitutes a major metabolite of ADR before its release into the extracellular fluid (Labrosse et al., 1958, Axelrod et al., 1959). Plasma metanephrine levels are roughly the same as plasma normetanephrine levels, although the levels of plasma NA are about 5- to 10-fold higher than the levels found for ADR. The levels of metanephrine result from the high rate of production of ADR in adrenomedullary chromaffin cells, the metabolism of adrenomedullary catecholamines by COMT (Goldstein et al., 2003), and the relatively high affinity of COMT for circulating ADR (Paiva and Guimarães, 1978, Eisenhofer and Finberg, 1994).

As already stated, 3-methoxy-4-hydroxy-phenylethylene glycol in human plasma has multiple sources, the main being *O*-methylation of DHPG after its uptake from the interstitial fluid but before its entrance into the circulation. The metabolic fate of the circulating 3-methoxy-4-hydroxy-phenylethylene glycol is complex and includes sulfation, glucuronidation, and specially conversion to VMA (Goldstein et al., 2003). 3-Methoxy-4-hydroxy-phenylethylene glycol and VMA constitute the major non sulphate catecholamine metabolites, reaching plasmatic values of 30 and 20 nM, respectively (Goldstein et al., 2003).

L-3,4-dihydroxyphenylalanine is the precursor of catecholamines and the product of the rate-limiting step of catecholamine synthesis. L-3,4-dihydroxyphenylalanine therefore occupies a crucial role in the catecholaminergic system. In humans, plasma levels of L-3,4-dihydroxyphenylalanine exceed those of NA about 10-fold, reaching 8.9 nM (Goldstein et al., 2003).

Some catecholamine storage vesicle elements are released during exocytosis like chromogranin A, DhB, and neuropeptide Y. Their plasma values can be used as an index of the neuroendrocrine system activation (Esler et al., 1990).

All catecholamines are ultimately excreted in urine, either in their native form or as metabolites (Esler et al., 1990, Goldstein et al., 2003). Nevertheless, in urine, only a small fraction of catecholamines is present in their unaltered form (Esler et al., 1990) and NA urinary excretion represents only 1-2% of the total NA synthesized. VMA is the major catecholamine metabolite excreted in the urine and 33 μM of VMA can be eliminated each 24 h (Gerlo and Sevens, 1994). The sulphate derivatives of 3-methoxy-4-hydroxy-phenylethylene glycol, normetanephrine, and metanephrine are the bulk of the other urinary metabolites (Eisenhofer et al., 2004). The use of urinary excretion levels of catecholamines and/or of their metabolites to estimate total body catecholamine turnover and plasma levels has to be very cautious. Urinary excretion depends on renal blood flow and renal function, thus it has some inter-individual variations (Fluck, 1972).

9.4 Another pathway to degrade catecholamines

The metabolization of catecholamines is generally attained either by deamination via MAO or *O*-methylation by COMT. However, the chemical alteration of catecholamines by other enzymes or through oxidative processes is also a probable pathway to the chemical alteration of the transmitters (Richter, 1940)(Figure 5). When the enzymes dealing with the catabolism of catecholamines are unable to cope efficiently, their levels rise and catecholamines can undergo oxidation. The oxidation rate is faster under enzymatic or metal catalysis (Heacock, 1959, Bindoli et al., 1992, Foppoli et al., 1997), in the presence of the superoxide anion ($O_2{\bullet}^-$) or high pH (West, 1947, Spencer et al., 1995, Costa et al., 2007). Although at physiological pH, the oxidation of catecholamines seems to occur very slowly, it has been found to occur *in vivo* namely in the septic shock (Macarthur et al., 2000). The oxidation of catecholamines ultimately produces a family of indole semiquinonic/quinonic species usually termed catecholaminochromes because of their orange-reddish colour (Heacock and Mahon, 1958). The oxidation of aqueous extracts of mammal suprarenal capsules was first reported by Vulpian (Vulpian, 1856). The oxidation products of ADR were crucial for the indirect quantification of ADR for many years, since adrenolutin and adrenochrome are easily detected by UV/VIS or by fluorometric methods (Annrsten et al., 1949, Fischer and Bacq, 1950, Ludemann et al., 1955, Remião et al., 2003, Ochs et al., 2004).

Generally speaking, catecholamines may be oxidized to an unstable *o*-semiquinone that, after deprotonation and loss of a second electron, gives rise to the corresponding *o*-quinone. For ADR, at physiological pH, partial deprotonation of the amine group of the side chain leads to an irreversible 1,4-intramolecular cyclization, a reaction that occurs through nucleophilic attack of the nitrogen atom at position 6 of the quinone ring, to form "leucoadrenochrome"; leucoadrenochrome is subsequently oxidized to form adrenochrome

(Heacock and Mahon, 1958, Bindoli et al., 1992, Bindoli et al., 1999). This indole is often represented as a zwitterionic structure in aqueous solutions (Heacock and Mahon, 1958, Remião et al., 2003, Costa et al., 2007) (Figure 5). In summary, the oxidation of catecholamines occurs through two-stages whereby a total of four electrons is removed and an indole is formed by cyclization (Costa et al., 2011).

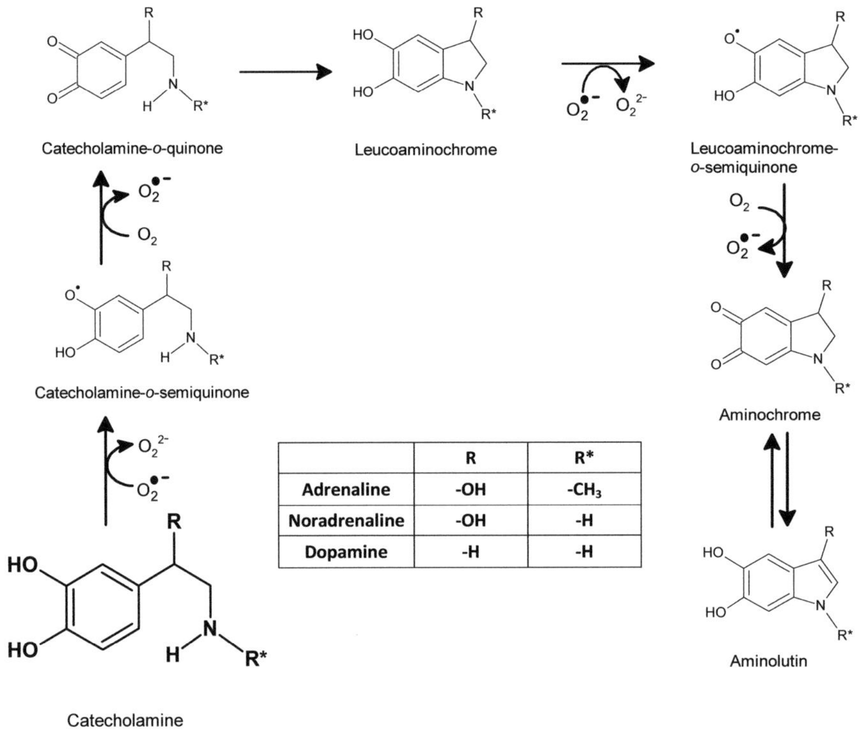

	R	R*
Adrenaline	-OH	$-CH_3$
Noradrenaline	-OH	-H
Dopamine	-H	-H

Fig. 5. Postulated pathway for the oxidation of catecholamines. The oxidation process of catecholamines initially involves their conversion to *o*-quinones through o-semiquinones intermediates. The *o*-semiquinone reduces oxygen resulting in superoxide anion (O_2•-). The *o*-quinone can undergo an irreversible 1, 4-intramolecular cyclization, forming leucoaminonochrome. The formation of aminochrome from leucoaminochrome is a reaction where a total of two electrons are removed and leucoaminochrome semiquinone is the intermediary with O_2•- as a by-product. Aminochrome formed can lead to the formation of aminolutins.

Adrenochrome is the most studied aminochrome due to its stability (Heacock, 1959, Rupp et al., 1994). When adrenochrome is formed and ADR still exists in solution, adrenochrome accelerates the oxidation process of the remaining ADR (Bindoli et al., 1999, Costa et al., 2007). Furthermore, the yield of adrenochrome increases if ADR semi-quinone reacts with O_2 to form O_2•- (Costa et al., 2007). This seems to be a general phenomenon of aminochromes, since it occurs also with the other catecholamines (Heacock, 1959, Bindoli et al., 1992).

Once formed, the aminochromes can be transformed into melanins, since they are reactive compounds that easily undergo a series of reactions among them. *In vivo*, this oxidation pathway may be more complex, since other factors such as metal ions or other nucleophilic groups can be involved (Spencer et al., 1998, Bindoli et al., 1999, Spencer et al., 2002, Costa et al., 2007, Costa et al., 2009a).

At physiological pH, the oxidation pathway of biogenic catecholamines is similar, as they share similar intermediates, however their stability is fairly different (Rupp et al., 1994). The rate of internal cyclization determines the probability of nucleophilic attack to the quinone intermediates (Rupp et al., 1994, Spencer et al., 1995, Alhasan and Njus, 2008). Thus, if the internal cyclization rate is low, the quinone is likely to be attacked by external nucleophilic groups such as sulfhydryl (-SH), hydroxyl (-OH), and amine (-NH_2) groups. The slowest cyclization rate is observed for dopamine, while ADR has the higher cyclization rate, 140 times higher than NA. Thus, the probability of external nucleophilic attack to occur is as following: dopamine > NA > ADR (Rupp et al., 1994). In fact, dopamine oxidized forms were found bound to proteins, as well as to other nucleophilic molecules, as cysteine or glutathione (Fornstedt et al., 1990, Patel et al., 1991, Segura-Aguilar et al., 1997, Byington, 1998, Spencer et al., 1998, Spencer et al., 2002, Miyazaki et al., 2006). Pathognomonic significance has been given to these products, namely in Parkinson's disease (Spencer et al., 1995, Shen et al., 1996, Spencer et al., 1998). As stated, the fastest cyclization rate occurs in ADR (Bindoli et al., 1992); however, GSH adducts and quinoproteins of ADR have been found in cells, thus showing that ADR quinone can also undergo attack from cellular nucleophiles (Costa et al., 2007, Costa et al., 2009a, Costa et al., 2009c). These changes can ultimately cause cellular injury (Costa et al., 2011).

10. Adrenergic receptors

10.1 Historic introduction and background

More than one hundred years ago, Langley proposed, for the first time, the idea of transmitter receptors, by stating "(...) neither the poisons nor the nervous impulse act directly on the contractile substance of the muscle but on some accessory substance. Since this accessory substance is the recipient of stimuli which it transfers to the contractile material, we may speak of it as the receptive substance (...)" (Langley, 1905).

The receptors for NA and ADR are nowadays called adrenoceptors. The adrenoceptors are the cell membrane sites where NA and ADR act. Several discoveries were performed before the concept of adrenoceptors was fully accepted. Dale in 1905 verified that the pressor effect of ADR was reversed by ergotoxine into a depressor effect. Later on, Barger and Dale verified that ADR when injected was able to dilate some vascular beds while constricting others (Barger and Dale, 1910). These facts were ignored until 1948 when Ahlquist performed a series of experiments with several sympathomimetic amines. He concluded that the variation in the pharmacological responses of several sympathomimetic agonists in different organs was related to the different types of receptors involved (Ahlquist, 1948). To the first type of adrenoceptors, he called α and to the second β (Ahlquist, 1948). The scientific contemporary community was not prompt to accept this idea and the theory of two different "sympathins" remained (Cannon and Rosenblueth, 1933). More than ten years later other works confirmed the theory by Ahlquist through the identification of selective antagonists for the two receptor families: phentolamine and ergotamine for α-adrenoceptors; dichloroisoprenaline (Powell et al., 1958) and propranolol for β-adrenoceptors (Black et al., 1964).

The development of more selective drugs and the use of molecular cloning technology showed that several adrenoceptor subtypes exist. As Ahlquist stated, two main classes are known, α- and β-adrenoceptors. Each group is further subdivided so that five subtypes are presently recognized: two main α-receptor subtypes (α_1 and α_2) and three β-receptor subtypes (β_1, β_2 and β_3) (Alexander et al., 2008). The α-receptor subtypes are nowadays accepted to be six subtypes in total (α_{1A}, α_{1B}, α_{1D}, $\alpha_{2A/D}$, α_{2B}, α_{2C}). Other two adrenoceptors candidates were described (α_{1L} and β_4), that may be conformational states of α_{1A} and β_1-adrenoceptors, respectively (Guimarães and Moura, 2001, Alexander et al., 2008) .

The pharmacological actions of NA and ADR have been extensively compared *in vivo* and *in vitro*. Both drugs are direct agonists on effectors cells and their actions differ mainly in their ability to stimulate α- and β-receptors. ADR and NA are approximately equipotent in stimulating β_1-receptors. NA is a potent α-agonist and has relatively little action on β_1-receptors; however, NA is somewhat less potent than ADR on α receptors in most organs (Westfall and Westfall, 2006). The rank order of potency is isoproterenol > ADR $\geq$ NA for β-adrenergic receptors and ADR $\geq$ NA >> isoproterenol for α-adrenergic receptors (Guimarães, 1975, Westfall and Westfall, 2006, Rang et al., 2007).

In the present review, the classical pharmacological point of view will be approached as it was historically the starting point in the study of the neurotransmission of catecholamines. Although not excluding neurotransmission plasticity and adaptation as key factors for the full understanding of the topic, these issues are still under debate, so they will not be addressed here.

The knowledge of the characteristics of adrenergic receptors and the biochemical and physiological pathways that they regulate increased the understanding of the seemingly contradictory and variable effects of catecholamines on different organs. Although structurally related, different receptors regulate distinct physiological processes by controlling the synthesis or release of a variety of second messengers. The adrenoceptors are coupled to second-messenger systems via G proteins. The responses that follow the activation of adrenergic receptors result from G protein-mediated effects with the generation of second messengers and/or the activation of ion channels (Guimarães and Moura, 2001) (Figure 3).

10.2 Alpha (α)-adrenoceptors

α_1-Adrenoceptors are found in the smooth muscle of the blood vessels, bronchi, gastrointestinal tract, uterus, and bladder. The activation of these receptors is mainly excitatory and results in the contraction of smooth muscle. However, the smooth muscle of the gut wall (but not that of the sphincters) becomes relaxed after activation of α_1-receptors. Overall, the α_1-adrenoceptors cause vasoconstriction, relaxation of gastrointestinal smooth muscle, salivary secretion, and hepatic glycogenolysis (Pocock and Richards, 2006, Rang et al., 2007). α_1-Adrenoceptors are mainly coupled to $G_{q/11}$-protein with consequent activation of phospholipase C. Phospholipase C promotes the hydrolysis of phosphatidylinositol bisphosphate producing inositol trisphosphate and diacylglycerol (Docherty, 1998, Zhong and Minneman, 1999, García-Sáinz et al., 2000, Guimarães and Moura, 2001), which act as second messengers. Inositol trisphosphate mediates intracellular Ca^{2+} release from non mitochondrial pools and, consequently, the activation of other Ca^{2+} and calmodulin sensitive pathways such as CaMKII, whilst diacylglycerol activates PKC (Guimarães and Moura, 2001, Westfall and Westfall, 2006). The three cloned α_1-adrenoceptor subtypes have significant differences in G protein coupling efficiency (α_{1A} > α_{1B} > α_{1D}) (Docherty, 1998, Zhong and Minneman, 1999, Guimarães and Moura, 2001).

Other signalling pathways are also activated by α_1-adrenoceptors, namely: stimulation of phospholipase A_2 leading to the release of free arachidonate, which is degraded by cyclooxygenase and lipoxygenase to form the bioactive prostaglandins and leukotrienes; Ca^{2+} influx via protein G; and phospholipase D activation (Docherty, 1998, Zhong and Minneman, 1999, Guimarães and Moura, 2001, Westfall and Westfall, 2006). Some of the responses induced by α_1-adrenoceptors are independent of Ca^{2+} and PKC but involve small G proteins and tyrosine kinases (Zhong and Minneman, 1999). Furthermore, α_1-adrenoceptors are able to activate mitogen-activated protein kinase pathways in many cells (Della Rocca et al., 1997). The mitogen-activated protein kinase superfamily, which consists of extracellular signal-regulated kinases 1/2 and three stress-responsive subfamilies, the c-Jun NH_2-terminal kinases, p38-mitogen-activated protein kinase (p38-MAPK), and extracellular signal-regulated kinases, is normally stimulated by growth factors and cellular stress or inflammatory cytokines (Zhang et al., 2005).

α_2-Adrenoceptors when located presynaptically are responsible for the inhibition of transmitter release (including NA and acetylcholine from autonomic nerves) and are considered modulators of neurotransmission (autoreceptors). The different α_2-receptors couple to a variety of effectors (Aantaa et al., 1995, Guimarães and Moura, 2001) and share about 50% in amino acid sequence in important domains (Aantaa et al., 1995). The importance of these receptors was well demonstrated in knockout mice for α_2-adrenoceptors (Vieira-Coelho et al., 2009). Brain tissue levels of L-3,4-dihydroxyphenylalanine, dopamine, and NA were significantly higher in the knockout mice for α_{2A}- and α_{2C}-adrenoceptors when compared to wild type. The activity of COMT was higher in all three knockout (α_{2A}-, α_{2B}- and α_{2C}-adrenoceptors), while the activities of MAO, dopamine β-hydroxylase or tyrosine hydroxylase were unchanged (Vieira-Coelho et al., 2009).

α_2-Adrenoceptors are predominantly coupled to the inhibitory G proteins, G_i and $G_{(o)}$, inhibiting the activity of adenylyl cyclase (Rouot et al., 1987, Cotecchia et al., 1990, Surprenant et al., 1992, Aantaa et al., 1995, Wise et al., 1997). The α_2-adrenoceptor stimulation leads to the activation of Na^+/H^+ exchange (Limbird, 1988), inhibition of the opening of voltage-gated Ca^{2+} channels (Cotecchia et al., 1990) or activation of K^+ channels (Surprenant et al., 1992), all resulting in membrane hyperpolarization.

α_2-Adrenoceptors are also found at postjunctional or nonjunctional sites in several tissues, thus their activation may also lead to the activation of other intracellular pathways. In peripheral tissues, postsynaptic α_2-receptors are found in vascular and other smooth muscle cells, in adipocytes, and in many types of secretory epithelial cells (intestinal, renal, and endocrine). The activation of α_2-adrenoceptors causes platelet aggregation, contraction of vascular smooth muscle, and inhibition of insulin release (Aantaa et al., 1995, Pocock and Richards, 2006, Rang et al., 2007). Intracellular pathways of postjunctional α_2-receptors are varied, with activation of phospholipase A_2, C, and D, with arachidonic acid mobilization, increase in phosphoinositide hydrolysis, and increase in the intracellular availability of Ca^{2+} (Limbird, 1988, Cotecchia et al., 1990, MacNulty et al., 1992, Kukkonen et al., 1998). In addition, α_2-adrenoceptors can activate mitogen-activated protein kinases (Della Rocca et al., 1997, Richman and Regan, 1998).

10.3 Beta (β)-adrenoceptors

The three β-adrenoceptor subtypes are encoded by three different genes located in human chromosomes 10 (β_1), 5 (β_2), and 8 (β_3). Approximately 60% of the amino acid sequence in membrane-spanning domains is the ligand-binding pocket for ADR and NA (Kobilka et al., 1987, Emorine et al., 1989, Guimarães and Moura, 2001).

β_1-Adrenoceptors are found in the heart where their activation results in increased rate and force of contraction. They are also present in the sphincter muscle of the gut where their activation leads to relaxation (Pocock and Richards, 2006, Westfall and Westfall, 2006, Rang et al., 2007).

The activation of β_2-adrenoceptors in the smooth muscle of certain blood vessels leads to vasodilatation. They are also present in the bronchial smooth muscle where they mediate bronchodilatation. Relaxation of visceral smooth muscle, hepatic glycogenolysis, and muscle tremor occur after β_2-adrenoceptors activation. Postsynaptic β_2-receptors can be found in the myocardium, as well as on vascular and some smooth muscle cells (Gauthier et al., 1996, Gauthier et al., 2000, Pocock and Richards, 2006, Rang et al., 2007). The stimulation of prejunctional β_2-adrenoceptors leads to NA release in neurons (Boehm and Kubista, 2002).

β_3-Adrenoceptors are present in adipose tissue, where they initiate lipolysis in white adipose tissue (Pocock and Richards, 2006, Rang et al., 2007). They are involved in the thermogenesis process that takes place in brown adipose tissue (Gauthier et al., 1996). β_3-Adrenoceptors are also present in the heart although their functions are not fully understood (Gauthier et al., 1996, Gauthier et al., 2000).

All β-receptor subtypes (β_1, β_2, and β_3) are coupled to the stimulatory G protein (G_s) leading to the activation of adenylyl cyclase and accumulation of the second messenger, cyclic adenosine monophosphate (cAMP) (Frielle et al., 1987, Emorine et al., 1989, Brown, 1990, Westfall and Westfall, 2006). Accumulation of cAMP leads to PKA activation with phosphorylation of several proteins, whose functions are changed as a result.

Curiously, several works indicate that, under certain circumstances, β-adrenoceptors can couple to G_i in addition to G_s. In fact, β_3-receptors interact with both G_s and G_i, whereas β_1-receptors couple predominantly to G_s (Asano et al., 1984, Chaudhry et al., 1994, Gauthier et al., 1996). β_2-Receptors usually bind to G_s but, after sustained activation, they couple to G_i (Xiao et al., 1995, Lefkowitz et al., 2002).

10.4 Location and regulation of adrenoceptors

The adrenoceptors are targets for many important drugs in therapeutics, including those used for treatment of cardiovascular diseases, asthma, prostatic hypertrophy, nasal congestion, obesity, and pain (Guimarães and Moura, 2001, Pocock and Richards, 2006). From a therapeutic standpoint, there are many occasions where the β-adrenoceptor selective stimulation (asthma, atrioventricular block, obesity) or blockage (hypertension, coronary insufficiency) is desired. α_2-Agonists are used in hypertension and α_1-agonist in nasal congestion (Aantaa et al., 1995, Guimarães and Moura, 2001, Westfall and Westfall, 2006, Rang et al., 2007). Inhibition of α_1-adrenoceptors has also proven useful to treat hypertension and prostate hypertrophy (Zhong and Minneman, 1999, Westfall and Westfall, 2006).

The α- and β-receptors appear to be located pre- and postsynaptically. The α_1- and β_1-receptors are mainly in the vicinity of sympathetic adrenergic nerve terminals in peripheral target organs, or distributed in the mammalian brain (Westfall and Westfall, 2006). The α_2- and β_2-receptors are heterogeneously distributed. Both α_2- and β_2-receptors may be situated at sites (vascular smooth muscle, platelets and leukocytes) that are relatively remote from nerve terminals and may be activated preferentially by circulating catecholamines (in particular ADR) (Westfall and Westfall, 2006). On the other hand, presynaptically located α_2- and β_2-adrenoceptors have important roles in the modulation of neurotransmitter release from sympathetic nerve endings (Figure 3).

Responses mediated by adrenoceptors are not static, as they can be modulated and adjusted. The number and function of adrenoceptors on the cell's surface and their elicited responses may be altered by catecholamines themselves, by other hormones and drugs but they can also change with age and disease. The release of neurotransmitters can be modulated by prejunctional autoreceptors. NA or ADR, neuropeptide Y, and ATP (the last two are frequent cotransmitters in the adrenergic transmission) elicit a feedback response on prejunctional receptors (Boehm and Kubista, 2002, Westfall et al., 2002). The most studied autoreceptors have been the prejunctional α_2-adrenergic receptors (Aantaa et al., 1995). The α_{2A}- (α_{2D}-, depending on the species investigated) and α_{2C}-adrenergic receptors are the principal prejunctional receptors that inhibit sympathetic neurotransmitter release, whereas the α_{2B}-adrenergic receptors may also inhibit the release of transmitters at selected sites (Boehm and Kubista, 2002). Antagonists of these receptors, in turn, can enhance the electrically evoked release of sympathetic neurotransmitters. Neuropeptide Y, acting on Y2 receptors (Chen et al., 1997), and ATP-derived adenosine, acting on P1 (A1) receptors, can also inhibit sympathetic neurotransmitter release, while nucleotides, acting on P2 receptors have inhibitory or facilitator effects, depending on the tissue evaluated (Driessen et al., 1994, Boehm and Kubista, 2002, Hoffmann, 2004). Other heteroreceptors present in sympathetic nerve varicosities can likewise inhibit the release of sympathetic neurotransmitters, namely through the activation of M_2 and M_4 muscarinic, 5-HT, prostaglandin E_2, histamine, enkephalin, and dopamine receptors (Lefkowitz et al., 1990, Gainetdinov et al., 2004, Hata et al., 2004).

Enhancement of sympathetic neurotransmitter release can occur after the activation of presynaptic β_2-adrenergic, angiotensin II, and nicotinic receptors. All of these receptors can be targets for agonists and antagonists (Boehm and Kubista, 2002).

The modulation of synaptic transmission is a crucial step in homeostasis, where receptors have key roles. The continuous exposure to adrenergic agonists causes a progressive decrease in the capacity to respond to those agents by catecholamine-sensitive cells. This phenomenon, often termed refractoriness, or desensitization, is another "check point" in neuroendrocrine regulation (García-Sáinz et al., 2000, Hoffmann, 2004). Two major types of desensitization have been distinguished: homologous and heterologous. In the homologous, reduced responsiveness is observed exclusively in the receptor originally stimulated. In heterologous desensitization, a decreased responsiveness is observed to an agent or agents unrelated to the initial stimulus. Certainly, this classification is only operational and both types of desensitization may occur simultaneously in the cells (García-Sáinz et al., 2000). Even so, the mechanisms are equally complex and need further characterization.

β-Adrenoceptor feedback regulation is common; however, β-receptors differ in the extent to which they can undergo such regulation, with the β_2-receptors being the most susceptible. Upon challenge with an agonist, the β_2-receptor couples to G_s and activates adenylyl cyclase to form cAMP. cAMP leads to stimulation of cyclic AMP-dependent protein kinases, like PKA, with consequent phosphorylation of β-receptor. That phosphorylation provides the signal for β-arrestin recruitment. Arrestins constitute a large family of widely expressed proteins (Baillie and Houslay, 2005, Westfall and Westfall, 2006). β-arrestin translocation from the cytosol to the activated β-receptor physically blocks the interaction of the receptor with its cellular effectors, presumably due to steric hindrance (Lefkowitz and Shenoy, 2005). The receptor phosphorylation followed by β-arrestin binding has been linked to subsequent endocytosis of the receptor. The capacity of β-arrestins to bind to the structural protein clathrin, initiating the internalization of phosphorylated receptors into vesicles, facilitates endocytosis (Goodman et al., 1996, Nelson et al., 2008). In addition to blunting responses that require the presence of the receptor on the surface of the cell, these regulatory processes may also contribute to novel mechanisms of receptor signalling via intracellular pathways (Baillie and Houslay, 2005).

Receptor desensitization may also be mediated by second messenger feedback. For example, β-adrenoceptor-mediated cAMP accumulation leads to activation of PKA, which can phosphorylate residues of β-receptors, which results in their own inhibition. For the β_2-receptor, phosphorylation occurs on serine residues both in the third cytoplasmic loop and in the carboxyl terminal tail of the receptor. β_3-Receptors do not suffer down regulation, since they lack recognition sites for the cAMP dependent kinases activated by stimulation of β-adrenoceptors (Gauthier et al., 1996).

Although less addressed, α-receptors desensitization has gained increased interest (García-Sáinz et al., 2000). Current data indicate that the decrease in receptor activity is associated with a homologous desensitization mechanism. The activation of PKC by Gq-coupled receptors may lead to phosphorylation of this class of G protein-coupled receptors. That phosphorylation constitutes a very substantial sterical impediment for the effective interaction of receptors with G proteins. Receptor phosphorylation is associated with receptor internalization and β-arrestins are involved (García- Sáinz et al., 2000).

In the case of α-receptors heterologous desensitization, it is not completely clear whether kinases, arrestins, or other molecules play the main role (García-Sáinz et al., 2000). However, activated PKA or PKC may phosphorylate any structurally similar receptor with the appropriate consensus sites for phosphorylation, a process which is considered a heterologous desensitization (Gainetdinov et al., 2004, Hoffmann, 2004).11. Summary

The autonomic nervous system is considered responsible for organ specific adjustments to the environment, while the endocrine system regulates more generalized adaptations by releasing hormones into the systemic circulation that act on "distant places" (Westfall and Westfall, 2006). NA and ADR play crucial roles in the interaction between the autonomic and endocrine systems when the body has to adjust to several and varied situations. It is of outmost importance that their roles and all the participants in the "adrenergic" system are well known. It is absolutely certain that, as it happened during the twentieth century, the new century will bring new and fascinating discoveries in this area that will challenge existing preconceptions. However, the knowledge gathered until this point resulted of the work of several notorious scientists whose work should not be forgotten but remembered and valued.

11. Abbreviations

Adrenaline; Epinephrine (ADR); Adenosine-5'-triphosphate (ATP); Adenosine triphosphatase (ATPase); Calcium ion (Ca^{2+}); Ca^{2+}/calmodulin-dependent protein kinase II (CaMKII); Cyclic adenosine monophosphate (cAMP); Catechol-*O*-methyltransferase (COMT); Dihydroxyphenylglycol (DHPG); Deoxyribonucleic acid (DNA); Inhibitory G protein (G_i); Stimulatory G protein (G_s); 5-Hydroxytriptamine; Serotonin (5-HT); Homovanillic acid (HVA); Potassium ion (K^+); Half-saturation constant; Michaelis constant (Km); Monoamine oxidase (MAO); Magnesium ion (Mg^{2+}); Sodium ion (Na^+); Noradrenaline; Norepinephrine (NA); Noradrenaline transporter (NET); Superoxide anion ($O_2^{\bullet -}$); Organic cation transporters (OCT); Hydroxyl radical (HO•); Phenylethanolamine N-methyltransferase; Noradrenaline N-methyltransferase (PMNT); Ribonucleic acid (RNA); Vanillylmandelic acid; Methoxy-4-hydroxymandelic acid (VMA); Vesicular monoamine transporter (VMAT).

12. Acknowledgments

This work received financial support from the Portuguese State through "Fundação para a Ciência e Tecnologia" (FCT) (project PPCDT/SAU-OBS/55849/2004 & POCI/SAU-OBS/55849/2004). Vera M. Costa acknowledges FCT for her Pos-Doc grant (SFRH/BPD/63746/2009). The authors acknowledge Joana Macedo for her technical assistance with figure 3 included in the manuscript.

13. References

Aantaa R, Marjamäki A, Scheinin M (1995) Molecular pharmacology of alpha 2-adrenoceptor subtypes. Ann Med 27:439-449.

Abel JJ, Crawford AC (1897) On the blood-pressure raising constituent of the suprarenal capsule. Bull Jonhs Hopkins Hosp 8.

Abell CW, Kwan SW (2001) Molecular characterization of monoamine oxidases A and B. Prog Nucleic Acid Res Mol Biol 65:129-156.

Ahlquist RP (1948) A study of the adrenotropic receptors. Am J Physiol 153:586-600.

Ahnert-Hilger G, Nürnberg B, Exner T, Schäfer T, Jahn R (1998) The heterotrimeric G protein Go2 regulates catecholamine uptake by secretory vesicles. EMBO J 17:406-413.

Akiyama T, Yamazaki T (2001) Myocardial interstitial norepinephrine and dihydroxyphenylglycol levels during ischemia and reperfusion. Cardiovasc Res 49:78-85.

Alexander SPH, Mathie A, Peters JA (2008) Guide to Receptors and Channels (GRAC) 3rd edn. Br J Pharmacol 153:S1-S209.

Alhasan R, Njus D (2008) The epinephrine assay for superoxide: Why dopamine does not work? Anal Biochem 381:142-147.

Annrsten S, Gronwall A, Koiw E (1949) Determination of adrenaline in blood plasma by the fluorescence method. Nature 163:136.

Apparsundaram S, Moore KR, Malone MD, Hartzell HC, Blakely RD (1997) Molecular cloning and characterization of an L-epinephrine transporter from sympathetic ganglia of the bullfrog, Rana catesbiana. J Neurosci 17:2691-2702.

Armstrong DM, Ross CA, Pickel VM, Joh TH, Reis DJ (1982) Distribution of dopamine-, noradrenaline-, and adrenaline-containing cell bodies in the rat medulla oblongata: demonstrated by the immunocytochemical localization of catecholamine biosynthetic enzymes. J Comp Neurol 212:173-187.

Asano T, Katada T, Gilman AG, Ross EM (1984) Activation of the inhibitory GTP-binding protein of adenylate cyclase, Gi, by beta-adrenergic receptors in reconstituted phospholipid vesicles. J Biol Chem 259:9351-9354.

Aunis D (1998) Exocytosis in chromaffin cells of the adrenal medulla. Int Rev Cytol 181:213-320.

Axelrod J (1958) Presence, formation, and metabolism of normetanephrine in the brain. Science 127:754-755.

Axelrod J (1962) Purification and properties of phenylethanolamine-N-methyl transferase. J Biol Chem 237:1657-1660.

Axelrod J, Kopin IJ (1969) The uptake, storage, release and metabolism of noradrenaline in sympathetic nerves. Prog Brain Res 31:21-32.

Axelrod J, Tomchick R (1958) Enzymatic *o*-methylation of epinephrine and other catechols. J Biol Chem 233:702-705.

Axelrod J, Weil-Malherbe H, Tomchick R (1959) The physiological disposition of H^3-epinephrine and its metabolite metanephrine. J Pharmacol Exp Ther 127:251-256.

Axelrod J, Whitby LG, Hertting G (1961) Effect of psychotropic drugs on the uptake of H^3-norepinephrine by tissues. Science 133:383-384.

Azuma T, Binia A, Visscher MB (1965) Adrenergic mechanisms in the bullfrog and turtle. Am J Physiol 209:1287-1294.

Baillie GS, Houslay MD (2005) Arrestin times for compartmentalised cAMP signalling and phosphodiesterase-4 enzymes. Curr Opin Cell Biol 17:129-134.

Bao X, Lu CM, Liu F, Gu Y, Dalton ND, Zhu B-Q, Foster E, Chen J, Karliner JS, Ross JJ, Simpson PC, Ziegler MG (2007) Epinephrine is required for normal cardiovascular responses to stress in the phenylethanolamine N-methyltransferase knockout mouse. Circulation 116:1024-1031.

Barger G, Dale HH (1910) Chemical structure and sympathomimetic action of amines. J Physiol 41:19-59.

Baynes JW, Dominiczak MH (2007) In Medical Biochemistry.

Behonick GS, Novak MJ, Nealley EW, Baskin SI (2001) Toxicology update: the cardiotoxicity of the oxidative stress metabolites of catecholamines (aminochromes). J Appl Toxicol 21 Suppl 1:S15-22.

Belfrage E, Fredholm BB, Rosell S (1977) Effect of catechol-*O*-methyl-transferase (COMT) inhibition on the vascular and metabolic responses to noradrenaline, isoprenaline and sympathetic nerve stimulation in canine subcutaneous adipose tissue. Naunyn Schmiedebergs Arch Pharmacol 300:11-17.

Betito K, Diorio J, Meaney MJ, Boksa P (1992) Adrenal phenylethanolamine N-methyltransferase induction in relation to glucocorticoid receptor dynamics: evidence that acute exposure to high cortisol levels is sufficient to induce the enzyme. J Neurochem 58:1853-1862.

Bindoli A, Rigobello MP, Deeble DJ (1992) Biochemical and toxicological properties of the oxidation products of catecholamines. Free Radic Biol Med 13:391- 405.

Bindoli A, Scutari G, Rigobello MP (1999) The role of adrenochrome in stimulating the oxidation of catecholamines. Neurotox Res 1:71-80.

Black JW, Crowther AF, Shanks RG, Smith LH, Dornhorst AC (1964) A new adrenergic betareceptor antagonist. Lancet 1:1080-1081.

Blaha CD, Coury A, Phillips AG (1996) Does monoamine oxidase inhibition by pargyline increase extracellular dopamine concentrations in the striatum? Neuroscience 75:543-550.

Bloom FE (2006) In Goodman & Gilman's The Pharmacological Basis of Therapeutics (Brunton, L. L. et al., eds), pp 283-304 New York: McGraw-Hill.

Boehm S, Kubista H (2002) Fine tuning of sympathetic transmitter release via ionotropic and metabotropic presynaptic receptors. Pharmacol Rev 54:43-99.

Bönisch H, Brüss M (2006) The norepinephrine transporter in physiology and disease. Handb Exp Pharmacol 175:485-524.

Bortolato M, Godar SC, Davarian S, Chen K, Shih JC (2009) Behavioral disinhibition and reduced anxiety-like behaviors in monoamine oxidase B-deficient mice. Neuropsychopharmacology 34:2746-2757.

Brown AM (1990) Regulation of heartbeat by G protein-coupled ion channels. Am J Physiol 259:H1621-1628.

Brunk I, Blex C, Rachakonda S, Höltje M, Winter S, Pahner I, Walther DJ, Ahnert-Hilger G (2006) The first luminal domain of vesicular monoamine transporters mediates G-protein-dependent regulation of transmitter uptake. J Biol Chem 281:33373-33385.

Brunner HG, Nelen M, Breakefield XO, Ropers HH, van Oost BA (1993) Abnormal behavior associated with a point mutation in the structural gene for monoamine oxidase A. Science 262:578-580.

Buck KJ, Amara SG (1994) Chimeric dopamine-norepinephrine transporters delineate structural domains influencing selectivity for catecholamines and 1-methyl-4-phenylpyridinium. Proc Natl Acad Sci U S A 91:12584-12588.

Burke WJ, Hanson DM, Chung H (1986) A highly sensitive assay for phenylethanolamine N-methyltransferase in human brain. Proc Soc Exp Biol Med 181:66-70.

Byington KH (1998) Detection of dopamine-tissue adducts. Life Sci 63:41-44.

Cannon WB, Rosenblueth A (1933) Studies on conditions of activity in endocrine organs: XXIX. Sympathin E and Sympathin I. Am J Physiol 104:557-574.

Capela JP, Carmo H, Remião F, Bastos ML, Meisel A, Carvalho F (2009) Molecular and cellular mechanisms of ecstasy-induced neurotoxicity: an overview. Mol Neurobiol 39:210-271.

Capela JP, Lautenschlager M, Dirnagl U, Bastos ML, Carvalho F, Meisel A (2008) 5,7-Dihydroxitryptamine toxicity to serotonergic neurons in serum free raphe cultures. Eur J Pharmacol 588:232-238.

Carlton SM, Honda CN, Denoroy L, Willis WDJ (1987) Descending phenylethanolamine-N-methyltransferase projections to the monkey spinal cord: an immunohistochemical double labeling study. Neurosci Lett 76:133-139.

Carlton SM, Honda CN, Willcockson WS, Lacrampe M, Zhang D, Denoroy L, Chung JM, Willis WDJ (1991) Descending adrenergic input to the primate spinal cord and its possible role in modulation of spinothalamic cells. Brain Res 543:77-90.

Carmo H, Remião F, Carvalho F, Fernandes E, de Boer D, dos Reys LA, Lourdes Bastos M (2003) 4-Methylthioamphetamine-induced hyperthermia in mice: influence of serotonergic and catecholaminergic pathways. Toxicol Appl Pharmacol 190:262-271.

Carroll JM, Evinger MJ, Goodman HM, Joh TH (1991) Differential and coordinate regulation of TH and PNMT mRNAs in chromaffin cell cultures by second messenger system activation and steroid treatment. J Mol Neurosci 3:75-83.

Carson RP, Robertson D (2002) Genetic manipulation of noradrenergic neurons. J Pharmacol Exp Ther 301:410-417.

Carvalho F, Duarte JA, Neuparth MJ, Carmo H, Fernandes E, Remião F, Bastos ML (2001) Hydrogen peroxide production in mouse tissues after acute d-amphetamine administration. Influence of monoamine oxidase inhibition. Arch Toxicol 75:465-469.

Carvalho F, Remiao F, Soares ME, Catarino R, Queiroz G, Bastos ML (1997) *d*-Amphetamine-induced hepatotoxicity: possible contribution of catecholamines and hyperthermia to the effect studied in isolated rat hepatocytes. Arch Toxicol 71:429-436.

Cases O, Seif I, Grimsby J, Gaspar P, Chen K, Pournin S, Müller U, Aguet M, Babinet C, Shih JC (1995) Aggressive behavior and altered amounts of brain serotonin and norepinephrine in mice lacking MAO-A. Science 268:1763-1766.

Chamba Gv, Renaud B (1983) Distribution of tyrosine hydroxylase, dopamine-β-hydroxylase and phenylethanolamine-N-methyltransferase activities in coronal sections of the rat lower brainstem. Brain Res 259:95-102.

Chaudhry A, MacKenzie RG, Georgic LM, Granneman JG (1994) Differential interaction of beta 1- and beta 3-adrenergic receptors with Gi in rat adipocytes. Cell Signal 6:457-465.

Chen X, Dimaggio DA, Han SP, Westfall TC (1997) Autoreceptor-induced inhibition of neuropeptide Y release from PC-12 cells is mediated by Y2 receptors. Am J Physiol Heart Circ Physiol 273:H1737-1744.

Costa VM, Carvalho F, Bastos ML, Carvalho RA, Carvalho M, Remião F (2011) Contribution of catecholamine reactive intermediates and oxidative stress to the pathologic features of heart diseases. Curr Med Chem 18:2272-2314.

Costa VM, Ferreira LM, Branco PS, Carvalho F, Bastos ML, Carvalho RA, Carvalho M, Remiao F (2009a) Cross-functioning between the extraneuronal monoamine transporter and multidrug resistance protein 1 in the uptake of adrenaline and export of 5-(glutathion-*S*-yl)adrenaline in rat cardiomyocytes. Chem Res Toxicol 22:129-135.

Costa VM, Silva R, Ferreira LM, Branco PS, Carvalho F, Bastos ML, Carvalho RA, Carvalho M, Remião F (2007) Oxidation process of adrenaline in freshly isolated rat cardiomyocytes: formation of adrenochrome, quinoproteins and GSH-adduct. Chem Res Toxicol 20:1183-1191.

Costa VM, Silva R, Ferreira R, Amado F, Carvalho F, Bastos ML, Carvalho RA, Carvalho M, Remião F (2009b) Adrenaline in pro-oxidant conditions elicits intracellular survival pathways in isolated rat cardiomyocytes. Toxicology 257:70-79.

Costa VM, Silva R, Tavares LC, Vitorino R, Amado F, Carvalho F, Bastos ML, Carvalho M, Carvalho RA, Remiao F (2009c) Adrenaline and reactive oxygen species elicit proteome and energetic metabolism modifications in freshly isolated rat cardiomyocytes. Toxicology 260:84-96.

Cotecchia S, Kobilka BK, Daniel KW, Nolan RD, Lapetina EY, Caron MG, Lefkowitz RJ, Regan JW (1990) Multiple second messenger pathways of alpha-adrenergic receptor subtypes expressed in eukaryotic cells. J Biol Chem 265:63-69.

Culman J, Torda T, Weise VK (1987) A radiometric assay for phenylethanolamine N-methyltransferase and catechol *O*-methyltransferase in a single tissue sample: application to rat hypothalamic nuclei, pineal gland, and heart. Anal Biochem 164:345-354.

Daubner SC, Lauriano C, Haycock JW, Fitzpatrick PF (1992) Site-directed mutagenesis of serine 40 of rat tyrosine hydroxylase. Effects of dopamine and cAMP-dependent phosphorylation on enzyme activity. J Mol Biol 267:12639-12646.

Della Rocca GJ, van Biesen T, Daaka Y, Luttrell DK, Luttrell LM, Lefkowitz RJ (1997) Ras-dependent mitogen-activated protein kinase activation by G protein-coupled receptors. Convergence of Gi- and Gq-mediated pathways on calcium/calmodulin, Pyk2, and Src kinase. J Biol Chem 272:19125-19132.

Docherty JR (1998) Subtypes of functional α_1- and α_2-adrenoceptors. Eur J Pharmacol 361:1-15.

Dooley TP (1998) Cloning of the human phenol sulfotransferase gene family: three genes implicated in the metabolism of catecholamines, thyroid hormones and drugs. Chem Biol Interact 109:29-41.

Driessen B, von Kügelgen I, Starke K (1994) P1-purinoceptor-mediated modulation of neural noradrenaline and ATP release in guinea-pig vas deferens. Naunyn Schmiedebergs Arch Pharmacol 350:42-48.

Duarte JA, Carvalho F, Fernandes E, Remião F, Bastos ML, Magalhães J, Appell HJ (2004) D-amphetamine-induced hydrogen peroxide production in skeletal muscle is modulated by monoamine oxidase inhibition. Int J Sports Med 25:446-449.

Eisenhofer G (1994) Plasma normetanephrine for examination of extraneuronal uptake and metabolism of noradrenaline in rats. Naunyn Schmiedebergs Arch Pharmacol 349:259-269.

Eisenhofer G (2001) The role of neuronal and extraneuronal plasma membrane transporters in the inactivation of peripheral catecholamines. Pharmacol Ther 91:35-62.

Eisenhofer G, Esler MD, Meredith IT, Dart A, Cannon ROr, Quyyumi AA, Lambert G, Chin J, Jennings GL, Goldstein DS (1992a) Sympathetic nervous function in human heart as assessed by cardiac spillovers of dihydroxyphenylglycol and norepinephrine. Circulation 85:1775-1785.

Eisenhofer G, Finberg JP (1994) Different metabolism of norepinephrine and epinephrine by catechol-*O*-methyltransferase and monoamine oxidase in rats. J Pharmacol Exp Ther 268:1242-1251.

Eisenhofer G, Keiser H, Friberg P, Mezey E, Huynh T-T, Hiremagalur B, Ellingson T, Duddempudi S, Eijsbouts A, Lenders JWM (1998) Plasma metanephrines are markers of pheochromocytoma produced by catechol-*O*-methyltransferase within tumors. J Clin Endocrinol Metab 83:2175-2185.

Eisenhofer G, Kopin IJ, Goldstein DS (2004) Catecholamine metabolism: a contemporary view with implications for physiology and medicine. Pharmacol Rev 56:331-349.

Eisenhofer G, Saigusa T, Esler MD, Cox HS, Angus JA, Dorward PK (1991) Central sympathoinhibition and peripheral neuronal uptake blockade after desipramine in rabbits. Am J Physiol Regulatory, Integrative and Comparative Physiology 260:R824-832.

Eisenhofer G, Smolich JJ, Esler MD (1992b) Disposition of endogenous adrenaline compared to noradrenaline released by cardiac sympathetic nerves in the anaesthetized dog. Naunyn Schmiedebergs Arch Pharmacol 345:160-171.

Emorine LJ, Marullo S, Briend-Sutren MM, Patey G, Tate K, Delavier-Klutchko C, Strosberg AD (1989) Molecular characterization of the human beta 3-adrenergic receptor. Science 245:1118-1121.

Erickson JD, Eiden LE, Hoffman BJ (1992) Expression cloning of a reserpine-sensitive vesicular monoamine transporter. Proc Natl Acad Sci U S A 89:10993-10997.

Esler M, Jennings G, Korner P, Blombery P, Sacharias N, Leonard P (1984a) Measurement of total and organ-specific norepinephrine kinetics in humans. Am J Physiol Endocrinology and Metabolism 247:E21-28.

Esler M, Jennings G, Lambert G, Meredith I, Horne M, Eisenhofer G (1990) Overflow of catecholamine neurotransmitters to the circulation: source, fate, and functions. Phys Rev 70:963-985.

Esler M, Jennings G, Leonard P, Sacharias N, Burke F, Johns J, Blombery P (1984b) Contribution of individual organs to total noradrenaline release in humans. Acta Physiol Scand Suppl 527:11-16.

Esler M, Kaye D (2000) Measurement of sympathetic nervous system activity in heart failure: the role of norepinephrine kinetics. Heart Fail Rev 5:17-25.

Fischer P, Bacq ZM (1950) The fluorescence of adrenaline and adrenochrome. Exp Med Surg 8:104-112.

Fluck DC (1972) Catecholamines. Br Heart J 34:869-873.

Foppoli C, Coccia R, Cini C, Rosei MA (1997) Catecholamines oxidation by xanthine oxidase. Biochim Biophys Acta 1334:200-206.

Fornstedt B, Pileblad E, Carlsson A (1990) In vivo autoxidation of dopamine in guinea pig striatum increases with age. J Neurochem 55:655-659.

Foster GA, Hökfelt T, Coyle JT, Goldstein M (1985) Immunohistochemical evidence for phenylethanolamine-N-methyltransferase-positive/tyrosine hydroxylase-negative neurones in the retina and the posterior hypothalamus of the rat. Brain Res 330:183-188.

Friedgen B, Halbrugge T, Graefe KH (1994) Roles of uptake1 and catechol-*O*-methyltransferase in removal of circulating catecholamines in the rabbit. Am J Physiol Endocrinology and Metabolism 267:E814-821.

Friedgen B, Wölfel R, Graefe K (1996) The contribution by monoamine oxidase and catechol-*O*-methyltransferase to the total-body and pulmonary plasma clearance of catecholamines. Naunyn Schmiedebergs Arch Pharmacol 353:193-199.

Frielle T, Collins S, Daniel KW, Caron MG, Lefkowitz RJ, Kobilka BK (1987) Cloning of the cDNA for the Human β1-adrenergic Receptor. Proc Natl Acad Sci U S A 84:7920-7924.

Fuller RW (1982) Pharmacology of brain epinephrine neurons. Annu Rev Pharmacol Toxicol 22:31-55.

Furchgott RF, Garcia PS (1968) Effects of inhibition of monoamino oxidase on the actions and interactions of norepinephrine, tyramine and other drugs on guinea-pig left atrium. J Pharmacol Exp Ther 163:98-122.

Gainetdinov RR, Premont RT, Bohn LM, Lefkowitz RJ, Caron MG (2004) Desensitization of G protein-coupled receptors and neuronal functions. Annu Rev Neurosci 27:107-144.

García-Sáinz JA, Vázquez-Prado J, del Carmen Medina L (2000) β1-Adrenoceptors: function and phosphorylation. Eur J Pharmacol 389:1-12.

Gauthier C, Langin D, Balligand J-L (2000) β3-Adrenoceptors in the cardiovascular system. Trends Pharmacol Sci 21:426-431.

Gauthier C, Tavernier G, Charpentier F, Langin D, Le Marec H (1996) Functional beta3-adrenoceptor in the human heart. J Clin Invest 98:556-562.

Gerlo E, Sevens C (1994) Urinary and plasma catecholamines and urinary catecholamine metabolites in pheochromocytoma: diagnostic value in 19 cases. Clin Chem 40:250-256.

Giros B, Wang YM, Suter S, McLeskey SB, Pifl C, Caron MG (1994) Delineation of discrete domains for substrate, cocaine, and tricyclic antidepressant interactions using chimeric dopamine-norepinephrine transporters. J Biol Chem 269:15985-15988.

Glover V, Sandler M, Owen F, Riley GJ (1977) Dopamine is a monoamine oxidase B substrate in man. Nature 265:80-81.

Godar SC, Bortolato M, Frau R, Dousti M, Chen K, Shih JC (2010) Maladaptive defensive behaviours in monoamine oxidase A-deficient mice. Int J Neuropsychopharmacol 1-13.

Gogos JA, Morgan M, Luine V, Santha M, Ogawa S, Pfaff D, Karayiorgou M (1998) Catechol-*O*-methyltransferase-deficient mice exhibit sexually dimorphic changes in catecholamine levels and behavior. Proc Natl Acad Sci U S A 95:9991-9996.

Goldstein DS (2003) Catecholamines and stress. Endocr Regul 37:69-80.

Goldstein DS, Brush JEJ, Eisenhofer G, Stull R, Esler M (1988) In vivo measurement of neuronal uptake of norepinephrine in the human heart. Circulation 78:41-48.

Goldstein DS, Eisenhofer G, Kopin IJ (2003) Sources and significance of plasma levels of catechols and their metabolites in humans. J Pharmacol Exp Ther 305:800-811.

Gonçalves J, Carvalho F, Guimarães S (1989) Uptake inhibitors do not change the effect of imidazoline alpha 2-adrenoceptor agonists on transmitter release evoked by single pulse stimulation in mouse vas deferens. Naunyn Schmiedebergs Arch Pharmacol 339:288-292.

Goodchild AK, Moon EA, Dampney RA, Howe PR (1984) Evidence that adrenaline neurons in the rostral ventrolateral medulla have a vasopressor function. Neurosci Lett 45:267-272.

Goodman OBJ, Krupnick JG, Santini F, Gurevich VV, Penn RB, Gagnon AW, Keen JH, Benovic JL (1996) Beta-arrestin acts as a clathrin adaptor in endocytosis of the beta2-adrenergic receptor. Nature 383:447-450.

Graefe KH, Henseling M (1983) Neuronal and extraneuronal uptake and metabolism of catecholamines. Gen Pharmacol 14:27-33.

Graefe KH, Trendelenburg U (1970) Influence of intraneuronal inactivating mechanisms on the membrane-amine pump. Naunyn Schmiedebergs Arch Pharmakol 266:336-337.

Grimsby J, Toth M, Chen K, Kumazawa T, Klaidman L, Adams JD, Karoum F, Gal J, Shih JC (1997) Increased stress response and beta-phenylethylamine in MAO B-deficient mice. Nat Genet 17:206-210.

Guimarães S (1975) Further study of the adrenoceptors of the saphenous vein of the dog: Influence of factors which interfere with the concentrations of agonists at the receptor level. Eur J Pharmacol 34:9-19.

Guimarães S, Moura D (2001) Vascular adrenoceptors: an update. Pharmacol Rev 53:319-356.

Haag C, Berkels R, Gründemann D, Lazar A, Taubert D, Schömig E (2004) The localisation of the extraneuronal monoamine transporter (EMT) in rat brain. J Neurochem 88:291-297.

Hadjiconstantinou M, Cohen J, Neff NH (1983) Epinephrine: a potential neurotransmitter in retina. J Neurochem 41:1440-1444.

Halliday GM, Li YW, Joh TH, Cotton RG, Howe PR, Geffen LB, Blessing WW (1988) Distribution of monoamine-synthesizing neurons in the human medulla oblongata. J Comp Neurol 273:301-317.

Hata JA, Williams ML, Koch WJ (2004) Genetic manipulation of myocardial beta-adrenergic receptor activation and desensitization. J Mol Cell Cardiol 37:11-21.

Heacock RA (1959) The chemistry of adrenochrome and related compounds. Chem Rev 59:181-237.

Heacock RA, Mahon ME (1958) The chemistry of the "aminochromes" II. The preparation, paper chromatography and spectroscopic properties of pure adrenolutin; the infared spectrum of adrenochrome. Can J Chem 36:1550.

Hoffmann BB (2004) Basic & Clinical Pharmacology. In: 10 th, vol. Adrenoceptor-Activating & Other Sympathomimetic Drugs (Katzung, B. G., ed) London: McGraw-Hill Medical.

Holtje M, von Jagow B, Pahner I, Lautenschlager M, Hortnagl H, Nurnberg B, Jahn R, Ahnert-Hilger G (2000) The neuronal monoamine transporter VMAT2 is regulated by the trimeric GTPase Go2. J Neurosci 20:2131-2141.

Holtje M, Winter S, Walther D, Pahner I, Hortnagl H, Ottersen OP, Bader M, Ahnert-Hilger G (2003) The vesicular monoamine content regulates VMAT2 activity through Galpha q in mouse platelets. Evidence for autoregulation of vesicular transmitter uptake. J Biol Chem 278:15850-15858.

Iversen LL (1963) The uptake of noradrenaline by the isolated perfused rat heart. Br J Pharmacol Chemother 21:523-537.

Iversen LL (1965a) The uptake of adrenaline by the rat isolated heart. Br J Pharmacol Chemother 24:387-394.

Iversen LL (1965b) The uptake of catecholamines at high perfusion concentrations in the rat isolated heart: a novel catecholamine uptake process. Brit J Pharmacol 24:18-33.

Iversen LL, De Champlain J, Glowinski J, Axelrod J (1967) Uptake, storage and metabolism of norepinephrine in tissues of the developing rat. J Pharmacol Exp Ther 157:509-516.

Jarrott B (1970) Uptake and metabolism of catecholamines in the perfused hearts of different species. Br J Pharmacol 38:810-821.

Johansson M, Rundqvist B, Eisenhofer G, Friberg P (1997) Cardiorenal epinephrine kinetics: evidence for neuronal release in the human heart. Am J Physiol Heart Circ Physiol 273:H2178-2185.

Johnson RG, Scarpa A (1979) Protonmotive force and catecholamine transport in isolated chromaffin granules. J Biol Chem 254:3750-3760.

Johnson RGJ (1988) Accumulation of biological amines into chromaffin granules: a model for hormone and neurotransmitter transport.. Physiol Rev 68:232-307.

Johnston JP (1968) Some observations upon a new inhibitor of monoamine oxidase in brain tissue. Biochem Pharmacol 17:1285-1297.

Kearney EB, Salach JI, Walker WH, Seng R, Singer TP (1971) Structure of the covalently bound flavin of monoamine oxidase. Biochem Biophys Res Commun 42:490-496.

Kelner KL, Pollard HB (1985) Glucocorticoid receptors and regulation of phenylethanolamine-N-methyltransferase activity in cultured chromaffin cells. J Neurosci 5:2161-2168.

Kennedy B, Elayan H, Ziegler MG (1990) Lung epinephrine synthesis. Am J Physiol Lung Cell Mol Physiol 258:L227-231.

Kennedy B, Elayan H, Ziegler MG (1993) Glucocorticoid elevation of mRNA encoding epinephrine-forming enzyme in lung. Am J Physiol Lung Cell Mol Physiol 265:117-120.

Kennedy B, Ziegler MG (1991) Cardiac epinephrine synthesis. Regulation by a glucocorticoid. Circulation 84:891-895.

Killingsworth CR, Wei C-C, Dell'Italia LJ, Ardell JL, Kingsley MA, Smith WM, Ideker RE, Walcott GP (2004) Short-acting beta-adrenergic antagonist esmolol given at reperfusion improves survival after prolonged ventricular fibrillation. Circulation 109:2469-2474.

Kim JJ, Shih JC, Chen K, Chen L, Bao S, Maren S, Anagnostaras SG, Fanselow MS, De Maeyer E, Seif I, Thompson RF (1997) Selective enhancement of emotional, but not motor, learning in monoamine oxidase A-deficient mice. Proc Natl Acad Sci U S A 94:5929-5933.

Kitahama K, Denoroy L, Goldstein M, Jouvet M, Pearson J (1988) Immunohistochemistry of tyrosine hydroxylase and phenylethanolamine N-methyltransferase in the human brain stem: description of adrenergic perikarya and characterization of longitudinal catecholaminergic pathways. Neuroscience 25:97-111.

Kitaichi Y, Inoue T, Nakagawa S, Boku S, Izumi T, Koyama T (2010) Combined treatment with MAO-A inhibitor and MAO-B inhibitor increases extracellular noradrenaline levels more than MAO-A inhibitor alone through increases in beta-phenylethylamine. Eur J Pharmacol 77-82.

Kjaer M (1998) Adrenal medulla and exercise training. Eur J Appl Physiol Occup Physiol 77:195-199.

Knoll J, Ecsery Z, Magyar K, Sátory E (1978) Novel (-)deprenyl-derived selective inhibitors of B-type monoamine oxidase. The relation of structure to their action. Biochem Pharmacol 27:1739-1747.

Kobilka BK, Frielle T, Collins S, Yang-Feng T, Kobilka TS, Francke U, Lefkowitz RJ, Caron MG (1987) An intronless gene encoding a potential member of the family of receptors coupled to guanine nucleotide regulatory proteins. Nature 329:75-79.

Kristufek D, Rudorfer W, Pifl C, Huck S (2002) Organic cation transporter mRNA and function in the rat superior cervical ganglion. J Physiol 543:117-134.

Krizanova O, Micutkova L, Jelokova J, Filipenko M, Sabban E, Kvetnansky R (2001) Existence of cardiac PNMT mRNA in adult rats: elevation by stress in a glucocorticoid-dependent manner. Am J Physiol Heart Circ Physiol 281:H1372-1379.

Kukkonen JP, Renvaktar A, Shariatmadari R, Akerman KEO (1998) Ligand- and subtype-selective coupling of human alpha-2 adrenoceptors to Ca^{2+} elevation in chinese hamster ovary cells. J Pharmacol Exp Ther 287:667-671.

Kumer SC, Vrana KE (1996) Intricate regulation of tyrosine hydroxylase activity and gene expression. J Neurochem 67:443-462.

Kuroko Y, Yamazaki T, Tokunaga N, Akiyama T, Kitagawa H, Ishino K, Sano S, Mori H (2007) Cardiac epinephrine synthesis and ischemia-induced myocardial epinephrine release. Cardiovasc Res 74:438-444.

Kvetnansky R, Micutkova L, Kubovcakova L, Sabban EL, Palkovits M, Krizanova O (2004) Localization and regulation of phenylethanolamine N-methyltransferase gene expression in the heart of rats and mice during stress. Ann N Y Acad Sci 1018:405-417.

Labrosse EH, Axelrod J, Kety SS (1958) O-Methylation, the principal route of metabolism of epinephrine in man. Science 128:593-594.

Lameris TW, Zeeuw S, Alberts G, Boomsma F, Duncker DJ, Verdouw PD, Man in 't Veld AJ, van den Meiracker AH (2000) Time course and mechanism of myocardial catecholamine release during transient ischemia in vivo. Circulation 101:2645-2650.

Langley JN (1905) On the reaction of cells and of nerve-endings to certain poisons, chiefly as regards the reaction of striated muscle to nicotine and to curari. J Physiol 33:374-413.

Lefkowitz RJ, Hausdorff WP, Caron MG (1990) Role of phosphorylation in desensitization of the β-adrenoceptor. Trends Pharmacol Sci 11:190-194.

Lefkowitz RJ, Pierce KL, Luttrell LM (2002) Dancing with different partners: protein kinase A phosphorylation of seven membrane-spanning receptors regulates their G protein-coupling specificity. Mol Pharmacol 62:971-974.

Lefkowitz RJ, Shenoy SK (2005) Transduction of receptor signals by beta-arrestins. Science 308:512-517.

Lenders JW, Eisenhofer G, Abeling NG, Berger W, Murphy DL, Konings CH, Wagemakers LM, Kopin IJ, Karoum F, van Gennip AH, Brunner HG (1996) Specific genetic deficiencies of the A and B isoenzymes of monoamine oxidase are characterized by distinct neurochemical and clinical phenotypes. J Clin Invest 97:1010-1019.

Lew JY, Matsumoto Y, Pearson J, Goldstein M, Hökfelt T, Fuxe K (1977) Localization and characterization of phenylethanolamine N-methyl transferase in the brain of various mammalian species. Brain Res 119:199-210.

Limbird LE (1988) Receptors linked to inhibition of adenylate cyclase: additional signaling mechanisms. FASEB J 2:2686-2695.

Loewi O (1921) Über humorale übertragbarkeit der herznervenwirkung. Pflügers Arch 189:239-242.

Loewi O (1936) Quantitative und qualitative intersuchugen über den sympaticusstoff. Pflügers Arch 237:505-514.

Lorang D, Amara SG, Simerly RB (1994) Cell-type-specific expression of catecholamine transporters in the rat brain. J Neurosci 14:4903-4914.

Ludemann HH, Filbert MG, Cornblath M (1955) Application of a fluorometric method for adrenaline-like substances in peripheral plasma. J Appl Physiol 8:59-66.

Macarthur H, Westfall TC, Riley DP, Misko TP, Salvemini D (2000) Inactivation of catecholamines by superoxide gives new insights on the pathogenesis of septic shock. Proc Natl Acad Sci 97:9753-9758.

MacNulty EE, McClue SJ, Carr IC, Jess T, Wakelam MJ, Milligan G (1992) Alpha 2-C10 adrenergic receptors expressed in rat 1 fibroblasts can regulate both adenylylcyclase and phospholipase D-mediated hydrolysis of phosphatidylcholine by interacting with pertussis toxin-sensitive guanine nucleotide-binding proteins. J Biol Chem 267:2149-2156.

Malmfors T (1967) Fluorescence histochemical studies on the uptake, storage, and release of catecholarnines. Circ Res XX-XXI: III25-III42.

Mannisto PT, Kaakkola S (1999) Catechol-*O*-methyltransferase (COMT): biochemistry, molecular biology, pharmacology, and clinical efficacy of the new selective COMT inhibitors. Pharmacol Rev 51:593-628.

Masson J, Sagné C, Hamon M, El Mestikawy S (1999) Neurotransmitter transporters in the central nervous system. Pharmacol Rev 51:439-464.

Mefford IN (1987) Are there epinephrine neurons in rat brain? Brain Res 434:383-395.

Meir A, Ginsburg S, Butkevich A, Kachalsky SG, Kaiserman I, Ahdut R, Demirgoren S, Rahamimoff R (1999) Ion channels in presynaptic nerve terminals and control of transmitter release. Physiol Rev 79:1019-1088.

Miyazaki I, Asanuma M, Diaz-Corrales FJ, Fukuda M, Kitaichi K, Miyoshi K, Ogawa N (2006) Methamphetamine-induced dopaminergic neurotoxicity is regulated by quinone formation-related molecules. FASEB J 20:571-573.

Moore KE, Phillipson OT (1975a) Effects of dexamethasone on phenylethanolamine N-methyl-transferase (PNMT) and adrenaline (A) in the brains of adult and neonatal rats. Br J Pharmacol 53:453P-454P.

Moore KE, Phillipson OT (1975b) Effects of dexamethasone on phenylethanolamine N-methyltransferase and adrenaline in the brains and superior cervical ganglia of adult and neonatal rats. J Neurochem 25:289-294.

Moore RY, Bloom FE (1979) Central catecholamine neuron systems: anatomy and physiology of the norepinephrine and epinephrine systems. Annu Rev Neurosci 2:113-168.

Nagatsu T (1991) Genes for human catecholamine-synthesizing enzymes. Neurosci Res 12:315-345.

Nagatsu T (2004) Progress in monoamine oxidase (MAO) research in relation to genetic engineering. Neurotoxicology 25:11-20.

Nelson CD, Kovacs JJ, Nobles KN, Whalen EJ, Lefkowitz RJ (2008) beta-arrestin scaffolding of phosphatidylinositol 4-phosphate 5-kinase Ialpha promotes agonist-stimulated sequestration of the beta 2-adrenergic receptor. J Biol Chem 21093-21101.

Nirenberg MJ, Chan J, Liu Y, Edwards RH, Pickel VM (1997) Vesicular monoamine transporter-2: immunogold localization in striatal axons and terminals. Synapse 26:194-198.

Nissinen E, Männistö PT (2010) Biochemistry and pharmacology of catechol-O-methyltransferase inhibitors. Int Rev Neurobiol 95:73-118.

Njus D, Kelley PM, Harnadek GJ (1986) Bioenergetics of secretory vesicles. Biochim Biophys Acta 853:237-265.

Nolte J (2009) The Human Brain: Elvesier Publisher.

Norberg KA, McIsaac RJ (1967) Cellular location of adrenergic amines in frog sympathetic ganglia. Experientia 23:1052.

Ochs S, Westfall TC, Macarthur H (2004) The separation and quantification of aminochromes using high- pressure liquid chromatography with electrochemical detection. J Neurosci Methods.

Oliver G, Schäfer EA (1895) The physiological effects of extracts of the suprarenal capsules. J Physiol 18:230-276.

Paiva MQ, Guimarães S (1978) A comparative study of the uptake and metabolism of noradrenaline and adrenaline by the isolated saphenous vein of the dog. Naunyn Schmiedebergs Arch Pharmacol 303:221-228.

Park DH, Teitelman G, Evinger MJ, Woo JI, Ruggiero DA, Albert VR, Baetge EE, Pickel VM, Reis DJ, Joh TH (1986) Phenylethanolamine N-methyltransferase-containing neurons in rat retina: immunohistochemistry, immunochemistry, and molecular biology. J Neurosci 6:1108-1113.

Patel N, Kumagai Y, Unger SE, Fukuto JM, Cho AK (1991) Transformation of dopamine and alpha-methyldopamine by NG108-15 cells: formation of thiol adducts. Chem Res Toxicol 4:421-426.

Pendleton RG, Gessner G, Sawyer J (1978) Studies on the distribution of phenylethanolamine N-methyltransferase and epinephrine in the rat. Res Commun Chem Pathol Pharmacol 21:315-325.

Peronnet F, Nadeau R, Boudreau G, Cardinal R, Lamontagne D, Yamaguchi N, De Champlain J (1988) Epinephrine release from the heart during left stellate ganglion stimulation in dogs. Am J Physiol Regulatory Integrative Comp Physiol 254:R659-662.

Pifl C, Hornykiewicz O, Giros B, Caron MG (1996) Catecholamine transporters and 1-methyl-4-phenyl-1,2,3,6-tetrahydropyridine neurotoxicity: studies comparing the cloned human noradrenaline and human dopamine transporter. J Pharmacol Exp Ther 277:1437-1443.

Pocock G, Richards CD (2006) Human Physiology: The Basis of Medicine. London: Oxford University Press.

Powell CE, Slater IH, LeCompte L, Jr, Waddell JE (1958) Blocking of inhibitory adrenergic receptors by a dichloro analog of isoproterenol. J Pharmacol Exp Ther 122:480-488.

Rang HP, Dale MM, Ritter JM, Flower RJ (2007) In Rang and Dale's Pharmacology: Churchill Livingstone.

Reis DJ, Ross CA, Ruggiero DA, Granata AR, Joh TH (1984) Role of adrenaline neurons of ventrolateral medulla (the C1 group) in the tonic and phasic control of arterial pressure. Clin Exp Hypertens A 6:221-241.

Remião F, Milhazes N, Borges F, Carvalho F, Bastos ML, Amado F, Domingues P, Ferrer-Correia A (2003) Synthesis and analyses of aminochromes by HPLC- photodiode array. Adrenochrome evaluation in rat blood. Biomed Chromatogr 17:6-13.

Richman JG, Regan JW (1998) alpha 2-Adrenergic receptors increase cell migration and decrease F-actin labeling in rat aortic smooth muscle cells. Am J Physiol Cell Physiol 274:C654-662.

Richter D (1940) The inactivation of adrenaline in vivo in man. J Physiol 98:361-374.

Ross CA, Ruggiero DA, Joh TH, Park DH, Reis DJ (1984a) Rostral ventrolateral medulla: selective projections to the thoracic autonomic cell column from the region containing C1 adrenaline neurons. J Comp Neurol 228:168-185.

Ross CA, Ruggiero DA, Park DH, Joh TH, Sved AF, Fernandez-Pardal J, Saavedra JM, Reis DJ (1984b) Tonic vasomotor control by the rostral ventrolateral medulla: effect of electrical or chemical stimulation of the area containing C1 adrenaline neurons on arterial pressure, heart rate, and plasma catecholamines and vasopressin. J Neurosci 4:474-494.

Ross ME, Evinger MJ, Hyman SE, Carroll JM, Mucke L, Comb M, Reis DJ, Joh TH, Goodman HM (1990) Identification of a functional glucocorticoid response element in the phenylethanolamine N-methyltransferase promoter using fusion genes introduced into chromaffin cells in primary culture. J Neurosci 10:520-530.

Roth JA (1992) Membrane-bound catechol-O-methyltransferase: a reevaluation of its role in the O-methylation of the catecholamine neurotransmitters. Rev Physiol Biochem Pharmacol 120:1-29.

Rottenberg H (1986) Energetics of proton transport and secondary transport. Methods Enzymol 125:3-15.

Rouot B, Brabet P, Homburger V, Toutant M, Bockaert J (1987) Go, a major brain GTP binding protein in search of a function: purification, immunological and biochemical characteristics. Biochimie 69:339-349.

Rupp H, Dhalla K, Dhalla N (1994) Mechanisms of cardiac cell damage due to catecholamines: significance of drugs regulating central sympathetic outflow. J Cardiovasc Pharmacol 24:S16-S24.

Schnaitman C, Erwin VG, Greenawalt JW (1967) The submitochondrial localization of monoamine oxidase. An enzymatic marker for the outer membrane of rat liver mitochondria. J Cell Biol 32:719-735.

Schömig E, Lazar A, Gründemann D (2006) Extraneuronal monoamine transporter and organic cation transporters 1 and 2: a review of transport efficiency. Handb Exp Pharmacol 175:151-180.

Schuldiner S (1994) A molecular glimpse of vesicular monoamine transporters. J Neurochem 62:2067-2078.

Schuldiner S, Fishkes H, Kanner BI (1978) Role of a transmembrane pH gradient in epinephrine transport by chromaffin granule membrane vesicles. Proc Natl Acad Sci U S A 75:3713-3716.

Segura-Aguilar J, Baez S, Widersten M, Welch CJ, Mannervik B (1997) Human class Mu glutathione transferases, in particular isoenzyme M2-2, catalyze detoxication of the dopamine metabolite aminochrome. J Biol Chem 272:5727-5731.

Shang T, Uihlein AV, Van Asten J, Kalyanaraman B, Hillard CJ (2003) 1-Methyl-4-phenylpyridinium accumulates in cerebellar granule neurons via organic cation transporter 3. J Neurochem 75:358-367.

Shen XM, Xia B, Wrona MZ, Dryhurst G (1996) Synthesis, redox properties, in vivo formation, and neurobehavioral effects of N-acetylcysteinyl conjugates of dopamine: possible metabolites of relevance to Parkinson's disease. Chem Res Toxicol 9:1117-1126.

Sonders MS, Quick M, Javitch JA (2005) How did the neurotransmitter cross the bilayer? A closer view. Curr Opin Neurobiol 15:296-304.

Spencer JPE, Jenner P, Daniel SE, Lees AJ, Marsden DC, Halliwell B (1998) Conjugates of catecholamines with cysteine and GSH in Parkinson's disease: possible mechanism of formation involving reactive oxygen species. J Neurochem 71:2112-2122.

Spencer JPE, Jenner P, Halliwel B (1995) Superoxide- dependent depletion of reduced glutathione by L-DOPA and dopamine. Neuroreport 6:1480-1484.

Spencer JPE, Whiteman M, Jenner P, Halliwel B (2002) 5-*S*-Cysteinyl-conjugates of catecholamines induce cell damage, extensive DNA base modication and increases in caspase-3 activity in neurons. J Neurochem 81:122-129.

Stachowiak MK, Rigual RJ, Lee PH, Viveros OH, Hong JS (1988) Regulation of tyrosine hydroxylase and phenylethanolamine N-methyltransferase mRNA levels in the sympathoadrenal system by the pituitary-adrenocortical axis. Brain Res 427:275-286.

Stolk JM, Vantini G, Perry BD, Guchhait RB, U'Prichard DC (1984) Assessment of the functional role of brain adrenergic neurons: chronic effects of phenylethanolamine N-methyltransferase inhibitors and alpha adrenergic receptor antagonists on brain norepinephrine metabolism. J Pharmacol Exp Ther 230:577-586.

Sun P, Bao X, Elayan H, Milic M, Liu F, Ziegler MG (2008) Epinephrine regulation of hemodynamics in catecholamine knockouts and the pithed mouse. Ann N Y Acad Sci 1148:325-330.

Surprenant A, Horstman DA, Akbarali H, Limbird LE (1992) A point mutation of the alpha 2-adrenoceptor that blocks coupling to potassium but not calcium currents. Science 257:977-980.

Takamine J (1902) The isolation of the active principle of the suprarenal gland. J Physiol 27:xxix- xxx.
Torda T, Culman J, Petriková M (1987) Distribution of phenylethanolamine-N-methyltransferase in the rat heart: effect of 6-hydroxydopamine. Eur J Pharmacol 141:305-308.
Trendelenburg U (1988) The extraneuronal uptake and metabolism of catecholamines. In: Catecholamines I (Trendelenburg, U. and Weiner, N., eds), pp 279-319 Berlin: Springer-Verlag.
Trendelenburg U (1990) The interaction of transport mechanisms and intracellular enzymes in metabolizing systems. J Neural Transm Suppl 32:3-18.
Trendelenburg U, Draskóczy PR, Graefe KH (1972) The influence of intraneuronal monoamine oxidase on neuronal net uptake of noradrenaline and on sensitivity to noradrenaline. Adv Biochem Psychopharmacol 5:371-377.
Vaarmann A, Gandhi S, Abramov AY (2010) Dopamine Induces Ca2+ Signaling in Astrocytes through Reactive Oxygen Species Generated by Monoamine Oxidase. J Biol Chem 285:25018-25023.
Valko M, Leibfritz D, Moncola J, Cronin MTD, Mazura M, Telser J (2007) Free radicals and antioxidants in normal physiological functions and human disease. Int J Biochem Cell Biol 39:44-84.
Vialou V, Amphoux A, Zwart R, Giros B, Gautron S (2004) Organic cation transporter 3 (Slc22a3) is implicated in salt-intake regulation. J Neurosci 24:2846-2851.
Vieira-Coelho MA, Serrão MP, Afonso J, Pinto CE, Moura E (2009) Catecholamine synthesis and metabolism in the central nervous system of mice lacking alpha-adrenoceptor subtypes. Br J Pharmacol 158:726-737.
von Euler U (1972) Pathophysiological aspects of catecholamine production. Clin Chem 18:1445-1448.
von Euler VS (1946) A specific sympathomimetic ergone in adrenergic nerve fibers (sympathin) and its relation to adrenaline and noradrenaline. Acta Physiologica Scandinavica 12.
Vulpian EF (1856) Note sur quelques reactions propes à la substance des capsules surrenales. C R Acad Sci 43:663- 665.
Wan DC, Livett BG (1989) Induction of phenylethanolamine N-methyltransferase mRNA expression by glucocorticoids in cultured bovine adrenal chromaffin cells. Eur J Pharmacol 172:107-115.
Wang Y-M, Xu F, Gainetdinov RR, Caron MG (1999) Genetic approaches to studying norepinephrine function: knockout of the mouse norepinephrine transporter gene. Biol Psychiatry 46:1124-1130.
West GB (1947) Oxidation of adrenaline in alkaline solution. Br J Pharmacol Chemother 2:121-130.
Westfall DP, Todorov LD, Mihaylova-Todorova ST (2002) ATP as a cotransmitter in sympathetic nerves and its inactivation by releasable enzymes. J Pharmacol Exp Ther 303:439-444.

Westfall TC, Westfall DP (2006) Adrenergic agonists and antagonists In: Goodman & Gilman's The pharmacological basis of therapeutics(Brunton, L. L. et al., eds), pp 215-264 New York: McGraw-Hill.

Wevers RA, de Rijk-van AJF, Bräutigam C, Geurtz B, van den Heuvel LP, Steenbergen-Spanjers GC, Smeitink JA, Hoffmann GF, Gabreëls FJ (1999) A review of biochemical and molecular genetic aspects of tyrosine hydroxylase deficiency including a novel mutation (291delC). J Inherit Metab Dis 22:364-373.

Wheatley AM, Thandroyen FT, Opie LH (1985) Catecholamine-induced myocardial cell damage: catecholamines or adrenochrome. J Mol Cell Cardiol 17:349-359.

Wise A, Watson-Koken MA, Rees S, Lee M, Milligan G (1997) Interactions of the alpha2A-adrenoceptor with multiple Gi-family G-proteins: studies with pertussis toxin-resistant G-protein mutants. Biochem J 321:721-728.

Wong DL, Lesage A, Siddall B, Funder JW (1992) Glucocorticoid regulation of phenylethanolamine N-methyltransferase in vivo. FASEB J 6:3310-3315.

Xiao RP, Ji X, Lakatta EG (1995) Functional coupling of the beta 2-adrenoceptor to a pertussis toxin-sensitive G protein in cardiac myocytes. Mol Pharmacol 47:322-329.

Xu F, Gainetdinov RR, Wetsel WC, Jones SR, Bohn LM, Miller GW, Wang Y-M, Caron MG (2000) Mice lacking the norepinephrine transporter are supersensitive to psychostimulants. Nat Neurosci 3:465-471.

Zhang G-X, Kimura S, Nishiyama A, Shokoji T, Rahman M, Yao L, Nagai Y, Fujisawa Y, Miyatake A, Abe Y (2005) Cardiac oxidative stress in acute and chronic isoproterenol-infused rats. Cardiovasc Res 65:230-238.

Zhong H, Minneman KP (1999) Alpha1-adrenoceptor subtypes. Eur J Pharmacol 375:261-276.

Zhou QY, Quaife CJ, Palmiter RD (1995) Targeted disruption of the tyrosine hydroxylase gene reveals that catecholamines are required for mouse fetal development. Nature 374:640-643.

Zigmond RE, Schwarzschild MA, Rittenhouse AR (1989) Acute regulation of tyrosine hydroxylase by nerve activity and by neurotransmitters via phosphorylation. Annu Rev Neurosci 12:415-461.

2

The Mystery of P2X7 Ionotropic Receptor: From a Small Conductance Channel to a Large Conductance Channel

R.X. Faria, L.G.B. Ferreira and L.A. Alves
Laboratory of Cellular Communication,
Oswaldo Cruz Institute,
Oswaldo Cruz Foundation,
Brazil

1. Introduction

1.1 Ion channels

Ion channels are aqueous pores which allow ions to pass based upon an electrochemical gradient. In order to conduct ions, these channels modify their shape by a process called gating, a shifting between opening and closing states. These channels are gated by various stimuli i.e. applied electric field, chemical transmitters, pH, heat and cold, among others. When an electrical potential is held constant in a cell, the gating process equilibriates rather than reaching an energy-dissipating position (a cyclic steady state). Ions diffuse through open channels very fast, involving an interaction between ions, the pore, and solvent that lead to ionic selectivity, saturation, block and flux coupling (Hille, 1975a; Läuger, 1973a).

The ion channel has generally been viewed as having unchanging selectivity strengthening the argument that there is a degree of specificity between ion and channel. Nevertheless, some classes of ion channels present a more varied selectivity of ions, allowing impermeable ions or molecules to permeate under certain circumstances. However, the there is no a systematic approach to distinguish different ion channels and in most cases, it is necessary to differentiate the channels by their kinetics, molecular sequence, pharmacological properties, and response to ionic substitution.

The diversity of channels continues to pose numerous areas to explore in physiology, molecular biology, pharmacology and biophysics.(Hille, 1991). Ion channels are generally classified into two groups: the channels that allow the passage of ions (Na+, K+, Ca2+) and those that allow the passage of large ions and solutes (ie ATP, glutamate, fluorescent dyes of low molecular weight). This second group is predominantly made up of large conductance ion channels which when activated change the permeability of cell membranes for molecules of up to 1000 Daltons (Ojcius, D. M. & Ding-E Young, J., 1990; Iacovache et al, 2010). These channels are and allow for the secretion of ATP and other intracellular molecules, not to mention implicated in various mechanisms of cell death.

2. Proteins that form large channels in mammal cells

These large channels are distinguished by their proteins which can be classified in accordance with their function, mechanism for membrane penetration, the size of their pores, its pore-forming subunits, and type of pore-forming proteins within the membrane plane (α- or β). By comparing the protein configuration in the plasma membrane it is possible to actually evolutionarily delineate the pore-forming protein of distinct organisms.

Proteins that form large conductance channels in the plasma membrane have been described in virus (Madan et al, 2007), bacteria (Huffman et al, 2004), fungi (Ojcius, D. M. & Young, J. D., 1991) and plantae (Klüsener & Weiler, 1999). Mostly due to these proteins being functionally linked to the mechanism of defense (plantae) or the invasion of the hosts (virus, bacteria, etc). These proteins are often secreted into the extracellular environment as monomers which then oligomerize and form the channel in the host membrane.

In humans and other mammals the secreted proteins, there have been found the antimicrobial peptide families of defensins (Kagan et al 1990) and cathelicidins (Scocchi et al, 1999; Skerlavaj et al, 2001). Other peptides, such as dermicidin (Boman et al 1993; Christensen et al, 1988) and anionic peptides (Brogden et al, 1996,1997,2003) are also found in tissue-specific areas. In the immune system, these pores cause physical damage to invading pathogens. In general, pore-forming proteins are monomeric molecules that interact with each other while they are inserted into membranes, where they continue to polymerize further to form large transmembrane pores, leading to a process of antimicrobial activity and cytotoxicity.

Generally, in vertebrates, more specifically in mammals, these pores are integral membrane proteins that are capable of opening under physiological or pathological condition. They can be found in several parts of the organism and may be associated with organism defense (release of pro-inflammatory agents, destruction of pathogens, cell death) or not (release of neurotransmissor, proliferation etc).

The main large conductance ion channels which are found in mammals, are the connexin hemichannels (Cx43, Cx32 and other), pannexins (pannexin-1), maxi anion channel, voltage-dependent anionic channel (VDAC), maxi-K channel, maitotoxin pore, transient receptor potential vanilloid type-1 (TRPV1), transient receptor potential ankhirin type-1 (TRPA1) and ATP-activated P2X pores (P2X2, P2X4 and P2X7 receptors). All of these permit the passage of mono and divalent ions and the flow of molecules of up to 1000 Da. The majority of these large conductance ion channels are preferentially permeable to cations, while VDAC and maxi anion are permeable to anions. In addition, they are all permeable to the anionic ATP4- molecule (Nagasawa et al, 2009; Pellegatti et al, 2005; Yip et al, 2009) and glutamate (Léon et al, 2008).

3. P2X7 receptor associated pore

Activation of the purinergic $P2X_7$ receptor (P2X7R) is rather unusual among ion channels. Brief agonist stimulation induces a non-selective cation-dependent pore, permitting the permeation of monovalent and divalent cations that leads to plasma membrane depolarization (Virginio et al, 1999b). By contrast, a prolonged and repetitive agonist application (at concentrations greater than 100 μM) promotes increased membrane permeability, allowing cellular uptake of fluorescent dyes such as propidium iodide (MW 639) or lucifer yellow (MW 457).

In the last years, some research groups have provided evidence that pannexin-1 (Panx1) hemichannel might be the protein associated with $P2X_7$ receptor pore formation. However, several cells allow the passage of dyes, despite having the pannexin-1 channel blocked (Faria et al, 2005, 2010; Schachter et al 2008; Yan et al 2008). This opens the possibility that other proteins may participate in the formation of the large channel associated with the $P2X_7$ receptor. As mentioned above, there are other proteins capable of forming large pores in plasma membrane.

In keeping with this idea, Faria and collaborators (2009) showed that calcium ionophores may massively increase the intracellular Ca^{2+} and induce dye uptake. They observed a pore with biophysical and pharmacological characteristics similar to $P2X_7$ receptor pore (Figure 1). In addition, Schilling and colleagues (1999) observed the Maitotoxin opening, a pore able to uptake fluorescent dyes. This pore was also biophysically similar to the $P2X_7$ receptor pore. Herein, we will address some questions about the possible protein candidate (or candidates) responsible for the $P2X_7$ receptor pore formation described above. Moreover, we will discuss the possible events which might be occurring to regulate the opening of these pores in mammalian cells.

4. Current methodologies to study large conductance channels

4.1 Patch clamp recordings

In patch-clamp recording, the microelectrode is a micropipette with a relatively large tip diameter. The microelectrode is placed next to a cell and a gentle suction is applied through the microelectrode to draw a piece of the cell membrane (the 'patch') into the microelectrode tip; the glass tip forms a high resistance 'seal' with the cell membrane. The suction causes the cell to form a tight and high-resistance seal around electrode, resulting in a resistance of approximately 10 giga Ohms, which is called a gigaseal. There are several variations of the patch-clamp technique, as depicted in Figure 2.

4.2 Cell permeabilization assays

This technique allows the detection of plasma membrane permeabilization in different cell types, by inducing the activation and opening of large conductance channels. In general, we use low molecular weight fluorescent dyes, such as fluorescein, lucifer yellow, calcein, ethidium bromide, propidium iodide, in order to observe the entrance of these impermeable dyes after the permeabilization phenomenon.

$P2X_7$ receptor pore-formation has been studied by several groups in different cell types. Most experiments associated with pore formation have centered around dye uptake experiments mediated by the $P2X_7$ receptor.

4.3 Flow cytometry assays

This is a technique for counting and examining microscopic particles, such as cells and chromosomes by suspending them in a stream of fluid and passing them through an

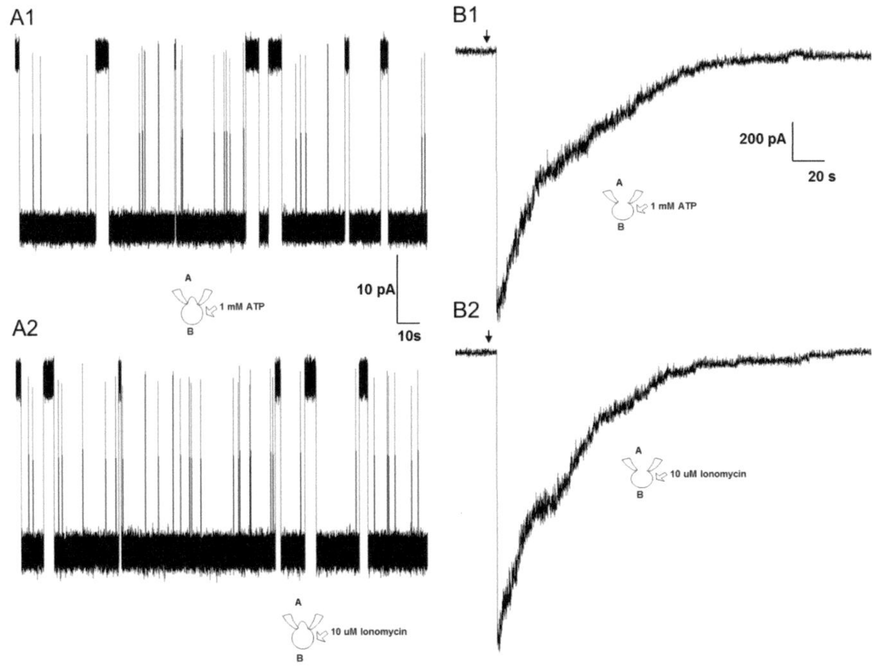

Fig. 1. Single channel and macroscopic currents in mouse peritoneal macrophages. The ionic currents were recorded at 37ºC and holding potential of -60mV using the cell attached configuration. A1- Single channel activity recorded after stimulation with 1mM ATP in the bath. A2- Single channel activity recorded after stimulation with 10uM Ionomycin in the bath. A3- Macroscopic current recorded after stimulation with 1mM ATP in the bath. A4- Macroscopic current recorded after stimulation with 10uM ioniomycin in the bath. Arrows in figure B represent the moment of application of the agonists. Under each recording there is a schematic representing the electrophysiological configuration, the localization and the agonist concentration used. A- Intracellular saline: 150mM KCl, 5mM NaCl, 0.1mM EGTA, 10mM HEPES, pH 7.4. B- Extracellular saline: 150mM NaCl, 5mM NaCl, 1mM MgC12+, 1mM CaC12+, 10mM Hepes, pH 7.4.

electron detection apparatus. It allows the simultaneous multiparametric analysis of the physical and chemical characteristics of thousands of particles per second. Clinical and research laboratories uses flow cytometry , to analyze multiple cell parameters such as cell cycle, cell membrane alterations and cell phenotype. Several studies have used flow cytometry in dye uptake assays stimulating the pore forming protein to open and permit the entry of fluorescent dyes.

4.4 Colorimetric assays

The measurement most commonly used to detect effects of P2X7 activation is colorimetric assays which are based on the absorbance of light. In according to Beer's Law, a solute absorbs light of a particular wavelength, and the absorbance is directly proportional to the substance concentration in solution. The measurement is done by a spectrophotometer, displaying and recording absorbance in quantifiable units. In general, the substance of

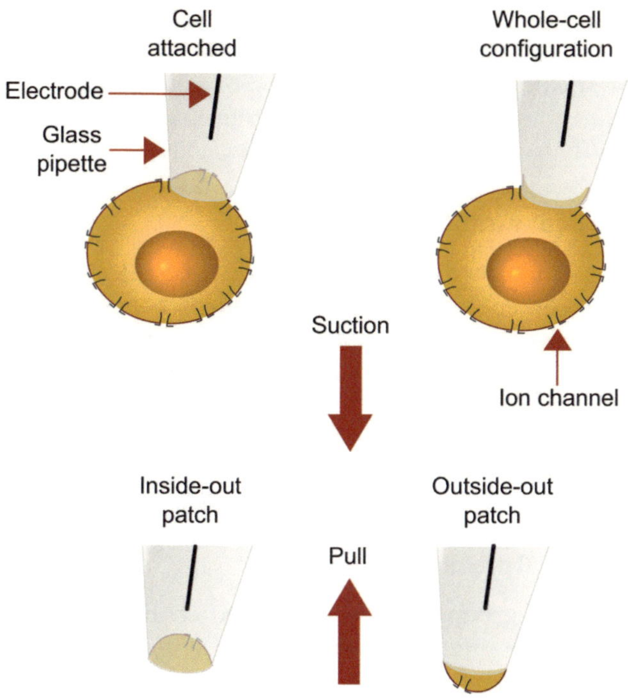

Fig. 2. Illustration of the different modes and configurations of the patch-clamp technique. In the cell-attached mode, the patch electrode remains sealed to the cell membrane, permitting the recording of currents through single-ion channels from the patch of membrane surrounded by the tip of the electrode. This configuration can be used for studying the activity of ion channels present in the membrane patch. In the whole cell mode, in the initial cell-attached configuration, additional suction is applied to rupture the cell membrane, thus providing access to the intracellular space. The larger opening at the tip of the patch electrode, compared with the sharp microelectrode, provides lower resistance and better electrical access to the cell- because the volume of the patch electrode is much bigger than the cell, cellular soluble contents will slowly be replaced by contents of the electrode, referred to as "dialyzing" the cell contents. Whole-cell mode records currents through all channels from the entire cell membrane at once. In the Inside-out patch mode, after the gigaseal are formed, the micropipette is quickly withdrawn from the cell, pulling off a patch of membrane from the cell, leaving the membrane patch attached to the micropipette, and exposing the intracellular surface of the membrane to the external media. This is useful when an experimenter wishes to pharmacologically manipulate the intracellular side of the ion channels. In the outside-out mode, after the whole-cell patch is formed, the electrode can be slowly withdrawn from the cell, allowing a bulb of membrane to bleb out from the cell. After the electrode to be pulled far enough away, this bleb will detach from the cell and reform as a convex membrane at the electrode end (like a ball open at the electrode tip), with the original outside of the membrane facing outward from the electrode. Single channel recordings are possible in this form if the membrane bleb is small enough. Outside-out patching gives the experimenter the opportunity to examine the properties of an ion channel when it is isolated from the cell, and exposed to different solutions on the extracellular membrane surface.

interest, by itself, does not absorb light in the wavelength used. We have to apply one or more reagents to produce colored compounds which are proportional to the substance concentration of the unknown. These methodologies may be used to measure cell death (LDH release, MTT assay), release of substances (neurotransmissors, cytokines and others), uptake of substances (fluorescent dyes) and enzymatic activity.

5. Electrophysiological studies of $P2X_7$

The first group which published a unitary current associated with the $P2X_7$ pore was Coutinho-Silva and coworkers in 1997. They used a cell attached configuration in mouse macrophages to show that the $P2X_7$ receptor when activated by ATP (in milimolar concentrations), is able to activate a large conductance channel with unitary conductance of about 400 pS (Coutinho-Silva et al, 1997). These pores were voltage dependent and had properties similar to P2Z permeabilization, such as uptake of large cations (N-methyl-D-glucamine) and anions (glutamate). Their opening is favored at temperatures higher than 30 degree Celsius and is blocked by oxidized ATP and Mg^{2+}. These authors did not record this conductance in excised patches which was the first clue for the participation of secondary messengers and cytoskeletal proteins.

After this discovery, other groups used cell attached configuration however only in low currents (~8pS) was the $P2X_7$ receptor recorded (Jiang et al, 2005; Ugur et al, 1997; Virginio et al, 1997). The large conductance activity was detected in dye uptake assays (Jiang et al, 2005; Hibell et al, 2000; Virginio et al, 1997;) or in whole cell experiments. In the whole cell, the macroscopic current induced by ATP or BzATP (a synthetic analog more potent than ATP) could be divided, according to some reports, into two distinct conductance (or components). The first component are the small channels opening and the second component is related to the large conductance of the $P2X_7$ receptor (Jiang et al, 2005; Virginio et al, 1999).

In 2005, our group, using cell attached configuration, recorded a unitary conductance of approximately 400 pS in murine macrophages and 2BH4 cells (Faria et al, 2005). We observed a linear response in positive and negative holding potential however this large conductance channel was never observed in excised patch, supporting that there is a dependence of intracellular signals as previously suggested by Coutinho-Silva's studies (Faria et al, 2005). In addition it was found that blockers of the $P2X_7$ receptor reduced the conductance and were modulated by the intracellular Ca^{2+} and MAPK. On the otherhand, Riedel's group in 2007, using the patch-clamp technique, studied the influence of external alkali and organic monovalent cations on the single-channel properties of the human $P2X_7$ receptor. In cell attached and excised patches, they observed activity only of the small conductance channel. Interestingly, they also reported an increased probability of $P2X_7$ small channel opening when extracellular Na^+ was substituted for other monovalent cations (Riedel et al, 2007a). This same group used human $P2X_7$ receptors expressed in *Xenopus laevis* oocytes and recorded single channels using the patch-clamp technique in the outside-out configuration. The result observed was similar to the previous paper as the large conductance channel was not observed (Riedel et al 2007b).

In 2008, Schachter and coworkers compared the $P2X_7$ receptor pore formation of macrophages and HEK-293 cells transfected with $P2X_7$ (HEK-P2X(7)) receptors using patch-clamp recordings. They did not record a unitary conductance activity in transfected HEK-293 cells. A pore with conductance of approximately 400 pS was recorded only in mouse peritoneal macrophages. Using dye uptake experiments, they also observed the differential uptake of cations and anions between the endogenous $P2X_7$ receptor pore formation in macrophages. The anionic pathways associated with the large conductance channel and the cationic pathway were unidentified (Schachter et al, 2008).

In 2009, based on previous data reporting that increasing intracellular Ca^{2+} is able to induce the opening of a pore biophysically similar to the $P2X_7$ receptor pore. Investigating this channel we found that calcium ionophores at micromolar concentrations induced dye uptake and ionic currents presented a unitary conductance of 400 pS, in the attached cell. This pore was unaffected by $P2X_7$ receptor blockers, but it had intracellular signaling components similar to the $P2X_7$ receptor large conductance channel and not observed in excised patches. However, we did not identify the entity responsible for inducing intracellular Ca^{2+} pore opening in mouse macrophages and 2BH4 cells (Faria et al, 2009).

In 2010, Yan and collaborators performed experiments to understand how the three binding site occupation for the ATP may affect the $P2X_7$ receptor gating. They showed that ATP concentrations in the milimolar range were able to biphasically activate and deactivate native receptors while micromolar concentrations responded monophasically. Both phases of response were abolished by the application of Az10606120, a $P2X_7R$-specific antagonist. This slow secondary growth of current in the biphasic response coincided temporally with pore dilation. This pore current was insensitive to Na^+ and Ca^{2+} influx and fully reestablished the initial gating properties after 30 min of washout. The complex pattern of gating exhibited by wild-type channels can be accounted for by the Markov state model that includes the negative cooperativity of agonist binding to unsensitized receptors caused by the occupancy of one or two binding sites, thus opening the channel pore to a low conductance state when the two sites are bound, and when three sites are occupied, triggering a high conductance state (pore dilation) (Yan et al, 2010). In contrast, Flittiger and collaborators while investigating the participation of protons in the activation of $hP2X_7Rs$ observed that human $P2X_7$ receptors expressed in *Xenopus laevis* oocytes were activated by ATP or BzATP at different pH values. The unitary currents were blocked by protonation and the large conductance channel not recorded (Flittiger et al, 2010).

In 2010, Roger and coworkers, used a whole cell configuration to characterize the functional properties of the biphasic ionic conductance recorded in human and rat $P2X_7$ receptors. They observed that in humans there was a Ca^{2+}/calmodulin independence of the secondary conductance (pore), while in rats there was dependency (Roger et al, 2010)

6. The search of large channels associated with $P2X_7$

In search of the $P2X_7$ receptor protein responsible for large unitary conductance and the pore that is induced rising intracellular Ca^{2+} (Faria et al, 2009) we compared the main biophysical properties of the other large conductance channels with these types of pores.

In cultured cells under resting conditions, hemichannels have a low open probability at negative membrane potentials, and the open probability is increased at positive potentials (Bukauskas & Verselis, 2004). Increases in hemichannel levels have been clearly associated with rises in intracellular-free Ca^{2+} concentration ($[Ca^{2+}]_i$) (Schalper et al, 2008, Sánchez et al, 2009). Normally, positive membrane potentials activate the fast gating, which corresponds to fast transitions between the fully open state and a substate. At negative membrane potentials, the loop gating activates slow transitions, perhaps involving multiple substates between the fully open state, substates and the fully closed state (Bukauskas & Verselis, 2004). Unitary conductance of the connexin hemichannel recorded in a cell attached configuration exhibited conductance values of approximately 300 pS for connexin 56 (Ebihara et al, 1999), for connexin 43 approximately of 200 pS (Contreras et al, 2003a, 2003b; Kang et al, 2008; Retamal et al, 2007b), 250 pS for connexin 46 (Ma & Dahl, 2006) and 200 pS for connexin 50 hemichannel (Liu et al, 2011).

Panx1 channels have been reported with different voltage dependence. In some cases, Panx1-mediated currents are outwardly rectifying and require a depolarization for activation (R. Bruzzone et al, 2003, Pelegrin et al, 2006). This observation is at odds with currents recorded in pyramidal neurons following Panx1 activation by ischemia or NMDAR stimulatio, where the current-voltage (I-V) relationship is clearly linear (Thompson et al, 2006, 2008a, 2008b) similar to Panx1 when it is conducting ATP (Bao et al, 2004). Upon activation, pannexons open into large non-selective pores, which are insensitive to physiological levels of extracellular Ca^{2+} but they are permeable to ions and small molecules as well as metabolites of up to 1000 Da and a wide range of membrane depolarization levels (S. Bruzzone et al, 2004). In addition, some groups have measured the unitary conductance of this large conductance channel, which is approximately 500 pS (Bao et al, 2004; Locovei et al, 2006; Thompson et al, 2006) which suggests that depolarization activates rectifying Panx1 currents and that other mechanisms lead to currents that are not significantly rectifying.

The presence of VDAC in the plasma membrane (pl-VDAC) would be expected to be lethal to the cell (Yu and Forte, 1996). However, considering the resting membrane potential across the plasma membrane of about -30 to -60 mV (Dermietzel et al, 1994), VDAC1 in the plasma membrane would be in a closed state most of the time (Mannella, 1997). Current events were recorded from excised patches of plasma membranes of a rat astrocytic cell line (RGCN)where it was found that the underlying channels exhibited a conductance from 401 to 250 pS. Open probability was the highest between 210 mV, and gradually approached zero beyond 225 mV. Activity induced by voltage ramps between 240 mV appeared after a several minute delay.

Several authors have reported the single-channel opening of the Maxi-anion with larger unitary conductance (300–400 pS) recorded in the cell-attached mode after cell swelling (Dutta et al, 2004; Liu et al, 2006, 2008a). Most authors noted that the maxi-anion channel has multiple subconductance states of various levels, such as 15, 50, 100, 150 and 200 pS (Dutta et al, 2004; Olesen & Bundgaard, 1992; Schwarze & Kolb, 1984; Akanda et al, 2008). When the extracellular Cl^- concentration varied, the single-channel conductance saturated at 640 pS with Km = 112 mM in L6 myoblasts (Hurnák & Zachar, 1994), at 581 pS with Km = 120 mM in T lymphocytes (Schlichter et al, 1990) and at 617 pS with Km = 77 mM in frog skeletal muscle "sarcoballs" (Hals et al, 1989). The maxi-anion channel presents roughly uniform behavior in different cell types. The current–voltage relationship of the fully open state is usually symmetrical and linear with no rectification when it is recorded by cell attached configuration. The channel has a maximal open channel probability at around 0 mV, but it readily closes when the voltage exceeds a range of ±15 to ± 30 mV. The macroscopic currents exhibit a time dependent inactivation at large positive and negative potentials over ±15 to +30 mV. The voltage dependence of open probability (Popen) remains bell-shaped with maximum at a voltage near 0 mV. These results indicate that the channel is highly selective to anions (Mitchell et al, 1997; Schlichter et al, 1990) but that the degree of anion selectivity may vary (Bajnath et al, 1993, Kemp et al, 1993) not only with cell types but also with the experimental conditions.

TRPV1 is a nonselective cation channel which is structurally related to the voltage-activated potassium (Kv) channels. The TRPV1 expressed alone in human embryonic kidney-derived HEK293 cells or *Xenopus* oocytes can account for the majority of the electrophysiological properties exhibited by native capsaicin receptors in sensory neurons, including ligand affinity, permeability sequence, current/voltage (I/V) relationship, conductance and open probability at both single-channel and whole-cell levels.

In whole cell configuration, I/V relationships have reversal potentials close to 0 mV, indicating the opening of non-selective cationic channels, and a substantial outwards rectification with a region of negative slope conductance at potentials negative to +70 mV (Gunthorpe et al, 2000).

In cell attached configuration, the single-channel amplitude histogram showed two well separated peaks representing open and closed states, without sub-conductance levels observed at +60 mV. The single-channel amplitude at +60 mV was 5.3 pA, corresponding to a conductance of 88.3 pS. Open probability depends on membrane potential as it has been shown in single-channel and whole-cell recordings (Premkumar *et al.* 2002; Voets *et al.* 2004b). At the molecular level, an extracellular Ca^{2+}-dependent reduction of TRPV1 responsiveness upon continuous vanilloid exposure (electrophysiological desensitization) may underlie this phenomenon, at least in part (Caterina et al, 1997; Szallasi & Blumberg, 1999). In relation to TRPV1 large conductance formation, some papers have published that this channel may mediate fluorescent dye uptake, however they did not characterize the biophysical properties related to this phenomenon (Blumberg, 2007; Hellwig et al, 2004; Myrdal & Steeiger, 2005). Since 2008, other research groups have now characterized this second stage of conductance of the TRPV1 channel.

MTX may initially induce the activation of a NSCC, which is permeable to Na+ and K+, but it has a low permeability to Ca2+ (Schilling et al., 1999; de la Rosa et al., 2007). MTX may also increase [Ca2+]i via various Ca^{2+} entry pathways following depolarization, including L-type voltage-sensitive Ca^{2+} channels (VSCCs), which are the predominant Ca^{2+} channel type in vascular smooth muscle (Sanders, 2001). The unitary conductance was 12 pS in the presence of 50 mM Ba^{2+}. Within a burst, the distribution of opening times was a single exponential with a mean open time of 10.4 ms (Kobayashi et al, 1987-Br J Pharmacol). GH4C1 rat pituitary cells were stimulated with independent currents of an MTX-induced steady-state voltage of nearly 400 pS/pF within seconds of addition to the bath. Ion substitution experiments demonstrated that these ionic currents are consistent with the conductance of sodium and chloride, but not calcium ions (Young et al, 1995).

7. Conclusion

In summary, Maxi anion and pl-VDAC had unitary conductance of 400 pS, but were voltage-dependent and anionic. In relation to Maitotoxin and TRPV1 pores which were not recorded in cell attached configuration yet their whole cell characteristics are similar. In addition, pannexin-1 hemichannels had unitary conductance of approximately 500 pS and could be activated by intracellular Ca^{2+}, though when this channel is activated by voltage its biophysical properties change. Altogether, these data show how complex and difficult is to characterize or rule out the participation of these proteins in the $P2X_7$ receptor large conductance.

A better understanding of the molecular mechanism for P2X7 pore formation might open new therapeutic strategies since this receptor is involved in several processes such as the killing of intracellular pathogens, chronic inflammation, neuropathic pain and rheumatoid arthritis.

So, despite the important efforts carried out in the studies of P2X7 receptor, the pore opening mechanism (large channel) is still unknown.

8. References

Akanda, N., Tofighi, R., Brask, J.,Tamm, C.,Elinder, F.& Ceccatelli, S. Voltage-dependent anion channels (VDAC) in the plasma membrane play a critical role in apoptosis in differentiated hippocampal neurons but not in neural stem cells. *Cell Cycle*, v. 7, n. 20, p. 3225-34, Oct 2008. ISSN 1551-4005.

Bajnath, R. B., Groot, J. A., de Jonge, H. R., Kansen, M. & Bijman, J.. Calcium ionophore plus excision induce a large conductance chloride channel in membrane patches of human colon carcinoma cells HT-29cl.19A. *Experientia*, v. 49, n. 4, p. 313-6, Apr 1993. ISSN 0014-4754.

Bao, L.; Locovei, S. & Dahl, G. Pannexin membrane channels are mechanosensitive conduits for ATP. *FEBS Lett*, v. 572, n. 1-3, p. 65-8, Aug 2004. ISSN 0014-5793.

Blumberg, P. M. Lighting a backfire to quench the blaze: a combined drug approach targeting the vanilloid receptor TRPV1. *Mol Interv*, v. 7, n. 6, p. 310-2, Dec 2007. ISSN 1534-0384.

Boman, H. G.; Agerberth, B.; Boman, A. Mechanisms of action on Escherichia coli of cecropin P1 and PR-39, two antibacterial peptides from pig intestine. *Infect Immun*, v. 61, n. 7, p. 2978-84, Jul 1993. ISSN 0019-9567. >.

Brogden, K. A., Ackermann, M., McCray, P. B. & Tack, B. F. Antimicrobial peptides in animals and their role in host defences. *Int J Antimicrob Agents*, v. 22, n. 5, p. 465-78, Nov 2003. ISSN 0924-8579.

Brogden, K. A., De Lucca, A. J., Bland, J. & Elliott, S. Isolation of an ovine pulmonary surfactant-associated anionic peptide bactericidal for Pasteurella haemolytica. Proc Natl Acad Sci U S A, v. 93, n. 1, p. 412-6, Jan 1996b. ISSN 0027-8424.

Brogden, K. A.; Ackermann, M.; Huttner, K. M. Small, anionic, and charge-neutralizing propeptide fragments of zymogens are antimicrobial. *Antimicrob Agents Chemother*, v. 41, n. 7, p. 1615-7, Jul 1997. ISSN 0066-4804.

Bruzzone, R., Hormuzdi, S. G.,Barbe, M. T.,Herb, A. & Monyer, H. Pannexins, a family of gap junction proteins expressed in brain. *Proc Natl Acad Sci U S A*, v. 100, n. 23, p. 13644-9, Nov 2003. ISSN 0027-8424.

Bruzzone, S., Verderio, C., Schenk, U., Fedele, E., Zocchi, E., Matteoli, M. & De Flora, A. Glutamate-mediated overexpression of CD38 in astrocytes cultured with neurones. *J Neurochem*, v. 89, n. 1, p. 264-72, Apr 2004. ISSN 0022-3042

Bukauskas, F. F. & Verselis, V. K. Gap junction channel gating. *Biochim Biophys Acta*, v. 1662, n. 1-2, p. 42-60, Mar 2004. ISSN 0006-3002.

Caterina, M. J., Schumacher, M. A., Tominaga, M., Rosen, T. A., Levine, J. D. & Julius, D. The capsaicin receptor: a heat-activated ion channel in the pain pathway. *Nature*, v. 389, n. 6653, p. 816-24, Oct 1997. ISSN 0028-0836.

Cavaliere, F.; Dinkel, K. & Reymann, K. Microglia response and P2 receptor participation in oxygen/glucose deprivation-induced cortical damage. *Neuroscience*, v. 136, n. 3, p. 615-23, 2005. ISSN 0306-4522.

Christensen, B., Fink, J., Merrifield, R. B. & Mauzerall, D.. Channel-forming properties of cecropins and related model compounds incorporated into planar lipid membranes. *Proc Natl Acad Sci U S A*, v. 85, n. 14, p. 5072-6, Jul 1988. ISSN 0027-8424.

Contreras, J. E., Sáez, J. C., Bukauskas, F. F. & Bennett, M. V. Functioning of cx43 hemichannels demonstrated by single channel properties. *Cell Commun Adhes*, v. 10, n. 4-6, p. 245-9, 2003 Jul-Dec 2003a. ISSN 1541-9061.

Contreras, J. E., Sáez, J. C., Bukauskas, F. F. & Bennett, M. V.. Gating and regulation of connexin 43 (Cx43) hemichannels. *Proc Natl Acad Sci U S A*, v. 100, n. 20, p. 11388-93, Sep 2003b. ISSN 0027-8424.

Coutinho-Silva, R. & Persechini, P. M. P2Z purinoceptor-associated pores induced by extracellular ATP in macrophages and J774 cells. *Am J Physiol*, v. 273, n. 6 Pt 1, p. C1793-800, Dec 1997. ISSN 0002-9513.

de la Rosa, L. A., Alavarez-Parrilla, E. & Martínez-Martínez, A. *Biochemistry of Maitotoxin, in Phycotoxins: Chemistry and Biochemistry*. Blackwell Publishing, Ames, Iowa, USA: 2007. ISBN 9780470277874.

Dermietzel, R., Hwang, T. K., Buettner, R., Hofer, A., Dotzler, E., Kremer, M., Deutzmann, R., Thinnes, F. P., Fishman, G. I. & Spray, D. C.. Cloning and in situ localization of a brain-derived porin that constitutes a large-conductance anion channel in astrocytic plasma membranes. *Proc Natl Acad Sci U S A*, v. 91, n. 2, p. 499-503, Jan 1994. ISSN 0027-8424.

Duan, S., Anderson, C. M., Keung, E. C., Chen, Y. & Swanson, R. A.. P2X7 receptor-mediated release of excitatory amino acids from astrocytes. *J Neurosci*, v. 23, n. 4, p. 1320-8, Feb 2003. ISSN 1529-2401.

Dutta, A. K., Sabirov, R. Z., Uramoto, H. & Okada, Y.. Role of ATP-conductive anion channel in ATP release from neonatal rat cardiomyocytes in ischaemic or hypoxic conditions. *J Physiol*, v. 559, n. Pt 3, p. 799-812, Sep 2004. ISSN 0022-3751.

Ebihara, L., Xu, X., Oberti, C., Beyer, E. C. & Berthoud, V. M.. Co-expression of lens fiber connexins modifies hemi-gap-junctional channel behavior. *Biophys J*, v. 76, n. 1 Pt 1, p. 198-206, Jan 1999. ISSN 0006-3495.

Faria, R. X., Cascabulho, C. M., Reis, R. A. & Alves, L. A.. Large-conductance channel formation mediated by P2X7 receptor activation is regulated through distinct intracellular signaling pathways in peritoneal macrophages and 2BH4 cells. *Naunyn Schmiedebergs Arch Pharmacol*, v. 382, n. 1, p. 73-87, Jul 2010. ISSN 1432-1912.

Faria, R. X., Reis, R. A., Casabulho, C. M., Alberto, A. V., de Farias, F. P., Henriques-Pons, A. & Alves, L. A.. Pharmacological properties of a pore induced by raising intracellular Ca2+. *Am J Physiol Cell Physiol*, v. 297, n. 1, p. C28-42, Jul 2009. ISSN 1522-1563.

Faria, R. X.; DeFARIAS, F. P. & Alves, L. A. Are second messengers crucial for opening the pore associated with P2X7 receptor? *Am J Physiol Cell Physiol*, v. 288, n. 2, p. C260-71, Feb 2005. ISSN 0363-6143.

Flittiger, B., Klapperstück, M., Schmalzing, G. & Markwardt, F.. Effects of protons on macroscopic and single-channel currents mediated by the human P2X7 receptor. *Biochim Biophys Acta*, v. 1798, n. 5, p. 947-57, May 2010. ISSN 0006-3002.

Gunthorpe, M.J., Harries, M.H., Prinjha, R.K., Davis, J.B., & Randall, A.. Voltage-and time-dependent properties of the recombinat rat vanilloid receptor. *Journal of Physiology*: 747-759 p. 2000.

Hals, G. D.; Stein, P. G. & Palade, P. T. Single channel characteristics of a high conductance anion channel in "sarcoballs". *J Gen Physiol*, v. 93, n. 3, p. 385-410, Mar 1989. ISSN 0022-1295.

Hellwig, N., Plant, T. D., Janson, W., Schäfer, M., Schultz, G. & Schaefer, M.. TRPV1 acts as proton channel to induce acidification in nociceptive neurons. *J Biol Chem*, v. 279, n. 33, p. 34553-61, Aug 2004. ISSN 0021-9258.

Hibell, A. D., Kidd, E. J., Chessell, I. P., Humphrey, P. P. & Michel, A. D.. Apparent species differences in the kinetic properties of P2X(7) receptors. *Br J Pharmacol*, v. 130, n. 1, p. 167-73, May 2000. ISSN 0007-1188.

Hille, B. . Ionic selectivity of Na and K channels of nerve membranes. *Membranes*, v. 3, p. 255-323, 1975. ISSN 0076-6356.

Huffman, D. L., Bischof, L. J., Griffitts, J. S. & Aroian, R. V.. Pore worms: using Caenorhabditis elegans to study how bacterial toxins interact with their target host. *Int J Med Microbiol*, v. 293, n. 7-8, p. 599-607, Apr 2004. ISSN 1438-4221.

Hurnák, O. & Zachar, J. Conductance-voltage relations in large-conductance chloride channels in proliferating L6 myoblasts. *Gen Physiol Biophys*, v. 13, n. 3, p. 171-92, Jun 1994. ISSN 0231-5882.

Iacovache, I.; Bischofberger, M. & Van der Goot, F. G. Structure and assembly of pore-forming proteins. *Curr Opin Struct Biol*, v. 20, n. 2, p. 241-6, Apr 2010. ISSN 1879-033X.

Jiang, L. H., Rassendren, F., Mackenzie, A., Zhang, Y. H., Surprenant, A. & North, R. A.. N-methyl-D-glucamine and propidium dyes utilize different permeation pathways at rat P2X(7) receptors. *Am J Physiol Cell Physiol*, v. 289, n. 5, p. C1295-302, Nov 2005. ISSN 0363-6143.

Kang, J., Kang, N., Lovatt, D., Torres, A., Zhao, Z., Lin, J. & Nedergaard, M.. Connexin 43 hemichannels are permeable to ATP. *J Neurosci*, v. 28, n. 18, p. 4702-11, Apr 2008. ISSN 1529-2401.

Kawamura, H., Aswad, F., Minagawa, M., Malone, K., Kaslow, H., Koch-Nolte, F., Schott, W. H., Leiter, E. H. & Dennert, G.. P2X7 receptor-dependent and -independent T cell death is induced by nicotinamide adenine dinucleotide. *J Immunol*, v. 174, n. 4, p. 1971-9, Feb 2005. ISSN 0022-1767.

Kemp, P. J. & Boyd, C. A. Anion exchange in type II pneumocytes freshly isolated from adult guinea-pig lung. *Pflugers Arch*, v. 425, n. 1-2, p. 28-33, Oct 1993. ISSN 0031-6768.

Klüsener, B. & Weiler, E. W. Pore-forming properties of elicitors of plant defense reactions and cellulolytic enzymes. *FEBS Lett*, v. 459, n. 2, p. 263-6, Oct 1999. ISSN 0014-5793.

Kobayashi, M. & Ochi, R.; Ohizumi, Y. Maitotoxin-activated single calcium channels in guinea-pig cardiac cells. *Br J Pharmacol*, v. 92, n. 3, p. 665-71, Nov 1987. ISSN 0007-1188.

Läuger, P. Ion transport through pores: a rate-theory analysis. *Biochim Biophys Acta*, v. 311, n. 3, p. 423-41, Jul 1973. ISSN 0006-3002.

León, D., Sánchez-Nogueiro, J., Marín-García, P. & Miras-Portugal, M. A.. Glutamate release and synapsin-I phosphorylation induced by P2X7 receptors activation in cerebellar granule neurons. *Neurochem Int*, v. 52, n. 6, p. 1148-59, May 2008. ISSN 0197-0186.

Lister, M. F., Sharkey, J., Sawatzky, D. A., Hodgkiss, J. P., Davidson, D. J., Rossi, A. G. & Finlayson, K.. The role of the purinergic P2X7 receptor in inflammation. *J Inflamm (Lond)*, v. 4, p. 5, 2007. ISSN 1476-9255.

Liu, H. T., Tashmukhamedov, B. A., Inoue, H., Okada, Y. & Sabirov, R. Z.. Roles of two types of anion channels in glutamate release from mouse astrocytes under ischemic or osmotic stress. *Glia*, v. 54, n. 5, p. 343-57, Oct 2006. ISSN 0894-1491.

Liu, H. T., Toychiev, A. H., Takahashi, N., Sabirov, R. Z. & Okada, Y. Maxi-anion channel as a candidate pathway for osmosensitive ATP release from mouse astrocytes in primary culture. *Cell Res*, v. 18, n. 5, p. 558-65, May 2008. ISSN 1748-7838.

Liu, J., Ek Vitorin, J. F., Weintraub, S. T., Gu, S., Shi, Q., Burt, J. M. & Jiang, J. X.. Phosphorylation of connexin 50 by protein kinase A enhances gap junction and hemichannel function. *J Biol Chem*, v. 286, n. 19, p. 16914-28, May 2011. ISSN 1083-351X.

Locovei, S.; Bao, L. & Dahl, G. Pannexin 1 in erythrocytes: function without a gap. *Proc Natl Acad Sci U S A*, v. 103, n. 20, p. 7655-9, May 2006. ISSN 0027-8424.

Ma, M. & Dahl, G. Cosegregation of permeability and single-channel conductance in chimeric connexins. *Biophys J*, v. 90, n. 1, p. 151-63, Jan 2006. ISSN 0006-3495.

Madan, R. P., Mesquita, P. M., Cheshenko, N., Jing, B., Shende, V., Guzman, E., Heald, T., Keller, M. J., Regen, S. L., Shattock, R. J. & Herold, B. C. Molecular umbrellas: a novel class of candidate topical microbicides to prevent human immunodeficiency virus and herpes simplex virus infections. *J Virol*, v. 81, n. 14, p. 7636-46, Jul 2007. ISSN 0022-538X.

Mannella, C. A. Minireview: on the structure and gating mechanism of the mitochondrial channel, VDAC. *J Bioenerg Biomembr*, v. 29, n. 6, p. 525-31, Dec 1997. ISSN 0145-479X.

Mariathasan, S., Weiss, D. S., Newton, K., McBride, J., O'Rourke, K., Roose-Girma, M., Lee, W. P., Weinrauch, Y., Monack, D. M. & Dixit, V. M.. Cryopyrin activates the inflammasome in response to toxins and ATP. *Nature*, v. 440, n. 7081, p. 228-32, Mar 2006. ISSN 1476-4687.

Milius, D., Gröger-Arndt, H., Stanchev, D., Lange-Dohna, C., Rossner, S., Sperlagh, B., Wirkner, K. & Illes, P.. Oxygen/glucose deprivation increases the integration of recombinant P2X7 receptors into the plasma membrane of HEK293 cells. *Toxicology*, v. 238, n. 1, p. 60-9, Aug 2007. ISSN 0300-483X.

Mitchell, C. H., Zhang, J. J., Wang, L. & Jacob, T. J.. Volume-sensitive chloride current in pigmented ciliary epithelial cells: role of phospholipases. *Am J Physiol*, v. 272, n. 1 Pt 1, p. C212-22, Jan 1997. ISSN 0002-9513.

Myrdal, S. E. & Steyger, P. S. TRPV1 regulators mediate gentamicin penetration of cultured kidney cells. *Hear Res*, v. 204, n. 1-2, p. 170-82, Jun 2005. ISSN 0378-5955.

Nagasawa, K.; Escartin, C. & Swanson, R. A. Astrocyte cultures exhibit P2X7 receptor channel opening in the absence of exogenous ligands. *Glia*, v. 57, n. 6, p. 622-33, Apr 2009. ISSN 1098-1136.

Ojcius, D. M. & Ding-E Young, J. A role for pore-forming proteins in the pathogenesis by parasites? *Parasitol Today*, v. 6, n. 5, p. 163-5, May 1990. ISSN 0169-4758.

Ojcius, D. M. & Young, J. D. Cytolytic pore-forming proteins and peptides: is there a common structural motif? *Trends Biochem Sci*, v. 16, n. 6, p. 225-9, Jun 1991. ISSN 0968-0004.

Olesen, S. P. & Bundgaard, M. Chloride-selective channels of large conductance in bovine aortic endothelial cells. *Acta Physiol Scand*, v. 144, n. 2, p. 191-8, Feb 1992. ISSN 0001-6772.

Papp, L., Vizi, E. S. & Sperlágh, B. Lack of ATP-evoked GABA and glutamate release in the hippocampus of P2X7 receptor-/- mice. *Neuroreport*, v. 15, n. 15, p. 2387-91, Oct 2004. ISSN 0959-4965.

Pelegrin, P. & Surprenant, A. Pannexin-1 mediates large pore formation and interleukin-1beta release by the ATP-gated P2X7 receptor. *EMBO J*, v. 25, n. 21, p. 5071-82, Nov 2006. ISSN 0261-4189.

Pellegatti, P., Falzoni, S., Pinton, P., Rizzuto, R. & Di Virgilio, F.. A novel recombinant plasma membrane-targeted luciferase reveals a new pathway for ATP secretion. *Mol Biol Cell*, v. 16, n. 8, p. 3659-65, Aug 2005. ISSN 1059-1524.

Premkumar, L. S.; Agarwal, S.; Steffen, D. Single-channel properties of native and cloned rat vanilloid receptors. *J Physiol*, v. 545, n. Pt 1, p. 107-17, Nov 2002. ISSN 0022-3751.

Retamal, M. A., Froger, N., Palacios-Prado, N., Ezan, P., Sáez, P. J., Sáez, J. C. & Giaume, C.. Cx43 hemichannels and gap junction channels in astrocytes are regulated oppositely by proinflammatory cytokines released from activated microglia. *J Neurosci*, v. 27, n. 50, p. 13781-92, Dec 2007. ISSN 1529-2401.

Riedel, T., Lozinsky, I., Schmalzing, G. & Markwardt, F.. Kinetics of P2X7 receptor-operated single channels currents. *Biophys J*, v. 92, n. 7, p. 2377-91, Apr 2007. ISSN 0006-3495.

Riedel, T., Schmalzing, G. & Markwardt, F. Influence of extracellular monovalent cations on pore and gating properties of P2X7 receptor-operated single-channel currents. *Biophys J*, v. 93, n. 3, p. 846-58, Aug 2007. ISSN 0006-3495.

Roger, S., Gillet, L., Baroja-Mazo, A., Surprenant, A. & Pelegrin, P.. C-terminal calmodulin-binding motif differentially controls human and rat P2X7 receptor current facilitation. *J Biol Chem*, v. 285, n. 23, p. 17514-24, Jun 2010. ISSN 1083-351X.

Sánchez, H. A., Orellana, J. A., Verselis, V. K. & Sáez, J. C.. Metabolic inhibition increases activity of connexin-32 hemichannels permeable to Ca2+ in transfected HeLa cells. *Am J Physiol Cell Physiol*, v. 297, n. 3, p. C665-78, Sep 2009. ISSN 1522-1563.

Sanders, K. M. Invited review: mechanisms of calcium handling in smooth muscles. *J Appl Physiol*, v. 91, n. 3, p. 1438-49, Sep 2001. ISSN 8750-7587.

Schachter, J., Motta, A. P., de Souza Zamorano, A., da Silva-Souza, H. A., Guimarães, M. Z. & Persechini, P. M.. ATP-induced P2X7-associated uptake of large molecules involves distinct mechanisms for cations and anions in macrophages. *J Cell Sci*, v. 121, n. Pt 19, p. 3261-70, Oct 2008. ISSN 0021-9533.

Schalper, K. A., Palacios-Prado, N., Retamal, M. A., Shoji, K. F., Martínez, A. D. & Sáez, J. C.. Connexin hemichannel composition determines the FGF-1-induced membrane permeability and free [Ca2+]i responses. *Mol Biol Cell*, v. 19, n. 8, p. 3501-13, Aug 2008. ISSN 1939-4586.

Schilling, W. P.; Sinkins, W. G. & Estacion, M. Maitotoxin activates a nonselective cation channel and a P2Z/P2X(7)-like cytolytic pore in human skin fibroblasts. *Am J Physiol*, v. 277, n. 4 Pt 1, p. C755-65, Oct 1999. ISSN 0002-9513.

Schlichter, L. C., Grygorczyk, R., Pahapill, P. A. & Grygorczyk, C.. A large, multiple-conductance chloride channel in normal human T lymphocytes. *Pflugers Arch*, v. 416, n. 4, p. 413-21, Jun 1990. ISSN 0031-6768.

Schwarze, W. & Kolb, H. A. Voltage-dependent kinetics of an anionic channel of large unit conductance in macrophages and myotube membranes. *Pflugers Arch*, v. 402, n. 3, p. 281-91, Nov 1984. ISSN 0031-6768.

Scocchi, M., Bontempo, D., Boscolo, S., Tomasinsig, L., Giulotto, E. & Zanetti, M. Novel cathelicidins in horse leukocytes(1). FEBS Lett, v. 457, n. 3, p. 459-64, Sep 1999. ISSN 0014-5793.

Skerlavaj, B., Scocchi, M., Gennaro, R., Risso, A. & Zanetti, M. Structural and functional analysis of horse cathelicidin peptides. *Antimicrob Agents Chemother*, v. 45, n. 3, p. 715-22, Mar 2001. ISSN 0066-4804.

Surprenant, A., Rassendren, F., Kawashima, E., North, R. A. & Buell, G.. The cytolytic P2Z receptor for extracellular ATP identified as a P2X receptor (P2X7). *Science*, v. 272, n. 5262, p. 735-8, May 1996. ISSN 0036-8075.

Szallasi, A. & Blumberg, P. M. Vanilloid (Capsaicin) receptors and mechanisms. *Pharmacol Rev*, v. 51, n. 2, p. 159-212, Jun 1999. ISSN 0031-6997.

Takenouchi, T., Sato, M. & Kitani, H. Lysophosphatidylcholine potentiates Ca2+ influx, pore formation and p44/42 MAP kinase phosphorylation mediated by P2X7 receptor activation in mouse microglial cells. *J Neurochem*, v. 102, n. 5, p. 1518-32, Sep 2007. ISSN 0022-3042.

Taylor, S. R., Gonzalez-Begne, M., Dewhurst, S., Chimini, G., Higgins, C. F., Melvin, J. E. & Elliott, J. I.. Sequential shrinkage and swelling underlie P2X7-stimulated lymphocyte phosphatidylserine exposure and death. *J Immunol*, v. 180, n. 1, p. 300-8, Jan 2008. ISSN 0022-1767.

Thompson, R. J. & Macvicar, B. A. Connexin and pannexin hemichannels of neurons and astrocytes. *Channels (Austin)*, v. 2, n. 2, p. 81-6, 2008 Mar-Apr 2008. ISSN 1933-6969.

Thompson, R. J., Jackson, M. F., Olah, M. E., Rungta, R. L., Hines, D. J., Beazely, M. A., MacDonald, J. F. & MacVicar, B. A.. Activation of pannexin-1 hemichannels augments aberrant bursting in the hippocampus. *Science*, v. 322, n. 5907, p. 1555-9, Dec 2008. ISSN 1095-9203.

Thompson, R. J., Zhou, N. & Macvicar, B. A. Ischemia opens neuronal gap junction hemichannels. *Science*, v. 312, n. 5775, p. 924-7, May 2006. ISSN 1095-9203.

Ugur, M., Drummond, R. M., Zou, H., Sheng, P., Singer, J. J. & Walsh, J. V.. An ATP-gated cation channel with some P2Z-like characteristics in gastric smooth muscle cells of toad. *J Physiol*, v. 498 (Pt 2), p. 427-42, Jan 1997. ISSN 0022-3751.

Virginio, C., Church, D., North, R. A. & Surprenant, A.. Effects of divalent cations, protons and calmidazolium at the rat P2X7 receptor. *Neuropharmacology*, v. 36, n. 9, p. 1285-94, Sep 1997. ISSN 0028-3908.

Virginio, C., MacKenzie, A., Rassendren, F. A., North, R. A. & Surprenant, A.. Pore dilation of neuronal P2X receptor channels. *Nat Neurosci*, v. 2, n. 4, p. 315-21, Apr 1999. ISSN 1097-6256.

Voets, T., Droogmans, G., Wissenbach, U., Janssens, A., Flockerzi, V. & Nilius, B.. The principle of temperature-dependent gating in cold- and heat-sensitive TRP channels. *Nature*, v. 430, n. 7001, p. 748-54, Aug 2004. ISSN 1476-4687.

Yan, Z., Khadra, A., Li, S., Tomic, M., Sherman, A. & Stojilkovic, S. S.. Experimental characterization and mathematical modeling of P2X7 receptor channel gating. *J Neurosci*, v. 30, n. 42, p. 14213-24, Oct 2010. ISSN 1529-2401.

Yip, L., Woehrle, T., Corriden, R., Hirsh, M., Chen, Y., Inoue, Y., Ferrari, V., Insel, P. A. & Junger, W. G.. Autocrine regulation of T-cell activation by ATP release and P2X7 receptors. *FASEB J*, v. 23, n. 6, p. 1685-93, Jun 2009. ISSN 1530-6860.

Young, R. C.; Mclaren, M. & Ramsdell, J. S. Maitotoxin increases voltage independent chloride and sodium currents in GH4C1 rat pituitary cells. *Nat Toxins*, v. 3, n. 6, p. 419-27, 1995. ISSN 1056-9014.

Yu, W. H. & Forte, M. Is there VDAC in cell compartments other than the mitochondria? *J Bioenerg Biomembr*, v. 28, n. 2, p. 93-100, Apr 1996. ISSN 0145-479X.

Yuan, B. S., Zhu, R. M., Braddock, M., Zhang, X. H., Shi, W. & Zheng, M. H.. Interleukin-18: a pro-inflammatory cytokine that plays an important role in acute pancreatitis. *Expert Opin Ther*

3

Facilitation of Neurotransmitter and Hormone Release by P2X Purinergic Receptors

Vojtech Vavra, Anirban Bhattacharya,
Marie Jindrichova and Hana Zemkova
*Institute of Physiology of the Academy of Sciences of the Czech Republic,
Czech Republic*

1. Introduction

Nucleotides are emerging as ubiquitous family of extracellular signaling molecules. Their effects are mediated through a specific class of plasma membrane receptors called purinergic P2 receptors that, according to the molecular structure, are further subdivided into two subfamilies: P2Y and P2X. Specifically, P2X receptors (P2XRs) are ligand-gated ion channels, whereas P2Y receptors (P2YRs) belong to the superfamily of G-protein-coupled receptors.

Purinergic P2XRs are expressed in a wide range of organisms from amoeba to humans (Fountain et al., 2007). In mammals, seven P2X subunits (termed P2X1-7) have been found (North, 2002). These receptors appeared early in evolution and have a widespread distribution on many neurons and non-neuronal cells. The P2XRs comprise the family of trimeric channels that use the energy of extracellular ATP binding to initiate a depolarizing flux of cations, including calcium, through the pore of channels. The extracellular actions of ATP are terminated by ectonucleotidases, leading to the generation of ADP, a primary agonist for some P2YRs, and adenosine, the common agonist for adenosine subtypes of receptor (Ralevic and Burnstock, 1998). Substantial progress has been made in elucidating the roles these receptors play under physiological and pathological conditions and in our understanding of the functional, structural, and pharmacological properties of seven P2X receptor subtypes. Purinergic signaling is involved in several basic physiological responses such as embryonic and stem cell development, pain sensation, regulation of renal blood flow, inflammatory responses, auditory neurotransmission etc., whereas pathophysiology of purinergic signalling includes stroke, thrombosis, osteoporosis, kidney failure, bladder incontinence, cystic fibrosis, dry eye, cancer and brain disorders (Khakh and North, 2006; Surprenant and North, 2009; Burnstock, 2011). In excitable cells, P2XR activation causes an increase in the cytosolic Ca^{2+} concentration via two distinct mechanisms: by membrane depolarization resulting in voltage-dependent Ca^{2+} entry and by Ca^{2+} entry through the P2XR itself. The role of P2XR involves fast synaptic transmission mediated by ATP in both the peripheral (Evans et al., 1992) and central nervous systems (Edwards et al., 1992), modulation of neuronal excitability (Khakh and Henderson, 1998), long-term potentiation (Sim et al., 2006), and stimulation of hormone secretion (luteinizing hormone, prolactin, oxytocin and vasopressin) (Kapoor and Sladek, 2000; Stojilkovic, 2009; Stojilkovic et al.,

2010b). ATP is also the dominant messenger for neuron-glia communication (Guthrie et al., 1999; Newman, 2003; Fields and Burnstock, 2006).

This review summarizes recent investigations and our contribution to the knowledge about the molecular structure and mechanism of function of P2X receptors, and also how do they facilitate neurotransmitter release in the brain and secretion of hormones in pituitary.

2. P2X receptors

The P2XRs are ATP-gated non-selective cation channels which are permeable to Na^+, K^+, Ca^{2+} and small organic cations (Valera et al., 1994; Egan and Khakh, 2004). The discovery of P2XRs introduced a third class of ligand-gated ion channels (North, 1996), distinct from the first class, represented by nicotinic acetylcholine receptors, γ-aminobutyric acid (GABA) receptors, glycine receptors and 5-hydroxytryptamine receptors, and the second class, represented by glutamate receptors, α-amino-3-hydroxy-5-methyl-4-isoxazole propionic acid receptors (AMPAR) and N-methyl-D-aspartate receptors (NMDAR). In mammals, seven genes encode the P2XR subunits (North, 2002) which can form functional channels as homo- and heterotrimers (Lewis et al., 1995; Nicke et al., 1998; Stoop et al., 1999). The distinct P2XR subtypes are functionally differentiated by comparisons in their sensitivity to ATP and its analogs, antagonists and allosteric modulators. Prolonged application of ATP causes a decrease in the conductivity of some P2XRs, a process termed receptor desensitization, which is also receptor-specific (North, 2002). For P2X1R and P2X3R the rate of desensitization is very fast - within milliseconds, the P2X4R desensitizes within seconds. The P2X2R and P2X7R do not desensitize, but their pore diameter increases in the continuous presence of agonist (Virginio et al., 1999). Subunit P2X6 does not form functional homomeric channels as it is retained in the endoplasmic reticulum in the monomeric form (Barrera et al., 2005; Ormond et al., 2006), but its heteromeric assemblies are functional (Le et al., 1998; King et al., 2000). So far, three combinations of heteromeric P2X6R channels have been characterized in functional and biochemical studies: P2X1+P2X6 (Nicke et al., 2005), P2X2+P2X6 (King et al., 2000) and P2X4+P2X6 (Le et al., 1998).

Various subclasses of P2XRs are activated with different potencies to ATP and its analogs. Low micromolar concentrations of ATP activate most of P2XRs, only the P2X7R requires millimolar concetrations of ATP. The P2X1R and P2X3R, are also potently activated by αβ-methylene ATP (αβmeATP) and the P2X7R by 2′,3′-0′,3′-O-(4-benzoylbenzoyl)-ATP (BzATP) in micromolar range (Jacobson et al., 2002); even though BzATP is also an agonist for P2X1, P2X3 and P2X4 receptors. P2XRs are inhibited by pyridoxalphosphate-6-azophenyl-2', 4'-disulfonic acid (PPADS) and suramin, which are both non-selective P2X antagonists (Coddou et al., 2011). Pharmacological experiments revealed two distinct features of P2X4R: relative resistance to suramin and PPADS (Buell et al., 1996), and robust sensitivity to positive modulatory effect of ivermectin, a high molecular weight lipophilic compound used as an antiparasitic agent in human and veterinary medicine (Burkhart, 2000), whereas other subtypes of P2XR family are ivermectin-insensitive (Khakh et al., 1999; Jelinkova et al., 2006). Among P2XRs, the P2X7R is unique as it gradually develops permeability to organic cations, causing a sustained current growth accompanied with cell blebbing and death (Surprenant et al., 1996; Di Virgilio et al., 1998; Mackenzie et al., 2005; Adinolfi et al., 2010; Yan et al., 2010). The P2X7Rs are blocked by KN62, and reactive blue-2, and also by a more potent and selective antagonists *N*-[2-[[2-[(2-hydroxyethyl)amino]ethyl] amino]-5-quinolinyl]-2-tricyclo[3.3.1.13,7]dec-1-ylacetamide dihydrochloride (AZ 10606120) (Michel et al., 2007) and 3-[[5-(2,3-dichlorophenyl)-1*H*-tetrazol-1-yl]methyl] pyridine hydrochloride (A 438079) (Nelson et al., 2006).

The P2XR subtypes are functionally differentiated also by comparisons in their calcium permeability which is relatively high, in the range from 2.7 % (P2X3R) to 12.4 % (P2X1R) of total ATP-induced current (Egan and Khakh, 2004).

2.1 Molecular structure of P2X receptors

Each P2XR subunit consists of a large extracellular domain which binds agonists, two α-helical transmembrane domains (TM1 and TM2) and cytoplasmic N- and C-termini (Valera et al., 1994; Egan et al., 2004). There are 10 conserved cysteine residues in the ectodomain that form five intrasubunit disulfide bonds (SS1-SS5) (Clyne et al., 2002; Ennion and Evans, 2002; Rokic et al., 2010). Using the baculovirus-Sf9 cell expression system, the P2X2R was expressed and purified, and its structure was observed using electron microscopy. These images showed that the P2X2R protein resembles an inverted three-sided pyramid 215 Å in height and 200 Å in side length (Mio et al., 2005), providing visual evidence of the trimeric composition of the P2XR family. This shape has been in principle confirmed by crystalization of zebrafish P2X4.1R (Kawate et al., 2009). Crystal structure shows that extracellular domain of P2XR trimer, rich in beta-strands, contains three non-canonical, intersubunit ATP-binding sites and three major subunit-to-subunit contacts, the role of which is still unknown. There are no contacts between the subunits at the base of the extracellular domain, proximal to the TM1 and TM2 domains; these lateral fenestration are suggested to provide a possible pathway for ions to enter and exit the channel pore (Kracun et al., 2010; Kawate et al., 2011). Crystal was solved in the absence of ATP and shows P2X4.1R in its closed state; subunit rearrangement after ATP binding and subsequent ion channel opening thus remains to be elucidated.

2.2 Role of TM2 in receptor function

Functional studies predict that both transmembrane helices move during gating (Li et al., 2004; Silberberg et al., 2005) and the P2XR apparently forms a parallel six-helix bundle, in the center of which is an aqueous cavity (Duckwitz et al., 2006; Li et al., 2011). While TM2 plays a key role in the formation of the ion pore and selectivity filter during receptor activation (Rassendren et al., 1997; Egan et al., 1998; Haines et al., 2001b; Haines et al., 2001a; Jiang et al., 2001; Migita et al., 2001; Li et al., 2004; Khakh and Egan, 2005; Silberberg et al., 2005; Kawate et al., 2009; Kracun et al., 2010) and is also critical as a hydrophobic anchor by which the receptor is fixed in the membrane (Torres et al., 1999), a contribution from TM1 to channel gating has also been suggested (Haines et al., 2001b; Haines et al., 2001a; Jiang et al., 2001; Samways et al., 2008; Jindrichova et al., 2009). In particular, TM2 residues Thr336, Thr339 and Ser340 (P2X2R numbering) contribute to formation of the selective filter, the narrow region in the channel pore, (Migita et al., 2001; Egan and Khakh, 2004). Conserved TM2 residue Asp355 (P2X5 numbering, human receptor form) has also been shown to be important for this function and it initiates oligomerization of subunits in the membrane (Duckwitz et al., 2006). It is clear that different residues are involved in the formation of selectivity filter of the other P2XR subtypes because their transmembrane helices are only 39-55% identical with the P2X2 subunit (North, 2002). For example, residues Gly340 and

Leu343 are important for P2X4R, in addition to Ser341 (position Thr336 in P2X2) and Ala344 (Thr339 in P2X2) (Jelinkova et al., 2008). The gating properties of P2X channels are affected by alanine mutation of conserved TM2 residue Gly342 that exhibited reduced sensitivity to ATP in the P2X2R (Li et al., 2004) and P2X4R (Jelinkova et al., 2008). This residue has been suggested to play a role in helix motion as a point of local flexibility, acting like a hinge between the lower and the upper part of TM2 (Khakh and Egan, 2005). The region between P2X2R residues Gly342 and Asp349 most probably contributes to formation of the channel pore gate (Egan et al., 1998). As mentioned above, the P2X2 and P2X7 receptors display a time- and activation-dependent increase in large cation permeability (Virginio et al., 1999). Dilation of the pore could proceed due to channel rearrangements that occur at the interface between TM1 and TM2 of neighboring subunits (Jiang et al., 2003; Khakh and Egan, 2005). Functional studies identified three TM1 residues (Phe31, Arg33 and Gln37) and six TM2 residues (Ile328, Ile332, Ser340, Gly342, Trp350 and Leu352) that might be involved in the increase of pore diameter at P2X2R (Khakh and Egan, 2005).

2.3 Role of TM1 and molecular basis of calcium conductivity

A study performed on several subtypes of P2X receptors revealed a key role for aromatic residues in the upper part of TM1 in sensitivity to agonist (Jindrichova et al., 2009). Out of several aromatic residues of TM1, Tyr42 (P2X4 numbering) is the only residue that is fully conserved among all species examined thus far (Bavan et al., 2009). Alanine or cysteine substitution of conserved TM1 tyrosine generated a constitutively active channel that exhibited enhanced ATP sensitivity in P2X2R (Haines et al., 2001a; Li et al., 2004), P2X3R (Jindrichova et al., 2009; Jindrichova et al., 2011) and P2X4R (Jelinkova et al., 2008; Jindrichova et al., 2009). This residue is important also for other receptor functions: it has been suggested to control Ca^{2+} permeability as an inter-pore binding site for Ca^{2+} in P2X2R (Samways and Egan, 2007), to link TM1 with TM2 of adjacent subunit to control P2X4R deactivation (Stojilkovic et al., 2010a) (Fig.1) or to stabilize desensitized states in P2X3R (Jindrichova et al., 2011). High Ca^{2+} permeability of P2X1R and P2X4R has been ascribed to negatively charged ectodomain residues glutamate and aspartate, localized near the membrane at the end of TM1 and at the beginning of TM2 (Samways and Egan, 2007). However, negatively charged residues are also present at the same positions in P2X3R and P2X7R which exhibit relatively low Ca^{2+} permeability (Samways and Egan, 2007) indicating that other residues are also involved in calcium conductivity of P2XRs. The dilatation of P2X2R and P2X7R channel pore is also accompanied by abnormal calcium influx.

These properties, particularly the high throughput for Ca^{2+} ions, account for numerous physiological functions stimulated by ATP and P2XR in the central nervous system. These involve an increase in neuronal activity (Khakh et al., 2003), potentiation of neurotransmitter release (Sperlagh et al., 2007) and stimulation of hormone secretion (luteinizing hormone, prolactin, oxytocin and vasopressin) (Kapoor and Sladek, 2000; Stojilkovic, 2009; Stojilkovic et al., 2010b).

A, Three-dimensional model and positions of the first transmembrane domains (C) and the second transmebrane domains (N) of the rat P2X4R as viewed from the extracellular side. Individual subunits are differentiated by color (gray, green and blue). The Tyr42 residue (red) is between TM1 and TM2 helices of adjacent subunits and its side chain is in close proximity to residues Ile333, I337 and Met336 (orange) from the adjacent subunit, forming a network of hydrophobic interactions B, The structural model shows Tyr42 side chain interactions with residues in TM2 helix of neighboring subunit (blue). The distance between OH:Tyr42 and TM2 atoms Ile333, Ile337 and Met336 are indicated using dashed lines. The figure was made using PyMOL (The PyMOL Molecular Graphics System, Version 1.2r3pre, Schrödinger, LLC.).

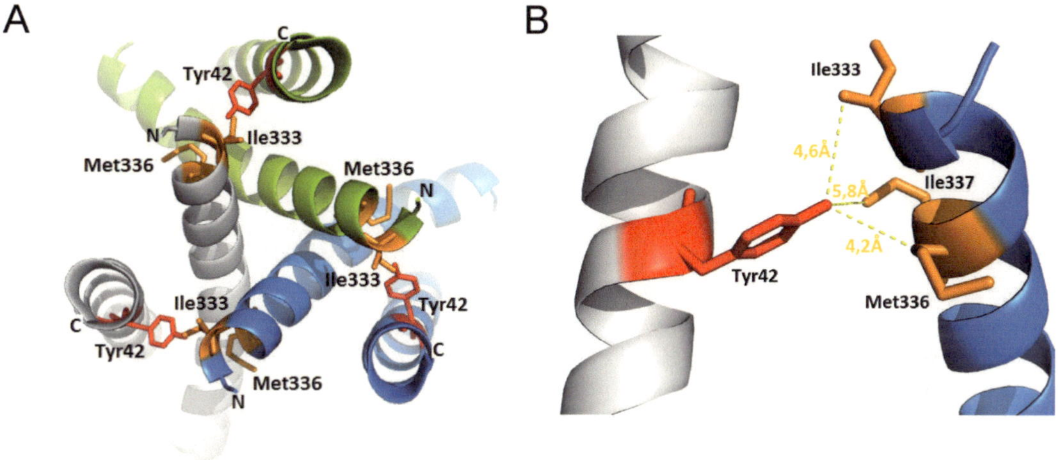

Fig. 1. Homology modeling of TM domains of P2X4 receptor.

3. Modulatory effect of P2X receptors on synaptic transmission

Following the discovery of purinergic neurotransmission in 1972 in non-adrenergic, non-cholinergic inhibitory nerves in guinea-pig taenia coli, ATP was identified as a co-transmitter in both sympathetic and parasympathetic peripheral nerves and latter also in the central nervous systems (Burnstock, 2011). Of all tissues investigated, the mammalian brain has the highest levels of purines and the greatest variety of the ATP-binding P2XRs (Buell et al., 1996; Collo et al., 1996; Seguela et al., 1996). Both neurons and glial cells release ATP and express P2XRs (Fields and Stevens, 2000; Raivich, 2005; Inoue et al., 2007) and it is common that several subtypes of P2XRs are expressed in the plasma membrane of one cell (Abbracchio et al., 2009). Neurons release ATP by exocytosis together with other neurotransmitters, such as GABA, glycine, glutamate and noradrenaline (Jo and Schlichter, 1999; Robertson et al., 2001; Sokolova et al., 2001; Jo and Role, 2002; Day et al., 1993). Glia have been shown to release ATP in response to mechanical and electrical stimulation (Newman, 2003; Burnstock, 2004), although the precise mechanisms have not been identified. The most frequent receptor forms in the brain are P2X2, P2X4, and P2X6 as well as heteromers composed of P2X2+X6, P2X4+X6, and perhaps P2X1+X4 receptors (Buell et al., 1996; Collo et al., 1996). Activation of P2X receptors by extracellular ATP acts mainly as a short-term signal but has also several long-term effects. The short-term effects involve fast synaptic transmission mediated by ATP in both the peripheral (Evans et al., 1992) and central nervous systems (Edwards et al., 1992), modulation of neuronal excitability (Khakh and Henderson, 1998) and long-term potentiation (Sim et al., 2006). Long-term (trophic) role comprise cell proliferation, differentiation and death, growth of axons during development and regeneration (Heine et al., 2006; Burnstock, 2011). Like other transmitters, ATP can mediate both reciprocal interactions between neurons and glia, and intercellular communication in astrocytic networks (Guthrie et al., 1999; Newman, 2003; Fields and Burnstock, 2006; Burnstock, 2007).

3.1 Expression of P2X receptor subtypes in hypothalamus

Purinergic P2X receptors are expressed throughout the hypothalamus where ATP, co-released with neuropeptides, appears to be involved in the regulation of hormone secretion (Troadec et al., 1998; Kapoor and Sladek, 2000) and control of specific autonomic functions including the central mechanism of body temperature regulation (Gourine et al., 2002), for example. P2X2, P2X4 and P2X6, but not P2X5 receptor mRNAs have been identified in the rat supraoptic nucleus (SON), ventromedial nucleus, paraventricular nucleus, arcuate nucleus, suprachiasmatic nucleus, and several other hypothalamic areas using in situ hybridization; the P2X1, P2X3 and P2X7 receptors were not tested in this study (Collo et al., 1996). Another PCR analysis revealed that P2X2, P2X3, P2X4, P2X6, and P2X7 receptor mRNAs are expressed in the rat SON neurons; P2X1 and P2X5 mRNAs were not found (Shibuya et al., 1999). In the preoptic area of the rhesus monkey, the P2X2, P2X4 and P2X7 receptor mRNAs, but not P2X1, P2X3 and P2X5 receptor mRNAs, were identified; subunit P2X6 was not examined (Terasawa et al., 2005). Immunohistochemistry shows local differences in P2XR protein distribution in the rat hypothalamus. For example, the P2X2R immunoreactive neurons and nerve fibers have been found to be localized in the paraventricular nucleus, arcuate nucleus, retrochiasmatic area, periventricular nucleus, the ventral part of tuber cinereum area, supraoptic, circular, and ventral tuberomammillary nuclei, organum vasculosum, and median eminence (Xiang et al., 1998; Yao et al., 2003), but are absent in the ventromedial nucleus (Vulchanova et al., 1996; Xiang et al., 1998). The magnocellular neurons from paraventricular and supraoptic nuclei synthesize vasopressin and oxytocin and transport them to the axonal terminals in the posterior pituitary where they are secreted into the general circulation. Double-labeling fluorescence immunohistochemistry has shown that both vasopressin- and oxytocin-containing neurons in the SON express P2X2, P2X4 and P2X5 receptor proteins (Guo et al., 2009). P2X2R-positive immunoreactivity has been found both on SON somata and nerve fibers (Yao et al., 2003; Vulchanova et al., 1996; Xiang et al., 1998; Shibuya et al., 1999; Loesch and Burnstock, 2001). Our quantitative reverse transcription-polymerase chain reaction (qRT-PCR) analysis showed the expression of mRNAs of all P2XR subunits and several P2YRs in SON-containing tissue; the expression of mRNAs for ionotropic P2X2R > P2X7R > P2X4R subunits was the most significant (Fig.2) (Vavra et al., 2011). Thus hypothalamus has a capacity to express both P2XR and P2YR.

Functional studies showed that application of ATP caused an increase in Ca^{2+} in cultured hypothalamic neurons (Chen et al., 1994), acutely isolated SON neurons and glial cells (Shibuya et al., 1999), SON neurons in hypothalamo-neurohypophyseal system explants (Song et al., 2007) and rat brain slices (Vavra et al., 2011). Application of ATP also stimulates the release of vasopressin and oxytocin in perfused explants of the hypothalamo-neurohypophyseal system (Gomes et al., 2009) and isolated neurohypophysial nerve terminals of the rat (Troadec et al., 1998). These ATP-induced effects were attenuated by the P2X receptor antagonists suramin and PPADS indicating that P2X2Rs or P2X3Rs play a role. Extracellular recordings showed that ATP application increases excitability of SON neurons in the hypothalamus (Day et al., 1993) and intracellular recordings from SON neurons in

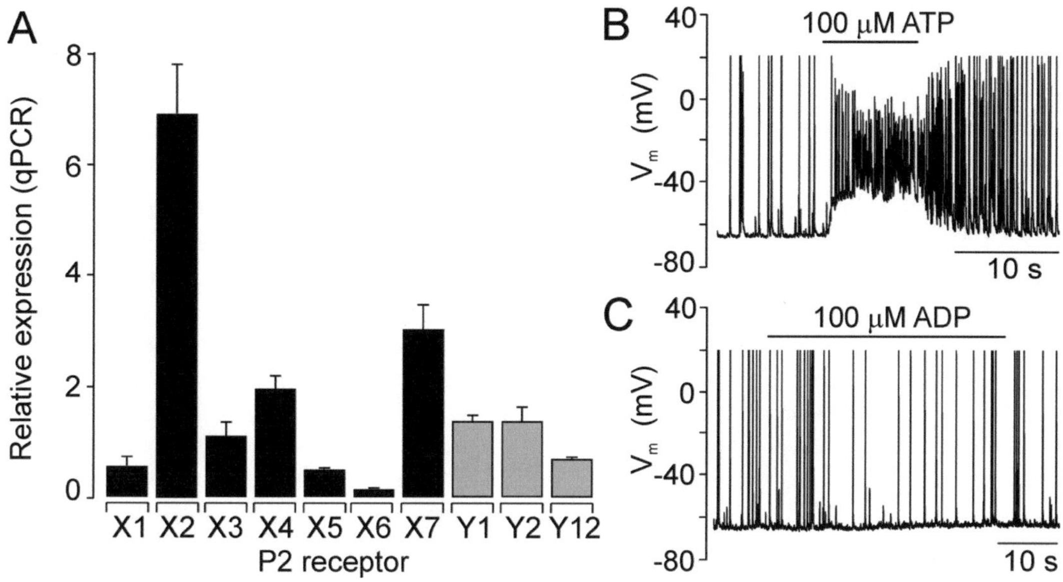

Fig. 2. Expression and function of P2X receptors in hypothalamus.

acute hypothalamic explants revealed that it was due to depolarization of membrane potential following exposure to ATP (Hiruma and Bourque, 1995). In voltage-clamped SON neurons of rat brain slices, application of ATP (10–100 μM) stimulated inward currents that were potentiated by acidic pH and attenuated by PPADS suggesting the involvement of P2X2R (Vavra et al., 2011). Similar ATP-evoked currents were recorded from neuronal somata of acutely dissociated SON neurons (Shibuya et al., 1999) and isolated terminals of the hypothalamic neurohypophysial system (Knott et al., 2005).

There are also evidences for the contribution of P2X4Rs, which are particularly prevalent in the central nervous system and hypothalamus (Illes and Ribeiro, 2004; Collo et al., 1996; Stojilkovic, 2009; Jo et al., 2011). Ivermectin, a receptor-specific allosteric modulator (Khakh et al., 1999) caused more than 2-fold augmentation of the maximum amplitude of ATP-evoked current and prolonged the ATP-stimulated calcium responses in SON neurons of slices (Vavra et al., 2011). A similar potentiating effect of ivermectin has been shown previously in neurons from the somato-sensory cortex (Lalo et al., 2007) and pituitary lactorophs that endogenously express homomeric or heteromeric P2X4Rs (Zemkova et al., 2010). The novel inhibitor of recombinant P2X4Rs, 5BDBD (Wu et al., 2011), failed to affect ATP-induced responses in neurons (Vavra et al., 2011), however, it may be ineffective on heteromeric P2X4Rs which prevail in the brain. The presence of the functional P2X2R and P2X4Rs on SON neurons was further corroborated by the qRT-PCR experiments, which demonstrated significant expression of mRNA transcripts for these receptors in SON tissue (Vavra et al., 2011). Significant level of mRNA for P2X7R was also observed but P2X1, P2X3, P2X5 and P2X6 mRNA expression levels were minor. The high mRNA level for P2X7 can be ascribed to P2X receptors expressed in non-neuronal cells, such as microglia (Collo et al., 1997), because the currents of SON neurons were not affected by BzATP, but non-neuronal SON cells in slices responded with an increase in intracellular calcium (Vavra et al., 2011).

ATP-evoked inward current mediated by P2X2 or P2X4 receptors, as observed in SON neurons, likely represents a particular example of a more general function of P2XRs: to make voltage-threshold more positive and to drive neurons to fire action potentials. We suppose the functional role of somatic P2XRs in the brain consists in controlling excitability close to the nominal resting potential of the neuron cell body, near − 60 mV (Vavra et al., 2011).

A, The presence of seven P2XRs (black columns) and three P2YRs (gray columns) mRNA transcripts in hypothalamic tissues from 16 day-old rats. Quantitative RT-PCR analysis shows significant expressions of ionotropic P2X2, P2X4 and P2X7 receptor mRNAs and moderate levels of mRNA for P2X3, P2Y1 and P2Y2 receptors. The mRNA levels of P2 receptor genes were related to the expression of GAPDH as a housekeeping gene /endogenous control. B,C Example recordings of action potentials from the SON neuron in slices before, during and after the application (bar) of 100 μM ATP (B) and 100 μM ADP (D). ATP induced depolarization and an increase in frequency of action potentials. Neither effect was observed after the application of ADP which had a tendency to decrease the frequency of action potentials. All neurons had resting membrane potential (Vm) lower than -50 mV when measured in current clamp mode. For details see: (Vavra et al., 2011).

3.2 Modulation of glutamate and GABA release by presynaptic P2XRs

ATP is viewed as a neurotransmitter in both the peripheral (Evans et al., 1992) and the central nervous system (Pankratov et al., 1998). It has been suggested that endogenously released ATP acts at postsynaptic P2XRs to mediate synaptic currents in the hippocampus (Edwards et al., 1992). This classical view, however, is challenged by a series of recent studies that showed that ATP acts rather as a modulator that stimulates the release of other neurotransmitters (Li et al., 1998; Sperlagh et al., 2002; Watano et al., 2004; Rodrigues et al., 2005; Kodama et al., 2007; Sperlagh et al., 2007; Donato et al., 2008). In the SON neurons, for instance, all spontaneous synaptic currents were inhibited by blockers of glutamate and GABAA receptors and application of ATP stimulated about 2300 % increase in frequency of both spontaneous inhibitory and excitatory postsynaptic currents without changes in their amplitude (Fig.3) (Vavra et al., 2011). This finding suggests that ATP does not act as a spontaneously released neurotransmitter, but as a modulator that stimulates the release of GABA or glutamate (or both) by activating purinergic receptors in the nerve terminals (Vavra et al., 2011). These experiments were performed in the presence of tetrodotoxin, which inhibits action potentials, thus P2XRs are implicated in presynaptic function by stimulating Ca^{2+} influx into the nerve terminals. Known presynaptic P2XR subtypes with a role in neurotransmission include P2X1, P2X2, P2X3 and possibly P2X4 and P2X7 receptors.

P2X1Rs have been localized and implicated in the function of sympathetic ganglion neurons (Calvert and Evans, 2004), cerebellum (Hervas et al., 2003) and spinal cord dorsal horn sensory neurons (Nakatsuka et al., 2003). Presynaptic P2X1R have been found to mediate agonist-evoked release of tritium-labeled glutamate from purified nerve terminals of the rat hippocampus (Rodrigues et al., 2005). Facilitation of both glutamate and GABA release mediated by presynaptic P2X1R was observed in the rat medial nucleus of the trapezoid body (Watano et al., 2004). Activation of presynaptic P2X1R elicits noradrenaline release from central catecholaminergic terminals in superfused rat hippocampal slices (Papp et al., 2004). These receptors are present in high concentrations on some smooth muscle cells

(Valera et al., 1994). Another role of the P2X1R in the brain thus might be in the smooth muscle of small arteries and arterioles, allowing the control of blood flow and pressure.

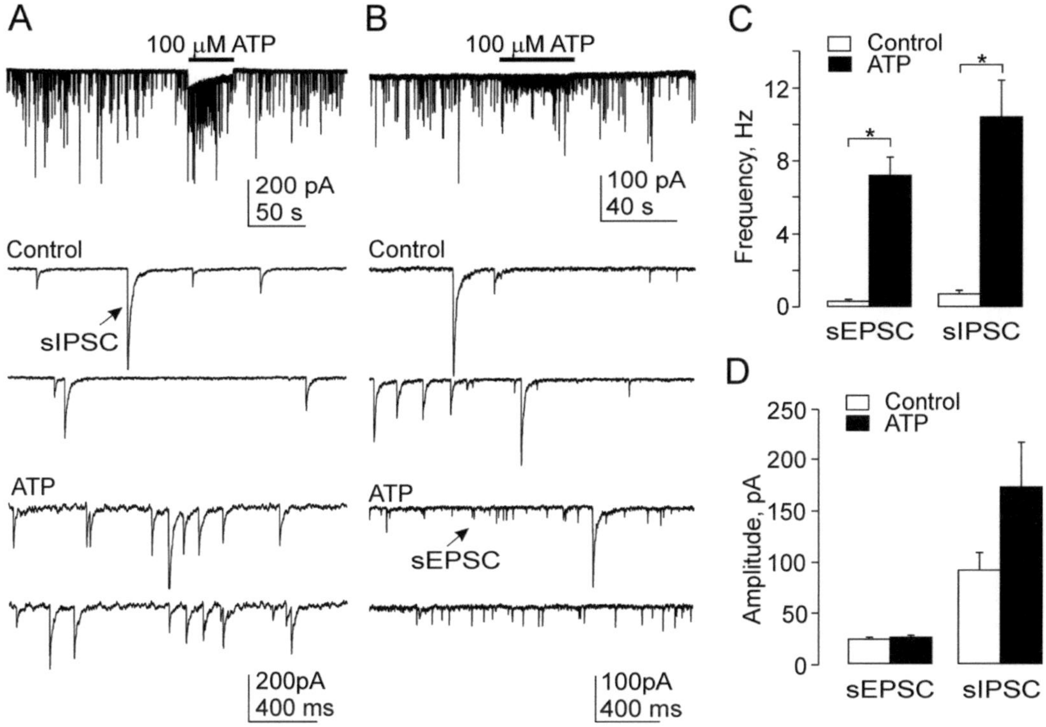

Fig. 3. Presynaptic effect of ATP on spontaneous glutamate and GABA release.

A, ATP (100 μM) induced inward current and increase in the frequency of spontaneous GABAergic inhibitory postsynaptic currents (sIPSC). B, ATP induced increases in the frequency of spontaneous glutamatergic excitatory postsynaptic currents (sEPSC). Traces in an expanded time scale show spontaneous synaptic currents before (Control) and after ATP application (ATP). Glutamatergic and GABAergic spontaneous postsynaptic currents differ in their amplitudes and duration. Experiments were performed on SON neurons voltage clamped at -60 mV. C,D, Summary histograms showing the effect of ATP on the frequency (C) and amplitude (D) of sEPSCs and sIPSCs. Analysis was performed on SON neurons in rat brain slices. (*) $P < 0.01$. For details see: (Vavra et al., 2011).

Numerous studies have shown that P2X2Rs act presynaptically to increase glutamate in several brain areas. Experiments with knockout mice showed that Ca^{2+} entry through presynaptic P2X2Rs increases the frequency of spontaneous AMPA receptor-mediated glutamatergic currents in GABAergic hippocampal interneurons (Khakh et al., 2003). Furthermore, inhibiting P2XRs by application of PPADS has been shown to abolish the glutamate-dependent postsynaptic currents evoked by focal application of ATP in dorsal horn neurons (Li et al., 1998 Nakatsuka and Gu, 2001). PPADS-sensitive P2X2Rs have been shown in glutamatergic terminals of neurons in trigeminal mesencephalic motor nucleus (Khakh and Henderson, 1998), the nucleus tractus solitari (Shigetomi and Kato, 2004) and the area postrema (Kodama et al., 2007). The presynaptic P2X2Rs have been shown to underlie increase in GABA release in a subset of GABAergic interneurons in the spinal cord (Hugel and Schlichter, 2000) and in Purkinje cells in rat cerebellar slices (Donato et al., 2008). In SON neurons, the ATP-induced increases in the frequency of spontaneous excitatory and inhibitory postsynaptic currents were also inhibited by PPADS and potentiated by pH 6.5, indicating the involvement of presynaptic P2X2Rs in the release of both neurotransmitters (Vavra et al., 2011).

The P2X3Rs are almost exclusively expressed in dorsal root ganglion (DRG) neuronal processes that are involved in acute pain (Vulchanova et al., 1997; Dunn et al., 2001; North, 2004). Immunocytochemistry for P2X3 subunits revealed that these receptors are expressed in small- and medium-sized neurons but are absent from large diameter neurons (Vulchanova et al., 1997; Vulchanova et al., 1998; Novakovic et al., 1999). Stimulation of presynaptic P2XRs in DRG neuronal processes by ATP application induced glutamate release that activated postsynaptic glutamatergic receptors expressed in the dorsal horn neurons (Gu and MacDermott, 1997) and that was inhibited by PPADS. Presynaptic P2X3R have been also found in other brain areas, including purified nerve terminals of the rat hippocampus (Rodrigues et al., 2005), in cranial afferent neurons in nodose ganglia (Kato and Shigetomi, 2001; Jin et al., 2004), in the midbrain periaqueductal gray (Xing et al., 2008), in the rat medial nucleus of the trapezoid body (Watano et al., 2004). ATP-stimulated GABA release from rat midbrain terminals are mediated through the activation of P2X receptors with an abundance of P2X3 subunits (Gomez-Villafuertes et al., 2001). Activation of presynaptic P2X3R receptors contributes to noradrenaline release in superfused rat hippocampal slices (Papp et al., 2004).

Evidence for the presence of P2X4Rs in the nerve terminals is less obvious because selective antagonists are lacking. We showed that the ATP-induced effect on frequency of spontaneous inhibitory postsynaptic currents in the SON declined during prolonged ATP application, which indicates the involvement of a desensitizing P2X4R (Vavra et al., 2011).

BzATP has been reported to enhance release of glutamate by acting at P2X7Rs in purified rat neocortex synaptosomes (Patti et al., 2006). Possible presynaptic mechanisms underlying enhancement of excitatory transmitter release by P2X7R has been also suggested for hypoglossal motoneurons in brainstem slices (Ireland et al., 2004). However, neuronal origin of P2X7R is still uncertain. The P2X7Rs are expressed on satellite glial cells enwrapping the peripheral neurons (e.g., DRG neurons) and on microglia, astrocytes and oligodendrocytes in the brain. After repeated or prolonged exposure to ATP, P2X7R are able to form pores permeable to small molecules, and could mediate release of cytokines from satellite glial and microglial cells (Ferrari et al., 1997b; Ferrari et al., 1997a; Ferrari et al., 2006; Matute et al., 2007) or release of neurotransmitters from astrocytes. Several reports have shown that the P2X7R, and not other P2XRs, is responsible for IL-1β release from activated myeloid cells (Mehta et al., 2001; Le Feuvre et al., 2002). LPS-primed macrophages from transgenic mice lacking P2X7 receptors fail to release IL-1β in response to ATP, although synthesis of pro-IL-1β and caspase-1 is unaltered (Solle et al., 2001; Labasi et al., 2002). Activation of P2X7Rs has been reported to elicit the release of glutamate (Duan et al., 2003), GABA (Wang et al., 2002), 2-arachidonoylglycerol (Walter et al., 2004), and purines (Ballerini et al., 1996) from cultured astrocytes. In neurological diseases or injuries extracellular ATP may activate P2X7Rs further enhancing purine release, with important pathophysiological consequences (Ballerini et al., 1996). In paraventricular nucleus of hypothalamus, P2X7 receptor activation results in insertion of AMPA receptors into postsynaptic neuronal membrane (Gordon et al., 2009).

In the rat suprachiasmatic nuclei, ATP content and extracellular ATP levels (Yamazaki et al., 1994; Womac et al., 2009) negatively correlate with electrical activity and arginine vasopressin (AVP) secretion rhythm: the frequency of action potentials and the level of AVP is high during the day and low during the night, but ATP release peaks during the night. This might indicate that ATP is primarily stored and released from distinct pool of vesicles and/or that ATP and AVP are released from different cells. How ATP release from hypothalamic cells is regulated and what is the reason for local differences in distribution of P2X receptor subtypes is still being elucidated.

4. Potentiation of hormone secretion in pituitary gland

Depolarization and Ca^{2+} influx stimulated by extracellular ATP has numerous functions also in endocrine cells. These involve stimulation of luteinizing hormone, prolactin, oxytocin and vasopressin hormone secretion by pituitary gland (Kapoor and Sladek, 2000; Stojilkovic, 2009; Stojilkovic et al., 2010b). The anterior pituitary is a heterogeneous gland with multiple cell types that secrete six major peptide hormones necessary for reproduction, lactation, growth, development, metabolic homeostasis, and the response to stress: FSH and LH-producing gonadotrophs, prolactin (PRL)-producing lactotrophs, GH-producing somatotrophs, TSH-producing thyrotrophs, and ACTH-producing corticotrophs. This lobe also contains the non-hormone-producing folliculostellate cells, which are glia-like cells, and endothelial cells that line the capillaries. Pituitary hormone secretion is under control of hypothalamic neurohormones and is also modulated by extracellular ATP (Chen et al., 1995) that is released by the anterior pituitary itself in a regulated manner, or coreleased with hypothalamic peptides (Tomic et al., 1996; Lazarowski et al., 2000; Stojilkovic and Koshimizu, 2001; He et al., 2005). The mRNA transcripts for several P2X subunits (P2X2R, P2X3R, P2X4R, and P2X7R) were identified in anterior pituitary cells from neonatal (Zemkova *et al.*, 2006) and adult rats (Koshimizu et al., 2000a; Koshimizu et al., 2000b; Stojilkovic and Koshimizu, 2001), including two spliced forms of the P2X2R subunit. Experiments with the plasma membrane-targeted luciferase expressed in HEK cells or ACN neuroblastoma cells indicated that endogenous extracellular ATP concentrations are in the range of 100-200 μM, which is more than sufficient to activate all types of P2X receptors (Pellegatti et al., 2005). *In vivo*, the ATP action on gonadotroph functions could be controlled by ectonucleotidases 1-3, which are expressed in pituitary cells (He et al., 2005) and provide an effective pathway for the control of extracellular ATP concentrations.

Detection and localization of mRNA transcripts for P2X2, P2X3 and P2X4 receptors in pituitary gland by in situ hybridization. *PP*, posterior pituitary, *AP*, anterior pituitary. For details see: (Stojilkovic et al., 2010b).

Most anterior pituitary cells express functional P2X receptors (Fig.4) (Carew et al., 1994; Villalobos et al., 1997; Koshimizu et al., 2000a). The P2X2Rs were identified in pituitary gonadotrophs (Tomic et al., 1996; Koshimizu et al., 2000b; Zemkova et al., 2006) and somatotrophs (Koshimizu et al., 2000a). Lactotrophs express functional P2X4Rs (Carew et al., 1994; He et al., 2003; Zemkova et al., 2010) as well as P2X7R subtypes (Chung et al., 2000; He et al., 2003). Corticotrophs seem not to respond to extracellular ATP directly by stimulation of any P2X receptor (Zhao et al., 2006), and identification of P2X receptors in remaining anterior pituitary cell type, thyrotrophs, has not yet been done. Functional studies showed that ATP application induces inward slowly desensitizig current and increases

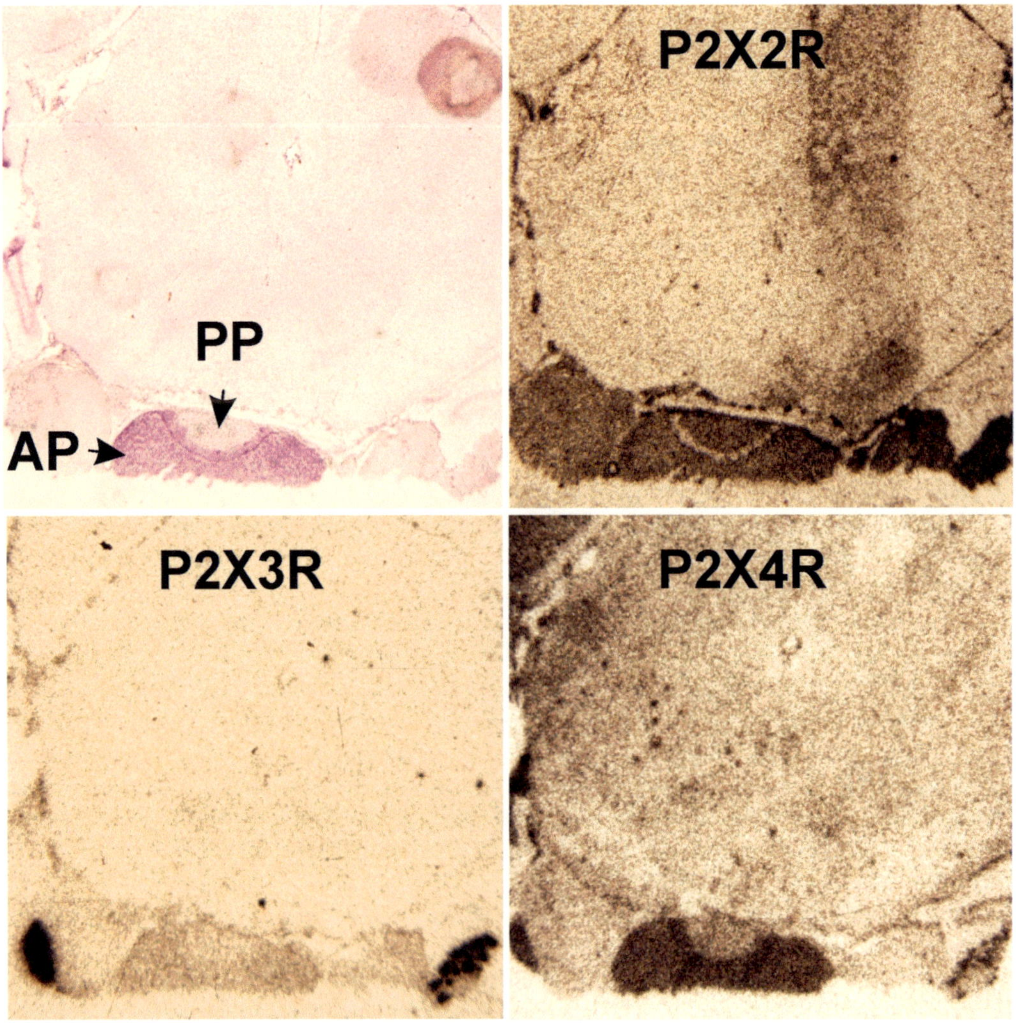

Fig. 4. Expression of P2XR in pituitary gland.

frequency of action potentials (Fig.5) in pituitary gonadotrophs. These responses were sensitive to PPADS indicating that P2X2Rs could operate as depolarizing channels in the pituitary (Zemkova et al., 2006). ATP could play the role of modulator in the anterior pituitary lactotrophs (Stojilkovic and Koshimizu, 2001), P2X4R potentiator ivermectin per se augmented ATP-induced prolactin secretion and slightly potentiated the effect of TRH in lactrotrophs which express P2X4Rs (Zemkova et al., 2006). Thus in pituitary, ATP may serve to synchronize of spontaneous electrical activity, to initiate intercellular Ca^{2+} waves, as observed in other cell types (Guthrie et al., 1999) and modulate G-protein coupled receptor-stimulated Ca^{2+} signaling by refilling of intracellular stores from calcium influx through P2XR pore (Zemkova et al., 2006). Such an action of extracellular ATP could provide a mechanism for the amplification of the effects of hypothalamic peptides on pituitary hormone secretion. Further experiments should clarify to what extent these capacities of P2X receptors are utilized *in vivo.*

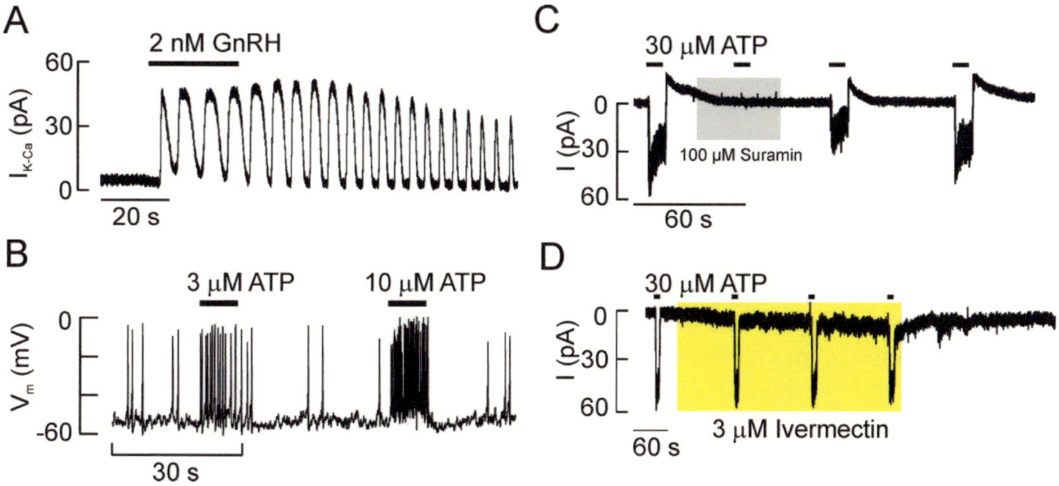

Fig. 5. Electrophysiological characterization of the P2X2R in pituitary gonadotrophs. A, Gonadotrophs can be identified in a mixed population of pituitary cells because of their specific GnRH-induced calcium oscillations monitored as outward calcium-activated potassium current ($I_{K\text{-}Ca}$). B, Stimulation of electrical activity by application of ATP to identified gonadotrophs. C, The sensitivity of ATP-induced current to suramine, general P2XR blocker. D, Insensitivity of ATP-induced current to ivermectin indicates that gonadotrophs express the P2X2 receptor. For details see: (Zemkova et al., 2006).

5. Conclusion

To summarize, the cellular actions of extracellular ATP and P2XRs in the brain range from modulation of resting membrane potential and electrical activity to stimulation of neurotransmitter and hormone release, including release of anterior pituitary hormones. It is clear that the effects of ATP and its analogs are realized by membrane depolarization resulting in voltage-dependent Ca^{2+} entry and by Ca^{2+} entry through the pore of P2XR itself. Nonetheless, the molecular and neurochemical mechanisms underlying these effects are far from being fully understood and likely involve multiple receptor systems and various signaling pathways. Experimental evidences gathered so far suggest that whereas neurotransmitter release seems to be linked to the activation of presynaptic P2X1, P2X2, P2X3 and perhaps P2X4 and P2X7 receptors expressed in nerve terminals, neuropeptide and hormone secretion more likely involves P2X2 and P2X4 receptors on the surface of neuronal somata and pituitary cells. Thus, extracellular ATP together with P2XRs comprise a new excitatory system in the mammalian central nervous system and an increasing number of studies support also an indirect role of P2XRs in inhibitory system owing to its ability to facilitate GABA release. However, surprisingly few studies confirmed the role of ATP as neurotransmitter in the central nervous system, whereas its modulatory roles are well established. Further studies aimed at analyzing the cellular and molecular actions of ATP in various brain regions and under different physiological states would be required for a comprehensive understanding.

6. Acknowledgements

This study was supported by the Internal Grant Agency of Academy of Sciences (Grant No. IAA500110910), the Grant Agency of the Czech Republic (305/07/0681, P304/12/P371, the Academy of Sciences of the Czech Republic (Research Project No. AVOZ 50110509) and the Centrum for Neuroscience (Research Project No. LC554).

7. References

Abbracchio MP, Burnstock G, Verkhratsky A, Zimmermann H (2009) Purinergic signalling in the nervous system: an overview. Trends Neurosci 32:19-29.

Adinolfi E, Cirillo M, Woltersdorf R, Falzoni S, Chiozzi P, Pellegatti P, Callegari MG, Sandona D, Markwardt F, Schmalzing G, Di Virgilio F (2010) Trophic activity of a naturally occurring truncated isoform of the P2X7 receptor. Faseb J 24:3393-3404.

Ballerini P, Rathbone MP, Di Iorio P, Renzetti A, Giuliani P, D'Alimonte I, Trubiani O, Caciagli F, Ciccarelli R (1996) Rat astroglial P2Z (P2X7) receptors regulate intracellular calcium and purine release. Neuroreport 7:2533-2537.

Barrera NP, Ormond SJ, Henderson RM, Murrell-Lagnado RD, Edwardson JM (2005) Atomic force microscopy imaging demonstrates that P2X2 receptors are trimers but that P2X6 receptor subunits do not oligomerize. J Biol Chem 280:10759-10765.

Bavan S, Straub VA, Blaxter ML, Ennion SJ (2009) A P2X receptor from the tardigrade species Hypsibius dujardini with fast kinetics and sensitivity to zinc and copper. BMC Evol Biol 9:17.

Buell G, Lewis C, Collo G, North RA, Surprenant A (1996) An antagonist-insensitive P2X receptor expressed in epithelia and brain. Embo J 15:55-62.

Burkhart CN (2000) Ivermectin: an assessment of its pharmacology, microbiology and safety. Vet Hum Toxicol 42:30-35.

Burnstock G (2004) Cotransmission. Curr Opin Pharmacol 4:47-52.

Burnstock G (2011) Introductory overview of purinergic signalling. Front Biosci (Elite Ed) 3:896-900.

Calvert JA, Evans RJ (2004) Heterogeneity of P2X receptors in sympathetic neurons: contribution of neuronal P2X1 receptors revealed using knockout mice. Mol Pharmacol 65:139-148.

Carew MA, Wu ML, Law GJ, Tseng YZ, Mason WT (1994) Extracellular ATP activates calcium entry and mobilization via P2U-purinoceptors in rat lactotrophs. Cell Calcium 16:227-235.

Clyne JD, Wang LF, Hume RI (2002) Mutational analysis of the conserved cysteines of the rat P2X2 purinoceptor. J Neurosci 22:3873-3880.

Coddou C, Stojilkovic SS, Huidobro-Toro JP (2011) Allosteric modulation of ATP-gated P2X receptor channels. Rev Neurosci 22:335-354.

Collo G, Neidhart S, Kawashima E, Kosco-Vilbois M, North RA, Buell G (1997) Tissue distribution of the P2X7 receptor. Neuropharmacology 36:1277-1283.

Collo G, North RA, Kawashima E, Merlo-Pich E, Neidhart S, Surprenant A, Buell G (1996) Cloning OF P2X5 and P2X6 receptors and the distribution and properties of an extended family of ATP-gated ion channels. J Neurosci 16:2495-2507.

Day TA, Sibbald JR, Khanna S (1993) ATP mediates an excitatory noradrenergic neuron input to supraoptic vasopressin cells. Brain Res 607:341-344.

Di Virgilio F, Chiozzi P, Falzoni S, Ferrari D, Sanz JM, Venketaraman V, Baricordi OR (1998) Cytolytic P2X purinoceptors. Cell Death Differ 5:191-199.

Donato R, Rodrigues RJ, Takahashi M, Tsai MC, Soto D, Miyagi K, Villafuertes RG, Cunha RA, Edwards FA (2008) GABA release by basket cells onto Purkinje cells, in rat cerebellar slices, is directly controlled by presynaptic purinergic receptors, modulating Ca2+ influx. Cell Calcium 44:521-532.

Duan S, Anderson CM, Keung EC, Chen Y, Chen Y, Swanson RA (2003) P2X7 receptor-mediated release of excitatory amino acids from astrocytes. J Neurosci 23:1320-1328.

Duckwitz W, Hausmann R, Aschrafi A, Schmalzing G (2006) P2X5 subunit assembly requires scaffolding by the second transmembrane domain and a conserved aspartate. J Biol Chem 281:39561-39572.

Dunn PM, Zhong Y, Burnstock G (2001) P2X receptors in peripheral neurons. Prog Neurobiol 65:107-134.

Edwards FA, Gibb AJ, Colquhoun D (1992) ATP receptor-mediated synaptic currents in the central nervous system. Nature 359:144-147.

Egan TM, Khakh BS (2004) Contribution of calcium ions to P2X channel responses. J Neurosci 24:3413-3420.

Egan TM, Haines WR, Voigt MM (1998) A domain contributing to the ion channel of ATP-gated P2X2 receptors identified by the substituted cysteine accessibility method. J Neurosci 18:2350-2359.

Egan TM, Cox JA, Voigt MM (2004) Molecular structure of P2X receptors. Curr Top Med Chem 4:821-829.

Ennion SJ, Evans RJ (2002) Conserved cysteine residues in the extracellular loop of the human P2X(1) receptor form disulfide bonds and are involved in receptor trafficking to the cell surface. Mol Pharmacol 61:303-311.

Evans RJ, Derkach V, Surprenant A (1992) ATP mediates fast synaptic transmission in mammalian neurons. Nature 357:503-505.

Ferrari D, Chiozzi P, Falzoni S, Hanau S, Di Virgilio F (1997a) Purinergic modulation of interleukin-1 beta release from microglial cells stimulated with bacterial endotoxin. J Exp Med 185:579-582.

Ferrari D, Chiozzi P, Falzoni S, Dal Susino M, Melchiorri L, Baricordi OR, Di Virgilio F (1997b) Extracellular ATP triggers IL-1 beta release by activating the purinergic P2Z receptor of human macrophages. J Immunol 159:1451-1458.

Ferrari D, Pizzirani C, Adinolfi E, Lemoli RM, Curti A, Idzko M, Panther E, Di Virgilio F (2006) The P2X7 receptor: a key player in IL-1 processing and release. J Immunol 176:3877-3883.

Fields RD, Stevens B (2000) ATP: an extracellular signaling molecule between neurons and glia. Trends Neurosci 23:625-633.

Fields RD, Burnstock G (2006) Purinergic signalling in neuron-glia interactions. Nat Rev Neurosci 7:423-436.

Fountain SJ, Parkinson K, Young MT, Cao L, Thompson CR, North RA (2007) An intracellular P2X receptor required for osmoregulation in Dictyostelium discoideum. Nature 448:200-203.

Gomes DA, Song Z, Stevens W, Sladek CD (2009) Sustained stimulation of vasopressin and oxytocin release by ATP and phenylephrine requires recruitment of desensitization-resistant P2X purinergic receptors. Am J Physiol Regul Integr Comp Physiol 297:R940-949.

Gomez-Villafuertes R, Gualix J, Miras-Portugal MT (2001) Single GABAergic synaptic terminals from rat midbrain exhibit functional P2X and dinucleotide receptors, able to induce GABA secretion. J Neurochem 77:84-93.

Gordon GR, Iremonger KJ, Kantevari S, Ellis-Davies GC, MacVicar BA, Bains JS (2009) Astrocyte-mediated distributed plasticity at hypothalamic glutamate synapses. Neuron 64:391-403.

Gourine AV, Melenchuk EV, Poputnikov DM, Gourine VN, Spyer KM (2002) Involvement of purinergic signalling in central mechanisms of body temperature regulation in rats. Br J Pharmacol 135:2047-2055.

Gu JG, MacDermott AB (1997) Activation of ATP P2X receptors elicits glutamate release from sensory neuron synapses. Nature 389:749-753.

Guo W, Sun J, Xu X, Bunstock G, He C, Xiang Z (2009) P2X receptors are differentially expressed on vasopressin- and oxytocin-containing neurons in the supraoptic and paraventricular nuclei of rat hypothalamus. Histochem Cell Biol 131:29-41.

Guthrie PB, Knappenberger J, Segal M, Bennett MV, Charles AC, Kater SB (1999) ATP released from astrocytes mediates glial calcium waves. J Neurosci 19:520-528.

Haines WR, Voigt MM, Migita K, Torres GE, Egan TM (2001a) On the contribution of the first transmembrane domain to whole-cell current through an ATP-gated ionotropic P2X receptor. J Neurosci 21:5885-5892.

Haines WR, Migita K, Cox JA, Egan TM, Voigt MM (2001b) The first transmembrane domain of the P2X receptor subunit participates in the agonist-induced gating of the channel. J Biol Chem 276:32793-32798.

He ML, Gonzalez-Iglesias AE, Stojilkovic SS (2003) Role of nucleotide P2 receptors in calcium signaling and prolactin release in pituitary lactotrophs. J Biol Chem 278:46270-46277.

He ML, A.E. GI, M. T, Stojilkovic SS (2005) Release and extracellular metabolism of ATP by ecto-nucleotidase eNTPDase 1-3 in hypothalamic and pituitary cells. Purinergic Signalling 1:135-144.

Heine C, Heimrich B, Vogt J, Wegner A, Illes P, Franke H (2006) P2 receptor-stimulation influences axonal outgrowth in the developing hippocampus in vitro. Neuroscience 138:303-311.

Hervas C, Perez-Sen R, Miras-Portugal MT (2003) Coexpression of functional P2X and P2Y nucleotide receptors in single cerebellar granule cells. J Neurosci Res 73:384-399.

Hiruma H, Bourque CW (1995) P2 purinoceptor-mediated depolarization of rat supraoptic neurosecretory cells in vitro. J Physiol 489:805-811.

Hugel S, Schlichter R (2000) Presynaptic P2X receptors facilitate inhibitory GABAergic transmission between cultured rat spinal cord dorsal horn neurons. J Neurosci 20:2121-2130.

Chen ZP, Levy A, Lightman SL (1994) Activation of specific ATP receptors induces a rapid increase in intracellular calcium ions in rat hypothalamic neurons. Brain Res 641:249-256.

Chen ZP, Kratzmeier M, Levy A, McArdle CA, Poch A, Day A, Mukhopadhyay AK, Lightman SL (1995) Evidence for a role of pituitary ATP receptors in the regulation of pituitary function. Proc Natl Acad Sci U S A 92:5219-5223.

Chung HS, Park KS, Cha SK, Kong ID, Lee JW (2000) ATP-induced [Ca(2+)](i) changes and depolarization in GH3 cells. Br J Pharmacol 130:1843-1852.

Illes P, Ribeiro JA (2004) Neuronal P2 receptors of the central nervous system. Curr Top Med Chem 4:831-838.

Inoue K, Koizumi S, Tsuda M (2007) The role of nucleotides in the neuron--glia communication responsible for the brain functions. J Neurochem 102:1447-1458.

Ireland MF, Noakes PG, Bellingham MC (2004) P2X7-like receptor subunits enhance excitatory synaptic transmission at central synapses by presynaptic mechanisms. Neuroscience 128:269-280.

Jacobson KA, Jarvis MF, Williams M (2002) Purine and pyrimidine (P2) receptors as drug targets. J Med Chem 45:4057-4093.

Jelinkova I, Yan Z, Liang Z, Moonat S, Teisinger J, Stojilkovic SS, Zemkova H (2006) Identification of P2X(4) receptor-specific residues contributing to the ivermectin effects on channel deactivation. Biochem Biophys Res Commun 349:619-625.

Jelinkova I, Vavra V, Jindrichova M, Obsil T, Zemkova HW, Zemkova H, Stojilkovic SS (2008) Identification of P2X(4) receptor transmembrane residues contributing to channel gating and interaction with ivermectin. Pflugers Arch 456:939-950.

Jiang LH, Rassendren F, Spelta V, Surprenant A, North RA (2001) Amino acid residues involved in gating identified in the first membrane-spanning domain of the rat P2X(2) receptor. J Biol Chem 276:14902-14908.

Jiang LH, Kim M, Spelta V, Bo X, Surprenant A, North RA (2003) Subunit arrangement in P2X receptors. J Neurosci 23:8903-8910.

Jin YH, Bailey TW, Li BY, Schild JH, Andresen MC (2004) Purinergic and vanilloid receptor activation releases glutamate from separate cranial afferent terminals in nucleus tractus solitarius. J Neurosci 24:4709-4717.

Jindrichova M, Vavra V, Obsil T, Stojilkovic SS, Zemkova H (2009) Functional relevance of aromatic residues in the first transmembrane domain of P2X receptors. J Neurochem 109:923-934.

Jindrichova M, Khafizov K, Skorinkin A, Fayuk D, Bart G, Zemkova H, Giniatullin R (2011) Highly Conserved Tyrosine 37 Stabilizes Desensitized States and Restricts Calcium Permeability of ATP-Gated P2X3 Receptor. J Neurochem 119:676-685.

Jo YH, Schlichter R (1999) Synaptic corelease of ATP and GABA in cultured spinal neurons. Nat Neurosci 2:241-245.

Jo YH, Role LW (2002) Coordinate release of ATP and GABA at in vitro synapses of lateral hypothalamic neurons. J Neurosci 22:4794-4804.

Jo YH, Donier E, Martinez A, Garret M, Toulme E, Boue-Grabot E (2011) Crosstalk between P2X4 and GABA-A receptors determines synaptic efficacy at central synapses. J Biol Chem 256:19993-20004.

Kapoor JR, Sladek CD (2000) Purinergic and adrenergic agonists synergize in stimulating vasopressin and oxytocin release. J Neurosci 20:8868-8875.

Kato F, Shigetomi E (2001) Distinct modulation of evoked and spontaneous EPSCs by purinoceptors in the nucleus tractus solitarii of the rat. J Physiol 530:469-486.

Kawate T, Michel JC, Birdsong WT, Gouaux E (2009) Crystal structure of the ATP-gated P2X(4) ion channel in the closed state. Nature 460:592-598.

Kawate T, Robertson JL, Li M, Silberberg SD, Swartz KJ (2011) Ion access pathway to the transmembrane pore in P2X receptor channels. J Gen Physiol 137:579-590.

Khakh BS, Henderson G (1998) ATP receptor-mediated enhancement of fast excitatory neurotransmitter release in the brain. Mol Pharmacol 54:372-378.

Khakh BS, Egan TM (2005) Contribution of transmembrane regions to ATP-gated P2X2 channel permeability dynamics. J Biol Chem 280:6118-6129.

Khakh BS, North RA (2006) P2X receptors as cell-surface ATP sensors in health and disease. Nature 442:527-532.

Khakh BS, Gittermann D, Cockayne DA, Jones A (2003) ATP modulation of excitatory synapses onto interneurons. J Neurosci 23:7426-7437.

Khakh BS, Proctor WR, Dunwiddie TV, Labarca C, Lester HA (1999) Allosteric control of gating and kinetics at P2X(4) receptor channels. J Neurosci 19:7289-7299.

King BF, Townsend-Nicholson A, Wildman SS, Thomas T, Spyer KM, Burnstock G (2000) Coexpression of rat P2X2 and P2X6 subunits in Xenopus oocytes. J Neurosci 20:4871-4877.

Knott TK, Velazquez-Marrero C, Lemos JR (2005) ATP elicits inward currents in isolated vasopressinergic neurohypophysial terminals via P2X2 and P2X3 receptors. Pflugers Arch 450:381-389.

Kodama N, Funahashi M, Mitoh Y, Minagi S, Matsuo R (2007) Purinergic modulation of area postrema neuronal excitability in rat brain slices. Brain Res 1165:50-59.

Koshimizu TA, Tomic M, Wong AO, Zivadinovic D, Stojilkovic SS (2000a) Characterization of purinergic receptors and receptor-channels expressed in anterior pituitary cells. Endocrinology 141:4091-4099.

Koshimizu TA, Van Goor F, Tomic M, Wong AO, Tanoue A, Tsujimoto G, Stojilkovic SS (2000b) Characterization of calcium signaling by purinergic receptor-channels expressed in excitable cells. Mol Pharmacol 58:936-945.

Kracun S, Chaptal V, Abramson J, Khakh BS (2010) Gated access to the pore of a P2X receptor: Structural implications for closed-open transitions. J Biol Chem 285:10110-10121.

Labasi JM, Petrushova N, Donovan C, McCurdy S, Lira P, Payette MM, Brissette W, Wicks JR, Audoly L, Gabel CA (2002) Absence of the P2X7 receptor alters leukocyte function and attenuates an inflammatory response. J Immunol 168:6436-6445.

Lalo U, Verkhratsky A, Pankratov Y (2007) Ivermectin potentiates ATP-induced ion currents in cortical neurones: evidence for functional expression of P2X4 receptors? Neurosci Lett 421:158-162.

Lazarowski ER, Boucher RC, Harden TK (2000) Constitutive release of ATP and evidence for major contribution of ecto-nucleotide pyrophosphatase and nucleoside diphosphokinase to extracellular nucleotide concentrations. J Biol Chem 275:31061-31068.

Le Feuvre RA, Brough D, Iwakura Y, Takeda K, Rothwell NJ (2002) Priming of macrophages with lipopolysaccharide potentiates P2X7-mediated cell death via a caspase-1-dependent mechanism, independently of cytokine production. J Biol Chem 277:3210-3218.

Le KT, Babinski K, Seguela P (1998) Central P2X4 and P2X6 channel subunits coassemble into a novel heteromeric ATP receptor. J Neurosci 18:7152-7159.

Lewis C, Neidhart S, Holy C, North RA, Buell G, Surprenant A (1995) Coexpression of P2X2 and P2X3 receptor subunits can account for ATP-gated currents in sensory neurons. Nature 377:432-435.

Li M, Kawate T, Silberberg SD, Swartz KJ (2011) Pore-opening mechanism in trimeric P2X receptor channels. Nat Commun 1:44.

Li P, Calejesan AA, Zhuo M (1998) ATP P2x receptors and sensory synaptic transmission between primary afferent fibers and spinal dorsal horn neurons in rats. J Neurophysiol 80:3356-3360.

Li Z, Migita K, Samways DS, Voigt MM, Egan TM (2004) Gain and loss of channel function by alanine substitutions in the transmembrane segments of the rat ATP-gated P2X2 receptor. J Neurosci 24:7378-7386.

Loesch A, Burnstock G (2001) Immunoreactivity to P2X(6) receptors in the rat hypothalamo-neurohypophysial system: an ultrastructural study with extravidin and colloidal gold-silver labelling. Neuroscience 106:621-631.

Mackenzie AB, Young MT, Adinolfi E, Surprenant A (2005) Pseudoapoptosis induced by brief activation of ATP-gated P2X7 receptors. J Biol Chem 280:33968-33976.

Matute C, Torre I, Perez-Cerda F, Perez-Samartin A, Alberdi E, Etxebarria E, Arranz AM, Ravid R, Rodriguez-Antiguedad A, Sanchez-Gomez M, Domercq M (2007) P2X(7) receptor blockade prevents ATP excitotoxicity in oligodendrocytes and ameliorates experimental autoimmune encephalomyelitis. J Neurosci 27:9525-9533.

Mehta VB, Hart J, Wewers MD (2001) ATP-stimulated release of interleukin (IL)-1beta and IL-18 requires priming by lipopolysaccharide and is independent of caspase-1 cleavage. J Biol Chem 276:3820-3826.

Migita K, Haines WR, Voigt MM, Egan TM (2001) Polar residues of the second transmembrane domain influence cation permeability of the ATP-gated P2X(2) receptor. J Biol Chem 276:30934-30941.

Michel AD, Chambers LJ, Clay WC, Condreay JP, Walter DS, Chessell IP (2007) Direct labelling of the human P2X7 receptor and identification of positive and negative cooperativity of binding. Br J Pharmacol 151:103-114.

Mio K, Kubo Y, Ogura T, Yamamoto T, Sato C (2005) Visualization of the trimeric P2X2 receptor with a crown-capped extracellular domain. Biochem Biophys Res Commun 337:998-1005.

Nakatsuka T, Gu JG (2001) ATP P2X receptor-mediated enhancement of glutamate release and evoked EPSCs in dorsal horn neurons of the rat spinal cord. J Neurosci 21:6522-6531.

Nakatsuka T, Tsuzuki K, Ling JX, Sonobe H, Gu JG (2003) Distinct roles of P2X receptors in modulating glutamate release at different primary sensory synapses in rat spinal cord. J Neurophysiol 89:3243-3252.

Nelson DW, Gregg RJ, Kort ME, Perez-Medrano A, Voight EA, Wang Y, Grayson G, Namovic MT, Donnelly-Roberts DL, Niforatos W, Honore P, Jarvis MF, Faltynek CR, Carroll WA (2006) Structure-activity relationship studies on a series of novel, substituted 1-benzyl-5-phenyltetrazole P2X7 antagonists. J Med Chem 49:3659-3666.

Newman EA (2003) Glial cell inhibition of neurons by release of ATP. J Neurosci 23:1659-1666.

Nicke A, Kerschensteiner D, Soto F (2005) Biochemical and functional evidence for heteromeric assembly of P2X1 and P2X4 subunits. J Neurochem 92:925-933.

Nicke A, Baumert HG, Rettinger J, Eichele A, Lambrecht G, Mutschler E, Schmalzing G (1998) P2X1 and P2X3 receptors form stable trimers: a novel structural motif of ligand-gated ion channels. Embo J 17:3016-3028.

North R (1996) P2X receptors: a third major class of ligand-gated ion channels. Ciba Found Symp 198:91-105.

North RA (2002) Molecular physiology of P2X receptors. Physiol Rev 82:1013-1067.

North RA (2004) P2X3 receptors and peripheral pain mechanisms. J Physiol 554:301-308.

Novakovic SD, Kassotakis LC, Oglesby IB, Smith JA, Eglen RM, Ford AP, Hunter JC (1999) Immunocytochemical localization of P2X3 purinoceptors in sensory neurons in naive rats and following neuropathic injury. Pain 80:273-282.

Ormond SJ, Barrera NP, Qureshi OS, Henderson RM, Edwardson JM, Murrell-Lagnado RD (2006) An uncharged region within the N terminus of the P2X6 receptor inhibits its assembly and exit from the endoplasmic reticulum. Mol Pharmacol 69:1692-1700.

Pankratov Y, Castro E, Miras-Portugal MT, Krishtal O (1998) A purinergic component of the excitatory postsynaptic current mediated by P2X receptors in the CA1 neurons of the rat hippocampus. Eur J Neurosci 10:3898-3902.

Papp L, Balazsa T, Kofalvi A, Erdelyi F, Szabo G, Vizi ES, Sperlagh B (2004) P2X receptor activation elicits transporter-mediated noradrenaline release from rat hippocampal slices. J Pharmacol Exp Ther 310:973-980.

Patti L, Raiteri L, Grilli M, Parodi M, Raiteri M, Marchi M (2006) P2X(7) receptors exert a permissive role on the activation of release-enhancing presynaptic alpha7 nicotinic receptors co-existing on rat neocortex glutamatergic terminals. Neuropharmacology 50:705-713.

Pellegatti P, Falzoni S, Pinton P, Rizzuto R, Di Virgilio F (2005) A novel recombinant plasma membrane-targeted luciferase reveals a new pathway for ATP secretion. Mol Biol Cell 16:3659-3665.

Raivich G (2005) Like cops on the beat: the active role of resting microglia. Trends Neurosci 28:571-573.

Ralevic V, Burnstock G (1998) Receptors for purines and pyrimidines. Pharmacol Rev 50:413-492.

Rassendren F, Buell G, Newbolt A, North RA, Surprenant A (1997) Identification of amino acid residues contributing to the pore of a P2X receptor. Embo J 16:3446-3454.

Robertson SJ, Ennion SJ, Evans RJ, Edwards FA (2001) Synaptic P2X receptors. Curr Opin Neurobiol 11:378-386.

Rodrigues RJ, Almeida T, Richardson PJ, Oliveira CR, Cunha RA (2005) Dual presynaptic control by ATP of glutamate release via facilitatory P2X1, P2X2/3, and P2X3 and inhibitory P2Y1, P2Y2, and/or P2Y4 receptors in the rat hippocampus. J Neurosci 25:6286-6295.

Rokic M, Tvrdonova V, Vavra V, Jindrichova M, Obsil T, Stojilkovic SS, Zemkova H (2010) Roles of Conserved Ectodomain Cysteines of the Rat P2X4 Purinoreceptor in Agonist Binding and Channel Gating. Physiol Res 59 59:927-935.

Samways DS, Egan TM (2007) Acidic amino acids impart enhanced Ca2+ permeability and flux in two members of the ATP-gated P2X receptor family. J Gen Physiol 129:245-256.

Samways DS, Migita K, Li Z, Egan TM (2008) On the role of the first transmembrane domain in cation permeability and flux of the ATP-gated P2X2 receptor. J Biol Chem 283:5110-5117.

Seguela P, Haghighi A, Soghomonian JJ, Cooper E (1996) A novel neuronal P2x ATP receptor ion channel with widespread distribution in the brain. J Neurosci 16:448-455.

Shibuya I, Tanaka K, Hattori Y, Uezono Y, Harayama N, Noguchi J, Ueta Y, Izumi F, Yamashita H (1999) Evidence that multiple P2X purinoceptors are functionally expressed in rat supraoptic neurones. J Physiol 514:351-367.

Shigetomi E, Kato F (2004) Action potential-independent release of glutamate by Ca2+ entry through presynaptic P2X receptors elicits postsynaptic firing in the brainstem autonomic network. J Neurosci 24:3125-3135.

Silberberg SD, Chang TH, Swartz KJ (2005) Secondary Structure and Gating Rearrangements of Transmembrane Segments in Rat P2X4 Receptor Channels. J Gen Physiol 125:347-359.

Sim JA, Chaumont S, Jo J, Ulmann L, Young MT, Cho K, Buell G, North RA, Rassendren F (2006) Altered hippocampal synaptic potentiation in P2X4 knock-out mice. J Neurosci 26:9006-9009.

Sokolova E, Nistri A, Giniatullin R (2001) Negative cross talk between anionic GABAA and cationic P2X ionotropic receptors of rat dorsal root ganglion neurons. J Neurosci 21:4958-4968.

Solle M, Labasi J, Perregaux DG, Stam E, Petrushova N, Koller BH, Griffiths RJ, Gabel CA (2001) Altered cytokine production in mice lacking P2X(7) receptors. J Biol Chem 276:125-132.

Song Z, Vijayaraghavan S, Sladek CD (2007) ATP increases intracellular calcium in supraoptic neurons by activation of both P2X and P2Y purinergic receptors. Am J Physiol Regul Integr Comp Physiol 292:R423-431.

Sperlagh B, Heinrich A, Csolle C (2007) P2 receptor-mediated modulation of neurotransmitter release-an update. Purinergic Signal 3:269-284.

Sperlagh B, Kofalvi A, Deuchars J, Atkinson L, Milligan CJ, Buckley NJ, Vizi ES (2002) Involvement of P2X7 receptors in the regulation of neurotransmitter release in the rat hippocampus. J Neurochem 81:1196-1211.

Stojilkovic SS (2009) Purinergic regulation of hypothalamopituitary functions. Trends Endocrinol Metab 20:460-468.

Stojilkovic SS, Koshimizu T (2001) Signaling by extracellular nucleotides in anterior pituitary cells. Trends Endocrinol Metab 12:218-225.

Stojilkovic SS, Yan Z, Obsil T, Zemkova H (2010a) Structural Insights into the Function of P2X4: An ATP-Gated Cation Channel of Neuroendocrine Cells. Cell Mol Neurobiol 30:1251-1258.

Stojilkovic SS, He ML, Koshimizu TA, Balik A, Zemkova H (2010b) Signaling by purinergic receptors and channels in the pituitary gland. Mol Cell Endocrinol 314:184-191.

Stoop R, Thomas S, Rassendren F, Kawashima E, Buell G, Surprenant A, North RA (1999) Contribution of individual subunits to the multimeric P2X(2) receptor: estimates based on methanethiosulfonate block at T336C. Mol Pharmacol 56:973-981.

Surprenant A, North RA (2009) Signaling at purinergic P2X receptors. Annu Rev Physiol 71:333-359.

Surprenant A, Rassendren F, Kawashima E, North RA, Buell G (1996) The cytolytic P2Z receptor for extracellular ATP identified as a P2X receptor (P2X7). Science 272:735-738.

Terasawa E, Keen KL, Grendell RL, Golos TG (2005) Possible role of 5'-adenosine triphosphate in synchronization of Ca2+ oscillations in primate luteinizing hormone-releasing hormone neurons. Mol Endocrinol 19:2736-2747.

Tomic M, Jobin RM, Vergara LA, Stojilkovic SS (1996) Expression of purinergic receptor channels and their role in calcium signaling and hormone release in pituitary gonadotrophs. Integration of P2 channels in plasma membrane- and endoplasmic reticulum-derived calcium oscillations. J Biol Chem 271:21200-21208.

Torres GE, Egan TM, Voigt MM (1999) Identification of a domain involved in ATP-gated ionotropic receptor subunit assembly. J Biol Chem 274:22359-22365.

Troadec JD, Thirion S, Nicaise G, Lemos JR, Dayanithi G (1998) ATP-evoked increases in [Ca2+]i and peptide release from rat isolated neurohypophysial terminals via a P2X2 purinoceptor. J Physiol 511:89-103.

Valera S, Hussy N, Evans RJ, Adami N, North RA, Surprenant A, Buell G (1994) A new class of ligand-gated ion channel defined by P2x receptor for extracellular ATP. Nature 371:516-519.

Vavra V, Bhattacharya A, Zemkova H (2011) Facilitation of glutamate and GABA release by P2X receptor activation in supraoptic neurons from freshly isolated rat brain slices. Neuroscience 188:1-12.

Villalobos C, Alonso-Torre SR, Nunez L, Garcia-Sancho J (1997) Functional ATP receptors in rat anterior pituitary cells. Am J Physiol 273:C1963-1971.

Virginio C, MacKenzie A, Rassendren FA, North RA, Surprenant A (1999) Pore dilation of neuronal P2X receptor channels. Nat Neurosci 2:315-321.

Vulchanova L, Riedl MS, Shuster SJ, Buell G, Surprenant A, North RA, Elde R (1997) Immunohistochemical study of the P2X2 and P2X3 receptor subunits in rat and monkey sensory neurons and their central terminals. Neuropharmacology 36:1229-1242.

Vulchanova L, Arvidsson U, Riedl M, Wang J, Buell G, Surprenant A, North RA, Elde R (1996) Differential distribution of two ATP-gated channels (P2X receptors) determined by immunocytochemistry. Proc Natl Acad Sci U S A 93:8063-8067.

Vulchanova L, Riedl MS, Shuster SJ, Stone LS, Hargreaves KM, Buell G, Surprenant A, North RA, Elde R (1998) P2X3 is expressed by DRG neurons that terminate in inner lamina II. Eur J Neurosci 10:3470-3478.

Wang CM, Chang YY, Kuo JS, Sun SH (2002) Activation of P2X(7) receptors induced [(3)H]GABA release from the RBA-2 type-2 astrocyte cell line through a Cl(-)/HCO(3)(-)-dependent mechanism. Glia 37:8-18.

Watano T, Calvert JA, Vial C, Forsythe ID, Evans RJ (2004) P2X receptor subtype-specific modulation of excitatory and inhibitory synaptic inputs in the rat brainstem. J Physiol 558:745-757.

Womac AD, Burkeen JF, Neuendorff N, Earnest DJ, Zoran MJ (2009) Circadian rhythms of extracellular ATP accumulation in suprachiasmatic nucleus cells and cultured astrocytes. Eur J Neurosci 30:869-876.

Wu T, Dai M, Shi X, Jiang ZG, Nuttall AL (2011) Functional expression of P2X(4) receptor in capillary endothelial cells of the cochlear spiral ligament and its role in regulating the capillary diameter. Am J Physiol Heart Circ Physiol.

Xiang Z, Bo X, Oglesby I, Ford A, Burnstock G (1998) Localization of ATP-gated P2X2 receptor immunoreactivity in the rat hypothalamus. Brain Res 813:390-397.

Xing J, Lu J, Li J (2008) Purinergic P2X receptors presynaptically increase glutamatergic synaptic transmission in dorsolateral periaqueductal gray. Brain Res 1208:46-55.

Yamazaki S, Ishida Y, Inouye S (1994) Circadian rhythms of adenosine triphosphate contents in the suprachiasmatic nucleus, anterior hypothalamic area and caudate putamen of the rat--negative correlation with electrical activity. Brain Res 664:237-240.

Yan Z, Khadra A, Li S, Tomic M, Sherman A, Stojilkovic SS (2010) Experimental characterization and mathematical modeling of P2X7 receptor channel gating. J Neurosci 30:14213-14224.

Yao ST, Gourine AV, Spyer KM, Barden JA, Lawrence AJ (2003) Localisation of P2X2 receptor subunit immunoreactivity on nitric oxide synthase expressing neurones in the brain stem and hypothalamus of the rat: a fluorescence immunohistochemical study. Neuroscience 121:411-419.

Zemkova H, Balik A, Jiang Y, Kretschmannova K, Stojilkovic SS (2006) Roles of purinergic P2X receptors as pacemaking channels and modulators of calcium-mobilizing pathway in pituitary gonadotrophs. Mol Endocrinol 20:1423-1436.

Zemkova H, Kucka M, Li S, Gonzalez-Iglesias AE, Tomic M, Stojilkovic SS (2010) Characterization of purinergic P2X4 receptor channels expressed in anterior pituitary cells. Am J Physiol Endocrinol Metab 298:E644-651.

Zhao LF, Iwasaki Y, Oki Y, Tsugita M, Taguchi T, Nishiyama M, Takao T, Kambayashi M, Hashimoto K (2006) Purinergic receptor ligands stimulate pro-opiomelanocortin gene expression in AtT-20 pituitary corticotroph cells. J Neuroendocrinol 18:273-278.

4

Assessment of Brain Monoaminergic Signaling Through Mathematical Modeling of Skin Conductance Response

Saša Branković
Clinic for Psychiatry,
Clinical Center of Serbia, Belgrade
Serbia

1. Introduction

The majority of mental disorders (schizophrenia and other psychotic disorders, mood and anxiety disorders) have become treatable for the last several decades mostly due to development of the agents which modulate function of the brain dopaminergic, noradrenergic, and serotonergic system. The art of pharmacological healing in psychiatry consists actually in a great part in choice of the monoaminergic agent (i.e. antipsychotic or antidepressant) or their combinations which will modify the brainstem monoaminergic systems in an appropriate way. In other words, a daily problem in psychiatric practice could be realized as the task of estimation of the actual "neurochemical status" of the patient mostly in respect to the three brainstem monoamines. In clinical setting the task is still accomplished relying on the clinical picture and identifying the dominant symptoms that the patient manifests (e.g. Nutt, 2008; Nutt et al., 2007).

The search for biological correlates (biomarkers) of neurochemical processes associated with mental disorders has not yet resulted in convincing and applicable findings (Bartova et al., 2010; Mössner et al., 2007). A reason that may account for the fail could be that attempts that have been made had been focused on a single neurotransmitter activity (Mössner et al., 2007). On the other hand, "Models which postulate too little or too much of a single neurotransmitter are not consistent with the complex regulation of neurotransmitter systems... There are major functional interactions among different neurotransmitter and neuropeptide systems which make single neurotransmitter theories simplisti A task for future investigations... is to develop clinically applicable biological tests that can assess the functional interactions among different neurotransmitter and neuropeptide systems and specific brain structures. Successful development of such paradigms could result in improved diagnostic classification and prediction of treatment response..." (Charney et al., 1995).

In our interpretation of the task set by Charney & colleagues "functional interactions among different neurotransmitter and neuropeptide systems" are viewed as neurobiological signals in control system theory meaning of the word 'signal'. With this interpretation the task appear to be "to develop clinically applicable biological tests" which will allow insight into the signal interactions among neurotransmitter systems. It means that we are interested in the signal properties of neurotransmission such as: strength of the signal, frequency of signal oscillations, signal amplification and integration, and feedback regulation of the neural signals. Although these signal properties are realized through chemical and electric neuronal activities our methodological approach is not based on the measurements at that level of the neurochemical events. Instead of direct measuring concentrations of released neurotransmitters, density, affinity, and activity of their membrane receptors and reuptake transporters we suggest a method that needs a shift in the perspective of looking at the brain neurochemistry. The twist is that we firstly examine signal processing and control system aspects of a relatively defined neurobiological mechanism. Then, informed with the system and the signals' properties we are able to infer about the underlying neurochemical activity of the involved neurotransmitter systems. In other words, we aim to estimate "interactions among different neurotransmitter and neuropeptide systems" looking at the signal processing in the examined neurobiological mechanism.

The method which enables to examine the underlying regulatory pattern and points to the way of signal processing during a neurobiological process is a mathematical tool, the system identification theory and technique (Ljung, 1999). As a neurobiological mechanism which is convenient for our task to reveal neurochemical signal processing involving the brain dopaminergic, noradrenergic, and serotonergic system we have employed an output of the process of emotional arousal, the phenomenon of emotional, palmar sweating measured as the skin conductance response (SCR), which is regarded as the most useful laboratory test for an autonomic response (Damasio, 1994).

The so-called electrodermal activity (EDA) was discovered at the end of the XIX century as two different phenomena which occur at the palmar and plantar skin surface. One is electrical resistance of the skin surface (Vigoroux, 1879, 1888) and its momentary decreases in response to variety of external stimuli (Féré, 1888). This phenomenon implies passing a small electrical current on the surface of the skin. The other phenomenon is a measurable electrical potential between two electrodes placed on the skin without applying an external current (Tarchanoff, 1890). Contemporary researchers use predominantly the first phenomenon as the method of choice whereby resistance is expressed as its reciprocal - conductance. From the earliest publications the tonic-phasic distinction in EDA has been implied. More about the phasic component speak other terms which have been used to refer to the EDA phenomena in the history, galvanic skin response (GSR), and psychogalvanic reflex (PGR). The phasic component of EDA is nowadays assigned as skin conductance response (SCR) as opposed to the tonic component of EDA which is referred to as skin conductance level (SCL).

Fluctuations in SCL occur at the time-scale of minutes while phasic SCRs appear at the time-scale of seconds. Both SCL and SCR activity refer to the activity of palmar and plantar sweat glands and myoepithelial cells of their ducts which are under neural control of the sympathetic branch of the autonomic nervous system (Dementienko et al., 2000). Palmar and plantar sweat glands are not involved in the process of thermoregulation until the ambient temperature does not exceed 30°C (Andreassi, 1989; Venables & Christie, 1980). On the other hand, palmar and plantar sweating is elicited by psychic, emotional stimuli.

The SCR is a sensitive measure, it could be evoked applying weaker psychic stimuli than it would be necessary for other physiological variables (e.g. heart rate, blood pressure, respiration, electromyography) (Lader, 1980; O'Gorman, 1971). We suppose that dealing with weaker emotional stimuli put more lights on usual everyday-life emotional responding and arousal fluctuations, a range where individuals with a mental disorder (e.g. depression) are altered presumably due to the alterations in the brainstem monoaminergic systems' activity. The second reason for choosing SCR as a neurobiological mechanism for system identification is continuous nature of the SCR signal. From mathematical point of view, heart rate and respiration rate are derived variables that cannot be computed for time periods shorter than beat-to-beat and respiration-to-respiration period. Therefore, they are to greater extent discreet and so less convenient, since less informative for analysis than a continuous biological signal such as SCR.

The goals of this chapter are: (1) to introduce the reader with the method of system identification of the SCR, (2) to point to the emerging metrics of the SCR process, and (3) to show how this metrics allow inferring about tonic and phasic functions of the brain monoaminergic signaling and about the central neural events - neural input for the SCR system.[1]

2. Mathematical model of the SCR process: A series of integrations with three feedback loops

System identification approach enables to look into the process of the SCR in a neurophysiologically meaningful way. Through this method we approximate the whole arousal process (from the initial central neural event to the SCR output) as a series of integrators, with the integration constant of 100 ms, which corresponds to the temporal scale of brain neural integrations (Varela et al., 2001; Koch et al., 1996; Koch, 2005). Knowing the dynamic model of the SCR process enables further examination of the neurochemical meaning of the system parameters and eventually association of the identified regulatory signals with the activity of specific neurotransmitter systems.

2.1 Solution for the "hidden input" problem in the SCR modeling

The prerequisite for the system identification procedure which is performed using the *System Identification Toolbox* included in the mathematical software MATLAB® is that both output and input signal of the system are known. But, while the output signal of the SCR system is observable and measurable, the input signal is not directly measurable. Therefore, a separate scientific task is to find an appropriate mathematical representation of the driving input to the SCR system, i.e. to solve the "hidden input" problem.

A hint to visualize the initial forcing event in the SCR process came from mathematical dealing with differential equations with discontinuous forcing functions: the highest derivative of the solution appearing in the differential equation has jump discontinuities at

[1] There is an aspect of the present approach which we want to point out. Many findings and concepts developed in neuroscience during the last two decades have not yet been operationalized for clinical use. The method which is presented here could contribute to lessen this gap translating some concepts of modern neuroscience and making them visible in everyday clinical work. The following concepts are involved: tonic and phasic function of neurotransmitters, gain modulation of neural activity by monoaminergic inervation, feedback regulation in the arousal process, resonance and frequency characteristics of neural systems, central neural code, and signal-to-noise ratio of neural signals.

the same points as the forcing function, but the solution itself and its lower derivatives are continuous even at those points (Boyce & DiPrima, 2001). Considering the SCR as an output (solution) of a serial integration (in both mathematical and neurophysiological (computation) meaning of the word) and having in mind this simple mathematical rule we assumed that a hidden neural input left its trace and had a fingerprint on the highest derivative of the SCR signal.

Indeed, an inspection of the SCR signal and its derivatives reveals that while the SCR signal and its first two derivates appear to be continuous, jump discontinuities features the third derivative of the SCR signal. This observation suggested that we could be able to read the traces of the discontinuous forcing function (the hidden input) in the third derivative of the SCR signal. The task is to determine an approximation of the unmeasured input signal looking at its fingerprints on the third derivative of the SCR (Figure 1). We approximated the hidden inputs with series of impulses and square pulses. The timing and duration of the pulses have been determined according to the jump discontinuities of the third derivative of the SCR signal. We also exploited the possibility to quantify the strength of the hidden input through measuring the magnitudes of these jump discontinuities. The height of the putative input pulses (the strength of the hidden neural input approximations) has been determined according to the height of the jump discontinuities of the third derivative of the SCR signal.

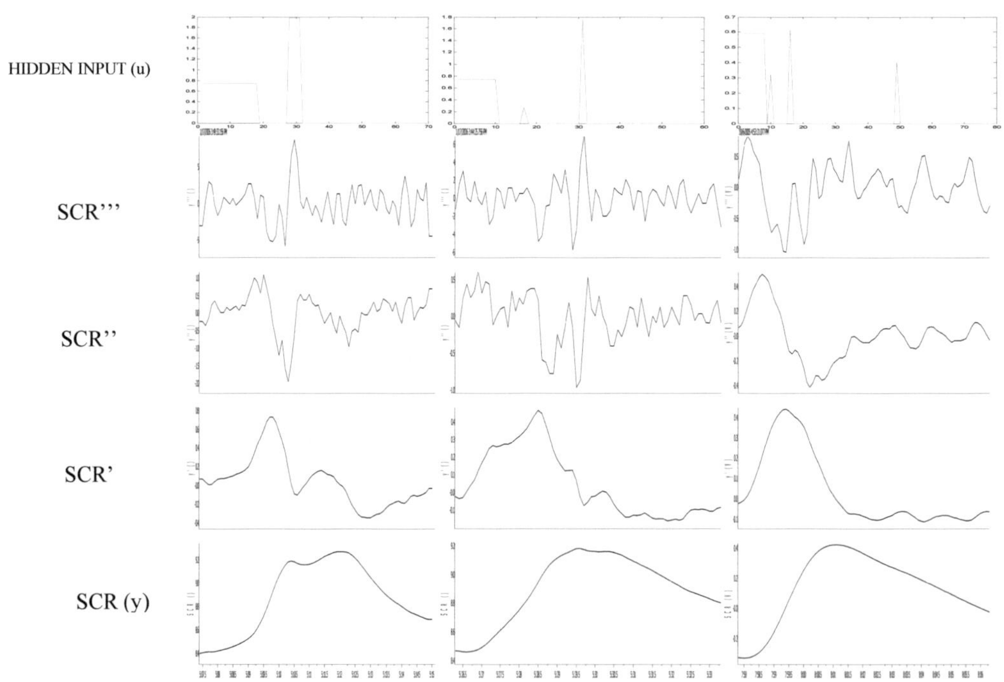

Fig. 1. Hidden-inputs to the SCR system determined observing the jump discontinuities in the third derivative of the SCR signal (SCR'''). Left column: the hidden-input consisting of two pulses of different strength and duration. Middle column: the input consisting of an initial pulse and two impulses of different strength. Right column: the input consisting of an initial pulse and three impulses.

The method showed simple to be performed and happened to be crucial for the feasibility and accuracy for the system identification approach to SCR. It enables easily obtaining almost perfect fit (>97%) between measured SCR and the corresponding simulated model's output. Recently we have automated the graphical procedure of estimating the neural input for the SCR system through a program application in the MATLAB® software environment (which will be available online at www.psychophysiological-computation.com and www.psychophysiological-computation.info). The tool could be regarded as a "temporal microscope" for the neural signals which had initiated the recorded SCRs (cf. Tyler & Likova, 2011).

2.2 Positive and negative feedback loops drive the SCR to pleasant emotional stimuli

System identification of the SCRs to pleasant emotional stimuli (textual fragments of short stories, see *Subjects and Methods* in Branković, 2011) has been performed using the *System Identification Toolbox* v. 6.0 included in the mathematical software MATLAB® v.7.0 (R14). We defined the model structure and set the fixed parameters and nominal (initial) values of the free parameters that enabled successful system identification of the SCRs to pleasant emotional stimuli for 27 healthy volunteers in the sample (see *Subjects and Methods* in Branković, 2011). The third-order state-space model appeared to be appropriate for two reasons. First, it yields accurate mathematical modeling of SCR providing high fit (>97%) between measured and simulated outputs, and second, it does it in a reliable, robust way, guarantying solution, convergence of the software algorithm dealing with the great variety of SCR input-output data.

Through the system identification procedure we estimate the parameters of the state-space models, which correspond to the coefficients in the equivalent linear differential equation of the system:

$$y''' + a \cdot y'' + b \cdot y' + c \cdot y = m \cdot u(t)$$

That enables us to regard the process of emotional arousal as an interaction among the following signals: 1) neural input to the SCR system, i.e. u(t), 2) the third derivative of the SCR signal (y'''), 3) the second derivative of the SCR signal (y''), 4) the first derivative of the SCR signal (y'), and 4) the SCR signal itself (y=SCR). Graphical representation of the interactions is shown in Figure 2.

Through modeling of over thousand SCRs to pleasant emotional stimuli we were consistently encountering the same resulting feedback structure: the fast positive feedback loop (occurring early in the feedback scheme), the negative (in the middle), and the slow positive feedback loop (originating at the peripheral end of the regulatory chain in the SCR process)[2].

[2] Interlinked positive and negative feedback loops have been identified in many biological systems as the key regulatory scheme (Tsai et al., 2008; Brandman et al., 2005; Brandman & Meyer, 2008). The wide occurrence of dual-time (fast and slow) positive feedback loops combined with a negative feedback loop has motivated investigations of properties and functions of that regulatory motif during the last decade. Mathematical simulations revealed that such coupled feedback circuits enable systems in noisy environment to produce perfect responses with respect to response duration and amplitude. The dual-time switch, consisting of interconnected fast and slow positive feedback loops, has been suggested as a

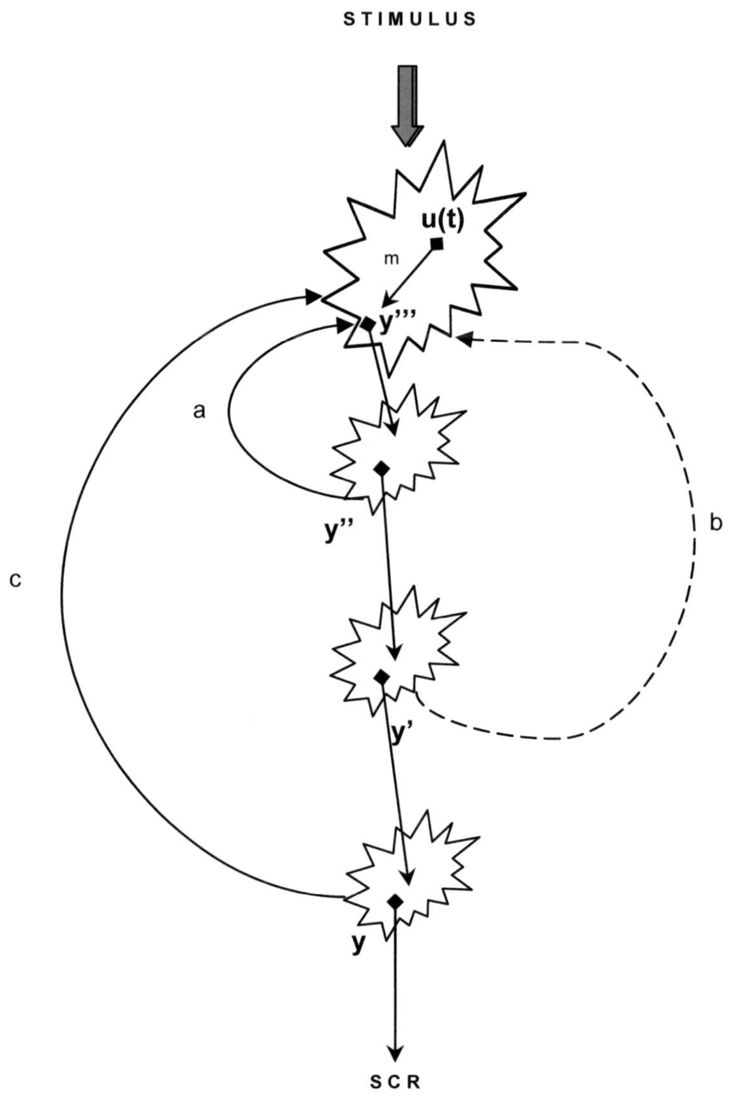

Fig. 2. State-diagram for the mathematical model of the skin conductance response (SCR): $y'''+a \cdot y''+b \cdot y'+c \cdot y=m \cdot u(t)$; y=SCR

ubiquitous regulatory motif performing sensitive robustness in biological systems (Zhang et al., 2007). The foremost activated positive feedback rapidly induces the "on" state transition of the signaling system, the delayed positive feedback robustly maintains this "on" state, while the negative feedback reinstates the system in the original "off" state, prevents excessive response due to multiple positive feedback loops, and suppresses noise effects (Kim et al., 2006; Pfeuty & Kaneko, 2009)

2.3 Emerging metrics of the SCR process

Since our mathematical dealing with the SCR process encompasses two steps - revealing the hidden input and system identification of the SCR - the approach yields to two sets of parameters. One set includes parameters which characterize the hidden initial neural input to the SCR system. The other set consists of parameters which characterize the SCR control system itself (Branković, 2011).

2.3.1 The hidden-input metrics

Through the graphical solving of the hidden input problem, relying on the jump discontinuities of the third derivative of the SCR signal (see 2.1), we approximated the initial neural event in the SCR process with series of impulses and square pulses (see Figure 1). The method enables quantification of the four features of the hidden input. In other words, we can define four dimensions in the hidden-input metrics: 1) number of pulses in the hidden input, 2) the amplitude (height, strength) of the pulses, 3) duration of the pulses, and 4) timing of the pulses (e.g. inter-pulse interval). This forms the hidden-input metrics.

The count of pulses in a hidden-input in our sample varied from 1 to 6. The amplitude of the pulses was in the range 0.023-7.74. The duration of the pulses in the hidden-inputs varied in the interval 0.1-2.8 s. The inter-pulse interval in the hidden-inputs was in the range 0.1-3.5 s.

Exploration of the within-subject distribution of values of the described hidden-input measures revealed normal distribution of *pulse duration* and log-normal distribution of *pulse amplitude* [3] (Figure 3).

2.3.2 System parameters of the SCR process

The set of the parameters which refer to the regulatory or control system aspect of the SCR process is composed of: *input gain, fast positive feedback loop gain, negative feedback loop gain, slow positive feedback loop gain, static system gain,* and *fidelity period* (Branković, 2011).

Input gain. This parameter corresponds to the constant "m" in the differential equation of the system. It reflects the initial step in the process of the regulation of emotional arousal. We have found the range of values 0.0013 - 0.025 for this parameter.

Fast positive feedback loop (FPFL) gain. Of the three feedback loops in the model (Figure 2) the first is proportional to the second derivative of the SCR signal (y'') and it is positive. We denote the parameter that characterizes this feedback loop as fast positive feedback loop gain. It equals the constant "-a" in the differential equation of the system. The found range of values of this parameter in healthy subject is 2.61 - 2.83. The within-subject coefficient of variation of this *fast enhancement* is about 1 %.

Negative feedback loop (NFL) gain. The second feedback loop in our model is proportional to the rate of change of the emotional arousal (y') and it is negative. It reflects a feedback inhibition in the arousal process. The parameter that characterizes this feedback inhibition equals the constant "-b" in the differential equation of the system. The found values of this

[3] It is interesting that within-subject variations of the pulse amplitudes sometimes manifested quantal nature (i.e. different values relate as integer multiplications to each other) (see Figure 3).

parameter are in the range from -2.44 to -2.68. The within-subject coefficient of variation of the *inhibition loop* in the SCR model is about 3 %.

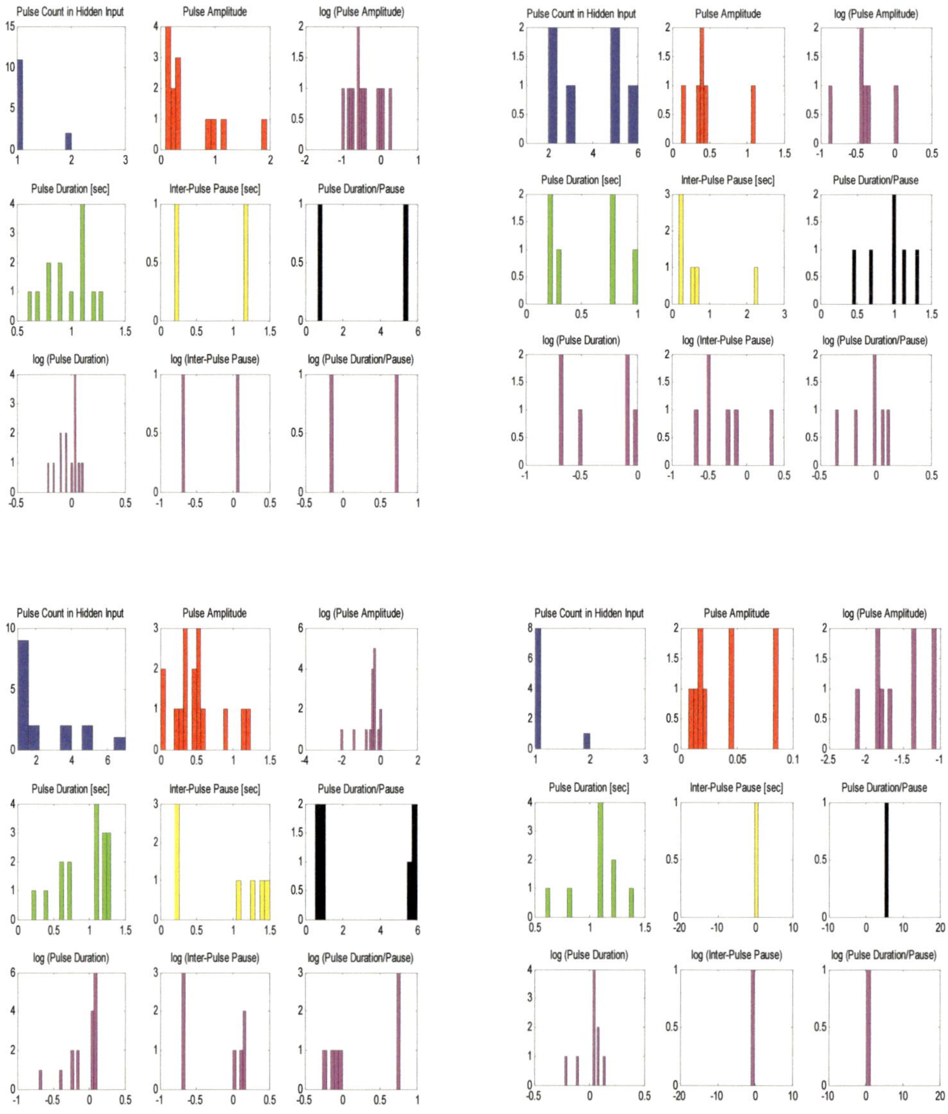

Fig. 3. Within-subject distributions of the hidden-input measures of four different subjects

Slow positive feedback loop (SPFL) gain. The third feedback loop in the model is proportional to the actual level of the emotional arousal, actual value of the SCR signal (y) and it is positive. The parameter that characterizes this feedback enhancement equals the constant "-c" in the differential equation of the system. The found range of values of this feedback loop gain is 0.65 - 0.86. The within-subject coefficient of variation of the *slow enhancement* is about 5 %.

Static system gain. The value of low frequency or static system gain of linear time-invariant system can be obtained as a direct result of the MATLAB® function "`dcgain`". The values of the *system gain* in our sample are 1.13 - 48.57.

Fidelity period. Some but not all models of the SCRs to pleasant emotional stimuli show potential for resonance. That is why we can not use resonant frequency as a parameter to characterize the all SCR models. Instead, we use the time period of periodic stimulation when the amplitude of response drops 3 dB below (or to 70.7% of) its zero-frequency value (amplitude of response which appears responding to a single stimulus). Expressed in seconds, *fidelity period* has a psychological meaning and face validity. Namely, with a further shortening of the inter-stimulus period in comparison with the *fidelity period* the amplitude of the SCR is rapidly diminishing. In that way, *fidelity period* gives an indication of the noise-filtering characteristics of the system. The found value of the fidelity period in our sample of the SCR models is about 13 seconds.[4]

Exploration of the within-subject distribution of values of the described system parameters revealed normal distribution of the three *feedback loops' gains* and *fidelity period,* and log-normal distribution of *input gain* and *overall static system gain* (Figure 4). The high intra-trial reliability of the estimations of the feedback loop gains (coefficients of variations: 1-5 %) points to the reliability of measurement of these parameters.

3. The mathematical model of the SCR in the context of neurobiological data

The stereotyped nature of the SCR waveform has recently inspired several dynamic modeling approaches to the process of SCR. The published models differ in the neurobiological interpretation of the system's parameters. While several research groups consider the peripheral sympathetic sudomotor nervous signal as the impulse input in their models of the SCR (Alexander et al., 2005; Bach et al., 2009, 2010a, 2010b, 2011; Benedek & Kaernbach, 2010), we assumed that the initial neural event and feedback regulatory mechanisms that we could comprise with our models took place in central brain structures (Branković, 2008). In the last case we would be able to derive much more information about the central neural processing from the SCR signal than we used to do, and, what is even more important, to infer about the brain mechanisms in a way that is not achievable by any other available method including invasive ones.

3.1 Evidence for the brain mechanisms involvement in the SCR model

We have recently found (Branković, 2011) that different types of SCRs (orienting response, SCR to pleasant emotional stimuli, weak movement, and respiratory SCR) have distinct regulation (i.e. different system parameters). This finding raises the question of adequacy of the assumption that mathematical models of the SCR process describe the sudomotor innervation and sweat gland activity (Alexander et al., 2005; Bach et al., 2009, 2010a, 2010b, 2011; Benedek & Kaernbach, 2010). The doubt has been recently expressed by Bach and

[4] The estimation of the duration of *fidelity period* of the SCR system in our sample corresponds well to the empirical data on breaking values of the interstimulus interval in the SCR measurement research (Breska et al., 2011; Benedek & Kaernbach, 2010).

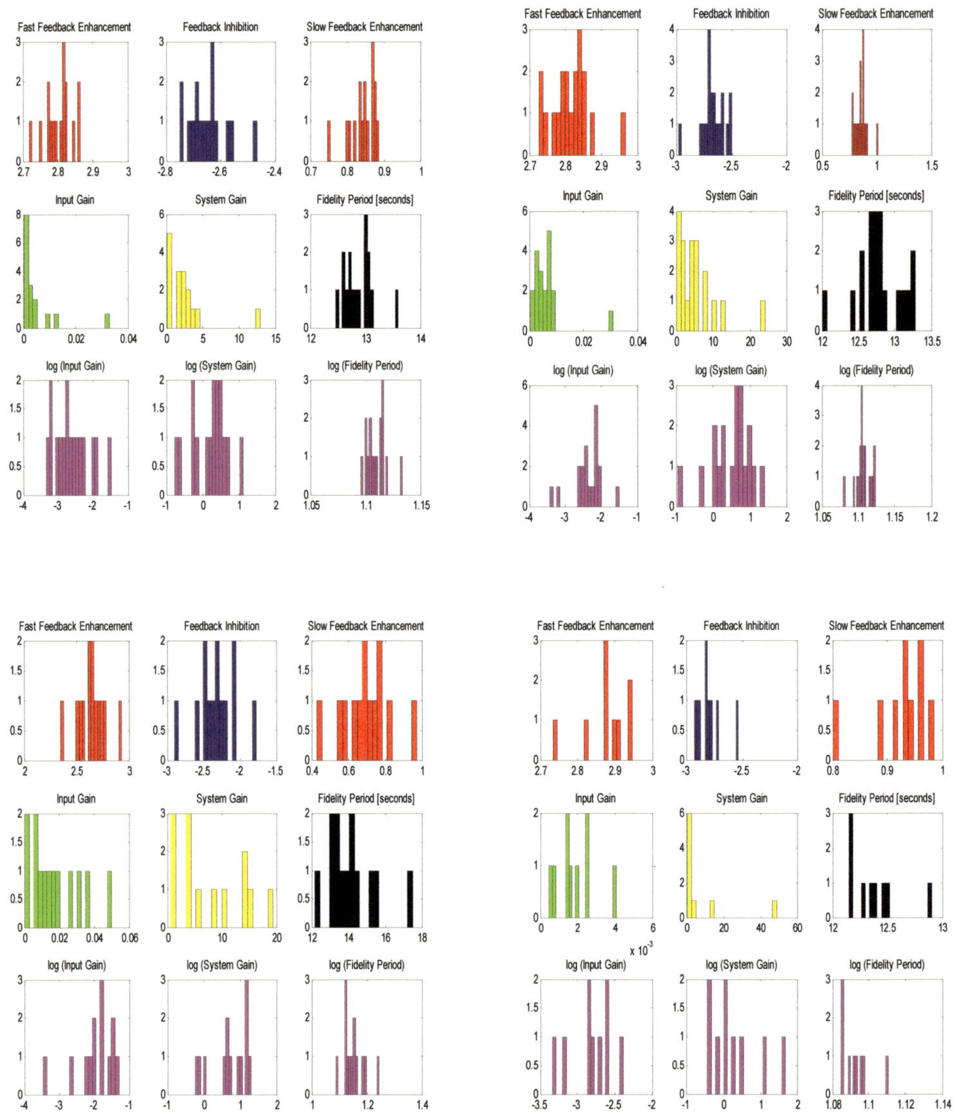

Fig. 4. Within-subject distributions of the SCR system parameters of four different subjects

colleagues (2010b) who found a difference of SCRs evoked by aversive pictures in comparison with other applied stimulus classes: "There is no reason why the peripheral output system should exhibit a different response to one stimulus class than to any other... The twist is that it might be possible to estimate characteristics of central nervous function by deconvolving the observed signal." Yet, the spark of this view we can trace back in the Edelberg's work on the so-called recovery limb of the SCR four decades ago. Edelberg (1970) proposed that rapid- and slow-recovery SCRs reflect qualitatively different psychological processes as a result of distinct neural control.

Different types of SCR lend support for the central interpretation of the identified model of the SCR process. This view has potentially significant implications. Namely, it follows that metrics of hidden-input and feedback loops in the SCR process could refer to the brain neurocircuitry and neurochemistry rather than to the biophysical properties of the sweat glands.

The shift from peripheral to central interpretation of the mathematical models of SCR challenges our understanding of the physiological nature of the SCR. Does the phasic electrodermal response reflect sweat secretion, passive diffusion, and reabsorption process? It would be difficult to explain precise influence and transmission of the central neural events on the distinct, stimulus specific SCR form if it would be realized through sluggish processes such as secretion, diffusion, and reabsorption. But there is evidence that formation of SCR could be better explained as determined by constriction of myoepithelial cells of ducts of the sweat glands (associated with vasomotor activity) on activation of the sympathetic nervous system than by long-time secretion, spreading and reabsorption of secretion (Dementienko et al., 2000).

3.2 Putative scenario of neural computations during the SCR process

Considering the results of the system identification studies of SCR (Branković, 2008, 2011) in the context of the data regarding the functional neuroanatomy of the SCR and emotional processing we suggest the following scenario during the process of generation and regulation of SCRs to pleasant emotional stimuli.

The initial step (generation of the initial neural event, i.e. the input neural signal for the SCR system) takes place in the interaction amygdala–hippocampus: "*Outcome* of the specific patterning of the match-mismatch process in the hippocampus/amygdala complex determines the precise constellation of signals to be either routed onward to the hypothalamus or aborted, and shapes the affective response or lack thereof to any stimulus event" (Hadley, 1989, p. 346; Laine et al., 2009; Phelps, 2004). In the amygdala-hippocampus interplay the role of the hippocampus is to detect novelty and unexpectedness of the stimulus (Kumaran & Maguire, 2007a, 2007b, 2008; Vinogradova, 1975). On the other hand, 'attachment of significance [emotional meaning] to a stimulus is critically dependent on the amygdala" (Mishkin & Aggleton, 1981, p. 412). We assumed that only unexpected pleasant emotional stimuli could elicit initial neural signal for pleasant emotional excitement (measured as the SCR) (Branković, 2001).

It is tempting to hypothesize that some features of the hidden-input to the SCR system could refer to novelty (or unexpectedness) aspect of the stimulus and some other hidden-input measures to significance (or emotional meaning) of the stimulus. It has been already suggested that different features of stimuli were represented through different dimensions of the neural pulse code in one neural system (Masuda & Aihara, 2007). Also, it has been realized that the neural code refers to population activity since individual neurons could not provide sufficient signal-to-noise ratio and speed to transmit information (Lestienne, 2001; Shadlen & Newsome, 1998; Eggermont, 1998). Relying on these findings we suggest that the dimension 'pulse amplitude' in our hidden-inputs metrics could correspond well to the 'population firing rate code' of the neural signal (Masuda & Aihara, 2007). Duration of the pulses in the hidden-input metrics fits the burst duration code (Kepecs & Lisman, 2004).

Finally, temporal distribution of the pulses in the 'hidden-input for the SCR' could refer to the temporal neural code (e.g. inter-burst interval) (Lestienne, 2001). Further work should be done to explore the statistics and semantics of the 'hidden-input code'. Probably, the neural code of the amigdalohippocampal circuit converts some subjective features (estimations) of stimuli ("stimulus attributes arrived at by computational process", and not physical attributes of stimuli (Eggermont, 1998)) into emotional (sympathetic) response. In other words, different dimensions of the hidden-input metrics could relate to different features (e.g. novelty vs. intensity (Barry, 2006)) of the stimulus that evokes the SCR.

The amigdalo-hippocampal interplay (resulting in the generation of neural input for the emotional SCR) is probably realized through the rhythmic, theta-related (5-11 Hz) modulation of neuronal activities in the amigdalo-hippocampal circuit which may provide adequate recurring time windows when synaptic interaction will be facilitated in this limbic network (Seidenbecher et al., 2003; Paré & Gaudreau, 1996). The theta self-synchronization of hippocampal and amygdala neurons (suggesting functional connectivity between those neurons) is not continuous but periodic process, which occurs both spontaneously every 5-30 seconds (mean 12.9 s) in brain slices maintained *in vitro* (Kano et al., 2005) and confronted with emotion-inducing stimuli (Pape et al., 2005; Seidenbecher et al., 2003). Interestingly, the periodicity of the amigdalo-hippocampal theta synchronization fits well with the fidelity period of the emotional SCR system - about 13 seconds (see 2.3.2). Moreover, the periodic theta amigdalo-hippocampal neural synchronizations last up to 2.5 seconds (Kano et al., 2005) what corresponds to the duration of the hidden-input pulses for the emotional SCR (see 2.3.1).

Along with the large amplitude theta synchronous oscillations both amygdala and hippocampal neurons generate action potentials at 24-45 Hz during the initial component of the periodic amigdalo-hippocampal synchronization (Kano et al., 2005). We speculate that postsynaptic integration of this early high frequency component of synchronous periodic events could be responsible for the strength (amplitude, height) of the "hidden" neural input for the emotional SCR (see 2.3.1). With this ends the first phase in the SCR process - generation of the neural input (the trigger of the emotional response).

The next phase is transmission and regulation of the SCR. This phase is realized through bidirectional connections among amygdala, hypothalamus, and the brain stem (cf. Pfaff, et al., 2005). In his neurobiological model of emotion regulation Lewis (2005) emphasized multiple positive and negative feedback components originating from brain stem which back up to amygdala and other cortical and subcortical systems increasing the activation of some systems while decreasing it in others. In the identified (central) control process of the SCR we detected three feedback loops (see 2.3.2). According to the known neurobiology of arousal the first candidates for the neurochemical substrate of the feedback loops could be brainstem originating monoaminergic inervation of amygdala and hippocampus: i.e. dopaminergic, noradrenergic, and serotonergic system.[5]

[5] "The activation of structures at different levels of the neuroaxis drives the brain into vertical integration. Reciprocal influences among brain stem, hypothalamic, and corticolimbic regions become coupled, perhaps through synchronization of independent oscillators, and this coupling may give rise to an emergent meta-synchronization that coordinates all lower-order couplings" (Lewis, 2005, p. 192).

4. Revealing the neurochemical meaning of the parameters in the model of the SCR process: Foundation for the psychophysiological probing of brain monoaminergic signaling

Considering the neurochemical meaning of the system parameters in the SCR model (e.g. feedback loops' gains) the following important issue should be clarified. Although the nodes in our dynamic model (Figure 2) could be realized as principal points on the path of integration and feedback regulation of the central neural signal conveying the information for emotional sweating we do not expect that the SCR signal which we measure at the skin surface and which figures as the slow positive feedback loop in the SCR model is actually transmitted back to the brain through some receptors and ascending neural pathways and takes part in the regulation of arousal. Rather, we suppose that in the central regulation of the arousal appears some neural signal (we assume a brain stem monoaminergic activity) with the similar and coherent temporal characteristics as the measured SCR which is the real slow positive feedback signal in the process of the SCR.[6] We hold the similar view on the fast positive feedback signal and the negative feedback signal in our SCR model. Mathematically they appear as the first and the second derivative of the measured SCR signal but neurobiologically they correspond to two earlier nodes in the neural integration chain during the SCR process.

Keeping in mind this notion we are equipped with a broader and more flexible perspective which could yield to a more accurate identification of the neurochemical meaning of the SCR system parameters than it would be the case if we would persist in trying to find real neuroanatomical pathways which convey the SCR signal (which we measure) back to the brain.

In order to reveal neurochemical meaning of the parameters obtained through mathematical modeling of the SCR process we have conducted a psychopharmacological intervention study. The basic idea had been to detect and follow the changes in the SCR system parameters in psychiatric patients receiving medication with well defined influence on certain brain neurotransmitter systems. The idea corresponds to that what Humble (2000) has assigned as "the psychopharmacological dissection". Although antidepressant exerts neither a single neurotransmitter effect nor a single action on a neurotransmission system (Leonard, 2000) there are differences among them. They differ in selectivity for both reuptake inhibition and receptor blockade. Among the most selective drugs for "the psychopharmacological dissection" are citalopram (the purest serotonin reuptake inhibitor available), reboxetin (the purest noradrenaline reuptake inhibitor), and maprotiline (which exerts considerably more receptor-blocking activity but also less inhibition of serotonin reuptake than other noradrenaline reuptake inhibitors) (Humble, 2000).

In agreement with the thesis that identified control process of SCR takes place in the neurocircuitry located between amygdala and brain stem speaks comparability of spectral characteristics of the signal components of the SCR system (SCR signal, its derivatives, and periodicity of the hidden input) on one side, with dominant oscillatory activity of the brain structures engaged in arousal process in that section of the neuroaxis (Branković, 2011).

[6] Similarity in temporal patterns displayed by a central measure of brain function (the N200 component of event-related potentials) and the measured peripheral SCR signal has been already detected, demonstrating dynamic relationship between the SCR signal and a brain neural process (Lim et al., 1999).

The neurochemical agents which we used to perform a kind of "the psychopharmacological dissection" of the SCR system were: (1) citalopram (daily dose 20 mg), a selective serotonin reuptake inhibitor (SSRI) - in revealing the serotonergic components of the SCR system (in 21 depressed patients); (2) maprotiline (daily dose 150 mg) - in revealing the noradrenergic SCR system's components (in 20 depressed patients); and (3) venlafaxin (daily dose 225 mg) or clomipramine (daily dose 150 mg) as dual acting (both serotonergic and noradrenergic) agents (in 18 depressed patients). The patients were diagnosed according to the DSM-IV criteria (American Psychiatric Association, 1994) for major depressive disorder currently in depressive episode. The mean score on the Hamilton (1960) rating scale for depression (HAMD) with 17 items was 21.4 (SD=6.7) on the day of the first psychophysiological measurement (the day before starting the pharmacological treatment) with non-significant differences among the treatment groups. All patients manifested significant clinical improvement after four weeks of the inter-trial period assessed as reduction of the HAMD score for more than 50 %.

One concept of the modern neuroscience should be mentioned before we continue with the results of the pharmacological intervention study. It deals with the distinction between the tonic and the phasic neurotransmitters' function. We find this distinction essentially for understanding the observed SCR system parameters' change in patients under psychopharmacological treatment. In the following we explain how some of the parameters refer to the tonic and others indicate the phasic function of serotonin and noradrenaline.

4.1 The hidden-input measures and the brain monoaminergic systems

According to the suggested scenario of neural computations during the SCR process (see 3.2) two features of the hidden input - pulse *amplitude* and *duration* - could be supposed as dependent not only on the characteristics of the encountering stimulus but also on the tonic monoaminergic innervation of the amygdalo-hippocampal circuit. For instance, it was shown that both dopamine agonists and antagonists alter the amygdala response to emotional stimuli (Salgado-Pineda et al., 2005; Takahashi et al., 2005; Exner et al., 2004). It is also known that noradrenaline modulates the filter function in the hippocampus causing an increase in the signal-to-noise ratio of the pyramidal cells such that the cells' response to stimuli near action potential threshold are inhibited, whereas the responses to larger stimuli are enhanced (Nicoll et al., 1987; Segal & Bloom, 1976).

Comparison between healthy subjects and acutely depressed patients of our sample regarding the amplitude and duration of the hidden-input and inter-pulse interval was performed using the t-test for independent samples with Bonferroni adjustment for multiple tests. The tests revealed significant lower amplitude of the hidden-input in depression and no difference regarding the duration and inter-pulse interval between healthy and depressed participants.

In order to test whether the diminution of the hidden-input amplitude in depression is due to deviant brain monoaminergic function we conducted an intervention study with antidepressants and probed the SCR system of the patients at the three times: 1) the day 0, i.e. the day before starting the antidepressant treatment, 2) the day 7, corresponding to the acute antidepressant treatment phase, and 3) the day 28, corresponding to the chronic antidepressant treatment phase. We tested the hypothesis that serotonergic and noradrenergic agents influence the process of generation of the initial neural input for the SCR system examining if there is any pattern of change in the amplitude and duration of the hidden-input in depressed patients before and during the treatment with antidepressants. The t-tests for dependent samples (using Bonferroni correction for multiple tests) revealed significant increase of the hidden-input amplitude and prolongation of the input pulse after four weeks of antidepressant treatment considering all applied agents together. The chronic antidepressant treatment did not significantly affect the timing of the pulses in the hidden-input, i.e. the inter-pulse interval remained unchanged.

In order to test if the monoaminergic agents show distinctive effect on the features of the hidden-input the following multivariate analysis of variance has been performed. We compared the relative change (in percents) of the hidden-input measures in the three groups of patients underwent to three different four weeks treatments: 1) citalopram group, 2) venlafaxin or clomipramine treated group, and 3) maprotiline group. The MANOVA revealed significant difference on the overall model between the treatment groups (Wilks' lambda=0.463, $F(6, 82)=6.42$, $p<0.0005$, multivariate eta-squared=0.32). The univariate analyses of variance revealed significant differences among the treatment groups regarding the hidden-input amplitude (eta-squared=0.438) and hidden-input duration (eta-squared=0.143) and non-significant differences regarding the inter-pulse pause. Pairwise comparisons revealed a stronger increasing effect on the hidden-input amplitude of the serotonergic agent (citalopram) than it was the case after venlafaxin or clomipramine treatment (Table 1). Interestingly, chronic treatment with maprotiline brought to lessening of the hidden-input amplitude. On the other hand, all three kinds of applied monoaminergic agents brought to prolongation of the hidden-input pulse but citalopram was significantly less effective than both venlafaxin/clomipramine and maprotiline. The last two kinds of treatment were not mutually significantly different regarding the effect on the hidden-input pulse prolongation.

Hidden-input feature	Citalopram	Venlafaxin/ Clomipramine	Maprotiline
Pulse Amplitude Change [%]	125.55 (19.98)	39.91 (22.89)	-83.33 (30.52)
Pulse Duration Change [%]	6.74 (36.64)	36.64 (9.98)	41.18 (13.31)
Inter-Pulse Pause Change [%]	28.53 (30.92)	79.68 (35.425)	-30.833 (42.23)

Table 1. Effects of a serotonergic agent (citalopram), dual acting agents (venlafaxin or clomipramine), and a noradrenergic antidepressant (maprotiline) on the hidden-input characteristics. The values represent means of the relative change in percents (SD).

4.2 Tonic and phasic functions of the brain monoaminergic signaling and the SCR system parameters

Relying on our neurobiological model of the SCR process (see 3.2) it follows that the parameter *input gain* appears as an indicator of the tonic function of the brain monoaminergic signaling. On the other hand, feedback loops' gains seem to refer to phasic functions of the brainstem monoaminergic systems conveying feedback enhancement and inhibition of the central neural signal which controls the output SCR signal.

Of the three feedback loops in the obtained mathematical model (Figure 2) the first one is proportional to the second derivative of the emotional arousal (SCR") and it is positive. It refers to some neural signal that backwards enhances the already initiated arousal process. Because of a proximal neuroanatomical position on the amygdala-brainstem axis in comparison with other monoaminergic systems, and similarity of the spectral characteristics of the SCR" and phasic dopaminergic activity (see Branković, 2011) we speculate that the fast feedback enhancement could relate to the phasic dopaminergic activation (Wanat et al., 2009; Redgrave et al., 2008; Lodge & Grace, 2006; Phillips et al., 2003) and positive feedback regulation of excitability in amygdala neurons through the process of slow afterdepolarization (Yamamoto et al., 2007).

The second feedback loop in the integration chain of our SCR model is negative one. It reflects the feedback inhibition in the arousal process. We speculate that for this feedback inhibition monoaminergic projections to the amygdala coming from the brainstem could be responsible - noradrenergic inhibition from the *locus coeruleus* (Buffalari & Grace, 2007; Schätze et al., 1987) and/or serotonergic inhibition from the raphe nuclei acting both directly on projection neurons and on interneurons (Stein et al., 2000; Rainnie, 1999).

One of the major outputs of the amygdala is the pathway from the medial amygdala to the paraventricular nucleus of the hypothalamus (PVN). This projection plays a critical role in expression of the autonomic response to stimulus (LeDoux, 1992). Beside the sympathetic projections of the PVN for the spinal cord, there is another arm of the PVN output that innervates *locus coeruleus* (LC) both directly (Reyes et al., 2005; Luppi et al., 1995) and indirectly through the innervation of the *nucleus paragigantocellularis*, which is the main input for the LC (Van Bockstaele et al., 1989; Aston-Jones et al., 1986). The majority of the axons of the PVN that directly innervate the LC release corticotrophin releasing factor (CRF) at their endings (Reyes et al., 2005). CRF activates the LC-noradrenergic system and increases the releasing of noradrenaline at the terminal projecting fields of the system (Dunn et al., 2004). The *locus coeruleus* does not innervate intermediolateral column of thoracic cord and, hence, is not directly involved in the transmission of the output of the sympathetic system to the periphery (Valentino & Aston-Jones, 1995; Fritschy et al., 1987). This refers to a different role of the LC activation that could lie in a feedback effect upon the higher brain structures. Indeed, it was shown that the noradrenegic projections from the LC have inhibitory influence on the kindling effect in the amygdala and the hippocampus (Giorgi et al., 2003). Beside that, the neurons in the amygdala that had been inhibited by the stimulation of the carotid sinus and baroreceptors were also inhibited by the stimulation of the LC (Schätze et al., 1987). For these reasons the projections of the hypothalamic PVN that innervate the LC (directly and through the *nucleus paragigantocellularis*) could be assigned as the regulatory output arm of the PVN.

In order to explore the neurochemical nature of the identified feedback loops and the parameter *input gain* in the SCR system we performed the following analyses. Comparison between healthy subjects and acutely depressed patients of our sample regarding the input gain and the three feedback loops gains was performed using the t-test for independent samples with Bonferroni adjustment for multiple tests. The tests revealed significantly weaker gains in all three feedback loops of the SCR system in depression and also a tendency in depression for lessening of the input gain although the found difference did not reach statistically significant level.

In order to test whether the weakening of the feedback loops' gains in depression is influenced by disturbed serotonergic and noradrenergic brain function we compared the SCR system parameters of depressed patients before, after 7 days, and after four weeks of the antidepressant treatment. The repeated measures MANOVA revealed significant effect for time of treatment (Wilks' lambda = 0.035, $F(8, 51) = 175.07$, $p < 0.0005$, multivariate eta squared = 0.965). The univariate analyses of variance revealed significant differences among the treatment phases regarding the three feedback loops' gains and also input gain (Figure 5). Pairwise comparisons (with Bonferroni adjustment for multiple tests) revealed significant strengthening of the feedback loops' gains during four weeks of antidepressant treatment. The applied antidepressants also changed the input gain of the SCR system.

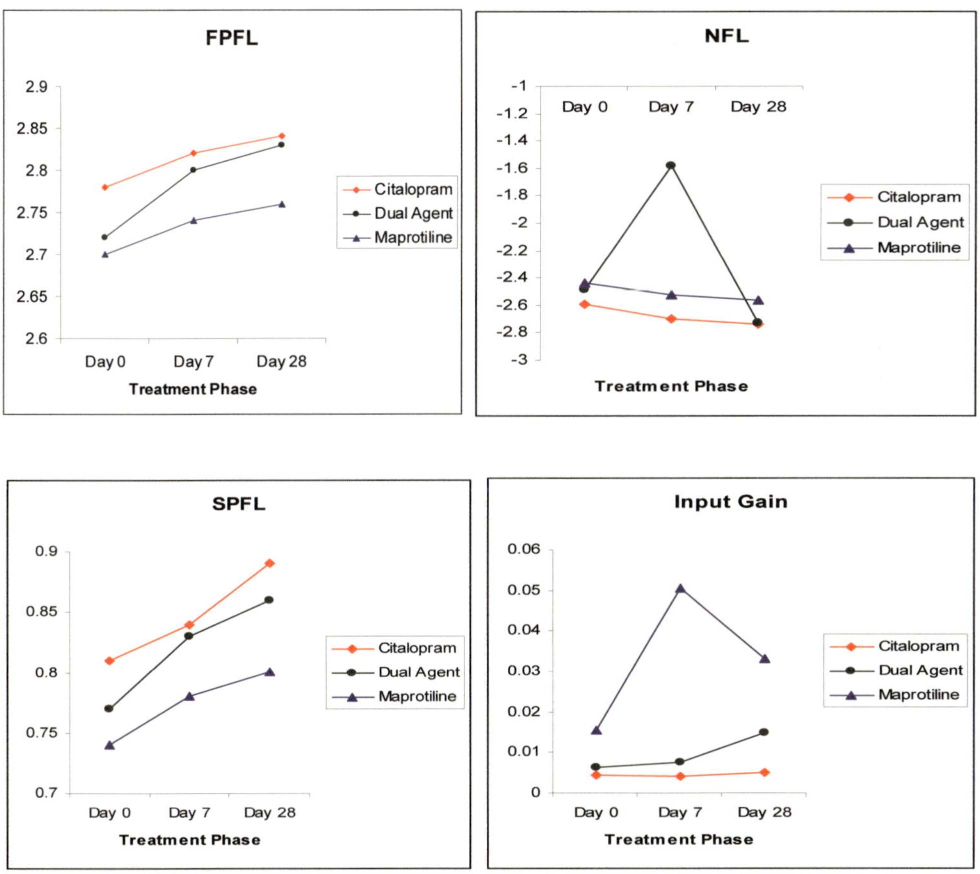

Fig. 5. Change of the SCR system parameters during the antidepressant treatment

In order to test whether the antidepressants have distinctive effect on the SCR system parameters the multivariate analysis of variance has been performed. We compared the relative increase (in percents) of the feedback loops' gains and of the input gain in the three groups of patients underwent to three different kinds of drug treatment. The MANOVA revealed significant difference on the overall model between the treatment groups (eta-squared=0.379). The univariate analyses of variance revealed significant differences among the treatment groups regarding the all three feedback loops' gains and non-significant differences in respect to input gain. Pairwise comparisons showed a stronger increasing effect of dual acting agents (venlafaxin/clomipramine) on the FPFL and the NFL gains than the effect of citalopram and maprotiline (Table 2). Citalopram and dual acting agents have similar strengthening effect on the SPFL gain and their effect is significantly stronger than the effect of maprotiline. The four weeks treatment with all three kinds of antidepressants was associated with similar increase of the input gain in the SCR system.

SCR System Parameter	Citalopram	Venlafaxin/ Clomipramine	Maprotiline
Fast Positive Feedback Loop Gain Increase [%]	2.61 (1.19)	4.01 (2.12)	2.49 (1.82)
Negative Feedback Loop Gain Increase [%]	5.79 (2.48)	9.59 (5.46)	4.91 (3.56)
Slow Positive Feedback Loop Gain Increase [%]	9.42 (4.01)	12.51 (6.73)	5.12 (4.25)
Input Gain Increase [%]	37.50 (114.58)	83.07 (120.11)	117.86 (18.37)

Table 2. Effects of a serotonergic agent (citalopram), dual acting agents (venlafaxin or clomipramine), and a noradrenergic antidepressant (maprotiline) on the SCR system characteristics. The values represent means of the relative increase in percents (SD).

4.3 Neurochemical meaning of the parameters in the SCR process model suggested by the results

Relying on the results (summarized in Tables 1 and 2) we suggest the following interpretation of the neurochemical meaning of the SCR model parameters. The finding of the strongest increasing effect of citalopram on the hidden-input amplitude could speak about the serotonergic nature of this hidden-input dimension. Since we assumed influence of the tonic function of the monoaminergic innervation on the strength and duration of the hidden neural input (see 4.1) it follows that the finding of 125% increase of the hidden-input amplitude after selective serotenergic treatment implicates responsibility of the tonic serotonergic function for this increase. Quantitatively this increase is in agreement with the prediction of the mathematical model of the neurochemistry of serotonin system where increase of 90% of the tonic serotonin activity is expected after chronic SSRI treatment (Best et al., 2011). The result is also in accordance with the finding of increased amygdala neural response to happy faces after citalopram treatment in an fMRI study on healthy volunteers (Norbury et al., 2009).

The 125% increase of the hidden-input amplitude after the four weeks citalopram treatment in our study is probably due to the evidenced a 75-80% decrease of serotonin reuptake transporters (SERT) binding site in the amygdala (Gould et al., 2003) and an internalization of SERT proteins from the cell surface, and redistribution of SERT from neurite extensions into the soma after a chronic SSRI treatment (Lau et al., 2008). A corollary of the result could be that depression associated with low hidden-input amplitude would be most effectively treated with a serotonegic agent (e.g. SSRI type antidepressant).

On the contrary, a weaker strengthening effect of citalopram on prolongation of the hidden-input pulse in comparison with the effect of maprotiline and venlafaxin/clomipramine could suggest a noradrenergic nature of the parameter 'hidden-input pulse duration'. It follows that depression associated with short hidden-input pulse would be most effectively treated with a noradrenergic agent.

The strongest increasing effect on the FPFL and NFL gains was shown by venlafaxin and clomipramine (dual acting serotonin/noradrenaline agents). The finding that maprotiline has a weaker strengthening effect on the SPFL gain in comparison with both citalopram and venlafaxin/clomipramine could suggest that the last feedback loop in the SCR control system is more directly associated with the phasic serotonergic than with noradrenergic neurotransmission. Corollary of this would be that depression associated with weakened feedback loops' gains would be most effectively treated with a dual acting agent. There is also possibility to combine knowledge about hidden-input parameters and feedback loops' gains in selecting antidepressant for the treatment of an individual depressed patient.

5. Limitations and future research

The approach which we have proposed is supposed to enable an insight into the neural signaling of the monoaminergic systems through measuring and processing of the behavioral variables such as skin conductance response. Although the monoaminergic neural signaling is a net result of the subtle neurochemical processes such as neurotransmitters' release, reuptake, and receptor binding the present method does not allow a direct insight into the relationship between our estimations of the neural signaling and the pharmacological actions such as processes of down- or up-regulation of receptors, inhibition of transporters, and intracellular changes (Leonard, 2000). But there is a possibility to overcome this limitation of the present method. It could be done through an integration of the present model with the existing mathematical models of the cellular mechanisms of the dopaminergic and serotonergic signaling (Best et al., 2009; Best, Nijhout & Reed, 2010; Best, Reed & Nijhout, 2010; Best et al., 2011). The later models are models of the processes of synthesis, release, and reuptake of brainstem monoamines. Establishing the link between the SCR model and these models could bring to a deeper insight into the monoaminergic processes specifying the deviation in the processes through knowing the vales of the SCR system parameters. It could enable even more informed choice of psychotropic drugs (e.g. is it more appropriate to intervene with a postsynaptic receptor agent or with a drug acting on the reuptake transporters). Agreement between our findings on the change of SCR system's indicators of tonic and phasic monoaminergic functions due to serotonergic treatment, and theoretical assumptions derived from the model of serotonergic signaling (Best at al., 2011) render the task feasible.

In this study we did not examine the effect of dopaminergic agents on the SCR system parameters what could be done in the future research. Further work could be also aimed to determine normative values of the hidden-input measures and the SCR system's parameters in larger samples of healthy individuals and to compare them with different populations of individuals currently experiencing an episode of a mental disorder.

6. Conclusion

In this contribution we introduced a methodological approach which appears promising for a possibility of establishing the bridge between the neurochemistry of the brain monoaminergic systems and psychophysiological measures such as skin conductance response. The SCR system in this perspective is viewed as a linear neurochemical oscillator suitable for mathematical modeling and estimation of the inherent control process. Through mathematical modeling of the SCR process two kinds of metrics emerged. One of them refers to the features of the hidden neural input for the SCR system generated in the amigdala-hippocamus interaction when an individual is encountered with an unexpected and significant stimulus. The other metrics specifies the regulatory (control system) aspect of the SCR process.

We presented the results of the first pharmacological intervention study aimed to reveal the neurochemical meaning of the parameters in the model of the SCR process. Future work on this issue could refine the method of the psychophysiological probing of the brain monoaminergic signaling systems and render it clinically applicable in: (1) the neurochemical characterization of an individual with a mental disorder and (2) a more informed choice of the psychotropic drugs for his or her treatment.

7. Acknowledgment

The author expresses great gratitude to Mr. Nenad Jeremić ("Blink N" Programming Agency) for the collaboration in development of the software tool for the automated analysis of the SCR signal. The publishing of the text was financially supported by Actavis-Serbia.

8. References

Alexander, D.M., Trengove, C., Johnston, P., Cooper. T., August, J.P. & Gordon, E. (2005). Separating individual skin conductance response in a short interstimulus-interval paradigm. *Journal of Neuroscience Methods,* Vol. 146, pp. 116-123.

American Psychiatric Association. (1994). *Diagnostic and Statistical Manual of Mental Disorders.* (the 4th edition), American Psychiatric Association, Washington, DC.

Andreassi, J.L. (1989). *Psychophysiology: Human Behavior and Physiological Response.* Lawrence Erlbaum Associates Publishers, Hillsdale, New Jersey, pp. 217-221.

Aston-Jones, G., Ennis, M., Pieribone, V.A., Nickell, W.T. & Shipley, M.T. (1986). The brain nucleus locus coeruleus: restricted afferent control of a broad efferent network. *Science,* Vol. 234, pp. 734-737.

Bach, D.R., Flandin, G., Friston, K.J. & Dolan, R.J. (2009). Time-series analysis for rapid event-related skin conductance responses. *Journal of Neuroscience Methods,* Vol. 184, pp. 224-234.

Bach, D.R., Friston, K.J. & Dolan, R.J. (2010a). Analytic measures for quantification of arousal from spontaneous skin conductance fluctuations. *International Journal of Psychophysiology,* Vol. 76, pp. 52-55.

Bach, D.R., Flandin, G., Friston, K.J. & Dolan, R.J. (2010b). Modelling event-related skin conductance responses. *International Journal of Psychophysiology,* Vol. 75, pp. 349-356.

Bach, D.R., Daunizeau, J., Kuelzow, N., Friston, K.J., & Dolan R.J. (2011). Dynamic causal modeling of spontaneous fluctuations in skin conductance. *Psychophysiology,* Vol. 48, pp. 252-257, doi: 10.1111/j.1469-8986.2010.01052.x

Benedek, M., Kaernbach, C. (2010). Decomposition of skin conductance data by means of nonnegative deconvolution. *Psychophysiology,* Vol. 47, pp. 647-658.

Barry, R.J. (2006). Promise versus reality in relation to the unitary orienting reflex: A case study examining the role of theory in psychophysiology. *International Journal of Psychophysiology,* Vol. 62, pp. 353-366.

Bartova L., Berger A. & Pezawas L. (2010). Is there a personalized medicine for mood disorders. *Eur. Arch. Psychiatry Clin. Neurosci.* Vol. 260, Suppl. 2, pp. S121-S126.

Best, J.A., Nijhout, H.F. & Reed, M.C. (2009). Homeostatic mechanisms in dopamine synthesis and release: a mathematical model. *Theoretical Biology and Medical Modelling,* Vol. 6, Retrieved from URL: http://www.tbiomed.com/content/6/1/21

Best, J.A., Nijhout, H.F. & Reed, M. (2010). Serotonin synthesis, release and reuptake in terminals: a mathematical model. *Theoretical Biology and Medical Modelling,* Vol. 7, Retrieved from URL: http://www.tbiomed.com/content/7/1/34

Best, J., Reed, M. & Nijhout, H.F. (2010). Models of dopaminergic and serotonergic signaling. *Pharmacopsychiatry,* Vol. 43, Suppl. 1, pp. S61-S66.

Best, J., Nijhout, H.F. & Reed, M.C. (2011). Bursts and the efficacy of selective serotonin reuptake inhibitors. *Pharmacopsychiatry,* Vol. 44, Suppl. 1, pp. S76-S83.

Boyce, W.E. & DiPrima, R.C. (2001). *Elementary Differential Equations* (7th edition), John Wiley & Sons: New York, USA, p. 319.

Brandman, O., Ferrell, J.E., Li, R. & Meyer, T. (2005). Interlinked fast and slow positive feedback loops drive reliable cell decisions. *Science,* Vol. 310, pp. 496-498.

Brandman, O. & Meyer, T. (2008). Feedback loops shape cellular signals in space and time. *Science,* Vol. 322, pp. 390-395.

Branković, S. (2001). What have the sexual, the attachment, and the exploratory motivation in common?: The theory of informational needs. *Psychiatria Danubina,* Vol. 13, No. 1-4, pp. 31-43.

Branković, S.B. (2008). System identification of skin conductance response in depression - an attempt to probe the neurochemistry of limbic system. *Psychiatria Danubina,* Vol. 20, No. 3, pp. 310-322.

Branković, S. (2011). Interlinked positive and negative feedback loops design emotional sweating. *Psychiatria Danubina,* Vol. 23, No. 1, pp 10-20.

Breska, A., Maoz, K. & Ben-Shakhar, G. (2011). Interstimulus intervals for skin conductance response measurement. *Psychophysiology,* Vol. 48, pp. 437-440.

Buffalary, D.M. & Grace A.A. (2007). Noradrenergic modulation of basolateral amygdala neuronal activity: opposing influences of α-2 and β receptor activation. (2007). *Journal of Neuroscience*, Vol. 27, No. 45, 12358-12366.

Charney, D.S., Bremner, J.D. & Redmond D.E. (1995). Noradrenergic neural substrates for anxiety and fear: clinical associations based on preclinical research. In: *Psychopharmacology: The Fourth Generation of Progress*, Bloom, F.E. & Kupfer, D.J. (Editors), pp. 387-395, Raven Press: New York.

Damasio, A,R. (1994). *Descartes' Error. Emotion, Reason, and the Human Brain.* Putnam Books, New York.

Dementienko, V.V., Dorokhov, V.B., Koreneva, L.G., Markov, A.G., Tarasov, A.V. & Shakhnarovich, V.M. (2000). The hypothesis of the nature of electrodermal reactions. *Human Physiology*, Vol. 26, pp. 232-239.

Dunn, A.J., Swiergiel, A.H. & Palamarchouk, V. (2004). Brain circuits involved in corticotropin–releasing factor - norepinephrine interactions during stress. *Ann NY Acad Sci*, Vol. 1018, pp. 25-34.

Edelberg, R. (1970). The information content of the recovery limb of the electrodermal response. *Psychophysiology*, Vol. 6, pp. 527-539.

Eggermont, J.J. (1998). Is there a neural code? *Neuroscience & Biobehavioral Reviews*, Vol. 22, No. 2, pp. 355-370.

Exner, C., Boucsein, K., Degner, D., Irle, E. & Weniger, G. (2004). Impaired emotional learning and reduced amygdala size in schizophrenia: a 3-month follow-up. *Schizophrenia Research*, Vol. 71, pp. 493-503.

Féré, C. (1888). Note sur des modifications de la résistance électrique sous l'influence des excitations sensorielles et des emotions. *Comptes Rendus des Seances de la Societe de Biologie (Ser. 9)*, Vol. 5, pp. 217-219.

Fritschy, J.M., Lyons, W.E., Mullen, C.A., Kosofsky, B.E., Molliver, M.E. & Grzanna, R. (1987). Distribution of locus coeruleus axons in the rat spinal cord: a combined anterograde transport and immunohistochemical study. *Brain Research*, Vol. 437, pp. 176-180.

Giorgi, F.S., Ferrucci, M., Lazzeri, G., Pizzanelli, C., Lenzi, P., Alessandri, M.G., Murri, L. & Fornai, F. (2003). A damage to locus coeruleus neurons converts sporadic seizures into self-sustaining limbic status epilepticus. *European Journal of Neuroscience*, Vol. 17, No. 12, pp. 2593-2601.

Gould, G.G., Pardon, M.C., Morilak, D.A. & Frazaer, A. (2003). Regulatory effects of reboxetine treatment alone, or following paroxetine treatment, on brain noradrenergic and serotonergic systems. *Neuropsychopharmacology*, Vol. 28, pp. 1633-1644.

Hadley, J.L. (1989). The neurobiology of motivational systems. In: *Psychoanalysis and Motivation*, Lichtenberg, J.D., pp. 337-372, The Analytic Press, Hove-London.

Hamilton, M. (1960). A rating scale for depression. *Journal of Neurology, Neurosurgery & Psychiatry*, Vol. 23, pp. 56-62.

Humble, M. (2000). Noradrenaline and serotonin reuptake inhibition as clinical principles: a review of antidepressant efficacy. *Acta Psychiatrica Scandinavica*, Vol. 101, Suppl. 402, pp. 28-36.

Kano, T., Inaba, Y. & Avoli, M. (2005). Periodic oscillatory activity in parahippocampal slices maintained in vitro. *Neuroscience*, Vol. 130, pp. 1041-1053.

Kepecs, A. & Lisman, J. (2004). How to read a burst duration code. *Neurocomputing*, Vol. 58-60, pp. 1-6.

Kim, D., Kwon, Y.K., Cho, K.H. (2006). Coupled positive and negative feedback circuits form an essential building block of cellular signaling pathways. *BioEssays*, Vol. 29, pp. 85-90.

Koch, C. (2005). *Biophysics of Computation: Information Processing in Single Neurons*, Oxford University Press, New York.

Koch, C., Rapp, M. & Segev, I. (1996). A breaf history of time (constants). *Cerebral Cortex*, Vol. 6, No. 2, pp. 93-101.

Kumaran, D. & Maguire, E.A. (2007a). Which computational mechanisms operate in the hippocampus during novelty detection. *Hippocampus*, Vol. 17, pp. 735-748.

Kumaran, D. & Maguire, E.A. (2007b). Match-mismatch process underliy human hippocampal response to associative novelty. *Journal of Neuroscience*, Vol. 27, No. 32, pp. 8517-8524.

Kumaran, D. & Maguire, E.A. (2008). Novelty signals: a window into hippocampal information processing. *Trends in Cognitive Neuroscience*, Vol. 13, No. 2, pp. 47-54.

Lader, M.H. (1980). The psychophysiology of anxiety. In: *Handbook of Biological Psychiatry Part II: Brain Mechanisms and Abnormal Behavior Psychophysiology*, Van Praag, H.M., Lader, M.H., Rafaelsen, O.J. & Sachar, E.J. (Editors), pp. 225-247, Marcel Dekker, New York.

Laine, C.M., Spitler, K.M., Mosher, C.P. & Gothard K.M. (2009). Behavioral Triggers of skin conductance response and their neural correlates in the primate amygdala. *Journal of Neurophysiology*, Vol. 101, April 2009, pp. 1749-1754.

Lau, T., Horschitz, S., Berger, S., Bartsch, D. & Schloss, P. (2008). Antidepressant-induced internalization of the serotonin transporter in serotonergic neurons. *FASEB J*, Vol. 22, 1702-1714.

LeDoux, J.E. (1992). Emotion and amygdala. In: *The Amygdala: Neurobiological Aspects of Emotion, Memory, and Mental Dysfunction*, Aggleton J.P. (Editor), pp. 339-351, Wiley-Liss, New York.

Leonard, B. (2000). Clinical implications of mechanisms of action of antidepressants. *Advances in Psychiatric Treatment*, Vol. 6, pp. 178-186.

Lestienne, R. (2001). Spike timing, synchronization and information processing on the sensory side of the central nervous system. *Progress in Neurobiology*, Vol. 65, pp. 545-591.

Lewis, M.D. (2005). Bridging emotion theory and neurobiology through dynamic systems modeling. *Behavioral and Brain Sciences*, Vol. 28, No. 2, pp. 169-245.

Lim, C.L., Gordon, E., Rennie, C., Wright, J.J., Bahramali, H., Li, W.M., Clouston, P. & Morris, J.G.L. (1999). Dynamics of SCR, EEG, and ERP activity in an oddball paradigm with short interstimulus intervals. *Psychophysiology*, Vol. 36, pp. 543-551.

Ljung, L. (1999). *System Identification – Theory for the User* (second edition), Prentice Hall, Upper Saddle River, N. J.

Lodge, D.J. & Grace, A.A. (2006). The hippocampus modulates dopamine neuron responsivity by regulating the intensity of phasic neuron activation. *Neuropsychopharmacology*, Vol. 31, pp. 1356-1361.

Luppi, P.H., Aston-Jones, G., Akaoka, H., Chouvet, G. & Jouvet, M. (1995). Afferent projections to the rat locus coeruleus demonstrated by retrograde and anterograde tracing with cholera-toxin B subunit and Phaseolus vulgaris leucoagglutinin. *Neuroscience*, Vol. 65, pp. 119-160.

Masuda, N. & Aihara, K. (2007). Dual coding hypotheses for neural information representation. *Mathematical Bioscience*, Vol. 207, pp. 312-321.

Mishkin, M. & Aggleton, J. (1981). Multiple functional contributions of the amygdala in the monkey, In: *The Amygdala Complex*, Ben-Ari, Y. (Editor), pp. 409-420, Elsevier/North Holland, New York.

Mössner, R. et al. (2007). Consensus paper of the WFSBP task force on biological markers: biological markers in depression. *World Journal of Biological Psychiatry*, Vol. 8, No. 3, pp. 141-174.

Nicoll, R.A., Madison, D.A., Lancaster, B. (1987). Noradrenergic modulation of neuronal excitability in mammalian hippocampus. In: *Psychopharmacology: The Third Generation of Progress*, Meltzer, H.Y. (Editor), pp. 105-112, Raven Press, New York.

Norbury, R., Taylor, M.J., Selvaraj, S., Murphy, S.E., Harmer, C.J. & Cowen, P.J. (2009). Short-term antidepressant treatment modulates amygdala response to happy faces. *Psychopharmacology*, doi: 10.1007/s00213-009-1597-1

Nutt, D. (2008). Relationship of neurotransmitters to the symptoms of major depressive disorder. *Journal of Clinical Psychiatry*, Vol. 69, Suppl. E1), pp. 4-7.

Nutt, D., Demyttenaere, K., Janka, Z., Aarre, T., Bourin, M., Canonico, P.L., Carrasco, J.L. & Stahl, S. (2007). The other face of depression, reduced positive affect: the role of catecholamines in causation and cure. *Journal of Psychopharmacology*, Vol. 21, No. 5, pp. 461-471.

O'Gorman, J.G. (1971). Habituation of the orienting reaction as a function of stimulus information. *Psichonomic Science*, Vol. 22, pp. 331-332.

Pape, H.C., Narayanan, R.T., Smid, J., Stork, O. & Seidenbecher, T. (2005). Theta activity in neurons and networks of the amygdala related to long-term fear memory. *Hippocampus*, Vol. 15, pp. 874-880.

Paré, D. & Gaudreau, H. (1996). Projection cells and interneurons of the lateral and basolateral amygdala: distinct firing patterns and differential relation to theta and delta rhythms in conscious cats. *Journal of Neuroscience*, Vol. 16, No. 10, pp. 3334-3350.

Pfaff, D., Westberg, L. & Kow, L.M. (2005). Generalized Arousal of Mammalian Central Nervous System. *Journal of Comparative Neurology*, Vol. 493, pp. 86-91.

Phelps, E.A. (2004). Human emotion and memory: interactions of the amygdala and hippocampal complex. *Current Opinion in Neurobiology*, Vol. 14, pp. 198-202.

Pfeuty, B. & Kaneko, K. (2009). The combination of positive and negative feedback loops confers exquisite flexibility to biochemical switches. *Physical Biology*, Vol. 6, pp. 46013, doi: 10.1088/1478-3975/6/4/046013

Phillips, A.G., Ahn, S. & Howland, J.G. (2003). Amygdalar control of the mesocorticolimbic dopamine system: parallel pathways to motivated behavior. *Neuroscience and Biobehavioral Reviews*, Vol. 27, pp. 543-554.

Rainnie, D.G. (1999). Serotonergic modulation of neurotransmission in the rat basolateral amygdala. *Journal of Neurophysiology*, Vol. 82, pp. 69-85.

Redgrave, P., Gurney, K. & Reynolds, J. (2008). What is reinforced by phasic dopamine signals? *Brain Research Reviews*, Vol. 58, pp.322-339.

Reyes, B.A., Valentino, R.J., Xu, G. & Van Bockstaele, E.J. (2005). Hypothalamic projections to locus coeruleus neurons in rat brain. *European Journal of Neuroscience*, Vol. 22, pp. 93-106.

Salgado-Pineda, P., Delaveau, P., Blin, O. & Nieoullon, A. (2005). Dopaminergic contribution to the regulation of emotional perception. *Clinical Neuropharmacology*, Vol. 28, pp. 228-237.

Shadlen, M.N. & Newsome, W.T. (1998). The variable discharge of cortical neurons: implications for connectivity, computation, and information coding. *Journal of Neuroscience*, Vol. 18, pp. 3870-3896.

Schätze, I., Knuepfer, M.M., Eismann, A., Stumpf, H. & Stock, G. (1987). Sensory input to single neurons in the amygdala of the cat. *Experimental Neurology*, Vol. 97, pp. 499-515.

Segal, M. & Bloom, F.E. (1976). The action of norepinephrine in the rat hippocampus. IV. The effects of locus coeruleus stimulation on evoked hippocampal activity. *Brain Research*, Vol. 107, pp. 513-525.

Seidenbecher, T., Laxmi, T.R., Stork, O. & Pape, H.C. (2003). Amygdalar and hippocampal theta rhythm synchronization during fear memory retrieval. *Science*, Vol. 301, pp. 846-850.

Stein, C., Davidowa, H. & Albrecht, D. (2000). 5-HT_{1A} receptor-mediated inhibition and 5-HT_2 as well as 5-HT_3 receptor-mediated excitation in different subdivisions of the rat amygdala. *Synapse*, Vol. 28, pp. 328-337.

Takahashi, H., Yahata, N., Koeda, M., Takano, A., Asai, K., Suhura, T. & Okubo, Y. (2005). Effects of dopaminergic and serotonergic manipulation on emotional processing: a pharmacological fMRI study. *Neuroimage*, Vol. 27, pp. 991-1001.

Tarchanoff, J. (1890). Über die galvanischen Erscheinungen an der Haut des Menschen bei Reizung der Sinnesorgane und bei verschidenen Formen der psychischen Tätigkeit. *Pflügers Archiv für die gesammte Physiologie des Menschen und der Tiere*, Vol. 46, pp. 46-55.

Tsai, T.Y.C., Choi, Y.S., Ma, W., Pomerening, J.R., Tang, C. & Ferrell J.E.Jr. (2008). Robust, tunable biological oscillations from interlinked positive and negative feedback loops. *Science*, Vol. 321, pp. 126-129.

Tyler, C.W. & Likova, L.T. (2011). Estimating neural signal dynamics in the human brain. *Frontiers in Systems Neuroscience*, Vol. 5, Article 33, doi: 10.3389/fnsys.2011.00033

Valentino, R.J. & Aston-Jones, G.S. (1995). Physiological and anatomical determinants of locus coeruleus discharge. Behavioral and clinical implikations. In: *Psychopharmacology: The Fourth Generation of Progress*, Bloom, F.E. & Kupfer, D.J. (Editors), pp. 373-385, Raven Press: New York.

Van Bockstaele, E.J., Pieribone, V.A. & Aston-Jones, G. (1989). Diverse afferents converge on the nucleus paragigantocellularis in the rat ventrolateral medulla: retrograde and anterograde tracing studies. *Journal of Comparative Neurology*, Vol. 290, No. 4, pp. 561-584.

Varela, F., Lachaux, J.P., Rodriguez, E. & Martinerie, J. (2001). The brainweb: phase sinchronization and large-scale integration. *Nature Neuroscience*, Vol. 2, pp. 229-239.

Venables, P.H. & Christie, M.J. (1980). Electrodermal activity. In: *Techniques in Psychophysiology*, Martin, I. & Venables, P.H. (editors), pp. 3-67, John Wiley & Sons, Chichester, New York, Brisbane, Toronto.

Vigoroux, R. (1879). Sur le role de la resistance electrique des tissues dans l'electro-diagnostic. *Comptes Rendus Societe de Biologie*, Vol. 31, pp. 336-339.

Vigoroux, R. (1888). The electrical resistance considered as a clinical sign. *Progres Medicale*, Vol. 3, pp. 87-89.

Vinogradova, O.S. (1975). The hippocampus and the orienting reaction. In: *Neuronal Mechanisms of the Orienting Reflex*, Sokolov, E.N. & Vinogradova, O.S. (editors), pp. 183-215, Lawrence Erlbaum Associates Publishers, Hillsdale, NJ.

Wanat, M.J., Willuhn, I., Clark, J.J. & Phillips, P.E.M. (2009). Phasic dopamine release in appetitive behaviors and drug addiction. *Current Drug Abuse Reviews*, Vol. 2, No. 2, pp. 195-213.

Yamamoto, R., Ueta, Y. & Kato, N. (2007). Dopamine induces a slow afterdepolarization in lateral amygdala neurons. *Journal of Neurophysiology*, Vol. 98, pp. 984-992.

Zhang, X.P., Cheng, Z., Liu, F. & Wang, W. (2007). Linking fast and slow positive feedback loops creates an optimal bistable switch in cell signaling. *Physical Review*, Vol. 76, pp. 031924, doi: 10.1103/PhysRevE.76.031924

5

Fatty Acids and Emotional Behavior

Carlos M. Contreras[1,2], Ana G. Gutiérrez-García[2,3]
and Diana Idania Vásquez-Hernández[2]
[1]*Unidad Periférica Xalapa, Instituto de Investigaciones Biomédicas, Universidad Nacional, Autónoma de México, Xalapa, Veracruz,*
[2] *Laboratorio de Neurofarmacología, Instituto de Neuroetología, Universidad Veracruzana,*
[3] *Facultad de Psicología, Universidad Veracruzana, Xalapa, Veracruz, Mexico*

1. Introduction

Fatty acids are widely distributed in nature. In addition to being found in plants and seeds, these organic compounds are present in other organisms, from unicellular protists to mammals, including humans. The anabolic and catabolic pathways of fatty acids have been identified. They have a well-known function as energy sources in metabolic processes and constitute a fundamental part of cellular membrane structures. Long-chain fatty acids also play a role in inflammatory process. Fatty acids exert their actions by modifying the fluidity of membranes, exerting marked actions on membrane ionic channels, and leading to a reduction in the excitability of cardiac myocytes, thus prompting interest in the study of fatty acids as protectors of cardiac function. Fatty acids exert similar actions on membrane neurons and the modulation of neurotransmission. The role of fatty acids in several psychiatric and neurologic conditions is a topic of current research. Fatty acid deficiency appears to be related to alterations in development, but the results from supplementary diet studies are far from conclusive. Interestingly, fatty acids are present in amniotic fluid, colostrum, and maternal milk in at least two mammalian species (i.e., pigs and humans) and according to both anecdotal and experimental reports appear to produce anxiolytic effects. Additionally, fatty acids exert effects when applied by the olfactory route. Odorant carrier proteins to olfactory receptors are present in maternal fluids and nasal mucosa epithelia. In newborns, fatty acids may also act as olfactory cues for feeding source seeking after exposure during prenatal life, which may constitute an additional function.

2. Overview

Lipids are organic compounds that are insoluble in water but soluble in nonpolar solvents, such as ether and chloroform. Some of these lipids naturally occur in the marine food chain. From an evolutionary ecological perspective, their presence in dinoflagelates, teleosts, amphibians, reptiles, birds, mammalians, and humans is important (Crawford et al., 2009).

In mammals, the highest lipid concentrations occur in adipose tissue, followed by the central nervous system (Carrié et al., 2000). However, lipids are present in all cell types, where they contribute to cell structure and energy storage and participate in many biological processes, such as gene transcription, the regulation of metabolic pathways, and other physiological processes (Gurr et al., 2002).

The biological functions of lipids are as diverse as their chemistry. Fats and oils are the main forms of energy storage in many organisms, and phospholipids and sterols are the major structural elements of biological membranes. Other lipids, although present in relatively small amounts, play a crucial role in the composition of enzymatic cofactors, electron carriers, light pigments, membrane protein folding, digestive tract emulsifiers, hormones, and intracellular messengers (Nelson & Cox, 2005). Fatty acids are the main component of phospholipids, triglycerides, and cholesterol esters (Agostoni & Bruzzese, 1992).

2.1 Definition and classification

Fatty acids are aliphatic carboxylic acids composed of four to 36 carbon chains and a variable degree of unsaturation, ending in a carboxyl group (Berg et al., 2003; Nelson & Cox, 2005). The moiety of carbon chains can be short (2-4 carbons), medium (6-12 carbons), long (14-18 carbons), and very long (derived from 18 carbon molecules; Agostoni & Bruzzese, 1992). The hydrocarbon chain can be saturated or may have one or more double unsaturated bonds (Bézard et al., 1994). Based on the number of unstaurations, the hydrocarbon chain may constitute monounsaturated fatty acids (MUFA) or polyunsaturated fatty acids (PUFA; Agostoni & Bruzzese, 1992; Bézard et al., 1994). The classification of PUFA is based on the location of the last double-bond near the methyl end, yielding the typical location n-3 or n-6. However, mammals cannot introduce double-bonds between C-9 and the methyl end of fatty acids; thus, mammals are not able to synthesize n-3 or n-6 PUFA or convert n-3 PUFAs into n-6 PUFAs or vice versa (Bézard et al., 1994; Colin et al., 2003; Dobryniewski et al., 2007). Instead, n-3 and n-6 PUFA are derived from other fatty acids that act as precursors (Stulnig, 2003). n-3 and n-6 PUFA can be synthesized from the precursors linoleic acid (18:2) and α-linolenic acid (18:3), which in turn may be synthesized from shorter-chain fatty acids, such as palmitic acid (C16:0; Cunnane et al., 1995). Similarly, saturated fatty acids (SFA) and MUFA can be synthesized from acetate precursors (e.g., carbohydrates, glycogenic amino acids) and PUFA (Brenna et al., 2009).

2.2 General properties

Fatty acids are esters in natural fats and oils but also exist in non-esterified forms, such as free fatty acids, that circulate in the blood of vertebrates via noncovalent bonds with the carrier protein serum albumin. Typically, the most abundant fatty acids have carbon chains from 14 to 24 atoms, although the most abundant fatty acids contain 16 to 18 atoms. In nature, the most abundant are unsaturated fatty acids, followed by saturated, with double-bonds and a *cis* configuration (Berg et al., 2003; Nelson & Cox, 2005). The *cis* configuration can be converted to the *trans* form by catalytic heating. Saturated fatty acids are very stable, whereas unsaturated acids are susceptible to oxidation (i.e., the more double-bonds, the higher susceptibility to oxidation; Gurr et al., 2002).

2.3 Physical and chemical properties

The physical properties of fatty acids are related to the length of their carbon chain and unsaturation. The nonpolar characteristics of the hydrocarbon chain explain the poor solubility of fatty acids in water. The polar carboxylic acid group (ionized at neutral pH) explains the poor solubility of short-chain fatty acids in water (Berg et al., 2003; Nelson & Cox, 2005). Likewise, longer chains have a higher melting point. Unsaturated fatty acids have a melting point that is lower than that of saturated fatty acids of the same length (Berg et al., 2003; Nelson & Cox, 2005).

2.4 Anabolic processes

The biotransformation process of fatty acids has been summarized by Nelson and Cox (2005). The synthesis of fatty acids may occur by *de novo* synthesis or modification of the carbon chain (Gurr et al., 2002). In *de novo* synthesis, fatty acids are synthesized from pyruvate, the final product of glycolysis, with the participation of a three-carbon intermediary and malonyl-CoA, an irreversible catalytic product of acetyl-CoA (Gurr et al., 2002).

The assembly of the carbon chains of fatty acids occurs through a four-step sequence. A saturated acyl group is the substrate for subsequent condensation with an activated malonyl group. With each step of the cycle, the acyl chain is extended by two carbons. The cycle is completed with the formation of a chain of 16 carbons (i.e., palmitic acid [C16:0], an SFA). Carbons C-16 and C-15 from palmitic acid are derived from the carboxyl and methyl carbons, respectively, of an acetyl-CoA. Other carbons are derived from acetyl-CoA via malonyl-CoA. NADPH acts as a reducing agent, and the two SH groups that are bound to the enzyme are the active group. All reactions in the synthesis are catalyzed by a multienzymatic complex, fatty acid synthase.

Palmitic acid is the terminal product in fatty acid synthesis in animal cells and is the precursor SFA and MUFA through elongation of the carbon chain. Palmitic acid (16:0) can be elongated to form stearate (18:0) or a longer carbon chain through the addition of acetyl groups with the participation of elongase enzymes. The process occurs via two elongation systems located in the mitochondria and smooth endoplasmic reticulum from the liver, brain, and some other tissues (Gurr et al., 2002).

One of the most important functions of elongation is the conversion of essential fatty acids into PUFA (Gurr et al., 2002). However, these fatty acids cannot be synthesized by mammalian cells and must be obtained from the diet as linoleic acid (18:2) and α-linolenic acid (18:3) to be transformed into PUFA, such as dihomo-γ-linolenic acid (18:3), arachidonic acid (20:4), eicosapentaenoic acid (20:5), and docosahexaenoic acid (DHA; 22:6; Haggarty, 2002).

A second mechanism for the synthesis of fatty acids is desaturation (Gurr et al., 2002). Palmitic acid and stearic acid serve as the precursors of two of the most common MUFA in animal tissues (i.e., palmitoleic acid [16:1] and oleic acid [18:1]), which have a *cis* double-bond between C-9 and C-10. The double-bond is introduced into the fatty acid chain by an oxidative reaction with the participation of O_2, NADH, and three proteins: cytochrome b5, a flavoprotein (cytochrome b5 reductase), and the enzyme acyl-CoA desaturase, which catalyzes the reaction and acts at specific positions in the fatty acid carbon chain (Sprecher et al., 1995). Mammals have two types of desaturases: stearoyl-CoA desaturase (which catalyzes the synthesis of MUFA) and A5D/A6D desaturases (which participate in the biosynthesis of PUFA; Sampath & Ntambi, 2005).

2.5 Catabolic processes

β-oxidation is the conversion of fatty acids to acetyl-CoA and is the main source of energy for most organisms. Its name derives from the position of the carbon attacked in the acyl chain, and the process occurs in the mitochondria and peroxisomes (Gurr et al., 2002). β-oxidation occurs in three stages. In the first stage, the fatty acids lose two carbon units by oxidative removal, starting from the carboxyl group and ending in the acyl chain. For example, palmitic acid undergoes seven steps in the oxidative sequence and at each step loses two carbons as acetyl-CoA. At the end of seventh cycle, the C-15 and C-16 palmitic acid carbons still remain as acetyl-CoA. The final result is the conversion of the 16-carbon chain of palmitic acid into eight two-carbon acetyl groups in acetyl-CoA molecules. The formation of acetyl-CoA requires the removal of four hydrogen atoms (two pairs of electrons and four H^+) in the middle of the acyl group by dehydrogenases.

In the second stage of oxidation, the acetyl groups of acetyl-CoA are oxidized in the mitochondrial matrix into CO_2 in the citric acid cycle. Thus acetyl-CoA derived from fatty acids enters the final stage of the oxidation of acetyl-CoA derived from glucose via glycolysis and pyruvate oxidation. The first two stages of oxidation produce NADH and FADH2, which in the third stage donate electrons to the respiratory chain, and electrons pass to oxygen, resulting in the phosphorylation of ADP to ATP; thus, the result of the β-oxidation of fatty acids is ATP.

2.6 Physiological role

Fatty acids are involved in energetic, metabolic, and structural processes. Short-chain fatty acids act as growth factors. Long saturated chains are a source of energy, and long-chain unsaturated chains participate in fundamental metabolic processes (Agostoni & Bruzzese, 1992), such as the synthesis of eicosanoids, which are closely related to inflammatory processes (Mesa-García et al., 2006; Zamaria, 2004), the modulation of enzymatic activity, the activation of nuclear transcription factors, and the formation of free radicals in response to oxidative stress (Zamaria, 2004).

Very long-chain molecules constitute biological membranes and participate in development (Agostoni & Bruzzese, 1992). n-3 PUFA (linolenic acid) and n-6 PUFA (linoleic acid; Bézard et al., 1994; Colin et al., 2003; Sardesai, 1992; Sinclair, 1984) are structural components of all tissues and indispensable for the synthesis of the cell membrane (Uauy et al., 2000).

2.7 Mechanism of action on excitable tissues

Fatty acids accumulate in membrane phospholipids near the ion channel, which alters the tension of the membrane, causes conformational changes in the ion channel, and consequently alters its conductance (Leaf et al., 2002). Two forms of Na^+/K^+-ATPase catalytic subunits are present in the nervous system. The α form is present in astrocytes, glial cells, and other tissues and is seemingly related to K^+ clearance. The α+ subunit is present in neuronal tissue, possesses high affinity for cardiac glycosides, is stimulated by biogenic amines, and participates in Na^+ and K^+ transport. In addition to the well known role of the Na^+/K^+ pump in resting membrane potential, it also participates in the differentiation of nerve cells during neurulation (Stahl, 1986). The modulation of membrane protein function by molecules that possess both hydrophilic and hydrophobic ends has been ascribed to changes in bilayer fluidity and alterations in bilayer stiffness. For example, *N*-type calcium channels may be modulated by a decrease in bilayer stiffness (Lundbaek et al., 1996).

Because of the reputation of PUFA as cardiac protectors, many studies have explored the action of fatty acids on cardiac myocytes. In these cells, n-3 and n-6 PUFA (DHA, α-linolenic acid, arachidonic acid, and linoleic acid) but not *trans* MUFA or SFA reduce Na^+ currents (Xiao et al., 1995). Free PUFA modulate voltage-sensitive Na^+ channels through the inhibition of agonist binding to the Na^+ channel protein in a dose-dependent, saturable, reversible, and allosteric manner (Kang & Leaf, 1996) but do not upregulate cardiac Na^+ channel expression in the long-term (Kang et al., 1997). Although PUFA may produce supraventricular and ventricular arrhythmias, its anti-arrhythmic properties are attributable to inhibition of Na^+ voltage-dependent currents, leading to hyperpolarization and reducing the availability and release of Ca^{2+} and sharing some actions with lidocaine (Lombardi & Terranova, 2007; Xiao et al., 1997, 1998). In other tissues, such as human fetal tracheal cells, *cis* PUFA and MUFA (e.g., arachidonic acid, linoleic acid, and oleic acid) but not SFA (e.g., stearic acid, palmitic acid, and myristic acid) modulate Cl^- channel activity by interrupting the open channel current (Hwang et al., 1990). In smooth muscle cells, arachidonic acid, oleic acid, myristic acid, and linoleic acid but not myristoleic acid, caprylic acid, or palmitic acid activate K^+ currents (Ordway et al., 1989; Robertson & Steinberg, 1990), also producing hyperpolarization.

The motor cortex of the human brain contains primarily long-chain fatty acids, such as arachidonic acid (C20:4n-6) and DHA (C22:6n-3). Other shorter-chain fatty acids are more likely to be involved in vascular blood flow, and eicosanoid activity involved in responses to injury. In animals, through alternative processes of desaturation and elongation, arachidonic acid may be formed from linoleic acid (18:2n-6), and DHA may be formed from α-linolenic acid (18:3n-3) but in a relatively inefficient manner because of the characteristics of being rate limited and very slow. Therefore, its ingestion in the diet seems to be crucial. Double-blind, controlled studies are needed before reaching conclusions about the properties of PUFA as cardiac protectors.

Intriguing results have been found regarding the actions of fatty acids in nervous tissue. Fatty acids regulate ion channels (Ordway et al., 1991) and can be delivered to the cells from extracellular sources, such as albumin and lipoproteins (Ordway et al., 1991). Fatty acids can enter the brain and exert their effects on neurons when administered systemically (Lauritzen et al., 2000). PUFA easily cross the blood-brain barrier and accumulate in neuronal membranes (Robinson & Rapoport, 1986). Arachidonic acid and other fatty acids regulate ion channels themselves through direct action or indirectly through their metabolites (Ordway et al., 1991). Likewise, at least one *cis* MUFA (oleic acid), one n-6 PUFA (arachidonic acid), and one n-3 PUFA (DHA) increase the binding of [^{3}H]diazepam to the benzodiazepine/γ-aminobutyric acid (GABA) receptor (Nielsen et al., 1988). Long-term ethanol or diazepam administration increases the proportions of plasma SFA and MUFA and decreases PUFA (Ristic et al., 1995). Therefore, some anxiolytic action may be expected.

The inhibition of GABA neurotransmission by arachidonic acid or its peroxidized metabolites contributes to the pathogenesis of ischemia-perfusion neuronal injury because the accumulation of these n-3 PUFA (but not SFA) inhibits GABA-mediated neuronal inhibition, leading to increased neuronal excitability (Schwartz & Yu, 1992). This may be related to the observation that barbiturates produce a Ca^{2+}-dependent decrease in Cl^- flux through the $GABA_A$ receptor, which is reduced by phospholipase A2 (Schwartz et al., 1988), leading to the increased formation of oxygen free radicals and consequently apoptosis. Interestingly, in the hippocampus, arachidonic acid helps maintain membrane fluidity (Fukaya et al., 2007) and enhances synaptic transmission (Williams et al., 1989). PUFA but not MUFA or SFA inactivate Na^+ currents, reducing neuronal firing and increasing their refractory period in CA1 neurons (Vreugdenhil et al., 1996).

In neuroblastoma/glioma hybrid cell culture studies, PUFA (e.g., linoleic acid, linolenic acid, and arachidonic acid) decrease Na^+ action potentials. One *trans* MUFA (i.e., oleic acid) does not produce such changes, and one SFA (i.e., palmitic acid) and one *trans* MUFA (i.e., elaidic acid) increase the frequency and amplitude of action potentials without influencing resting membrane potentials, Ca^{2+} action potentials, or membrane capacitance (Love et al., 1985).

Arachidonic acid also appears to modulate the activity of cytosolic protein kinase C by selective induction of phosphorylation, modulating transmembrane signaling (Khan et al., 1991). The fluidity of the acyl chains of fatty acids present in the bulk of membrane phospholipids modulates enzymatic activity (Harris, 1985).

In summary, n-3 PUFA modify some membrane functions, such as ion channel modulation, by increasing membrane fluidity (Simopoulos, 1999). The ion channel modulation exerted by fatty acids is very similar to that produced by local anesthetics, such lidocaine (Bean et al., 1983), and some anticonvulsant drugs, such as phenytoin (Rogawski & Porter, 1990; Schwartz & Grigat, 1989). The activation of several neurotransmitter receptors, such as dopamine D_2, 5-hydroxytryptamine-3, and opioids, alters the membrane flux of K^+ (Drukarch et al., 1989; Miyake et al., 1989). Some of the known effects of DHA include changes in membrane fluidity and stability (Litman et al., 2001), changes in dopaminergic and serotonergic transmission (Chalon et al., 2001; Zimmer et al., 2000, 2002), and the regulation of membrane-bound enzymes and cellular signal transduction (McNamara et al., 2006; Vaidyanathan et al., 1994).

2.8 Clinical aspects

The role of essential fatty acids in mammals was long been unknown, but more similarities than discrepancies appear to exist between the general actions of SFA, MUFA, and PUFA on diet pleasantness, visual appearance, smell, taste, aftertaste, and palatability, subjective hunger ratings, and energy intake in healthy males (Strik et al., 2010). Differences can be found with regard to undesirable effects. With regard to cholesterolemia, no differences were found between diets rich in MUFA and PUFA, but a SFA-rich diet produced the highest cholesterol concentrations (Trautwein et al., 1999). Decades ago, fatty acids were perceived as precursors for the biosynthesis of other substances (e.g., those related to inflammatory processes) and other fatty acids (Friesen & Innis, 2006) that are components of the cell membrane (Carrié et al., 2000) may participate in many functional processes (Kidd, 2007).

2.9 Development

Docosahexaenoic acid is the main n-3 PUFA found in the phospholipid fraction of the brain and has been implicated in the prenatal and postnatal development of the retina and brain (Hamazaki et al., 1996; McCann & Ames, 2005; SanGiovanni et al., 2000). Deficiencies in DHA during development are related to deficits in the structure of the retina, impairing visual acuity and cognitive function (Crawford, 1993; Neuringer et al., 1986; Reisbick et al., 1997).

During pregnancy, dietary *trans* fatty acids (e.g., elaidic acid) produce deleterious effects on health. The most abundant long-chain fatty acids in breast milk are DHA and arachidonic acid. Supplementation with marine oil products does not produce adverse effects and improves sensorial function and other cognitive functions after birth (Brenna & Lapillonne, 2009). Supplementation with DHA in infants that are less than 1 year old improves seeking behavior that later it is related to increased exploratory activity and less distractibility (Colombo et al., 2004). A DNA microarray study of the brain in rats subjected to different diets that contained different amounts of n-3 PUFA found some deficiencies in the expression of several genes, which became up- or downregulated and were related to the expression of cytochrome c and tumor necrosis factor (Kitajka et al., 2004). Maternal dietary SFA may produce persistent alterations in Na^+,K^+-ATPase function in the offspring, which could increase the risk of adulthood disease (Armitage et al., 2008).

2.10 Cognitive impairment

Decreased plasma levels of n-6 PUFA have been associated with physical rather than cognitive or behavioral ailments (Richardson, 2006). Deficiencies in DHA and eicosapentaenoic acid are involved in behavioral problems, such as attention deficit hyperactivity disorder, autism, dyspraxia, dyslexia, and aggression (Richardson, 2006; Stevens et al., 1996), and affective disorders, such as major depressive disorder, bipolar disorder, schizophrenia, and personality disorder. Evidence of altered PUFA status in mental illness, however, is weak. Reports of symptom improvement after PUFA consumption included patients with previous generalized dietary deficiencies of fatty acids (Liperoti et al., 2009; Milte et al., 2009) or other deleterious lifestyle habits (Suominen-Taipale et al., 2010), thus contaminating the interpretation of the data. n-3 PUFA supplementation appears to be effective only in depressive or Alzheimer's carriers of non-apolipoprotein E epsilon4 (Solfrizzi et al., 2010). In animal models of Alzheimer's disease, SFA and n-3 PUFA, including arachidonic acid, produced higher secretion of both Aβ-40 and -42 peptides compared with long-chain downstream omega-3 and MUFA. Lower levels of Aβ and amyloid plaques in the brain were observed when the subjects were fed a low-fat diet enriched with DHA (Amtul et al., 2011).

Some promising reports of the beneficial effects of n-3 PUFA on Alzheimer's disease and Huntington's disease showed that fatty acids appear to be devoid of any effect on cognition, aggression, hostility, and social behavior (Crawford et al., 2009).

2.11 Depression

Reports of the effects of fatty acids on depression have been controversial. For example, in an open-label study, juvenile bipolar disorder patients received supplementary eicosapentaenoic acid and DHA in their diet and exhibited a reduction in their clinical symptoms (Clayton et al., 2009). However, diets enriched with DHA failed to prevent postpartum depression in a randomized controlled trial (Makrides et al., 2010).

However, some intriguing results have been found. Membrane viscosity plays a role in the molecular bases of depression and other disorders and mediates the pharmacology of serotonin. Depression has been associated with low lipid raft viscosity (Cocchi et al., 2010a). The hydroxytrytophan transporter responsible for serotonin reuptake may be the functional locus for depression (Rosen, 2009), and an inverse relationship has been found between arachidonic acid content in neural tissue and the accessibility of serotonin to its receptors. However, an increase in arachidonic acid in brain tissue reduced membrane viscosity (i.e., increased fluidity; Cocchi et al., 2010b), reducing the accessibility of serotonin to its receptors (Heron et al., 1980). The brains of Flinders Sensitive rats, an animal model of depression, contain high concentrations of arachidonic acid (Green et al., 2005).

2.12 Calming effects of maternal biological fluids

Some odors can elicit a sense of family and home safety in adult mammals. Schapiro and Salas (1970) demonstrated that exposure to maternal odors in rat pups before weaning reduced the movements of pups. Oswalt and Meier (1975) found that infant rats reduce their emission of ultrasonic vocalizations when exposed to maternal odors. Therefore, maternal litter or home odors produce signs of calm. In contrast, kittens, pups, and human babies exhibit increased agitation and vocalizations when placed in an unfamiliar environment, but when they return to their nest or close proximity to their mother, both familiar odors, they calm down (Christensson et al., 1995; Michelsson et al., 1996; Schaal, 1988). The application of amniotic fluid odor to the nose significantly reduced crying in human babies when they were separated from their mothers (Varendi et al., 1998). Sullivan and Toubas (1998) suggested that maternal odors could be used to calm and reduce crying in babies. These fluids may be used to promote the acceptance of nipple feeding (Sullivan & Toubas, 1998) because breast milk odors (Rattaz et al., 2005) and milk odor (Nishitani et al., 2009) produce signs of calm. Olfactory exposure to maternal biological fluids (i.e., amniotic fluid, colostrum, and breast milk) appears to promote breastfeeding (Winberg & Porter, 1998).

Any odorant molecule requires a binding carrier protein with high affinity for membrane olfactory receptor neurons (Pelosi, 2001). Guiraudie-Capraz et al. (2005) used gas chromatography-mass spectrometry (GC-MS) to identify seven fatty acids (i.e., linoleic acid, palmitic acid, lauric acid, capric acid, myristic acid, palmitoleic acid, and oleic acids) in breast milk, colostrum, and amniotic fluid in pigs. Three carrier proteins were found not only in amniotic fluid, colostrum, and milk, but also in nasal mucosa and the vomeronasal organ, which seemingly mediate the fatty acid-induced initiation of perception (Guiraudie-

Capraz et al., 2003; Tegoni et al., 2000) with different affinities (Guiraudie-Capraz et al., 2003). Therefore, these proteins participate in the detection of chemical and biochemical signals, at least in pigs (Guiraudie-Capraz et al., 2005). Notably, these proteins have also been found in human amniotic fluid (Liberatori et al., 1997) and colostrum (Murakami et al., 1998), suggesting the stimulation of olfactory receptors very early in life, even during intrauterine life.

2.13 Fatty acids and anxiety

Few studies have compared the effects of n-3 and n-6 fatty acids on behavior. Although better results have been found in animals that received n-3 fatty acids than n-6 fatty acids (Wainwright, 1992), the absence of control groups prevents the acceptance of the results. Another study sought to find a relationship between essential fatty acids and behavior. Nakashima et al. (1993) used the elevated plus maze to assess anxiolytic-like behavior in rodents. In this study, linoleic acid produced a trend toward anxiolysis compared with α-linolenic acid, but this study also lacked a control group.

In humans, Mamalakis et al. (1998) did not find any relationship between linoleic acid and myristic acid and anxiety measured with the Spielberg scale or trait anxiety measured and Zung scales. However, they detected a positive relationship between trait anxiety scores and the linoleic acid + α-linolenic acid / DHA + arachidonic acid ratio (Mills et al., 1994). However, a mixture of PUFA may reduce anxiety scores, reflected by increased appetite, increased sense of humor, increased strength, decreased fatigue, increased academic performance, decreased lack of sleep, and decreased plasma cortisol (Yehuda et al., 2005).

Pageat (2001) patented a product whose active ingredient is a mixture of fatty acids that has been used to decrease stress, anxiety, and aggression in mammals, such as pigs, dogs, cats, and even children, and reduce anxiety signs when the animals are separated from their mother or in an unfamiliar place. The same formulation was tested by McGlone and Anderson (2002) on weight gain, feeding efficiency, and agonistic behavior in piglets.

We recently used GC-MS to demonstrate that human amniotic fluid, colostrum, and maternal milk consistently contain eight fatty acids (Mendoza-López et al., 2010). Both human amniotic fluid and an artificial mixture of the same proportion of fatty acids produced anxiolytic effects comparable to diazepam in Wistar rats subjected to validated tests that measure anxiety, including the defensive burying test and elevated plus maze. We concluded that amniotic fluid and its fatty acids have anxiolytic effects (Contreras et al., 2011).

2.14 Fatty acids as feeding cues

Newborns are attracted to odors that come from their mother's breast (Porter & Winberg, 1999), milk, colostrum (Nowak et al., 2000), and amniotic fluid (Porter & Winberg, 1999; Schaal et al., 1998). This behavior could be related to the fact that during the last trimester, the odorants in amniotic fluid are in close contact with nasal chemoreceptors. Newborn infants may retain an olfactory memory of these odors and later respond to these signals during the early postnatal period (Hepper, 1995).

Amniotic fluid is a complex mixture of fetal and maternal fluid (Lev & Orlic, 1972). Its composition varies according to gestational age and the evolution of maternal-fetal exchange. During early pregnancy, amniotic fluid is predominantly an ultrafiltrate of maternal serum. During late pregnancy, fetal urine is the main constituent of amniotic fluid (Loughhead et al., 2006).

Newborns oriented longer time to the odor of their own amniotic fluid compared with an unscented control (Schaal et al., 1995; Varendi et al., 1996). Recently, Contreras et al. (2011) analyzed the amniotic fluid, colostrum, and breast milk of 15 volunteer women. Eight fatty acids were consistently found in measurable amounts in the three biological fluids, including lauric acid, myristic acid, palmitic acid, palmitoleic acid, stearic acid, oleic acid, elaidic acid, and linoleic acid. The total amounts of fatty acids were different in each fluid, with the lowest amount found in amniotic fluid, followed by colostrum and milk. These results suggest that similar to other mammalian species (Guiraudie-Capraz et al., 2005; Pageat, 2001), some fatty acids present in biological fluids could serve as sensory cues of maternal and child identification. Additionally, newborns younger than 24 h preferentially orientated toward their own amniotic fluid and an artificial mixture of similar fatty acids (Díaz-Marte et al., 2010). This suggests that the first recognition of odors occurs during intrauterine life. Some of the fatty acids present in amniotic fluid could be a source of prenatal sensory stimulation, and colostrum odor is a bridge between amniotic fluid and milk (Contreras et al., 2011), thus leading to feeding behavior. Therefore, fatty acids could act as feeding cues, leading to appetitive behavior.

3. Conclusions

1. The functions of fatty acids as energy sources and their structural role in cellular membranes and as precursors of inflammatory processes are well known.
2. Fatty acids may modify the fluidity of the lipid membrane of cardiac and neuronal cells, impinging on ion channel permeability and decreasing cellular excitability. These conformational changes in the membrane may also modulate some neurotransmitter functions.
3. Decreased excitability produced by long-chain PUFA is related to some beneficial effects on cardiac function.
4. Similar actions on cardiac cell membranes appear to occur in neurons, in addition to neurotransmitter modulation. Some clinical studies of the therapeutic effects of fatty acids on neurological and psychiatric diseases have been conducted, but most of these studies need to be replicated using double-blind controlled designs before definitive conclusions can be made.
5. Fatty acids are components of amniotic fluid, colostrum, and milk and produce some anxiolytic effects.
6. The sensorial process of odor recognition related to fatty acids has been identified.
7. Fatty acids in maternal-fetal fluids appear to act as feeding cues that guide newborns to the maternal breast.

4. Acknowledgments

The authors thank Michael Arends for revising and editing the English of this manuscript. This study was partially supported by a grant from the Consejo Nacional de Ciencia y Tecnología, México (CONACyT: CB-2006-1, 61741) and Proyecto PAPITT-UNAM IN211111.

5. References

Agostoni, C. & Bruzzese, M.G. (1992). Fatty acids: their biochemical and functional classification. *La Pediatria Medica e Chirurgica: medical and surgical pediatrics,* Vol.14, No.5, (September-October 1992), pp. 473-479, ISSN 0391-5387

Amtul, Z.; Uhring, M.; Rozmahel, R.F. & Bevreuther, K. (2011). Structural insight into the differential effects of omega-3 and omega-6 fatty acids on the production of Aβ peptides and amyloid plaques. *Journal of Biological Chemistry,* Vol. 286, No.8, (February 2011), pp. 6100-6107, ISSN 1083-351X

Armitage, J.A.; Gupta, S.; Wood, C.; Jensen, R.I; Samuelsson, A.M; Fuller, W.; Shattock, M.J.; Poston, L. & Taylor, P.D. (2008). Maternal dietary supplementation with saturated, but not monounsaturated or polyunsaturated fatty acids, leads to tissue-specific inhibition of offspring Na^{+},K^{+}-ATPase. *Journal of Physiology,* Vol. 586, No.Pt 20, (October 2008), pp. 5013-5022, ISSN 1469-7793

Bean, B.P.; Cohen, C.J. & Tsien, R.W. (1983). Lidocaine block of cardiac sodium channels. *Journal of General Physiology,*Vol. 81, No. 5, (May 1983), pp. 613-642, ISSN 1540-7748

Berg, J.M.; Tymoczko, J.L. & Stryer, L. (2003). *Bioquímica,* 5th ed, Reverté, ISBN 0-06-097550-4, Barcelona, España

Bézard, J.; Blond, J.P.; Bernard, A. & Clouet, P. (1994). The metabolism and availability of essential fatty acids in animal and human tissues. *Reproduction Nutrition Development,* Vol.34, No.6, pp. 539-568, ISSN 1297-9708

Brenna, J.T. & Lapillonne, A. (2009). Background paper on fat and fatty acid requirements during pregnancy and lactation. *Annals of Nutrition & Metabolism,* Vol.55, No.1-3, (September 2009), pp. 97-122, ISSN 1421-9697

Brenna, J.T.; Salem, N. Jr.; Sinclair, A.J. & Cunnane, S.C. (2009). α-Linolenic acid supplementation and conversion to n-3 long-chain polyunsaturated fatty acids in humans. *Prostaglandins Leukotrienes &Essential Fatty Acids (PLEFA),* Vol.80, No.2-3, (February & March 2009), pp. 85-91, ISSN 0952-3278

Carrié, I.; Clément, M.; de Javel, D.; Francès, H. & Bourre, J.M. (2000). Phospholipid supplementation reverses behavioral and biochemical alterations induced by n-3 polyunsaturated fatty acid deficiency in mice. *Journal of Lipid Research,* Vol.41, No.3, (March 2000), pp. 473-480, ISSN 1539-7262

Chalon, S.; Vancassel, S. ; Zimmer, L. ; Guilloteau, D. & Durand, G. (2001). Polyunsaturated fatty acids and cerebral function: focus on monoaminergic neurotransmission. *Lipids,* Vol.36, No.9, (September 2001), pp. 937-944, ISSN 1558-9307

Christensson, K.; Cabrera, T.; Christensson, E.; Uvnäs-Moberg, K. & Winberg, J. (1995). Separation distress call in the human neonate in the absence of maternal body contact. *Acta Paediatrica,* Vol.84, No.5, (May 1992), pp. 468-473, ISSN 1651-2227

Clayton, E.H.; Hanstock, T.L.; Hirneth, S.J.; Kable, C.J.; Garg, M.L. & Hazell, P.L. (2009). Reduced mania and depression in juvenile bipolar disorder associated with long-chain omega-3 polyunsaturated fatty acid supplementation. *European Journal of Clinical Nutrition,* Vol.63, No.8, (August 2009), pp. 1037-1040, ISSN 0954-3007

Cocchi, M.; Gabrielli, F.; Tonello, L. & Pregnolato, M. (2010a). The interactome hypothesis of depression. *NeuroQuantology,* Vol.8, No.4, (December 2010), pp. 603-613, ISSN 1303-5150

Cocchi, M.; Tonello, L. & Lercker, G. (2010b). Fatty acids, membrane viscosity, serotonin and ischemic heart disease. *Lipids in Health &Disease,* Vol.8, No.9, (September 2010), pp. 97, ISSN 1476-511X

Colin, A.; Reggers, J.; Castronovo, V. & Ansseau, M. (2003). Lipids, depression and suicide. *L'Encéphale,* Vol.29, No.1, (January & Febrary 2003), pp. 49-58, ISSN 0013-7006.

Colombo, J.; Kannass, K.N.; Shaddy, D.J.; Kundurthi, S.; Maikranz, J.M.; Anderson, C.J.; Blaga, O.M. & Carlson, S.E. (2004). Maternal DHA and the development of attention in infancy and toddlerhood. *Child Development,* Vol.75, No.4, (July & August 2004), pp. 1254-1267, ISSN 1467-8624

Contreras, C.M.; Rodríguez-Landa, J.F.; Gutiérrez-García, A.G.; Mendoza-López, R.; García-Ríos, R.I. & Cueto-Escobedo, J. (2011). Anxiolytic-like effects of human amniotic fluid and its fatty acids in Wistar rats. *Behavioural Pharmacology,* Vol.22, No.7, (October 2011), pp. 655-662, , ISSN 1473-5849

Crawford, M.A.; Bazinet, R.P. & Sinclair, A.J. (2009). Fat intake and CNS functioning: ageing and disease. *Annals of Nutrition & Metabolism,* Vol.55, No.1-3, (September 2009), pp. 202-228, ISSN 1421-9697

Crawford, M.A. (1993). The role of essential fatty acids in neural development: implications for perinatal nutrition. *The American Journal of Clinical Nutrition,* Vol.57, No.5 Suppl, (May 1993), pp. 703S-709S, ISSN 1938-3207

Cunnane, S.C.; Ryan, M.A.; Craig, K.S.; Brookes, S.; Koletzko, B.; Demmelmair, H.; Singer, J. & Kyle, D.J. (1995). Synthesis of lnoleate and α-linoleated by chain elongation in the rat. *Lipids,* Vol.30, No.8, (August 1995), pp. 781-783, ISSN 1558-9307

Díaz-Marte, C.; Gutiérrez-García, A.G.; Mendoza-López, M.R. & Contreras, C.M. (2010). Recién nacidos despliegan movimientos de orientación hacia su líquido amniótico y algunos ácidos grasos. *Rev Med UV,* Vol.10, No.2, (July-December 2010), pp. 6-10, ISSN 1870-3267

Dobryniewski, J.; Szajda, S.D.; Waszkiewicz, N. & Zwierz, K. (2007). Biology of essential fatty acids (EFA). *Przeglad Lekarski,* Vol.64, No.2, pp. 91-99, ISSN 0033-2240

Drukarch, B.; Schepens, E.; Schoffelmeer, A.N. & Stoof, J.C. (1989). Stimulation of D-2 dopamine receptors decreases the evoked in vitro release of [^{3}H]acetylcholine from rat neostriatum: role of K^+ and Ca^{2+}. *Journal of Neurochemistry,* Vol.52, No.6, (June 1989), pp. 1680-1685, ISSN 1471-4159

Friesen, R. & Innis S.M. (2006). Maternal dietary fat alters amniotic fluid and fetal intestinal membrane essential n-6 and n-3 fatty acids in the rat. *American Journal of Physiology Gastrointestinal & Liver Physiology,* Vol.290, No.3, (March 2006), pp. G505-G510, ISSN 1522-1547

Fukaya, T.; Gondaira, T.; Kashiyae, Y.; Kotani, S.; Ishikura, Y.; Fujikawa, S.; Kiso, Y. & Sakakibara, M. (2007). Arachidonic acid preserves hippocampal neuron membrane fluidity in senescent rats. *Neurobiology of Aging,* Vol.28, No.8, (August 2007), pp. 1179-1186, ISSN 0197-4580

Green, P.; Gispan-Herman, I. & Yadid, G. (2005). Increased arachidonic acid concentration in the brain of Flinders Sensitive Line rats, an animal model of depression. *Journal of Lipid Research,* Vol.46, No.6, (June 2005), pp. 1093-1096, ISSN 1539-7262

Guiraudie-Capraz, G. ; Pageat, P. ; Cain, A.H. ; Madec, I. & Nagnan-Le Meillour, P. (2003). Functional characterization of olfactory binding proteins for appeasing compounds and molecular cloning in the vomeronasal organ of pre-pubertal pigs. *Chemical Senses*, Vol.28, No.7, (September 2003), pp. 609-619, ISSN 1464-3553

Guiraudie-Capraz, G. ; Slomianny, M.C. ; Pageat, P. ; Malosse, C. ; Cain, A.H. ; Orgeur, P. & Nagnan-Le Meillour, P. (2005). Biochemical and chemical supports for a transnatal olfactory continuity through sow maternal fluids. *Chemical Senses*, Vol.30, No.3, (March 2005), pp. 241-251, ISSN 1464-3553

Gurr, M.I.; Harwood, J.L. & Frayn, K,N. (2002). *Lipid biochemistry: an introduction*, 5th ed, Blackwell Science, ISBN 0632054093, Oxford, United Kingdom

Haggarty, P. (2002). Placental regulation of fatty acid delivery and its effect on fetal growth: a review. *Placenta*, Vol.23, No.Suppl A, (April 2002), pp. S28-S38, ISSN 0143-4004

Hamazaki, T.; Sawazaki, S.; Itomura, M.; Asaoka, E.; Nagao, Y.; Nishimura, N.; Yazawa, K., Kuwamori, T. & Kobayashi, M. (1996). The effect of docosahexaenoic acid on aggression in young adults: a placebo-controlled double-blind study. *Journal of Clinical Investigation*, Vol.97, No.4, (February 1996), pp. 1129-1133, ISSN 00219738

Harris, W.E. (1985). Modulation of (Na^+,K^+)-ATPase activity by the lipid bilayer examined with dansylated phosphatidylserine. *Biochemistry*, Vol.24, No.12, (June 1985), pp. 2873-2883, ISSN 0264-6021

Hepper P.G. (1995). Human fetal olfactory learning. *International Journal of Prenatal &Perinatal Psychology and Medicine*, Vol.7, No.2, (June 1993-2002), pp. 147-151, ISSN 0943-5417

Heron, D.S.; Shinitzky, M.; Hershkowitz, M. & Samuel, D. (1980). Lipid fluidity markedly modulates the binding of serotonin to mouse brain membranes. *Proceeding of the National Academic of Sciences of the United States of the American*, Vol.77, No.12, (December 1980), pp. 7463-7467, ISSN 1091-6490

Hwang, T.C.; Guggino, S.E. & Guggino, W.B. (1990). Direct modulation of secretory chloride channels by arachidonic and other cis unsaturated fatty acids. *Proceeding of the National Academic of Sciences of the United States of the American*, Vol.87, No.15, (August 1990), pp. 5706-5709, ISSN 1091-6490

Kang, J.X. & Leaf, A. (1996). Evidence that free polyunsaturated fatty acids modify Na^+ channels by directly binding to the channel proteins. *Proceeding of the National Academic of Sciences of the United States of the American*, Vol.93, No.8, (April 1996), pp. 3542-3546, ISSN 1091-6490

Kang, J.X.; Li, Y. & Leaf, A. (1997). Regulation of sodium channel gene expression by class I antiarrhythmic drugs and n - 3 polyunsaturated fatty acids in cultured neonatal rat cardiac myocytes. *Proceeding of the National Academic of Sciences of the United States of the American*, Vol.94, No.6, (March 1997), pp. 2724-2728, ISSN 1091-6490

Khan, W.; el Touny, S. & Hannun, Y.A. (1991). Arachidonic and cis-unsaturated fatty acids induce selective platelet substrate phosphorylation through activation of cytosolic protein kinase C. *FEBS Letters*, Vol.292, No.1-2, (November 1991), pp. 98-102, ISSN 0014-5793

Kidd, P.M. (2007). Omega-3 DHA and EPA for cognition, behavior, and mood: clinical findings and structural-functional synergies with cell membrane phospholipids.

Alternative Medicine Review, Vol.12, No.3, (September 2007), pp. 207-227, ISSN 1089-5159

Kitajka, K.; Sinclair, A.J.; Weisinger, R.S.; Weisinger, H.S.; Mathai, M.; Jayasooriya, A.P.; Halver, J.E. & Puskás, L.G. (2004). Effects of dietary omega-3 polyunsaturated fatty acids on brain gene expression. *Proceeding of the National Academic of Sciences of the United States of the American,* Vol.101, No.30, (July 2004), pp. 10931-10936, ISSN 1091-6490

Lauritzen, I.; Blondeau, N.; Heurteaux, C.; Widmann, C.; Romey, G. & Lazdunski, M. (2000). Polyunsaturated fatty acids are potent neuroprotectors. *The EMBO Journal*, Vol.19, No.8, (April 2000), pp. 1784-1793, ISSN 0261-4189

Leaf, A.; Xiao, Y.F. & Kang, J.X. (2002). Interactions of n-3 fatty acids with ion channels in excitable tissues. *Prostaglandins Leukotrienes &Essential Fatty Acids (PLEFA),* Vol.67, No.2-3, (August-September 2002), pp. 113-120, ISSN 0952-3278

Lev, R. & Orlic, D. (1972). Protein absorption by the intestine of the fetal rat in utero. *Science,* Vol.177, No.48, (August 1972), pp. 522-524, ISSN 1095-9203

Liberatori, S.; Bini, L.; De Felice, C.; Magi, B.; Marzocchi, B.; Raggiaschi, R.; Frutiger, S.; Sanchez, J.C.; Wilkins, M.R.; Hughes, G.; Hochstrasser, D.F.; Bracci, R. & Pallini, V. (1997). A two-dimensional protein map of human amniotic fluid at 17 weeks' gestation. *Electrophoresis*, Vol.18, No.15, (December 1997), pp. 2816-2822, ISSN 1522-2683

Liperoti, R.; Landi, F.; Fusco, O.; Bernabei, R. & Onder, G. (2009). Omega-3 polyunsaturated fatty acids and depression: a review of the evidence. *Current PharmaceuticalDesing*, Vol.15, No.36, (December 2009), pp. 4165-4172, ISSN 1381-6128

Litman, B.J.; Niu, S.L.; Polozova, A. & Mitchell, D.C. (2001). The role of docosahexaenoic acid containing phospholipids in modulating G protein-coupled signaling pathways: visual transduction. *Journal of Molecular Neuroscience,* Vol.16, No.2-3, (April-June 2001), pp. 237-242, ISSN 0895-8696

Lombardi, F. & Terranova, P. (2007). Anti-arrhythmic properties of N-3 poly-unsaturated fatty acids (n-3 PUFA). *Current Medicine Chemistry*, Vol.14, No.19, (December 1994), pp. 2070-2080, ISSN 0929-8673

Loughhead, A.M.; Fisher, A.D.; Newport, D.J.; Ritchie, J.C.; Owens, M.J.; DeVane, C.L. & Stowe, Z.N. (2006). Antidepressants in amniotic fluid: another route of fetal exposure. *American Journal of Psychiatry*, Vol.163, No.1, (January 2006), pp. 145-147, ISSN 1535-7228

Love, J.A.; Saum, W.R. & McGee, R.Jr. (1985). The effects of exposure to exogenous fatty acids and membrane fatty acid modification on the electrical properties of NG108-15 cells. *Cellular and Molecular Neurobiology*, Vol.5, No.4, (December 1985), pp. 333-352, ISSN 1573-6830

Lundbaek, J.A.; Birn, P.; Girshman, J.; Hansen, A.J. & Andersen, O.S. (1996). Membrane stiffness and channel function. *Biochemistry*, Vol.35, No.12, (March 1996), pp. 3825-3830, ISSN 0264-6021

Makrides, M.; Gibson, R.A.; McPhee, A.J.; Yelland, L.; Quinlivan, J. & Ryan P. (2010). Effect of DHA supplementation during pregnancy on maternal depression and neurodevelopment of young children: a randomized controlled trial. *The Journal of*

American Medical Association, Vol.304, No.15, (October 2010), pp. 1675-1683, ISSN 0098-7484

Mamalakis, G.; Kafatos, A.; Tornaritis, M. & Alevizos, B. (1998). Anxiety and adipose essential fatty acid precursors for prostaglandin E1 and E2. *Journal of the American College of Nutrition*, Vol.17, No. 3, (June, 1998), pp. 239-243, ISSN 0731-5724

McCann, J.C. & Ames, B.N. (2005). Is docosahexaenoic acid, an n-3 long-chain polyunsaturated fatty acid, required for development of normal brain function? An overview of evidence from cognitive and behavioral tests in humans and animals. *American Journal of Clinical Nutrition*, Vol.82, No.2, (August 2005), pp. 281-295, ISSN 0002-9165

McGlone, J.J. & Anderson, D.L. (2002). Synthetic maternal pheromone stimulates feeding behavior and weight gain in weaned pigs. *Journal of Animal Science*, vol.80, No.12, (December 2002), pp.3179-3183, ISSN 0021-8812

McNamara, R.K.; Ostrander, M.; Abplanalp, W.; Richtand, NM.; Benoit, SC. & Clegg, D.J. (2006). Modulation of phosphoinositide-protein kinase C signal transduction by omega-3 fatty acids: implications for the pathophysiology and treatment of recurrent neuropsychiatric illness. *Prostaglandins, Leukotrienes, and Essential Fatty Acids*, vol.75, No.4-5, (October-November 2006), pp.237-257, ISSN 0952-3278

Mendoza-López, M.R.; Contreras, C.M.; Gutiérrez-García, A.G. & Díaz-Marte, C. (2010). ¿Los ácidos grasos presentes en líquidos maternos participan en la comunicación materno-infantil? *Procesos Psicológicos y Sociales*, Vol.6, No.1-2, (July-December 2010), pp.1-25, ISSN 1870-5618

Mesa-García, M.D.; Aguilera-García, C.M. & Gil-Hernández, A. (2006). Importance of lipids in the nutritional treatment of inflammatory diseases. *Nutrición Hospitalaria*, Vol.21, (May 2006), pp.28-41, ISSN 0212-1611

Michelsson, K.; Christensson, K.; Rothgänger, H. & Winberg, J. (1996). Crying in separated and non-separated newborns: sound spectrographic analysis. *Acta Paediatrica*, Vol.85, No.4, (April 1996), pp. 471-475, ISSN 0803-5253

Mills, D.E. ; Huang, Y.S. ; Narce, M. & Poisson, J.P. (1994). Psychosocial stress, catecholamines and essential fatty acid metabolism in rats. *Proceedings of the Society for Experimental Biology and Medicine*, Vol.205, No.1, (January 1994), pp.56-61, ISSN 0037-9727

Milte, C.M.; Sinn, N. & Howe, P.R. (2009). Polyunsaturated fatty acid status in attention deficit hyperactivity disorder, depression, and Alzheimer's disease: towards an omega-3 index for mental health? *Nutrition Reviews*, Vol.67, No.10, (October 2009), pp. 573-590, ISSN 1753-4887

Miyake, M.; Christie, M.J. & North, R.A. (1989). Single potassium channels opened by opioids in rat locus ceruleus neurons. *Proceedings of the National Academy of Sciences of the United States of America*, Vol.86, No.9, (May 1989), pp.3419-3422, ISSN 0027-8424

Murakami, K.; Lagarde, M. & Yuki, Y. (1998). Identification of minor proteins of human colostrum and mature milk by two-dimensional electrophoresis. *Electrophoresis*, Vol.19, No.14, (October 1998), pp. 2521-2527, ISSN 0173-0835

Nakashima, Y.; Yuasa, S.; Hukamizu, Y.; Okuyama, H.; Ohhara, T.; Kameyama, T. & Nabeshima, T. (1993). Effect of a high linoleate and a high α-linolenate diet on general behavior and drug sensitivity in mice. *Journal of Lipid Research,* Vol.34, No.2, (February 1993), pp.239-247, ISSN 0022-2275

Nelson, D.L. & Cox, M.M. (2005). *Lehninger Principles of Biochemistry*, Omega, ISBN 0-7167-4339-6, Barcelona, España

Neuringer, M.; Connor, W.E.; Lin, D.S.; Barstad L. & Luck, S. (1986). Biochemical and functional effects of prenatal and postnatal omega 3 fatty acid deficiency on retina and brain in rhesus monkeys. *Proceedings of the National Academy of Sciences of the United States of America*, Vol.83, No.11, (June 1986), pp.4021-4025, ISSN 0027-8424

Nielsen, M.; Witt, M.R. & Thøgersen, H. (1988). [^{3}H]diazepam specific binding to rat cortex in vitro is enhanced by oleic, arachidonic and docosahexenoic acid isolated from pig brain. *European Journal of Pharmacology*, Vol.146, No.2-3 (February 1988), pp.349-353, ISSN 0014-2999

Nishitani, S.; Miyamura, T.; Tagawa, M.; Sumi, M.; Takase, R.; Doi, H.; Moriuchi, H. & Shinohara K. (2009). The calming effect of a maternal breast milk odor on the human newborn infant. *Neuroscience Research,* Vol.63, No.1, (January 2009), pp.66-71, ISSN 0168-0102

Nowak, R.; Porter, RH.; Lévy, F.; Orgeur, P. & Schaal, B. (2000). Role of mother-young interactions in the survival of offspring in domestic mammals. *Reviews Reproduction*, Vol.5, No.3, (September 2000), pp.153-163, ISSN 1359-6004

Ordway, R.W.; Singer, J.J. & Walsh, J.V. Jr. (1991). Direct regulation of ion channels by fatty acids. *Trends in Neurosciences*, Vol.14, No.3, (Mach 1991), pp.96-100, ISSN 0166-2236

Ordway, R.W.; Walsh, J.V.Jr. & Singer, J.J. (1989). Arachidonic acid and other fatty acids directly activate potassium channels in smooth muscle cells. *Science*, Vol.244, No.4909, (June 1989), pp.1176-1179, ISSN 0036-8075

Oswalt, G.L. & Meier, G.W. (1975). Olfactory, thermal, and tactual influences on infantile ultrasonic vocalization in rats. *Developmental Psychobiology*, Vol.8, No.2, (May 1975), pp.129-135, ISSN 0012-1630

Pageat, P. (2001). Pig appeasing pheromones to decrease stress, anxiety and aggressiveness. *US Patent No. 6*,169,113.

Pelosi, P. (2001). The role of the perireceptor events in vertebrates olfaction. *Cell and Molecular Life Sciences,* Vol.58, No.4, (April 2001), pp.503-509, ISSN 1420-682X

Porter, R.H. & Winberg, J. (1999). Unique salience of maternal breast odors for newborn infants. *Neuroscience and Biobehavioral Reviews*, Vol.23, No.3, (*January 1999)*, pp.439-449, ISSN 0149-7634

Rattaz, C.; Goubet, N. & Bullinger, A. (2005). The calming effect of a familiar odor on full-term newborns. *Journal of Developmental and Behavioral Pediatrics,* Vol.26, No.2, (April 2005), pp.86-92, ISSN 0196-206X

Reisbick, S.; Neuringer, M.; Gohl, E.; Wald, R. & Anderson, G.J. (1997). Visual attention in infant monkeys: effects of dietary fatty acids and age. *Developmental Psychology,* Vol.33, No.3, (May 1997), pp.387-395, ISSN 0012-1649

Richardson, A.J. (2006). Omega-3 fatty acids in ADHD and related neurodevelopmental disorders. *International Review of Psychiatry*, Vol.18, No.2, (April 2006), pp.155-172, ISSN 0954-0261

Ristic, V.; Vrbaski, S.; Lalic, Z. & Miric, M. (1995). The effect of ethanol and diazepam on the fatty acid composition of plasma and liver phospholipids in the rat. *Biological & Pharmaceutical Bulletin*, Vol.18, No.6, (June 1995), pp.842-845, ISSN 0918-6158

Robertson, D.W. & Steinberg, M.I. (1990). Potassium channel modulators: scientific applications and therapeutic promise. *Journal of Medicine Chemistry*, Vol.33, No.6, (June 1990), pp.1529-1541, ISSN 0022-2623

Robinson, P.J. & Rapoport, S.I. (1986). Kinetics of protein binding determine rates of uptake of drugs by brain. *The American Journal of Physiology*, Vol.251, No.6, (December 1986), pp.R1212-R1220, ISSN 0002-9513

Rogawski, M.A. & Porter, R.J. (1990). Antiepileptic drugs: pharmacological mechanisms and clinical efficacy with consideration of promising developmental stage compounds. *Pharmacology Reviews*, Vol.42, No.3, (September 1990), pp.223-286, ISSN 0031-6997

Rosen, C.J. (2009). Breaking into bone biology: serotonin's secrets. *Nature Medicine*, Vol.15, No.2, (February 2009), pp.145-146, ISSN 0031-6997

Sampath, H. & Ntambi, JM. (2005). Polyunsaturated fatty acid regulation of genes of lipid metabolism. *Annual Review of Nutrition*, Vol.25, (2005), pp.317-340, ISSN 0199-9885

SanGiovanni, J.P.; Parra-Cabrera, S.; Colditz, G.A.; Berkey, C.S. & Dwyer, J.T. (2000). Meta-analysis of dietary essential fatty acids and long-chain polyunsaturated fatty acids as they relate to visual resolution acuity in healthy preterm infants. *Pediatrics*, Vol.105, No.6, (June 2000), pp.1292-1298, ISSN 1098-4275

Sardesai, V.M. (1992). The essential fatty acids. *Nutrition in Clinical Practice*, Vol.7, No.4, (August 1992), pp.179-186, ISSN 0884-5336

Schaal, B. ; Marlier, L. & Soussignan, R. (1995). Responsiveness to the odour of the amniotic fluid in the human neonate. *Biology of the Neonate*, Vol.67, No.6, (September 2009), pp.397-406, ISSN 0006-3126

Schaal, B.; Marlier, L. & Soussignan, R. (1998). Olfactory function in the human fetus: evidence from selective neonatal responsiveness to the odor of amniotic fluid. *Behavioral Neuroscience*, Vol.112, No.6, (December 1998), pp.1438-1449, ISSN 0735-7044

Schaal, B. (1988). Olfaction in infants and children: developmental and functional perspectives. *Chemical Senses*, Vol.13, No.2, (June 1988), pp.145-190, ISSN 0379-864X

Schapiro, S. & Salas, M. (1970). Behavioral response of infant rats to maternal odor. *Physiology and Behavior*, Vol.5, No.7, (July 1970), pp.815-817, ISSN 0031-9384

Schwartz, R.D.; Skolnick, P. & Paul, S.M. (1988). Regulation of γ-aminobutyric acid/barbiturate receptor-gated chloride ion flux in brain vesicles by phospholipase A_2: possible role of oxygen radicals. *Journal of Neurochemistry*, Vol.50, No.2, (February 1988), pp.65-71, ISSN 0022-3042

Schwartz, R.D. & Yu, X. (1992). Inhibition of GABA-gated chloride channel function by arachidonic acid. *Brain Research*, Vol.585, No.1-2, (July 1992), pp.405-410, ISSN 0006-8993

Schwarz, J.R. & Grigat, G. (1989). Phenytoin and carbamazepine: potential- and frequency-dependent block of Na currents in mammalian myelinated nerve fibers. *Epilepsia*, Vol.30, No.3, (May-June 1989), pp.286-294, ISSN 0013-9580

Simopoulos, A.P. (1999). Essential fatty acids in health and chronic disease. *The American Journal of Clinical Nutrition*, Vol.70 No.3, (September 1999), pp.560S-569S, ISSN 0002-9165

Sinclair, H.M. (1984). Essential fatty acids in perspective. *Human Nutrition. Clinical Nutrition*, Vol.38, No.4, (July 1984), pp.245-260, ISSN 0263-8290

Solfrizzi, V.; Frisardi, V.; Capurso, C.; D'Introno, A.; Colacicco, A.M.; Vendemiale, G.; Capurso, A. & Panza, F. (2010). Dietary fatty acids in dementia and predementia syndromes: epidemiological evidence and possible underlying mechanisms. *Ageing Research Reviews*, Vol.9, No.2, (April 2010), pp.184-189, ISSN 1568-1637

Sprecher, H.; Luthria, D.L.; Mohammed, B.S. & Baykousheva, S.P. (1995). Reevaluation of the pathways for the biosynthesis of polyunsaturated fatty acids. *Journal of Lipid Research*, Vol.36, No.12, (December 1995), pp.2471-2477, ISSN 0022-2275

Stahl, W.L. (1986). The Na,K-ATPase of nervous tissue. *Neurochemistry International*, Vol.8, No.4, (March 1986), pp.449-476, ISSN 0197-0186

Stevens, L.J.; Zentall, S.S.; Abate, M.L.; Kuczek, T. & Burgess, J.R. (1996). Omega-3 fatty acids in boys with behavior, learning, and health problems. *Physiology and Behavior*, Vol.59, No.4-5, (April-May 1996), pp.915-920, ISSN 0031-9384

Strik, C.M.; Lithander, F.E.; McGill, A.T.; MacGibbon, A.K.; McArdle, B.H. & Poppitt, S.D. (2010). No evidence of differential effects of SFA, MUFA or PUFA on post-ingestive satiety and energy intake: a randomised trial of fatty acid saturation. *Nutrition Journal*, Vol.9, (May 2010), pp.24, ISSN 1475-2891

Stulnig, T.M. (2003). Immunomodulation by polyunsaturated fatty acids: mechanisms and effects. *International Archives of Allergy and Immunology*, Vol.132, No.4, (December 2003), pp.310-321, ISSN 1018-2438.

Sullivan, R.M. & Toubas, P. (1998). Clinical usefulness of maternal odor in newborns: soothing and feeding preparatory responses. *Biology of the Neonate*, Vol.74, No.6, (December 1998), pp.402-408, ISSN 0006-3126

Suominen-Taipale, A.L.; Partonen, T.; Turunen, A.W.; Männistö, S.; Jula, A. & Verkasalo, P.K. (2010). Fish consumption and omega-3 polyunsaturated fatty acids in relation to depressive episodes: a cross-sectional analysis. *Pediatrics*, Vol.5, No.5, (August 2010), pp.e10530, ISSN 0031-4005

Tegoni, M.; Pelosi, P. ; Vincent, F. ; Spinelli, S. ; Campanacci, V. ; Grolli, S. ; Ramoni, R. & Cambillau, C. (2000). Mammalian odorant binding proteins. *Biochimica Biophysica Acta*, vol.1482, No.1-2, (October 2000), pp.229-240, ISSN 0006-3002

Trautwein, E.A.; Rieckhoff, D.; Kunath-Rau, A. & Erbersdobler, H.F. (1999). Replacing saturated fat with PUFA-rich (sunflower oil) or MUFA-rich (rapeseed, olive and high-oleic sunflower oil) fats resulted in comparable hypocholesterolemic effects in cholesterol-fed hamsters. *Annals of Nutrition & Metabolism*, Vol.43, No.3, (May-June 1999), pp.159-172, ISSN 0250-6807

Uauy, R.; Mena, P. & Rojas, C. (2000). Essential fatty acids in early life: structural and functional role. *The Proceedings of the Nutrition Society*, Vol.59, No.1, (February 2000), pp.3-15, ISSN 0029-6651

Vaidyanathan, V.V.; Rao, K.V. & Sastry, P.S. (1994). Regulation of diacylglycerol kinase in rat brain membranes by docosahexaenoic acid. *Neuroscience Letters*, Vol.179, No.1-2, (September 1994), pp.171-174, ISSN 0304-3940

Varendi, H. ; Christensson, K. ; Porter, R.H. & Winberg, J. (1998). Soothing effect of amniotic fluid smell in newborn infants. *Early Human Development*, Vol.51, No.1, (April 1998), pp.47-55, ISSN 0378-3782

Varendi, H.; Porter, R.H. & Winberg, J. (1996). Attractiveness of amniotic fluid odor: evidence of prenatal learning? *Acta Pediatrica*, Vol.85, No.10, (October 1996), pp.1223-1227, ISSN 0803-5253

Vreugdenhil, M.; Bruehl, C.; Voskuyl, R.A.; Kang, J.X.; Leaf, A. & Wadman, W.J. (1996). Polyunsaturated fatty acids modulate sodium and calcium currents in CA1 neurons. *Proceedings of the National Academy of Sciences of the United States of America*, Vol.93, No.22, (October 1996), pp.12559-12563, ISSN 0027-8424

Wainwright, P.E. (1992). Do essential fatty acids play a role in brain and behavioral development? *Proceedings of the Nutrition Society*, Vol.61, No.2, (November 2005), pp.61-69, ISSN 2001130

Williams, J.H.; Errington, M.L.; Lynch, M.A. & Bliss, T.V. (1989). Arachidonic acid induces a long-term activity-dependent enhancement of synaptic transmission in the hippocampus. *Nature*, Vol.341, No.6244, (October 1989), pp.739-742, ISSN 0028-0836.

Winberg, J. & Porter, R.H. (1998). Olfaction and human neonatal behaviour: clinical implications. *Acta Paediatrica*, Vol.87, No.1, (January 1998), pp.6-10, ISSN 0803-5253

Xiao, Y.F.; Gomez, A.M.; Morgan, J.P.; Lederer, W.J. & Leaf, A. (1997). Suppression of voltage-gated L-type Ca2+ currents by polyunsaturated fatty acids in adult and neonatal rat ventricular myocytes. *Proceedings of the National Academy of Sciences of the United States of America*, Vol.94, No.8, (April 1997), pp.4182-1487, ISSN 0027-8224

Xiao, Y.F.; Kang, J.X.; Morgan, J.P. & Leaf, A. (1995). Blocking effects of polyunsaturated fatty acids on Na+ channels of neonatal rat ventricular myocytes. *Proceedings of the National Academy of Sciences of the United States of America*, Vol.92, No.24, (November 1995), pp.11000-11004, ISSN 0027-8224

Xiao, Y.F.; Wright, S.N.; Wang, G.K.; Morgan, J.P. & Leaf, A. (1998). Fatty acids suppress voltage-gated Na^+ currents in HEK293t cells transfected with the α-subunit of the human cardiac Na^+ channel. *Proceedings of the National Academy of Sciences of the United States of America*, Vol.95, No.5, (March 1998), pp.2680-2685, ISSN 0027-8424

Yehuda, S.; Rabinovitz, S. & Mostofsky, D.I. (2005). Mixture of essential fatty acids lowers test anxiety. *Nutritional Neuroscience*, Vol.8, No.4, (August 2005), pp.265-267, ISSN 1028-415X

Zamaria, N. (2004). Alteration of polyunsaturated fatty acid status and metabolism in health and disease. *Reproduction, Nutrition, Development*, Vol.44, No.3, (May-June 2004), pp.273-282, ISSN 0926-5287

Zimmer, L.; Delion-Vancassel, S.; Durand, G.; Guilloteau, D.; Bodard, S.; Besnard, J.C. & Chalon, S. (2000). Modification of dopamine neurotransmission in the nucleus accumbens of rats deficient in n-3 polyunsaturated fatty acids. *Journal of Lipid Research*, Vol.41, No.1, (January 2000), pp.32-40, ISSN 0022-2275

Zimmer, L.; Vancassel, S.; Cantagrel, S. ; Breton, P. ; Delamanche, S. ; Guilloteau, D. ; Durand, G. & Chalon, S. (2002). The dopamine mesocorticolimbic pathway is affected by deficiency in n-3 polyunsaturated fatty acids. *The American Journal of Clinical Nutrition*, Vol.75, No.4, (April 2002), pp.662-667, ISSN 0002-9165

6

Transforming Growth Factor Beta in the Central Nervous System

Arpád Dobolyi
*Neuromorphological and Neuroendocrine Research Laboratory,
Department of Anatomy, Histology and Embryology,
Hungarian Academy of Sciences and Semmelweis University,
Hungary*

1. Introduction

By definition, growth factors are polypeptides that modulate the proliferation of mammalian cells by acting on their receptors at low concentration. Based on similarities in their sequences and their receptors, growth factors can be divided into several superfamilies including platelet-derived growth factors, epidermal growth factors, insulin-like growth factors, the transforming growth factor-beta (TGF-β) family, fibroblast growth factors, nerve growth factors (neurotrophins), erythropoietin, and hemopoietic colony stimulating factors. Transforming growth factors were originally named by their capacity to induce oncogenic transformation in rat kidney fibroblasts (Roberts et al., 1981). Transforming growth factor alpha has a structure and action similar to epidermal growth factor (Wells, 1999) and is not a subject of the present chapter. The TGF-β superfamily includes products of over 25 distinct genes. Comparison of the deduced amino acid sequences led to the definition of several groups within the superfamily, such as TGF-βs, bone morphogenetic proteins, multiple isoforms of activins and inhibins, anti-Mullerian hormone, decapentaplegic protein in *Drosophila*, and Vg1 protein in *Xenopus* (Burt & Law, 1994). There are five TGF-β sequences including three mammalian isoforms (TGF-β1, β2 and β3), which are encoded by unique genes located on different chromosomes (Lawrence, 1996). Besides the regulation of cell growth and division, *TGF-βs* can control the proliferation, survival, differentiation, migration, or function of cells depending on the circumstance. The best established activities of TGF-βs are the following: they inhibit proliferation of most cells, but can stimulate the growth of some mesenchymal cells; they enhance the formation of extracellular matrix; and they exert immunosuppressive effects (Roberts, 1998). Based on their effects on cells of the immune system, TGF-βs can also be considered cytokines (Kiefer et al., 1995).

2. Biochemistry of transforming growth factor-βs (TGF-βs)

2.1 Release and activation of TGF-βs

A characteristic feature in the biology of TGF-βs is that they are usually secreted from cells in latent forms. TGF-βs are synthesized as homodimeric proproteins (proTGF-βs). These precursor proteins are modified intracellularly prior to secretion. The C-terminal pro-regions are cleaved from the N-terminal portion of the protein and in the trans Golgi to provide mature TGF-β and the latency-associated protein (LAP) which remain non-covalently associated to form the small latent complex (Clark & Coker, 1998; Khalil, 1999). In turn, disulfide bridges bind the so-called latent TGF-β binding proteins (LTBPs) to this complex to result the TGF-β large latent complex, in which TGF-βs are present in the extracellular space (Koli et al., 2001; Saharinen et al., 1999). LTBPs are large multidomain proteins belonging to the fibrillin-LTBP family of extracellular matrix proteins. LTBPs have a typical repeated domain structure consisting mostly of epidermal growth factor (EGF)-like repeats and characteristic eight cysteine (8-Cys) repeats. They are required for the proper folding and secretion of TGF-βs (Sinha et al., 1998; Todorovic et al., 2005). Following secretion, TGF-β is deposited to the extracellular matrix in the pericellular space covalently via the N-termini of the LTBPs. LTBPs contain multiple proteinase sensitive sites, providing means to solubilize the large latent complex from the extracellular matrix structures (Keski-Oja et al., 2004; Rifkin, 2005).

2.2 Latent TGF-β binding proteins

There are four mammalian LTBP isoforms encoded by distinct genes, including LTBP-1, -2, -3, and -4 and different splice variants for each of them (Mangasser-Stephan & Gressner, 1999; Oklu & Hesketh, 2000). The significance of this structural diversity is mostly unclear at present. The potential selective binding of different LTBPs to different proTGF-β types is not well characterized yet. *In vitro* studies suggest that LTBP-1, and -3 can bind to all three types of proTGF-β types efficiently whereas LTBP-2 does not bind to proTGF-βs (Saharinen & Keski-Oja, 2000). TGF-β associated with the large latent complex cannot interact with its receptor and has no biological effect. Therefore, TGF-β activity is regulated by the release of mature TGF-β from the large latent complex. Alternatively, the large latent complex undergoes a conformational change, which exposes the TGF-βs to their receptor binding sites. Many potential activators of the extracellular TGF-βs have been proposed (Annes et al., 2003; Gumienny & Padgett, 2002) including proteases, thrombospondin-1, integrins, reactive oxygen species, and pH. The activation of the 3 different isoforms of TGF-βs may be different. Furthermore, the type of LTBPs may affect the way of activation of TGF-βs (Rifkin, 2005).

2.3 Release of TGF-βs from neurons

Apart from various peripheral cell types, the model neuron chromaffin cell has also been demonstrated to possess regulated secretion of TGF-β and LTBPs (Krieglstein & Unsicker, 1995). Cholinergic stimulation of bovine chromaffin cells leads to the release of storage vesicles. The released content of the vesicles was shown to contain TGF-β but not other members of the TGF-β superfamily suggesting that TGF-β is stored in chromaffin granules and can be released by exocytosis (Krieglstein & Unsicker, 1995). In addition, the level of active TGF-β has been suggested to be increased by elevated neuronal activity (Lacmann et al., 2007). In primary cell culture of embryonic hippocampal neurons, various treatments leading to increased neuronal activity resulted in tetrodotoxon-dependent elevation of active TGF-β levels (Lacmann et al., 2007).

2.4 Receptors and signal transduction pathways

With regard to mediation of TGF-β actions, different TGF-β receptors have been identified (Massague, 1992). Type I and type II TGF-β receptors bind TGF-βs with high-affinity. Ligand binding induces the assembly of type I and type II receptors into complexes. The exact stoichiometry in the TGF-β-induced heteromeric type I and type II receptor complex is likely to be a heterotetramer comprising two TGF-β type I and two TGF-β type II receptors. Following activation, type II receptors phosphorylate type I receptors in the juxtamembrane region. This phosphorylation is both essential and sufficient for TGF-β signalling (ten Dijke & Hill, 2004). In addition, the type III TGF-β receptor also binds TGF-βs with high affinity. However, it is an extracellular protein, which does not lead to signal transduction. In fact, it may be a negative regulator of TGF-β function (Chu et al., 2011).

Both type I and type II receptors are single-pass transmembrane proteins with a serine/threonine kinase domain on the cytosolic side of the plasma membrane (Arighi et al., 2009; Attisano & Wrana, 2002). The activated type I kinase propagates the signal inside the cell through the phosphorylation of receptor-regulated Smads (R-Smads: Smad1, Smad2, Smad3, Smad5 and Smad8). Access of the R-Smads to the type I receptors is facilitated by auxiliary proteins such as Smad anchor for receptor activation. Activated R-Smads form heteromeric complexes with Smad4. These complexes accumulate in the nucleus, where they control gene expression in a cell-type-specific and ligand dose-dependent manner. Inhibitory Smads (I-Smads: Smad6 and Smad7) form a distinct subclass of Smads that act in an opposing manner to R-Smads and antagonize signalling (Padgett et al., 1998; Schmierer & Hill, 2007).

TGF-β also uses non-Smad signaling pathways such as the p38 and Jun N-terminal kinase (JNK) mitogen-activated protein kinase (MAPK) pathways to convey its signals. Other potential TGF-β-induced non-Smad signaling pathways include the phosphoinositide 3-kinase-Akt-mTOR pathway, the small GTPases Rho, Rac, and Cdc42, and the Ras-Erk-MAPK pathway (Mu et al., 2011).

3. Distribution of TGF-βs, their binding proteins and receptors in the central nervous system

The distribution pattern of TGF-βs established using immunohistochemistry at the protein level (Unsicker et al., 1991) and by means of in situ hybridization histochemistry at the mRNA level (Vincze et al., 2010) was similar in several brain regions. TGF-β2 and β3 immunoreactivities were present constitutively in cerebral cortical layers II, III and V and their expression depended on the cortical layer rather than the areas within the cerebral cortex. Furthermore, different regions of hippocampus, as well as widely distributed cells in the hypothalamus and amygdala contained both TGF-ß2 and ß3. Intense labeling of these isoforms was also described in brainstem monoaminergic neurons, and motor nuclei (Unsicker et al., 1991; Vincze et al., 2010). In turn, the striatum, most thalamic nuclei, and the superior colliculus were almost devoid of TGF-β2 and ß3 mRNA and immunoreactivities. However, considerable differences between the distribution of mRNAs and immunoreactivities of TGF-βs have also been reported. Most importantly, TGF-β1 immunoreactivity was reported to be constitutively present only in meninges and the choroid plexus in the brain (Komuta et al., 2009 ; Unsicker et al., 1991) while a more widespread expression of the mRNA of this isoform was described including intense labeling in some cortical and hippocampal cells, the medial preoptic area, the paraventricular hypothalamic nucleus, the central amygdaloid nucleus, and the superior olive. Furthermore, TGF-β2 and β3 immunoreactivities entirely overlapped and, in general, were found in large multipolar neurons (Unsicker et al., 1991) with the level of TGF-ß2 being considerably higher (Bottner et al., 2000). In some areas, including brainstem motoneurons and the area postrema, the 2 isoforms had similar mRNA expression patterns with high intensity labeling suggesting that different isoforms of TGF-βs may be co-expressed in the same cell. In most brain areas, however, the distributions of TGF-ß2 and-ß3 mRNAs were markedly different. In the cerebral cortex, TGF-βs were expressed in different layers. In the hippocampus, TGF-β2 was abundantly expressed only in the dentate gyrus while TGF-β3 in the CA2 region and the dentate gyrus. In the cerebellum, TGF-β2 was present in the Purkinje cell layer while TGF-β3 mRNA was absent in the cerebellum. In addition, the medial mamillary nucleus, the parafascicular thalamic nucleus and the choroid plexus expressed predominantly TGF-β2 while the reticular thalamic nucleus, the superior colliculus, and the inferior olive contained almost exclusively TGF-β3 mRNA (Vincze et al., 2010). An important future question is the type of cells that express TGF-β in the central nervous system. Most previous studies examined the cell type of TGF-β expression following some type of induction. TGF-β1 upregulation in astrocytes and microglia has been reported to be a predominant response to lesion and during pathology (Krohn, 1999; Wu et al., 2007; Wu et al., 2008) that results in the induction of reactive phenotypes (Flanders et al., 1998; Morgan et al., 1993). Under basal conditions, astrocytes were also shown to express TGF-β1 in the preoptic area (Bouret et al., 2004; Dhandapani & Brann, 2003). However, neuronal expression of TGF-β1 has also been reported (Battaglia et al., 2011; Lacmann et al., 2007; Wu et al., 2007). The available data on the cell type specific expression of other TGF-β isoforms is scarce. However, their distributions suggest a dominant neuronal expression (Unsicker et al., 1991; Vincze et al., 2010).

The four types of LTBPs also had distinct distribution patterns in the brain based on the localization of their mRNAs (Dobolyi & Palkovits, 2008). The dominant form in the brain was LTBP3 while LTBP4 also had high level of expression in a variety of forebrain areas. LTBP1 had considerable level of expression in only some brain regions including the choroid plexus, the cerebral cortex, the medial amygdaloid nucleus, the anteromedial and midline thalamic nuclei, the medial preoptic area, the arcuate and dorsomedial hypothalamic nuclei, the superior olive and the area postrema. LTBP2 expression was restricted to the cerebral cortex, the hippocampus, and the lateral hypothalamus (Dobolyi & Palkovits, 2008). Comparison of the distribution of TGF-β and LTBP subtypes suggested that all 3 isoforms of TGF-βs are co-expressed with LTBP3 in the brain. In addition, TGF-βs might also bind to other types of LTBPs in certain brain regions. For example, the distribution of TGF-β1 and LTBP-4 is similar in the supraoptic nucleus and the central nucleus of the amygdala. The choroid plexus, where TGF-β2 expression is dominant contains LTBP1 and 3. The inferior olive and the arcuate nucleus, brain areas with dominant TGF-β3 expression contain large amount of LTBP4 and LTBP1, respectively (Dobolyi & Palkovits, 2008). Nevertheless, further double labeling studies are needed to actually establish co-expression of different isoforms of TGF-βs and LTBPs in single cells of the nervous system.

Although the topographical distribution of TGF-β receptors in the central nervous system has not been systematically described, the available data suggest widespread localization. When TGF-β receptor mRNA was detected by RT-PCR in rats at different stages of development similar levels were found in several regions of the CNS, including cortex, midbrain, cerebellum, brain stem and hippocampus (Bottner et al., 1996).

4. The role of TGF-βs in neural functions

Many of the investigations of TGF-β functions did not differentiate between the isoforms of TGF-βs. In many cases, TGF-β1 was applied, which, when exogenously applied, can mimick the effects of other endogenous TGF-β isoforms. Therefore, we will only mention TGF-β in these cases.

4.1 Neuronal differentiation and survival

Distributional data were the first to suggest a role of TGF-βs in the regulation of neuronal differentiation. During the development of the central nervous system, TGF-β immunostaining was most prominent in zones where neuronal differentiation occurs and less intense in zones of active proliferation (Flanders et al., 1991). Subsequent in vitro experiments using quail neural crest cell demonstrated that TGF-β inhibits proliferation of neural crest cells while neurogenesis increased significantly in the presence of TGF-β (Zhang et al., 1997). Subsequent experiments using brains supported an inhibitory role of TGF-βs on neuronal stem cell proliferation (Aigner & Bogdahn, 2008). TGF-β had an antimitotic effect on progenitors and increased expression of neuronal markers in hippocampal and cortical primary cell cultures of developing mouse (Vogel et al., 2010). These effects were dependent upon Smad4. Furthermore, in vivo loss-of-function analyses using TGF-β2(-/-)/TGF-β3(-/-) double mutant mice showed the opposite effect of increased cell proliferation and fewer neurons in the cerebral cortex and hippocampus (Vogel et al., 2010). TGF-β may also play a role in the regulation of adult neurogenesis as it had a pro-neurogenic effect in the dentate gyrus in a model of increased neurogenesis by adrenalectomy as well as in the subventricular zone when administered chronically with adenoviral vectors expressing TGF-β (Mathieu et al., 2011). Furthermore, adrenalectomy increased TGF-β levels in the dentate gyrus while blockade of TGF-β biological activity by administration of an anti-TGF-β type II receptor antibody diminished neurogenesis (Battista et al., 2006).

Apart from playing a role in the adoption of neuronal cell fate, TGF-β may also be involved in the differentiation of selected neuronal isoforms at the expense of other isoforms. Within the intermediate and ventral domains, Smad3 promoted differentiation of ventral interneurons at the expense of motoneuron generation. Consequently, the absence of Smad3 expression from the motoneuron progenitor domain during pattern formation of the neural tube was a prerequisite for the correct generation of spinal motoneurons (Garcia-Campmany & Marti, 2007). In turn, the survival of motoneurons may also depend on TGF-βs as a potentially continous trophic support factor from muscle fibres or other cell types. Using cultures of purified chick embryonic motoneurons, TGF-βs acted synergistically with basic fibroblast growth factor to keep motoneurons alive (Gouin et al., 1996). Indeed, motoneurons were shown to synthesize TGF-β receptors and to transport them anterogradely, where they were inserted into the axonal membrane and nerve terminal

(Jiang et al., 2000a) Furthermore, TGF-β2 was detected in the synaptic portions of muscle fibres, motoneurons and in injured nerves, indicating that motoneurons may be exposed to multiple and potentially redundant sources of transforming growth factor-beta 2 (Jiang et al., 2000a). In addition, double-ligation experiments were used to demonstrate that motoneurons transport transforming growth factor-beta 2 up and down their axons (Jiang et al., 2000a). To test the effect of TGF-β on motoneuron survival in vivo, TGF-β2 was administered to the hypoglossal nucleus following the avulsion of the hypoglossal nerve in adult rats, which caused a significant attenuation of the motoneuron cell death in a low dose (Jiang et al., 2000b). TGF-β2 was, however, unable to prevent or reduce the axotomy-induced down regulation of choline acetyltransferase suggesting that TGF-β2 is only one of the growth factors regulating the homeostasis of motoneurons (Jiang et al., 2000b).

In addition to motoneurons, TGF-βs may also be required for the differentiation of midbrain dopaminergic neurons influencing motor activity, emotional behavior, and cognition and being involved in the generation of Parkinson's disease, a neurodegenerative disorder of dopaminergic neurons (Markus, 2007). Treatment of cells dissociated from the rat embryonic day 12 midbrain floor with TGF-β significantly increased the number of tyrosine hydroxylase (TH)-positive dopaminergic neurons within 24 h. Neutralization of TGF-β in vitro completely abolished the induction of dopaminergic neurons (Farkas et al., 2003). In addition to the development, the survival of midbrain dopaminergic neurons may also depend on TGF-β. Administration of TGF-β2 and TGF-β3, prevented the death of cultured rat embryonic midbrain dopaminergic neurons at picomolar concentrations (Poulsen et al., 1994). Furthermore, they provided protection against N-methyl-4-phenylpyridinium ion (MPP+) toxicity of dopaminergic neurons (Krieglstein et al., 1995). In contrast to some other cytokines affecting dopaminergic neurons the mechanism of action of the TGF-βs did not involve cell proliferation or delivery of growth factors from astroglial cells (Krieglstein et al., 1995).

Since TGF-β is only one of the factors regulating the differentiation and survival of motoneurons and midbrain dopaminergic cells, their interactions with other regulatory molecules has been examined. For example, glial cell line-derived neurotrophic factor (GDNF) is also a potent survival factor for dopaminergic neurons in culture whose effect can be potentiated by TGF-βs (Poulsen et al., 1994). However, while TGF-β is required for the induction of dopaminergic neurons, GDNF is only required for regulating and/or maintaining a differentiated neuronal phenotype (Roussa et al., 2008). A cooperative role of TGF-β2 and GDNF with regard to promotion of survival has also been demonstrated within the peripheral motor system (Rahhal et al., 2009).

Finally, it has to be emphasized that motoneurons and midbrain dopaminergic cells are 2 neuronal cell types whose development has been demonstrated to be affected by TGF-β. A role of TGF-β in the differentiation and survival of other, as yet unexplored neuronal cell types might also be possible. As far as glial cells, data are available that in the peripheral nervous system, TGF-β regulates the degree of Schwann cell proliferation induced by neuronal contact (Guenard et al., 1995; Parkinson et al., 2001).

TGF-βs are also involved in apoptosis, the genetically regulated form of cell death. Apoptosis enables the balance between growth and elimination of cells and occurs physiologically during the embryonal development or involution processes. Furthermore, infectious agents and other cell-damaging circumstances (e.g., traumatic or ischemic conditions) can lead to apoptosis. TGF-β1 has been recently characterized as an antiapoptotic factor in a model of staurosporine-induced neuronal death through a mechanism involving activation of the extracellular signal-regulated kinase 1/2 and a concomitant increase phosphorylation of the antiapoptotic protein Bad. 5 (Buisson et al., 2003). This action of TGF-β may be involved in its neuroprotective actions (see below).

4.2 Synaptic transmission and plasticity

TGF-β2 was demonstrated to influence synaptic transmission, rather than synaptogenesis, at some central synapses (Heupel et al., 2008). TGF-β2 was found to be essential for proper synaptic function in the pre-Botzinger complex, a central rhythm organizer located in the brainstem while it was not crucial for the morphology and function of the neuromuscular junction of the diaphragm muscle. Genetic deletion of TGF-β2 in mice strongly impaired both GABA/glycinergic and glutamatergic synaptic transmission in the pre-Botzinger complex area, while numbers and morphology of central synapses of knock-out animals were indistinguishable from their wild-type littermates at embryonic day 18.5 (Heupel et al., 2008). The role of TGF-β in synaptic transmission might be the basis of its proposed function in synaptic facilitation. Prolonged treatment with TGF-β2 induced facilitation of evoked postsynaptic currents in hippocampal neurons suggesting that it may play a role in the cascade of events underlying long-term synaptic facilitation (Fukushima et al., 2007). The long-term electrophysiological changes may be associated with cAMP response element-binding protein (CREB) because TGF-β2 enhanced the phosphorylation of CREB previously implicated in long-term potentiation (Fukushima et al., 2007).

The effect of TGF-β on synaptogenesis has also been proposed. In particular, TGF-β1 was identified as the molecule responsible for the synaptogenesis promiting effect of Schwann cell-conditioned medium in Xenopus nerve-muscle cocultures (Feng & Ko, 2008). TGF-β1 increased agrin expression and synaptogenesis were along nerve-muscle contacts while immunodepletion of TGF-β1 with a specific antibody abolished the synaptogenic effect of Schwann cell-conditioned medium (Feng & Ko, 2008). These results indicate that TGF-β1 may be a glial signal that instructs neurons to switch from a "growth state" to a "synaptogenic state".

4.3 Involvement in inflammatory and neuroendocrine functions

In an induced inflammatory model, the concentration of TGF-β increased in cerebrospinal fluid. This increase occurred earlier than those in the concentrations of other proinflammatory cytokines (Matsumura et al., 2008). In another inflammatory model, systemic injection of complete Freund's adjuvant, TGF-β1 and TGF-β receptor II both markedly increased in the leptomeninges and the parenchymal cells (Wu et al., 2007). Double-staining immunohistochemistry demonstrated TGF-β1 to be induced in both glial cells and cortical neurons, whereas TGF-βRII was induced only in cortical neurons. The intracisternal administration of an anti-TGF-β antibody partially inhibited the resulting fever (Matsumura et al., 2007). Furthermore, intracisternal administration of TGF-β dose-dependently raised the body temperature (Matsumura et al., 2008). These findings suggest a novel function of TGF-β as a proinflammatory cytokine in the central nervous system

The potential involvement of TGF-β in central reproductive regulation is also an emerging topic. Gonadotropin-releasing hormone neurons in the preoptic area contain TGF-β receptors as well as SMAD2/3 suggesting that they are fully capable of responding directly to TGF-β1 stimulation (Prevot et al., 2000). Subsequent double-labeling experiments showed that astrocytes in the preoptic area expressed TGF-β1 mRNA and that GnRH perikarya were often found in close association with TGF-β1 mRNA-expressing cells (Bouret et al., 2004). Incubation of preoptic explants with TGF-β1 caused a significant, dose-dependent decrease in GnRH mRNA expression in individual neurons. This effect was inhibited by addition of the soluble form of TGF-β-RII to the incubation medium (Bouret et al., 2004). These results support that astrocyte-derived TGF-β1 may directly influence GnRH expression and/or secretion in vivo by acting on the perikarya of GnRH neurons.

Intracisternal administration of TGF-β induces an increase in fat oxidation while intracisternal administration of anti-TGF-β antibody partially inhibits an increase in fat oxidation during treadmill running in rats indicating a regulatory role of TGF-β in the brain on fat oxidation during exercise (Fujikawa et al., 2007). Since TGF-β3 increased noradrenaline levels in the paraventricular and ventromedial hypothalamic nuclei and chemical lesion of noradrenaline input to these nuclei completely abolished the regulatory effect of TGF-β on fat oxidation it has been suggested that TGF-β in the brain enhances fat oxidation via noradrenergic neurons in the paraventricular and ventromedial hypothalamic nuclei (Fujikawa et al., 2007). An inhibitor of FA oxidation could induce an activation of TGF-β in the CSF suggesting that shortage of energy derived from fatty acids leads to the activation of TGF-β (Fujikawa et al., 2011).

TGF-β1 and 3 also co-localize with arginine vasopressin in magnocellular neurons of the supraoptic and paraventricular nuclei of the hypothalamus suggesting that TGF-β secreted by the neurohypophysis might regulate the proliferation and secretion of certain anterior pituitary cells (Fevre-Montange et al., 2004). So far, the regulatory role of TGF-β on hormone secretion, gene transcription, and cellular growth of prolactin-producing cells has been shown. TGF-β inhibited the transcriptional activity of the estrogen receptor although estrogens had no effect on TGF-β-specific Smad protein transcriptional activity (Giacomini et al., 2009). A diurnal pattern of expression of TGF-β as well as SMAD3 was found in the suprachiasmatic and paraventricular nuclei of young animals, a rhythm that was not onserved in older mice suggesting a diurnal and age-dependent function of the TGF-β system in these nuclei (Beynon et al., 2009). These expressional data indicate numerous yet unexplored functions of TGF-βs in the hypothalamus. Therefore, promising future investigations on the role of TGF-βs in endocrine regulations are eagerly awaited.

5. Pathophysiological functions of TGF-βs in the nervous system

In addition to their role in normal functioning of the nervous system, TGF-βs have also been implicated in different mechanisms under pathophysiological conditions. TGF-βs have been shown to be injury-related proteins. They were suggested to be neuroprotective following ischemia as well as in various neurological diseases. Furthermore, TGF-βs were implicated in glial scar formation. Finally, their role in brain tumor formation will be discussed.

5.1 Neuroprotective function in brain ischemia

A number of studies have documented that TGF-β1 levels are enhanced in the brain following cerebral ischemia (Dhandapani & Brann, 2003). The expressions of other isoforms are also enhanced albeit with a different pattern around a focal lesion. Following middle cerebral artery occlusion, TGF-β1 expression was elevated in the penumbra around the lesion site while TGF-β2 and 3 expressions showed increases in particular cortical layers throughout the ipsilateral cerebral cortex (Vincze et al., 2010).

TGF-β1 administered into the brain reduced the infarct size dose dependently in experimental models of ischemia including permanent occlusion of the left middle cerebral artery by microbipolar electrocoagulation in mice (Prehn et al., 1993), autologous clot embolus injection into the right internal carotid artery in rabbit (Gross et al., 1993), and transient middle cerebral artery occlusion in rat (Zhu et al., 2002). In turn, antagonizing the endogenous action of TGF-β1 with a soluble TGF-β type II receptor resulted in a dramatic increase in infarct area (Ruocco et al., 1999). An intracortical injection of the soluble antagonsi in rats subjected to a 30-minute reversible cerebral focal ischemia aggravated the volume of infarction (Ruocco et al., 1999). These results suggest that, in response to an ischemic insult, brain tissue responds by the synthesis of TGF-β1, which is involved in the limitation of the extent of the injury.

Despite the accumulating knowledge on the signal transduction of TGF-βs, the signaling pathway mediating its protective effect is not fully understood. Bad is a proapoptotic member of the Bcl-2 family and is inactivated on phosphorylation via mitogen-activated protein kinase (MAPK). A gradual activation of extracellular signal-regulated kinase 1/2 and MAPK-activated protein kinase-1 and a concomitant increase in Bad phosphorylation in mouse brains after adenovirus-mediated TGF-β1 transduction under nonischemic and ischemic conditions induced by transient middle cerebral artery occlusion (Zhu et al., 2002). Consistent with these effects, the ischemia-induced increases in Bad protein level and caspase-3 activation were suppressed in TGF-β1-transduced brain. Consequently, DNA fragmentation, ischemic lesions, and neurological deficiency were significantly reduced. Furthermore, inhibitors of the MAPK signal transduction pathway abolished the neuroprotective activity of TGF-β1 in staurosporine-induced apoptosis, indicating that activation of MAPK is necessary for the antiapoptotic effect of TGF-β1 (Zhu et al., 2002). These data suggest that TGF-β1 regulates the expression and ratio of apoptotic (Bad) and antiapoptotic proteins, creating an environment favorable for cell survival of death-inducing insults (Dhandapani & Brann, 2003).

5.2 TGF-β in astrogliosis

The physiological role of astrogliosis remains controversial with respect to the beneficial or detrimental influence of reactive astrocytes on CNS recovery. On the one hand, the very dense network of processes built up in the scar by reactive astrocytes suggests that the scar tissue may fulfill important functions as a barrier isolating and protecting the intact tissue from the lesions, from which toxic molecules could be released. On the other hand, molecules expressed in lesion scars on the astroglial cell surface or secreted molecules render the reactive astrocyte a less favorable substrate, which could be inhibitory to neuritic outgrowth. Nevertheless, scar formation in the nervous system begins within hours after traumatic injury and is characterized primarily by reactive astrocytes depositing proteoglycans that inhibit regeneration. A fundamental question in CNS repair has been the identity of the initial molecular mediator that triggers glial scar formation. Recent evidence suggests that one of the gliosis signaling molecules is TGF-β. TGF-β up-regulates the biosynthesis of keratin sulphate and chondroitin sulphate (Yin et al., 2009). Local injection of TGF-β antagonists into cerebral wounds reduces glial scarring (Lagord et al., 2002). Inhibition of the TGF-β receptor pathway abolished the fibrinogen-induced effects on glial scar formation in vivo and in vitro (Schachtrup et al., 2011) pointing to TGF-β as a molecular link between vascular permeability and scar formation. Furthermore, TGF-β expression increases immediately after injury e.g. in the injured segment in an animal model using an impactor (Wang et al., 2009). There are, however, differences in the expression pattern of individual TGF-β isoforms. Levels of TGF-β1 mRNA were most elevated over the acute inflammatory phase after transection of the dorsal funiculi in the spinal cord, while TGF-β2 mRNA levels were raised locally about the wound, particularly in astrocytes and neovascular endothelial cells, over the subacute period of scarring. TGF-β protein production also increased after injury. Both TGF-β1 and TGF-β2 were found in hematogenous inflammatory cells, while TGF-β1 was also neuron-associated, and high levels of TGF-β2 were localized to multiple cell types in the wound, including reactive astrocytes, during the period of glial/collagen scar formation (Lagord et al., 2002). More recently, TGF-β levels were also reported in the human spinal cord after traumatic injury. Sections from human spinal cords from 4 control patients and from 14 patients who died at different time points after traumatic spinal cord injury were investigated immunohistochemically. In control cases, TGF-β1 was confined to occasional blood vessels, intravascular monocytes and some motoneurons, whereas TGF-β2 was only found in intravascular monocytes (Buss et al., 2008). After traumatic spinal cord injury, TGF-β1 immunoreactivity was dramatically upregulated by 2 days after injury and was detected within neurons, astrocytes and invading macrophages. The staining was most intense over the first weeks after injury but gradually declined by 1 year. TGF-β2 immunoreactivity was first detected 24 days after injury. It was located in macrophages and astrocytes and remained elevated for up to 1 year. In white matter tracts undergoing Wallerian degeneration, there was no induction of either isoform (Buss et al., 2008). The conclusion from these studies is that TGF-β1 modulates the acute inflammatory and neural responses and formation of the glial scar, while the later induction of TGF-β2 may indicate a role in the maintenance of the scar.

5.3 The role of TGF-βs in brain tumor formation

TGF-β reveals anti-proliferative control on most cell types including an inhibitory effect on the proliferation of normal astrocytes. Thus, upon TGF-β treatment, primary rat astrocytes show a significant decrease in DNA synthesis upon thymidine incorporation with a cell cycle arrest in the G(1) phase and the expression of the cyclin-dependent kinase inhibitor (CdkI) p15(INK4B) is up-regulated (Rich et al., 1999). The SMAD signal transduction pathway is likely to be involved as Smad3 null mouse astrocytes show a loss of both TGF-β-mediated inhibition of growth (Rich et al., 1999). Analysis of Smad3 null mouse astrocytes showed a significant loss of both TGF-β-mediated growth inhibition and p15(INK4B) induction compared with wild-type mouse astrocytes.

Paradoxically, many brain tumors escape from normal TGF-β inhibitory control. High-grade human gliomas secrete TGF-β and can activate latent TGF-β (Sasaki et al., 2001). Yet, they are resistant to its growth inhibitory effects. In fact, they develop mechanisms that change the anti-proliferative influence of TGF-β into oncogenic cues. Thus, TGF-β is involved in tumor progression (Aigner & Bogdahn, 2008). The dominant hypothesis of TGF-β's pathogenetic association with malignant transformation has been predicated upon acquisition of resistance to its growth inhibitory effects. However, the lack of obvious correlation with TGF-β receptor expression between hyperdiploid glioblastoma multiforme and TGF-β-inhibited glioblastoma cultures suggests the existence of intrinsically opposed regulatory mechanisms influenced by TGF-β (Jennings & Pietenpol, 1998). The mechanism of conversion might be explained either by the loss of a putative tumor suppressor gene, which mediates TGF-β's inhibition of growth or by enhancement of an active oncogenic pathway among hyperdiploid glioblastoma multiforme. Experimental evidence supports the involvement of several factors including inactivating mutation/loss of the TbetaR type II, alterations in post-receptor signal transmission or the cyclin/cyclin dependent kinase system. The expression of the Smad2 and Smad3 proteins is lowered in many glioma cell lines. The phosphorylation and nuclear translocation of Smad2 and Smad3 are also impaired (Zhang et al., 2006). The loss of p15(INK4B) may also explain the selective loss of growth inhibition by TGF-β in gliomas to form a more aggressive tumor phenotype (Rich et al., 1999). TGF-β also induced expression of Sox2, a stemness gene, and this induction was mediated by Sox4, a direct TGF-β target gene. Inhibitors of TGF-β signaling drastically deprived tumorigenicity of glioblastoma cells identifying the relevance of the TGF-β-Sox4-Sox2 pathway, too (Ikushima et al., 2009). Among TGF-β isoforms, TGF-β2 has been identified as the most important factor in the progression of malignant gliomas. TGF-β2, originally described as "glioblastoma-derived T-cell suppressor factor", was particularly associated with the immuno-suppressed status of patients with glioblastoma. Furthermore, elevated TGF-β2 levels in tumors and in the plasma of patients have been associated with advanced disease stage and poor prognosis (Hau et al., 2011).

High-grade gliomas are the most common primary tumors in the central nervous system (CNS) in adults. Despite efforts to improve treatment by combination therapies (neurosurgery, radio- and chemotherapy), high-grade glioma patients still have a grim prognosis, indicating an urgent need for new therapeutic approaches. Since TGF-β is intimately involved in the regulation of several processes characteristic of human malignant glioma including excessive proliferation, infiltrative growth, angiogenesis and suppression of anti-tumor immune surveillance, TGF-β promises to become a novel target for the experimental therapy of human malignant glioma (Platten et al., 2001). Several in vitro paradigms and rodent glioma models have been used to demonstrate that the antagonism of TGF-β holds promise for the treatment of glioblastoma, employing antisense strategies, inhibition of pro-TGF-β processing, scavenging TGF-β by decorin, or blocking TGF-β activity by specific TGF-β receptor I kinase antagonists (Naumann et al., 2008; Wick et al., 2006). Among these possibilites, the antisense oligonucleotide trabedersen (AP 12009) that specifically blocks TGF-β2 mRNA has the highest potential at present to treat gliobastomas (Hau et al., 2011). In three phase I/II studies and a randomized, active-controlled dose-finding phase IIb study, trabedersen treatment of high-grade glioma patients with recurrent or refractory tumor disease led to long-lasting tumor responses and so far promising survival data. On the basis of these data the currently ongoing phase III study SAPHIRRE was initiated (Hau et al., 2011). In addition, TGF-β inhibition may also be used as a supplementary treatment as it can enhance the therapeutic efficacy of glioma-associated antigen vaccines (Ueda et al., 2009).

5.4 Neuroprotective function in additional neurological diseases

Apart from ischemia, trauma, or tumors, deafferentation and neurodegeneration also induce TGF-β expression in the central nervous system (Morgan et al., 1993). Therefore, it is not surprising that TGF-βs were implicated in a variety of neurodegenerative diseases.

Alzheimer's disease (AD) is characterized by the presence of amyloid (Abeta) plaques, neurofibrillary tangles, and neuronal loss. The disorder is also frequently associated with cerebrovascular changes, including perivascular astrocytosis, amyloid deposition, and microvascular degeneration, but it is not known whether these pathological changes contribute to functional deficits in AD. TGF-β1 expressed in the astrocytes of transgenic mice induced a prominent perivascular astrocytosis, followed by the accumulation of basement membrane proteins in microvessels, thickening of capillary basement membranes, and later, around 6 months of age, deposition of amyloid in cerebral blood vessels. At 9 months of age, various AD-like degenerative alterations were observed in endothelial cells and pericytes. These results suggest that chronic overproduction of TGF-β1 triggers a pathogenic cascade leading to AD-like cerebrovascular amyloidosis, microvascular degeneration, and local alterations in brain metabolic activity (Wyss-Coray et al., 2000). A specific impairment of TGF-β1 signaling pathway has also been demonstrated in AD brain. The deficiency of TGF-β1 signaling has been shown to increase both Abeta accumulation and Abeta-induced neurodegeneration in AD models. The loss of function of TGF-β pathway also seems to contribute to tau pathology and neurofibrillary tangle formation (Caraci et al., 2009). Growing evidence suggests a neuroprotective role for TGF-β1 against Abeta toxicity both in vitro and in vivo models of AD. Different drugs, such as lithium or group II mGlu receptor agonists are able to increase TGF-β1 levels in the central nervous system. The combined Abeta- and TGF-β1-driven pathology recapitulates salient cerebrovascular, neuronal, and cognitive AD landmarks and yields a versatile model toward highly anticipated diagnostic and therapeutic tools for patients featuring Abeta and TGF-β1 increments (Ongali et al., 2011). Thus, TGF-β1 might be considered as new neuroprotective tools against Abeta-induced neurodegeneration.

A defective expression or activity of neurotrophic factors, such as brain- and glial-derived neurotrophic factors, is known to contribute to neuronal damage in Huntington's disease (HD). Asymptomatic HD patients also showed a reduction in TGF-β1 levels in the peripheral blood, which was related to trinucleotide mutation length and glucose hypometabolism in the caudate nucleus. Immunohistochemical analysis in post-mortem brain tissues showed that TGF-β1 was reduced in cortical neurons in HD patients. In mouse models of HD, the animals showed a reduced expression of TGF-β1 in the cerebral cortex, localized in neurons, but not in astrocytes. In these mice, glutamate receptor agonist failed to increase TGF-β1 formation in the cerebral cortex and corpus striatum, suggesting that a defect in the regulation of TGF-β1 production is associated with HD. Accordingly, reduced TGF-β mRNA and protein levels were found in cultured astrocytes transfected with mutated exon 1 of the human huntingtin gene, and in striatal knock-in cell lines expressing full-length huntingtin with an expanded glutamine repeat (Battaglia et al., 2011). These data suggest that serum TGF-β1 levels are potential biomarkers of HD development during the asymptomatic phase of the disease, and raise the possibility that strategies aimed at rescuing TGF-β1 levels in the brain may influence the progression of HD.

Additional neurodegenerative diseases were also associated with an alteration of the TGF-βs. Using immunohistochemistry, the expression of TGF-β2 appeared in neurofibrillary tangle bearing neurons and tangle-bearing glial cells in progressive supranuclear palsy and in neurons with age-related neurofibrillary tangle formation (Lippa et al., 1995). Widespread staining of reactive astrocytes for TGF-β2 was observed in all degenerative diseases. TGF-β1 and -3 staining was not selectively altered in these diseases (Lippa et al., 1995). These data suggest that the induction of TGF-β2 may be an intrinsic part of the processes that underlie neurofibrillary tangle formation and reactive gliosis in a variety of neurodegenerative diseases.

Activation of the TGF-β pathway was identified as the underlying mechanism behind the epileptogenic effect of albumin following the compromise of the blood brain barrier (Cacheaux et al., 2009). TGF-β1 resulted in epileptiform activity similar to that after exposure to albumin. Coimmunoprecipitation revealed binding of albumin to TGF-β receptor II, and Smad2 phosphorylation confirmed downstream activation of this pathway. Transcriptome profiling demonstrated similar expression patterns after blood brain barrier breakdown, albumin, and TGF-β1 exposure, including modulation of genes associated with the TGF-β pathway, early astrocytic activation, inflammation, and reduced inhibitory transmission. Importantly, TGF-β pathway blockers suppressed most albumin-induced transcriptional changes and prevented the generation of epileptiform activity. Based on these data, the TGF-β pathway was suggested to be a novel putative epileptogenic signaling cascade and therapeutic target for the prevention of injury-induced epilepsy (Cacheaux et al., 2009).

6. Conclusion

TGF-βs are a class of growth factors and cytokines with a special biochemistry and range of actions thoughout the organs of the body. Our knowledge on their roles in the central nervous system is accumulating fast in the last years. Neverthless, their neurochemistry is not well described, and often we can only anticipate that their synthesis, activation, and signal transduction pathways is similar to that in other tissues. The potential differences are to be determinded in future studies. Our understanding of the physiological functions of endogenous TGF-βs is also limited despite recent significant progress in the field. An increasing body of evidence suggests the otherwise logical assumption that TGF-βs play a role in the development of the nervous tissue. Recent studies revelased that TGF-βs are also involved in the physiological functions of the adult nervous system as well. So far, the best established functions include synaptic transmission and neuronal plasticity. Somewhat surprisingly, however, the direct involvement of TGF-βs in neuroendocrine functions has also been supported. The experiments often did not differentiate between the 3 different isoforms of TGF-β. Therefore, future studies are needed to elaborate their specific functions. Based on differences in the distribution of TGF-β1, TGF-β2, and TGF-β3, they possess separate neural functions.

TGF-βs also participate in a number of pathophysiological processes. It has been long established that they are neuroprotective during excitotoxicity and ischemia. Strong evidence supports that TGF-βs constitute part of an endogenous neuroprotective system involved in ischemic preconditioning. This action of TGF-βs may or may not be related to their role in astroglial scar formation following injury. Nevertheless, the pharmacologic potentiation of this endogenous defensive mechanism might represent an alternative and novel strategy for the therapy of hypoxic-ischemic cerebral injury. TGF-β also play a pivotal role in brain tumor formation. The anti-proliferative actions of TGF-βs on astrocytes can be converted in tumor cells. Therefore, TGF-β-antagonistic treatment strategies are among the most promising of the current innovative approaches for glioblastoma, particularly in conjunction with novel approaches of cellular immunotherapy and vaccination.

7. Acknowledgements

Grant support was provided by the Bolyai János Grant from the Hungarian Academy of Sciences, as well as NFM-OTKA NNF2 85612, OTKA K100319, and NKTH TECH_09_A1 grants.

8. References

Aigner, L. & Bogdahn, U. (2008). TGF-beta in neural stem cells and in tumors of the central nervous system. *Cell and Tissue Research*, 331, pp. 225-241, ISSN 0302-766X (Print)

Annes, J.P.; Munger, J.S. & Rifkin, D.B. (2003). Making sense of latent TGFbeta activation. *Journal of Cellular Science*, 116, pp. 217-224

Arighi, C.N.; Liu, H.; Natale, D.A.; Barker, W.C.; Drabkin, H.; Blake, J.A.; Smith, B. & Wu, C.H. (2009). TGF-beta signaling proteins and the Protein Ontology. *BMC Bioinformatics*, 10 Suppl 5, pp. S3, ISSN 1471-2105 (Electronic)

Attisano, L. & Wrana, J.L. (2002). Signal transduction by the TGF-beta superfamily. *Science*, 296, pp. 1646-1647

Battaglia, G.; Cannella, M.; Riozzi, B.; Orobello, S.; Maat-Schieman, M.L.; Aronica, E.; Busceti, C.L.; Ciarmiello, A.; Alberti, S.; Amico, E.; Sassone, J.; Sipione, S.; Bruno, V.; Frati, L.; Nicoletti, F. & Squitieri, F. (2011). Early defect of transforming growth factor beta1 formation in Huntington's disease. *Journal of Cellular and Molecular Medicine*, 15, pp. 555-571, ISSN 1582-4934 (Electronic), 1582-1838 (Linking)

Battista, D.; Ferrari, C.C.; Gage, F.H. & Pitossi, F.J. (2006). Neurogenic niche modulation by activated microglia: transforming growth factor beta increases neurogenesis in the adult dentate gyrus. *European Journal of Neuroscience*, 23, pp. 83-93

Beynon, A.L.; Thome, J. & Coogan, A.N. (2009). Age and time of day influences on the expression of transforming growth factor-beta and phosphorylated SMAD3 in the mouse suprachiasmatic and paraventricular nuclei. *Neuroimmunomodulation*, 16, pp. 392-399, ISSN 1423-0216 (Electronic), 1021-7401 (Linking)

Bottner, M.; Krieglstein, K. & Unsicker, K. (2000). The transforming growth factor-betas: structure, signaling, and roles in nervous system development and functions. *Journal of Neurochemistry*, 75, pp. 2227-2240

Bottner, M.; Unsicker, K. & Suter-Crazzolara, C. (1996). Expression of TGF-beta type II receptor mRNA in the CNS. *NeuroReport*, 7, pp. 2903-2907

Bouret, S.; De Seranno, S.; Beauvillain, J.C. & Prevot, V. (2004). Transforming growth factor beta1 may directly influence gonadotropin-releasing hormone gene expression in the rat hypothalamus. *Endocrinology*, 145, pp. 1794-1801

Buisson, A.; Lesne, S.; Docagne, F.; Ali, C.; Nicole, O.; MacKenzie, E.T. & Vivien, D. (2003). Transforming growth factor-beta and ischemic brain injury. *Cellular and Molecular Neurobiology*, 23, pp. 539-550, ISSN 0272-4340 (Print), 0272-4340 (Linking)

Burt, D.W. & Law, A.S. (1994). Evolution of the transforming growth factor-beta superfamily. *Progress in Growth Factor Research*, 5, pp. 99-118

Buss, A.; Pech, K.; Kakulas, B.A.; Martin, D.; Schoenen, J.; Noth, J. & Brook, G.A. (2008). TGF-beta1 and TGF-beta2 expression after traumatic human spinal cord injury. *Spinal Cord*, 46, pp. 364-371, ISSN 1362-4393 (Print), 1362-4393 (Linking)

Cacheaux, L.P.; Ivens, S.; David, Y.; Lakhter, A.J.; Bar-Klein, G.; Shapira, M.; Heinemann, U.; Friedman, A. & Kaufer, D. (2009). Transcriptome profiling reveals TGF-beta signaling involvement in epileptogenesis. *Journal of Neuroscience*, 29, pp. 8927-8935, ISSN 1529-2401 (Electronic), 0270-6474 (Linking)

Caraci, F.; Battaglia, G.; Bruno, V.; Bosco, P.; Carbonaro, V.; Giuffrida, M.L.; Drago, F.; Sortino, M.A.; Nicoletti, F. & Copani, A. (2009). TGF-beta1 Pathway as a New Target for Neuroprotection in Alzheimer's Disease. *CNS Neuroscience Ther*, pp., 1755-5949 (Electronic)

Chu, W.; Li, X.; Li, C.; Wan, L.; Shi, H.; Song, X.; Liu, X.; Chen, X.; Zhang, C.; Shan, H.; Lu, Y. & Yang, B. (2011). TGFBR3, a potential negative regulator of TGF-beta signaling, protects cardiac fibroblasts from hypoxia-induced apoptosis. *Journal of Cellular Physiology*, 226, pp. 2586-2594, ISSN 1097-4652 (Electronic), 0021-9541 (Linking)

Clark, D.A. & Coker, R. (1998). Transforming growth factor-beta (TGF-beta). *International Journal of Biochemistry and Cellular Biology*, 30, pp. 293-298

Dhandapani, K.M. & Brann, D.W. (2003). Transforming growth factor-beta: a neuroprotective factor in cerebral ischemia. *Cellular Biochemistry and Biophysics*, 39, pp. 13-22

Dobolyi, A. & Palkovits, M. (2008). Expression of latent transforming growth factor beta binding proteins in the rat brain. *Journal of Comparative Neurology*, 507, pp. 1393-1408, ISSN 1096-9861 (Electronic)

Farkas, L.M.; Dunker, N.; Roussa, E.; Unsicker, K. & Krieglstein, K. (2003). Transforming growth factor-beta(s) are essential for the development of midbrain dopaminergic neurons in vitro and in vivo. *Journal of Neuroscience*, 23, pp. 5178-5186

Feng, Z. & Ko, C.P. (2008). Schwann cells promote synaptogenesis at the neuromuscular junction via transforming growth factor-beta1. *Journal of Neuroscience*, 28, pp. 9599-9609, ISSN 1529-2401 (Electronic), 0270-6474 (Linking)

Fevre-Montange, M.; Dumontel, C.; Chevallier, P.; Isnard, A.K.; Guigard, M.P. & Trouillas, J. (2004). Localization of transforming growth factors, TGFbeta1 and TGFbeta3, in hypothalamic magnocellular neurones and the neurohypophysis. *Journal of Neuroendocrinology*, 16, pp. 571-576

Flanders, K.C.; Ludecke, G.; Engels, S.; Cissel, D.S.; Roberts, A.B.; Kondaiah, P.; Lafyatis, R.; Sporn, M.B. & Unsicker, K. (1991). Localization and actions of transforming growth factor-beta s in the embryonic nervous system. *Development*, 113, pp. 183-191

Flanders, K.C.; Ren, R.F. & Lippa, C.F. (1998). Transforming growth factor-betas in neurodegenerative disease. *Progress in Neurobiology*, 54, pp. 71-85

Fujikawa, T.; Fujita, R.; Iwaki, Y.; Matsumura, S.; Fushiki, T. & Inoue, K. (2011). Inhibition of fatty acid oxidation activates transforming growth factor-beta in cerebrospinal fluid and decreases spontaneous motor activity. *Physiology and Behavior*, 101, pp. 370-375, ISSN 1873-507X (Electronic), 0031-9384 (Linking)

Fujikawa, T.; Matsumura, S.; Yamada, H.; Inoue, K. & Fushiki, T. (2007). Transforming growth factor-beta in the brain enhances fat oxidation via noradrenergic neurons in the ventromedial and paraventricular hypothalamic nucleus. *Brain Research*, 1173, pp. 92-101, ISSN 0006-8993 (Print), 0006-8993 (Linking)

Fukushima, T.; Liu, R.Y. & Byrne, J.H. (2007). Transforming growth factor-beta2 modulates synaptic efficacy and plasticity and induces phosphorylation of CREB in hippocampal neurons. *Hippocampus*, 17, pp. 5-9

Garcia-Campmany, L. & Marti, E. (2007). The TGFbeta intracellular effector Smad3 regulates neuronal differentiation and cell fate specification in the developing spinal cord. *Development*, 134, pp. 65-75

Giacomini, D.; Paez-Pereda, M.; Stalla, J.; Stalla, G.K. & Arzt, E. (2009). Molecular interaction of BMP-4, TGF-beta, and estrogens in lactotrophs: impact on the PRL promoter. *Molecular Endocrinology*, 23, pp. 1102-1114, ISSN 1944-9917 (Electronic), 0888-8809 (Linking)

Gouin, A.; Bloch-Gallego, E.; Tanaka, H.; Rosenthal, A. & Henderson, C.E. (1996). Transforming growth factor-beta 3, glial cell line-derived neurotrophic factor, and fibroblast growth factor-2, act in different manners to promote motoneuron survival in vitro. *Journal of Neuroscience Research*, 43, pp. 454-464

Gross, C.E.; Bednar, M.M.; Howard, D.B. & Sporn, M.B. (1993). Transforming growth factor-beta 1 reduces infarct size after experimental cerebral ischemia in a rabbit model. *Stroke*, 24, pp. 558-562

Guenard, V.; Rosenbaum, T.; Gwynn, L.A.; Doetschman, T.; Ratner, N. & Wood, P.M. (1995). Effect of transforming growth factor-beta 1 and -beta 2 on Schwann cell proliferation on neurites. *Glia*, 13, pp. 309-318, ISSN 0894-1491 (Print), 0894-1491 (Linking)

Gumienny, T.L. & Padgett, R.W. (2002). The other side of TGF-beta superfamily signal regulation: thinking outside the cell. *Trends in Endocrinology and Metabolism*, 13, pp. 295-299

Hau, P.; Jachimczak, P.; Schlaier, J. & Bogdahn, U. (2011). TGF-beta2 Signaling in High-Grade Gliomas. *Current Pharm Biotechnol*, pp., ISSN 1873-4316 (Electronic), 1389-2010 (Linking)

Heupel, K.; Sargsyan, V.; Plomp, J.J.; Rickmann, M.; Varoqueaux, F.; Zhang, W. & Krieglstein, K. (2008). Loss of transforming growth factor-beta 2 leads to impairment of central synapse function. *Neural Development*, 3, pp. 25, ISSN 1749-8104 (Electronic)

Ikushima, H.; Todo, T.; Ino, Y.; Takahashi, M.; Miyazawa, K. & Miyazono, K. (2009). Autocrine TGF-beta signaling maintains tumorigenicity of glioma-initiating cells through Sry-related HMG-box factors. *Cell Stem Cell*, 5, pp. 504-514, ISSN 1875-9777 (Electronic)

Jennings, M.T. & Pietenpol, J.A. (1998). The role of transforming growth factor beta in glioma progression. *Journal of Neurooncology*, 36, pp. 123-140, ISSN 0167-594X (Print), 0167-594X (Linking)

Jiang, Y.; McLennan, I.S.; Koishi, K. & Hendry, I.A. (2000a). Transforming growth factor-beta 2 is anterogradely and retrogradely transported in motoneurons and up-regulated after nerve injury. *Neuroscience*, 97, pp. 735-742, ISSN 0306-4522 (Print), 0306-4522 (Linking)

Jiang, Y.; Zhang, M.; Koishi, K. & McLennan, I.S. (2000b). TGF-beta 2 attenuates the injury-induced death of mature motoneurons. *Journal of Neuroscience Research*, 62, pp. 809-813, ISSN 0360-4012 (Print), 0360-4012 (Linking)

Keski-Oja, J.; Koli, K. & von Melchner, H. (2004). TGF-beta activation by traction? *Trends in Cell Biology*, 14, pp. 657-659

Khalil, N. (1999). TGF-beta: from latent to active. *Microbes in Infection*, 1, pp. 1255-1263

Kiefer, R.; Streit, W.J.; Toyka, K.V.; Kreutzberg, G.W. & Hartung, H.P. (1995). Transforming growth factor-beta 1: a lesion-associated cytokine of the nervous system. *Internal Journal of Developmental Neuroscience,* 13, pp. 331-339, ISSN 0736-5748 (Print), 0736-5748 (Linking)

Koli, K.; Saharinen, J.; Hyytiainen, M.; Penttinen, C. & Keski-Oja, J. (2001). Latency, activation, and binding proteins of TGF-beta. *Microscopic Research Techniques*, 52, pp. 354-362

Komuta, Y.; Teng, X.; Yanagisawa, H.; Sango, K.; Kawamura, K. & Kawano, H. (2009). Expression of transforming growth factor-beta receptors in meningeal fibroblasts of the injured mouse brain. *Cellular and Molecular Neurobiology,* 30, pp. 101-111, ISSN 1573-6830 (Electronic), 0272-4340 (Linking)

Krieglstein, K.; Suter-Crazzolara, C.; Fischer, W.H. & Unsicker, K. (1995). TGF-beta superfamily members promote survival of midbrain dopaminergic neurons and protect them against MPP+ toxicity. *Embo Journal*, 14, pp. 736-742

Krieglstein, K. & Unsicker, K. (1995). Bovine chromaffin cells release a transforming growth factor-beta-like molecule contained within chromaffin granules. *Journal of Neurochemistry*, 65, pp. 1423-1426

Krohn, K. (1999). TGF-beta1-dependent differential expression of a rat homolog for latent TGF-beta binding protein in astrocytes and C6 glioma cells. *Glia*, 25, pp. 332-342

Lacmann, A.; Hess, D.; Gohla, G.; Roussa, E. & Krieglstein, K. (2007). Activity-dependent release of transforming growth factor-beta in a neuronal network in vitro. *Neuroscience*, 150, pp. 647-657, ISSN 0306-4522 (Print)

Lagord, C.; Berry, M. & Logan, A. (2002). Expression of TGFbeta2 but not TGFbeta1 correlates with the deposition of scar tissue in the lesioned spinal cord. *Molecular and Cellular Neuroscience,* 20, pp. 69-92, ISSN 1044-7431 (Print), 1044-7431 (Linking)

Lawrence, D.A. (1996). Transforming growth factor-beta: a general review. *European Cytokine Network*, 7, pp. 363-374

Lippa, C.F.; Smith, T.W. & Flanders, K.C. (1995). Transforming growth factor-beta: neuronal and glial expression in CNS degenerative diseases. *Neurodegeneration*, 4, pp. 425-432, ISSN 1055-8330 (Print), 1055-8330 (Linking)

Mangasser-Stephan, K. & Gressner, A.M. (1999). Molecular and functional aspects of latent transforming growth factor-beta binding protein: just a masking protein? *Cell and Tissue Research*, 297, pp. 363-370

Markus, A. (2007). How dopamine neurons survive. *Nature Neuroscience,* 10, pp. 12

Massague, J. (1992). Receptors for the TGF-beta family. *Cell*, 69, pp. 1067-1070

Mathieu, P.; Piantanida, A.P. & Pitossi, F. (2011). Chronic expression of transforming growth factor-beta enhances adult neurogenesis. *Neuroimmunomodulation*, 17, pp. 200-201, ISSN 1423-0216 (Electronic), 1021-7401 (Linking)

Matsumura, S.; Shibakusa, T.; Fujikawa, T.; Yamada, H.; Inoue, K. & Fushiki, T. (2007). Increase in transforming growth factor-beta in the brain during infection is related to fever, not depression of spontaneous motor activity. *Neuroscience*, 144, pp. 1133-1140

Matsumura, S.; Shibakusa, T.; Fujikawa, T.; Yamada, H.; Matsumura, K.; Inoue, K. & Fushiki, T. (2008). Intracisternal administration of transforming growth factor-beta evokes fever through the induction of cyclooxygenase-2 in brain endothelial cells. *American Journal of Physiology Regulation of Integral Comparative Physiology*, 294, pp. R266-275, ISSN 0363-6119 (Print)

Morgan, T.E.; Nichols, N.R.; Pasinetti, G.M. & Finch, C.E. (1993). TGF-beta 1 mRNA increases in macrophage/microglial cells of the hippocampus in response to deafferentation and kainic acid-induced neurodegeneration. *Experimental Neurology*, 120, pp. 291-301, ISSN 0014-4886 (Print), 0014-4886 (Linking)

Mu, Y.; Gudey, S.K. & Landstrom, M. (2011). Non-Smad signaling pathways. *Cell and Tissue Research*, pp., ISSN 1432-0878 (Electronic), 0302-766X (Linking)

Naumann, U.; Maass, P.; Gleske, A.K.; Aulwurm, S.; Weller, M. & Eisele, G. (2008). Glioma gene therapy with soluble transforming growth factor-beta receptors II and III. *International Journal of Oncology*, 33, pp. 759-765, ISSN 1019-6439 (Print), 1019-6439 (Linking)

Oklu, R. & Hesketh, R. (2000). The latent transforming growth factor beta binding protein (LTBP) family. *Biochemical Journal*, 352, pp. 601-610

Ongali, B.; Nicolakakis, N.; Lecrux, C.; Aboulkassim, T.; Rosa-Neto, P.; Papadopoulos, P.; Tong, X.K. & Hamel, E. (2011). Transgenic mice overexpressing APP and transforming growth factor-beta1 feature cognitive and vascular hallmarks of Alzheimer's disease. *Am J Pathol*, 177, pp. 3071-3080, ISSN 1525-2191 (Electronic), 0002-9440 (Linking)

Padgett, R.W.; Cho, S.H. & Evangelista, C. (1998). Smads are the central component in transforming growth factor-beta signaling. *Pharmacological Therapeutics*, 78, pp. 47-52, ISSN 0163-7258 (Print), 0163-7258 (Linking)

Parkinson, D.B.; Dong, Z.; Bunting, H.; Whitfield, J.; Meier, C.; Marie, H.; Mirsky, R. & Jessen, K.R. (2001). Transforming growth factor beta (TGFbeta) mediates Schwann cell death in vitro and in vivo: examination of c-Jun activation, interactions with survival signals, and the relationship of TGFbeta-mediated death to Schwann cell differentiation. *Journal of Neuroscience*, 21, pp. 8572-8585, ISSN 1529-2401 (Electronic), 0270-6474 (Linking)

Platten, M.; Wick, W. & Weller, M. (2001). Malignant glioma biology: role for TGF-beta in growth, motility, angiogenesis, and immune escape. *Microscopic Research Techniques*, 52, pp. 401-410, ISSN 1059-910X (Print), 1059-910X (Linking)

Poulsen, K.T.; Armanini, M.P.; Klein, R.D.; Hynes, M.A.; Phillips, H.S. & Rosenthal, A. (1994). TGF beta 2 and TGF beta 3 are potent survival factors for midbrain dopaminergic neurons. *Neuron*, 13, pp. 1245-1252

Prehn, J.H.; Backhauss, C. & Krieglstein, J. (1993). Transforming growth factor-beta 1 prevents glutamate neurotoxicity in rat neocortical cultures and protects mouse neocortex from ischemic injury in vivo. *Journal of Cerebral Blood Flow and Metabolism*, 13, pp. 521-525

Prevot, V.; Bouret, S.; Croix, D.; Takumi, T.; Jennes, L.; Mitchell, V. & Beauvillain, J.C. (2000). Evidence that members of the TGFbeta superfamily play a role in regulation of the GnRH neuroendocrine axis: expression of a type I serine-threonine kinase receptor for TGRbeta and activin in GnRH neurones and hypothalamic areas of the female rat. *Journal of Neuroendocrinology*, 12, pp. 665-670

Rahhal, B.; Heermann, S.; Ferdinand, A.; Rosenbusch, J.; Rickmann, M. & Krieglstein, K. (2009). In vivo requirement of TGF-beta/GDNF cooperativity in mouse development: focus on the neurotrophic hypothesis. *International Journal of Developmental Neuroscience*, 27, pp. 97-102, ISSN 0736-5748 (Print)

Rich, J.N.; Zhang, M.; Datto, M.B.; Bigner, D.D. & Wang, X.F. (1999). Transforming growth factor-beta-mediated p15(INK4B) induction and growth inhibition in astrocytes is SMAD3-dependent and a pathway prominently altered in human glioma cell lines.

Journal of Biological Chemistry, 274, pp. 35053-35058, ISSN 0021-9258 (Print), 0021-9258 (Linking)

Rifkin, D.B. (2005). Latent transforming growth factor-beta (TGF-beta) binding proteins: orchestrators of TGF-beta availability. *Journal of Biological Chemistry*, 280, pp. 7409-7412

Roberts, A.B. (1998). Molecular and cell biology of TGF-beta. *Mineral and Electrolyte Metabolism*, 24, pp. 111-119

Roberts, A.B.; Anzano, M.A.; Lamb, L.C.; Smith, J.M. & Sporn, M.B. (1981). New class of transforming growth factors potentiated by epidermal growth factor: isolation from non-neoplastic tissues. *Proceedings in the North Atlantic Academy of Sciences United States of America*, 78, pp. 5339-5343, ISSN 0027-8424 (Print), 0027-8424 (Linking)

Roussa, E.; Oehlke, O.; Rahhal, B.; Heermann, S.; Heidrich, S.; Wiehle, M. & Krieglstein, K. (2008). Transforming growth factor beta cooperates with persephin for dopaminergic phenotype induction. *Stem Cells*, 26, pp. 1683-1694, ISSN 1549-4918 (Electronic)

Ruocco, A.; Nicole, O.; Docagne, F.; Ali, C.; Chazalviel, L.; Komesli, S.; Yablonsky, F.; Roussel, S.; MacKenzie, E.T.; Vivien, D. & Buisson, A. (1999). A transforming growth factor-beta antagonist unmasks the neuroprotective role of this endogenous cytokine in excitotoxic and ischemic brain injury. *Journal of Cerebral Blood Flow and Metabolism*, 19, pp. 1345-1353

Saharinen, J.; Hyytiainen, M.; Taipale, J. & Keski-Oja, J. (1999). Latent transforming growth factor-beta binding proteins (LTBPs) - structural extracellular matrix proteins for targeting TGF-beta action. *Cytokine and Growth Factor Reviews*, 10, pp. 99-117

Saharinen, J. & Keski-Oja, J. (2000). Specific sequence motif of 8-Cys repeats of TGF-beta binding proteins, LTBPs, creates a hydrophobic interaction surface for binding of small latent TGF-beta. *Molecular Biololgy of the Cell*, 11, pp. 2691-2704

Sasaki, A.; Naganuma, H.; Satoh, E.; Kawataki, T.; Amagasaki, K. & Nukui, H. (2001). Participation of thrombospondin-1 in the activation of latent transforming growth factor-beta in malignant glioma cells. *Neurological and Medicinal Chirurgie (Tokyo)*, 41, pp. 253-258; discussion 258-259, ISSN 0470-8105 (Print), 0470-8105 (Linking)

Schachtrup, C.; Ryu, J.K.; Helmrick, M.J.; Vagena, E.; Galanakis, D.K.; Degen, J.L.; Margolis, R.U. & Akassoglou, K. (2011). Fibrinogen triggers astrocyte scar formation by promoting the availability of active TGF-beta after vascular damage. *Journal of Neuroscience*, 30, pp. 5843-5854, ISSN 1529-2401 (Electronic), 0270-6474 (Linking)

Schmierer, B. & Hill, C.S. (2007). TGFbeta-SMAD signal transduction: molecular specificity and functional flexibility. *Nature Reviews in Molecular and Cellular Biology*, 8, pp. 970-982, ISSN 1471-0080 (Electronic), 1471-0072 (Linking)

Sinha, S.; Nevett, C.; Shuttleworth, C.A. & Kielty, C.M. (1998). Cellular and extracellular biology of the latent transforming growth factor-beta binding proteins. *Matrix Biology*, 17, pp. 529-545

ten Dijke, P. & Hill, C.S. (2004). New insights into TGF-beta-Smad signalling. *Trends in Biochemical Science*, 29, pp. 265-273, ISSN 0968-0004 (Print), 0968-0004 (Linking)

Todorovic, V.; Jurukovski, V.; Chen, Y.; Fontana, L.; Dabovic, B. & Rifkin, D.B. (2005). Latent TGF-beta binding proteins. *International Journal of Biochemistry and Cell Biology*, 37, pp. 38-41

Ueda, R.; Fujita, M.; Zhu, X.; Sasaki, K.; Kastenhuber, E.R.; Kohanbash, G.; McDonald, H.A.; Harper, J.; Lonning, S. & Okada, H. (2009). Systemic inhibition of transforming growth factor-beta in glioma-bearing mice improves the therapeutic efficacy of glioma-associated antigen peptide vaccines. *Clinical Cancer Research*, 15, pp. 6551-6559, ISSN 1078-0432 (Print), 1078-0432 (Linking)

Unsicker, K.; Flanders, K.C.; Cissel, D.S.; Lafyatis, R. & Sporn, M.B. (1991). Transforming growth factor beta isoforms in the adult rat central and peripheral nervous system. *Neuroscience*, 44, pp. 613-625

Vincze, C.; Pal, G.; Wappler, E.A.; Szabo, E.R.; Nagy, Z.G.; Lovas, G. & Dobolyi, A. (2010). Distribution of mRNAs encoding transforming growth factors-beta1, -2, and -3 in the intact rat brain and after experimentally induced focal ischemia. *Journal of Comparative Neurology*, 518, pp. 3752-3770, ISSN 1096-9861 (Electronic), 0021-9967 (Linking)

Vogel, T.; Ahrens, S.; Buttner, N. & Krieglstein, K. (2010). Transforming growth factor beta promotes neuronal cell fate of mouse cortical and hippocampal progenitors in vitro and in vivo: identification of Nedd9 as an essential signaling component. *Cerebral Cortex*, 20, pp. 661-671, ISSN 1460-2199 (Electronic), 1047-3211 (Linking)

Wang, X.; Chen, W.; Liu, W.; Wu, J.; Shao, Y. & Zhang, X. (2009). The role of thrombospondin-1 and transforming growth factor-beta after spinal cord injury in the rat. *Journal of Clinical Neuroscience*, 16, pp. 818-821, ISSN 0967-5868 (Print), 0967-5868 (Linking)

Wells, A. (1999). EGF receptor. *International Journal of Biochemistry and Cell Biology*, 31, pp. 637-643, ISSN 1357-2725 (Print), 1357-2725 (Linking)

Wick, W.; Naumann, U. & Weller, M. (2006). Transforming growth factor-beta: a molecular target for the future therapy of glioblastoma. *Current Pharmacological Research*, 12, pp. 341-349, ISSN 1381-6128 (Print), 1381-6128 (Linking)

Wu, Z.; Hayashi, Y.; Zhang, J. & Nakanishi, H. (2007). Involvement of prostaglandin E2 released from leptomeningeal cells in increased expression of transforming growth factor-beta in glial cells and cortical neurons during systemic inflammation. *Journal of Neuroscience Research*, 85, pp. 184-192, ISSN 0360-4012 (Print)

Wu, Z.; Tokuda, Y.; Zhang, X.W. & Nakanishi, H. (2008). Age-dependent responses of glial cells and leptomeninges during systemic inflammation. *Neurobiology of Disease*, 32, pp. 543-551, ISSN 1095-953X (Electronic)

Wyss-Coray, T.; Lin, C.; von Euw, D.; Masliah, E.; Mucke, L. & Lacombe, P. (2000). Alzheimer's disease-like cerebrovascular pathology in transforming growth factor-beta 1 transgenic mice and functional metabolic correlates. Annals of the New York Academy of Sciences, 903, pp. 317-323, ISSN 0077-8923 (Print), 0077-8923 (Linking)

Yin, J.; Sakamoto, K.; Zhang, H.; Ito, Z.; Imagama, S.; Kishida, S.; Natori, T.; Sawada, M.; Matsuyama, Y. & Kadomatsu, K. (2009). Transforming growth factor-beta1 upregulates keratan sulfate and chondroitin sulfate biosynthesis in microglias after brain injury. *Brain Research*, 1263, pp. 10-22, ISSN 1872-6240 (Electronic)

Zhang, J.M.; Hoffmann, R. & Sieber-Blum, M. (1997). Mitogenic and anti-proliferative signals for neural crest cells and the neurogenic action of TGF-beta1. *Developmental Dynamics*, 208, pp. 375-386, ISSN 1058-8388 (Print), 1058-8388 (Linking)

Zhang, L.; Sato, E.; Amagasaki, K.; Nakao, A. & Naganuma, H. (2006). Participation of an abnormality in the transforming growth factor-beta signaling pathway in resistance of malignant glioma cells to growth inhibition induced by that factor. *Journal of Neurosurgery*, 105, pp. 119-128, ISSN 0022-3085 (Print), 0022-3085 (Linking)

Zhu, Y.; Yang, G.Y.; Ahlemeyer, B.; Pang, L.; Che, X.M.; Culmsee, C.; Klumpp, S. & Krieglstein, J. (2002). Transforming growth factor-beta 1 increases bad phosphorylation and protects neurons against damage. *Journal of Neuroscience*, 22, pp. 3898-3909

7

Neurochemistry in the Pathophysiology of Septic Encephalopathy

Yukio Imamura[1,3,4], Huan Wang[1,2], Naoya Matsumoto[1], Hiroshi Ogura[1], Takeshi Shimazu[1], Takashi Jin[5] and Akitoshi Seiyama[3,4]
[1]*Department of Trauma and Acute Critical Care Center, Osaka University Hospital*
[2]*Department of Molecular Oncology, Kyoto University Graduate School of Medicine*
[3]*Unit for Liveable Cities, Kyoto University Graduate School of Medicine*
[4]*Human Health Science, Kyoto University Graduate School of Medicine*
[5]*Laboratory for Nano-Bio Probes, Quantitative Biology Center,*
Japan

1. Introduction

Neurochemical studies clarify scientific mechanisms for neurochemicals in the nervous system. These include identification and characterization of neurotransmitters and neuromodulators supportive for neurotransmission in neuronal and glial cells networks in the brain. Neurochemicals based on neural mechanisms have been explained by the ongoing evolution of scientific techniques. These neurochemical techniques include immunohistochemistry, immunoblotting using species' specific antibodies or radio-labeled substances, etc. And these techniques with electrophysiological methods will be powerful tools to describe the pathophysiological mechanisms of sepsis-related brain dysfunction.

Neurochemical techniques are useful to examine the physiological mechanism of normal brain function such as synaptic transmission, plasticity and neurogenesis. On the other hand, these techniques are available to find pathogenesis of the brain. In this chapter, we'd like to focus on the brain pathophysiology, which is often confronted in an intensive care unit, **'septic encephalopathy'**.

In normal condition, our brain is protected for its environment such as neurochemical balance by the barrier called 'blood brain barrier (guardian of the brain)'. However, sepsis leads to be the impairment of blood brain barrier function (i.e., enhancement of permeability through blood brain barrier) and imbalance of neurotransmission. In addition, following sepsis, apoptotic signaling pathway is activated (Hotchkiss RS & Nicholson DW, 2006) and/ or chemical mediators passing through disrupted blood brain barrier lead to necrotic neuronal cell death accompanying with ischemia (Sharshar T et al, 2004) and edema (Kafa IM et al, 2007). These phenomena finally lead to the imbalance of brain activity after septic encephalopathy.

Next section, we introduce the neurochemical techniques in terms of the contents: 1) what are pathophysiological phenomena in sepsis and its related encephalopathy in combination of inflammatory response, 2) how to examine the aberrant brain function, 3) what is the future for sepsis research.

2. Sepsis

2.1 Pathogenesis of sepsis

2.1.1 Symptoms

Sepsis is a systemic inflammatory state in the whole body by bacteria infection in the blood stream (i.e., systemic inflammatory response syndrome) (Bone RC et al, 1992). In systemic inflammatory response syndrome, the innate immune systems are overactivated. The systemic inflammatory response syndrome is characterized by the symptoms such as fever and hypotension in patients. In severe sepsis pathology, immunohistochemical studies using both of postmortem human and an animal model of sepsis in rodents reveal the brain ischemia (Sharshar T et al, 2004), edema (Pfister D et al, 2008), hemorrhage (Casanova E et al, 2001) after sepsis. On the other hand, following sepsis, several kinds of symptoms such as polyneuropathy are also observed. These symptoms enhance complexity of the septic pathophysiology (Bolton CF et al, 1993; Nauwynck M & Huyghens L, 1998). Hence, the septic conditions include neurological symptoms.

2.1.2 Molecular mechanisms

Molecular mechanism of immunology for sepsis is investigated. When pathogen (bacteria etc.) is invaded into the blood stream, it is recognized to be pathogen-associated molecular pattern such as lipopolysaccaride, bacterial component in immunological dendritic cells and T cells. When the pathogen-associated molecular pattern binds to toll-like receptor, the toll-like receptor facilitates cytokine release (Kim KD et al, 2007). After the cytokine release, the septic condition triggers downstream signaling pathways. These pathways translocate and activate NF-kappa B in the nucleus through I-kappaB degradation and mitogen-activated protein kinase (MAPK) and JUN kinase activation. Finally, NF-kappaB drives transcription of interleukin family (interleukin -1, 2, 6, 8 and 12) and tumor necrosis factor-α.

2.1.3 Cytokine storm

These activations lead to be **cytokine storm** (Harrison C, 2010). In fact, 30% of septic patients have serious symptoms without bacteremia in their blood (Sprung CL et al, 1990). The result suggests that after removal of bacteria, cytokine storm is a major factor for the tissue injury after severe sepsis. What is a player for accelerating cytokine storm? Recent finding suggests that small protein 'complement' creates cytokine storm (Ward PA, 2010). The complement serves as a supportive factor to enhance the efficacy of antibodies in order to clear pathogen in the blood. The complement C5a has their receptors, C5aR and C5L2, in the pituitary and their receptors are up-regulated after sepsis. C5a is also performed as a central hub to activate various inflammatory responses including disseminated intravascular coagulation, systemic inflammatory response syndrome, lethal bacteremia, immunosuppression, septic shock and heart failure (Rittirsch D et al, 2008). Conversely, when the C5a is neutralized by specific antibody, blood brain barrier disruption and pituitary dysfunction in severe sepsis is alleviated in the rat (Flierl MA et al, 2009). Hence, C5a will be a hopeful target for cytokine storm regulation after sepsis.

2.1.4 Multiple organ dysfunction syndrome

Because of the amplification of systemic inflammatory states after sepsis, without appropriate intensive care including antibiotic therapy, vasopressor medications, mechanical dialysis (Dellinger RP et al, 2008), systemic inflammatory response syndrome and cytokine storm then lead to be multiple organ dysfunction syndrome. Once sepsis is reached to multiple organ dysfunction syndrome, the patients are destined to be coma or delirium. Multiple organ dysfunction syndrome implicates in the pathogenesis of septic encephalopathy.

2.2 Septic encephalopathy

Septic encephalopathy is devastating syndrome results from systemic inflammatory response syndrome in sepsis. In patients after multiple organ dysfunction syndrome, septic encephalopathy is appeared. The symptoms of septic encephalopathy patients are characterized as long-term cognitive impairment including deficits in memory, attention, concentration of consciousness (Streck EL et al, 2008). Why do these symptoms occur?

A lot of research groups have performed to tackle and continue the challenging to uncover the mystery of septic encephalopathy. Typical characteristic in septic encephalopathy is that the chemical substances in the whole body can access to the neuronal function in the brain after blood brain barrier (a guardian of brain) disruption. In fact, we find that occludin, the marker for tight junction, is drastically reduced in the mouse brain after septic encephalopathy (Imamura Y et al, 2011). This may cause the edema after septic encephalopathy (Papadopoulos MC et al, 1999). Then, what is the pathophysiology in the neurochemical substances related to septic encephalopathy?

Several decade ago, several lines of research reports have been addressed for the possibility of neurotransmitters imbalance in septic encephalopathy. One of the possible suggestions to septic encephalopathy-induced abnormalities stems from amino acid derangements in septic patients (Freund HR et al, 1978). The altered patterns of plasma amino acids are well correlated between non- septic encephalopathy and severe septic encephalopathy groups (Freund H et al, 1979). For example, several amino acids including glutamate, aspartate and tryptophan are altered in septic encephalopathy patient. These amino acids serve as neurotransmitters or are utilized for synthesization of neurotransmitters. Furthermore, using an animal model of septic encephalopathy, it is also suggested that these amino acid alteration affect the neurotransmitter in the brain. After cecal ligation and puncture, an animal model of septic encephalopathy, in rat, neurotransmitters serotonin and norepinephrine are altered and the altered patterns are correlated with these differences of amino acids (Freund HR et al, 1986). Hence, monoamine neurotransmitters are aberrant in septic encephalopathy. In addition, as shown in the following section, glutamatergic neurotransmission may be also affected and synaptic plasticity is disturbed (Imamura Y et al, 2011). Altogether, a whole body inflammation after sepsis 1) leads to blood brain barrier disruption, 2) affects the neurotransmitter levels and 3) may lead to be the symptoms of septic encephalopathy.

3. Scientific techniques of neurochemistry: How to see synaptic mechanism in septic brain

3.1 General mechanism of synaptic transmission in the brain

Neurochemical studies have been performed to clarify the temporal and spatial distribution of substances (i.e., proteins, enzymes, etc.) in brain. In the brain, neuronal cells which are major components of nervous system including brain, spinal cord constitute synapses. When the neurons are electrically excitable, neurotransmitters are released from the terminal of neuronal synapses (i.e., pre-synaptic terminals). On the other hand, the other neurons which receive the neurotransmitters possess receptors (i.e., post-synaptic terminals). The receptors binding to neurotransmtters activate electrically post-synaptic neurons and thereby the neuronal information is processed in the brain (i.e., synaptic transmission). Furthermore, the synaptic transmission is modulated by various chemical mediators (i.e., carbon monooxide (CO), nitric oxide (NO) etc.). These mediators are also critical to induce synaptic plasticity (i.e., plastic changes of electrical strength or efficacy in synaptic transmission). Hence, the neurotransmitters such as glutamate, acethylcholine and monoamine are major neurochemical substances, furthermore, these chemical mediators are necessary for normal synaptic transmission and synaptic plasticity. Aberrant expressions of these neurochemicals impede on the synaptic functions.

3.2 Sepsis affects synaptic receptor and its modulator

After sepsis, synaptic transmission seems to be affected. Although, to date, no reports are found for the direct evidence for the aberrant synaptic transmission by sepsis, sepsis-induced inflammatory cytokine alters the synaptic function. For example, interleukin-1β, which is up-regulated after sepsis, inhibits the expression of excitatory neurotransmitter receptors such as N-methyl-d-aspartate (NMDA) receptor (Coogan A & O'Connor JJ, 1997) and α-amino-3-hydoxy-5-methyl-4-isoxazolepropionic acid (AMPA) receptor (Lai AY et al, 2006). Conversely, interleukin -1β enhances the expression level of inhibitory neurotransmitter receptor, gamma-aminobutyric acid (GABA) receptor (Serantes R et al, 2006). In addition, NO synthase (NOS) were up-regulated after endotoxemia (El-Mas MM et al, 2011). These neurochemicals and their receptors are critical for synaptic transmission and plasticity. These findings suggest that the sepsis-induced downstream effects such as interleukin (i.e, cytokine) are possibly associated with imbalance of synaptic transmission and its plasticity.

3.3 Neuochemical methods to uncover the effect of sepsis

Our research group is challenging to tackle this issue (Imamura Y et al, 2011). To examine this, an animal model of sepsis is used. The methods are 'cecal ligation and puncture' and 'intraperitoneal injection of lipopolysaccharide (i.e., cell wall of gram negative bacteria)'. Compared to sham-operated animals (i.e., surgical operation without cecal ligation and puncture or intraperitoneally injected saline', the difference is determined by biochemical assays.

To visualize the dynamics of neurochemicals between the sham-operated mice and septic mice, our methods are 1) immunohistochemistry, 2) immunoblotting, 3) electrophysiology. These methods are well-established to examine the pathological condition by comparing with normal condition and its effect in animal models. For 1) immunohistochemistry, the procedure is summarized in Figure 1A. In brief, immunohistochemical staining is usually performed in following steps: 1) septic brain is fixed in 1-4% paraformaldehyde solution in

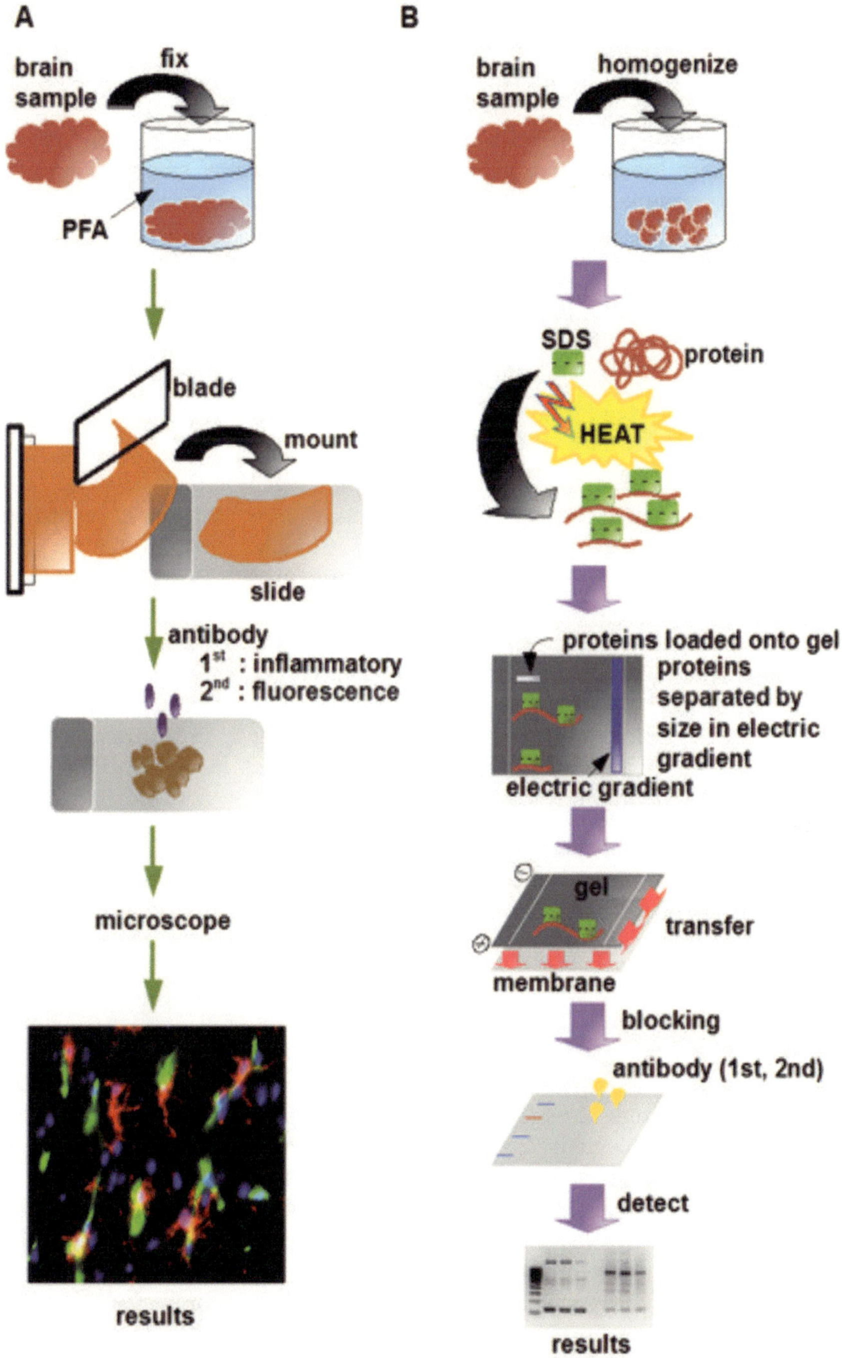

Fig. 1. Experimental procedure. A, immunohitochemistry. B, immunoblotting

phosphate buffered saline (PBS, pH = 7.2-7.4), 2) the brain is immersed in sucrose suspension for dehydration, embedded in optical cutting temperature compound and frozen in -80° C until use, 3) incubation with bovine serum albumin or serum solution to prevent non-specific binding of antibody which augments the background noise, 4) very thin brain slices (10 μm thick) are incubated with suspension including 1/100 -1/500 concentration (it depends on the specificity of antibody) of primary antibodies, 4) secondary antibodies which illuminate specific wavelength (usually 300-700nm) to visualize the spatial distribution of the proteins. Statistical analyses are performed between sham-operated groups and septic groups under normalization of each signal intensity and area by the number of cells (using nuclei staining).

Difference of amount of specific proteins after sepsis can be determined by immunoblotting (Figure 1B). Following suspension of tissue samples with homogenizer, the amount of total proteins in the brain mixture is measured by bradford protein assay for normalization between sample amounts. Then, the proteins are loaded with polyacrylamide gel electrophoresis. Amount of the subject protein samples transferred to PVDF membrane are determined by the specific primary antibody and the band intensities visualized by the enzyme, horse radish peroxidase, secondary antibody.

Brain function was determined by electrophysiology. Field excitatory post-synaptic potentials (fEPSPs) recordings detect population neuronal activity from recording electrode placed in extracellular neurons. Since, the method is available when neurons are arranged coordinately, it is useful for study of long-potentiation (LTP). For LTP study, our research group uses following methods: 1) making brain slices including hippocampus (300 μm thick) and maintaining them in perfusing solution (2-3 ml/min) of artificial cerebrospinal solution (ACSF) saturated with mixture gas of 95% oxygen and 5% carbon dioxide, 2) the hippocampal slices are transferred to the recording chamber and placed, 3) stimulation electrode is placed on perforant path fiber and recording is performed from neurons in dentate gyrus, 4) LTP is induced by the high frequency stimulation (100 Hz for 1sec x 4times, interval 5min)(Figure 2).

As a result, we find that endotoxemia after cecal ligation and puncture results in occludin (i.e., a marker for blood brain barrier) disruption (Figure 3), increased interleukin-1β on microglial cells in the hippocampus of the brain (Figure 4) and up-regulated interleukin-1β receptor on neurons (Figure 5).

Importantly, LTP is unable to induce in a group of septic mice (Figure 6B). Several lines of studies indicate that interleukin-1β inhibits LTP (Katsuki H et al, 1990; Ross FM et al, 2003). Due to these suggestions, we apply interleukin-1β antagonist before LTP induction. Interleukin-1β antagonist effectively cancels LTP deficiency after cecal ligation and puncture (Figure. 6C). These findings strongly suggest that increased interleukin in the brain after sepsis results in synaptic plasticity deficiency. Our approach successfully demonstrates the synaptic functional deficiency in septic encephalopathy and relevance of interleukin antagonist for the deficiency. However, there are still unclear for the following points: 1) effects of other inflammatory mediators, such as high mobility group box (HMGB)-1 (Zhao X et al, 2011) and tumor necrosis factor (Clark IA et al, 2010) which are expressed abundantly in the brain, to synaptic function, 2) How is the consequence of sepsis on the other brain regions except hippocampus. In following section, relevance of autonomic nervous system and a novel technology for the treatment and prescription of septic encephalopathy in the future are discussed.

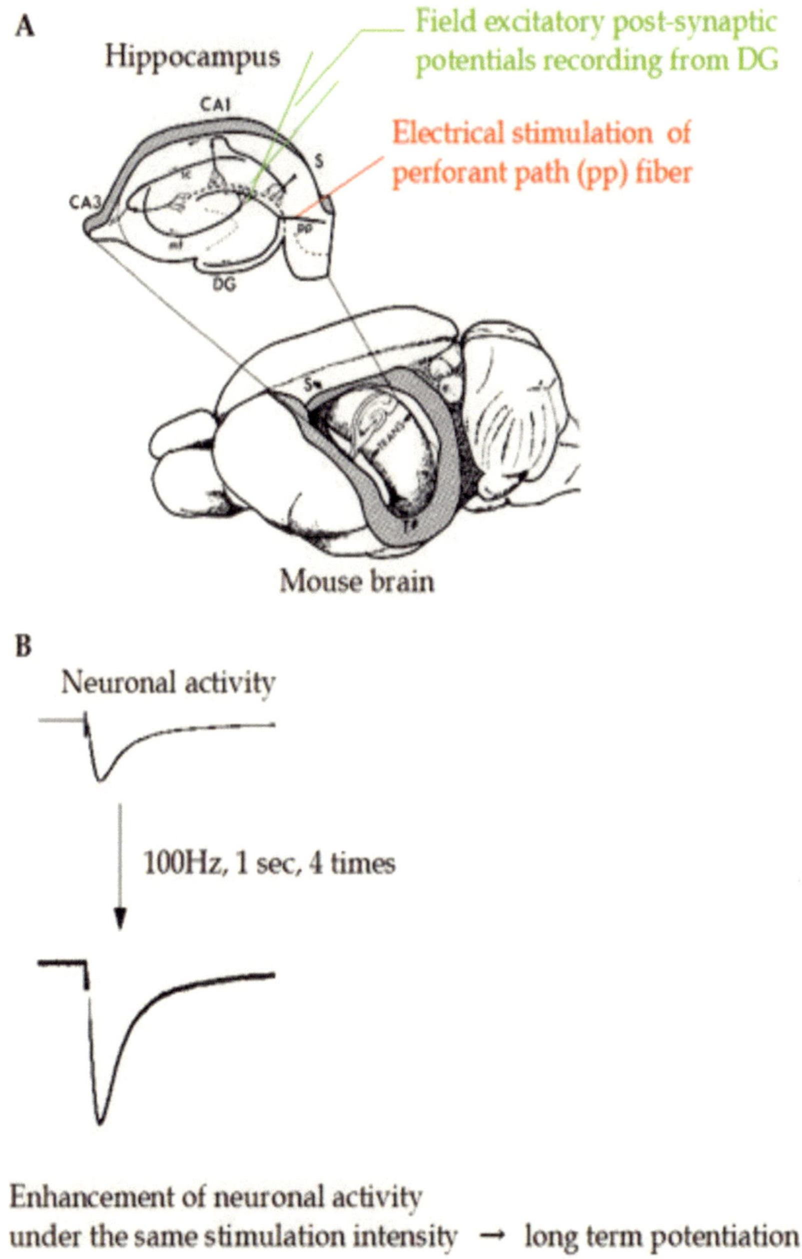

Fig. 2. Long-term potentialtion (LTP) in the hippocampal slices. A, hippocampal slices from mouse brain. B, LTP is induced by high frequency stimulation (100Hz for 1sec x 4 times, 5 min interval).

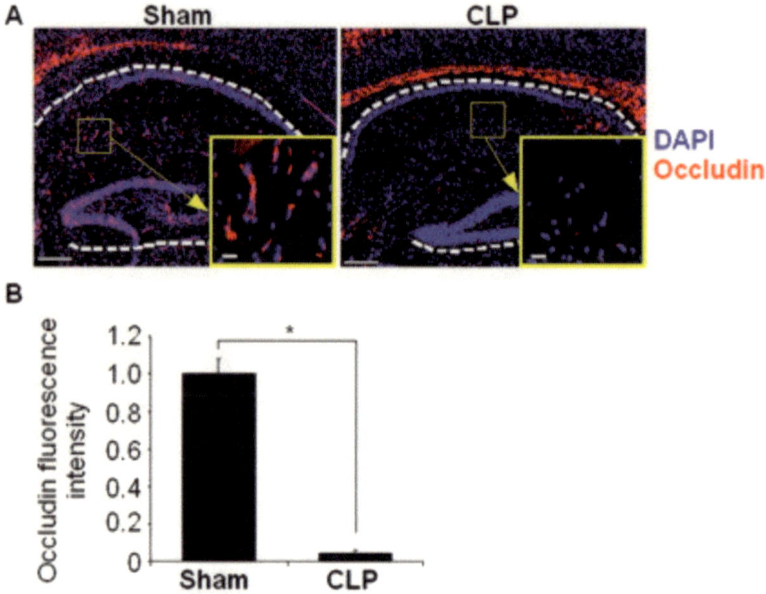

Fig. 3. Blood brain barrier disruption after cecal ligation and puncture. Occludin: a marker of blood brain barrier component. (A) Occludin immunoreactivity (a marker for blood brain barrier) in hippocampus from sham-operated mice (left panel) and cecal ligation and puncture (CLP) -treated mice (right panel). Magnified view shown in the lower right-hand corner. Red: occludin, blue: DAPI. (B) Lower intensity of occludin immunoreactivity in mice after cecal ligation and puncture (CLP). In subsequent experiments, areas of hippocampus surrounded by dashed white lines were analyzed. Exposure time of UV laser for immunodetection using each marker was normalized by DAPI signal intensities. Scale bar: 200 µm (lower magnification), 50 µm (higher magnification). Bar represents mean±SEM; (n = 7: sham, n = 6: cecal ligation and puncture). * $P < 0.01$ (Student t-test). (from Imamura et. al, (2011))

4. Cholinergic anti-inflammatory pathway

Sepsis affects autonomic systems (Tracey KJ, 2002). In lipopolysaccharide-injected rat (i.e., an animal model of sepsis), electrical threshold to induce action potentials are increased (i.e., hard neuronal firing) in vagus nerve (Huang J et al, 2010). This finding suggests that the vagus nerve activity is reduced after sepsis. Conversely, when the vagus nerve is electrically charged by external stimulation electrode, sepsis is alleviated (Huston JM et al, 2006; Rosas-Ballina M et al, 2008; Vida G et al, 2011). The vagus nerve projects parasympathetic neurons to all organs except adrenal gland and controls acetylcholinergic synaptic transmission. Wang and colleagues ,using α7-subunit of acetylcholine receptor knockout mice, demonstrate that vagus nerve stimulation inhibits excess release of tumor necrosis factor (i.e., activator of inflammatory mediator) in wild-type mice but not in acetylcholine knockout mice (Wang H et al, 2003). In addition, vagus nerve stimulation inhibits organ injury in the lung (Boland C et al, 2011), gut (Eisner F et al, 2011), spleen (Vida G et al, 2011) after sepsis. Furthermore, excess release of high mobility group box (HMGB)-1

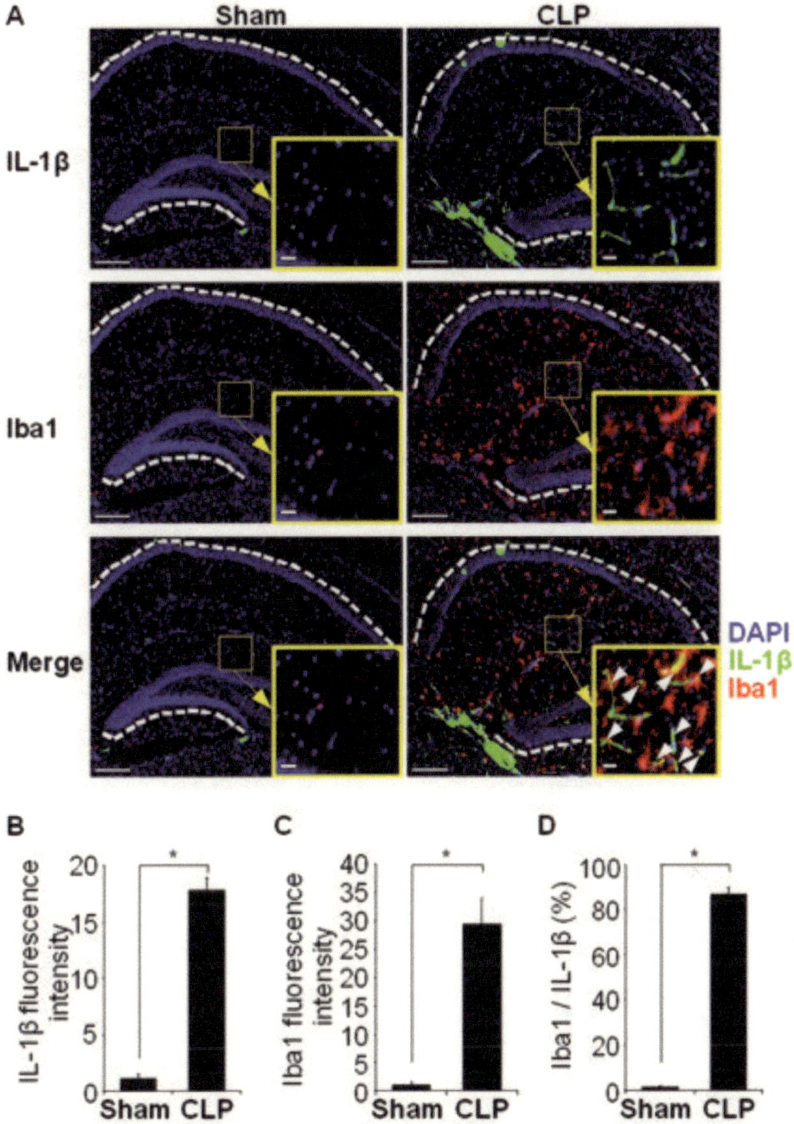

Fig. 4. Up-regulation of interleukin (IL)-1 on Iba1-positive cells after cecal ligation and puncture (CLP). (A) Staining of IL-1β immunoreactivity (green), Iba1 (marker for microglial and/or macrophage phagocytosis) immunoreactivity (red), and DAPI (nuclei, blue) in hippocampus from sham-operated mice (left panels) and CLP-treated mice (right panels). Magnified view shown in the lower right-hand corner. Merge: white arrow heads in higher magnification indicate Iba1 positive cells in the IL-1β positive cells. Scale bar: 200 μm (lower magnification), 50 μm (higher magnification). Higher intensity of IL-1β (B) and Iba1 (C) is seen in CLP mice. (D) The ordinate shows the percentage of Iba1-positive cells in the IL-1-positive cells. The numbers of immunopositive cells were counted between slices, respectively. Almost all (>80%) IL-1-positive cells are Iba1-positive after CLP. Bar represents mean±SEM; (n=7: sham, n=6: CLP-treated). * P<0.01 (Student t-test). (from Imamura et. al, (2011))

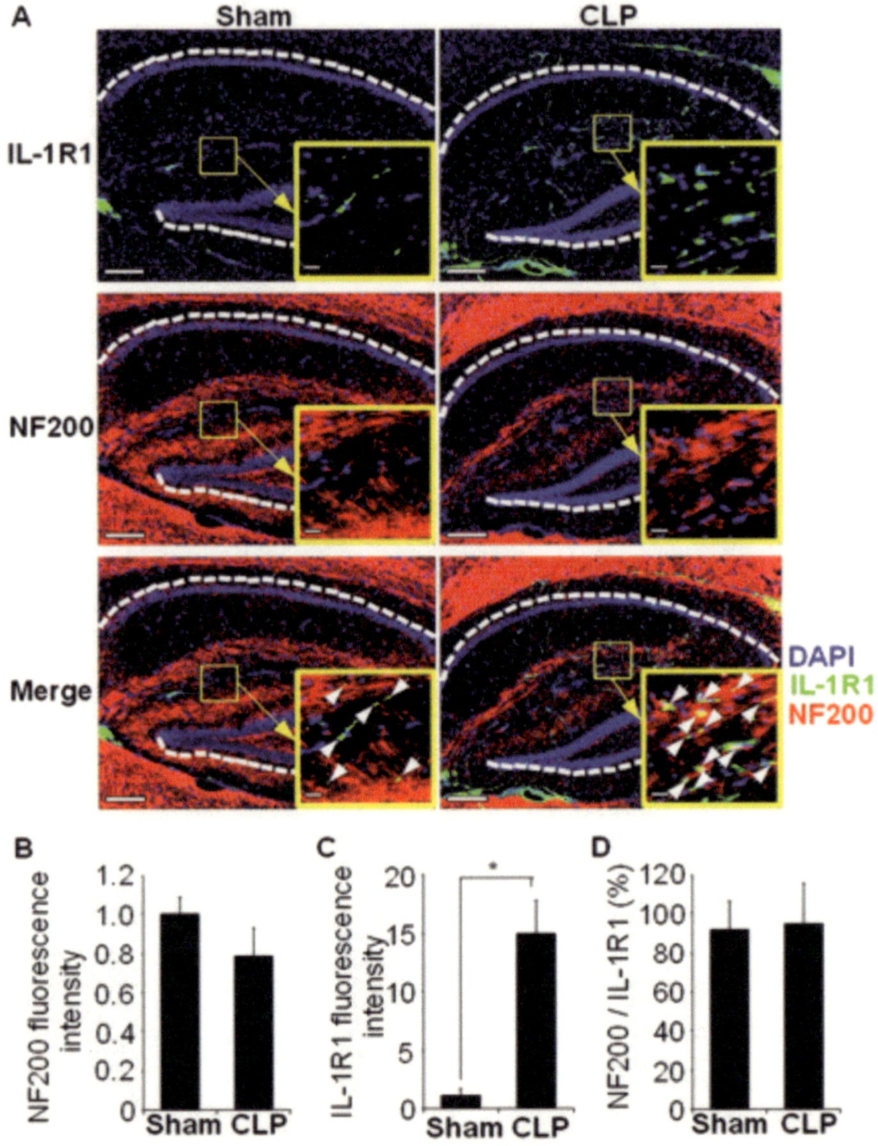

Fig. 5. Increased interleukin (IL)-1 receptor on hippocampal neurons after cecal ligation and puncture (CLP). (A) Triple staining of DAPI, type 1 IL-1 receptor (IL-1R1) and NF200. Blue: DAPI, green: IL-1R1, red: NF200. Magnified view shown in the lower right-hand corner. Merge: white arrow heads in higher magnification indicate NF200 positive cells in the IL-1R1 positive cells. Scale bar: 200 µm (lower magnification), 50 µm (higher magnification). (B) Slight decrease in neuronal fibers after CLP. (C) Increased IL-1R1 intensity after CLP. (D) Almost all (>90%) IL-1R1s are distributed on neurons. Bar represents mean±SEM; (n=7: sham, n=6: CLP-treated). * P<0.01 (Student t-test). (from Imamura Y et. al, (2011))

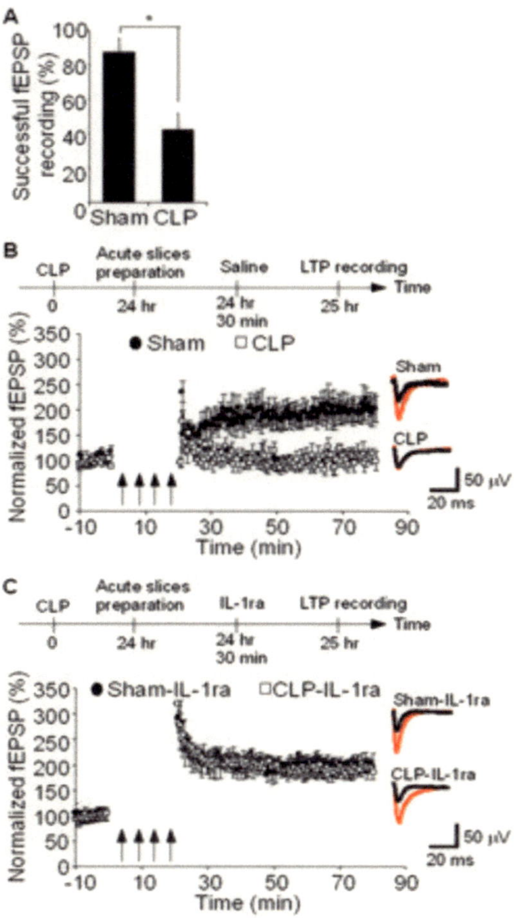

Fig. 6. Septic encephalopathy (SE) results in long-term potentiation (LTP) deficiency by interleukin (IL)-1β. (A) Successful rates of recording of field excitatory post-synaptic potentials (fEPSP) from sham-operated mice and cecal ligation and puncture (CLP)-treated mice. Hippocampal perforant-path fibers were stimulated with test pulse stimulation (30-s intervals, 200-µs duration, half-maximum intensity). fEPSP was recorded at the dentate gyrus at a distance of 300 µm from the stimulation electrode ($P<0.002$, Student *t*-test). (B) Schematic showing LTP deficiency after CLP. LTP experiments after CLP were performed according to the schematic, which shows the time course of the experimental procedure. LTP was induced by high-frequency stimulation (100 Hz x 1 s, four times, at 5-min intervals indicated by the arrows). Representative traces of baseline at $t = 0$ min and LTP at $t = 80$ min are shown. Black trace: baseline fEPSP, red trace: fEPSP after LTP. (C) Schematic showing cancelation of LTP deficiency in CLP-treated mice by IL-1R antagonist (IL-1ra). Brain slices were incubated in the presence of IL-1ra for 30 min before LTP recording. Note that IL-1ra is effective for LTP recovery after CLP, and IL-1ra reagent has no effect on fEPSP amplitudes. Bar represents mean±SEM; ($n = 7$: sham, $n = 7$: CLP-treated). * $p < 0.01$ (Student *t*-test). (from Imamura et. al, (2011))

(i.e., inflammatory mediator) from macrophage is also inhibited by vagus nerve stimulation (Wang H et al, 2004). The neural mechanism of vagus nerve stimulation is summarized in review (Tracey KJ, 2009). The review describes the mechanisms as follows: when sepsis is induced by endotoxemia, a site of infection imposes cytokine release through NF-kappaB (nuclear factor kappa-light-chain enhancer of activated B cells) activation. This signaling pathway accelerates cytokine production and thereby cell death via cytokine storm. When the vagus nerve from the brain stem is stimulated, it activates cholinergic anti-inflammatory pathway (efferent arc) and inhibits innate immune response in the spleen via activation of nicotinic acetylcholine receptor. The nicotinic acetylcholine receptor activation suppresses NF-kappaB activation via JAK2 (Janus kinase 2, cytokine receptor) - STAT3 (signal transducer and activator of transcription 3, transcription activator) pathway and the cytokine release.

Hence, vagus nerve stimulation may employ a high potential for the therapeutics of the clinical treatment of sepsis-related systemic inflammatory symptoms of septic encephalopathy.

5. Future prospect: A novel technology for tracking one molecule imaging in living organism

The findings we introduce are mainly resulted from neurochemical research assays using dissected tissues and cells. Recently, non-invasive methods such as functional magnetic resonance imaging (fMRI) are utilized to examine the brain dysfunction in living organism (rodents and human, etc). For example, in a mouse model of sepsis, accumulation of effusion by vasogenic edema is observed using fMRI in hippocampus and cortex (Bozza FA et al, 2010). Thus, fMRI is a powerful tool to find the damaged region in the brain because of the high spatial resolution. However, since fMRI detects the alteration of blood stream and estimates this as brain functional alteration, there is a limitation of the fMRI study. For example, it is hard to distinguish excitatory or inhibitory neurotransmission without a tag of each. In addition, because action potentials propagation between synapses in the brain is conducted within 100 msec (Wu JY et al, 2008), it is hard to track the temporal alteration of fast synaptic transmission with the time resolution (later than 1s) of fMRI (Tsao J, 2010). To reinforce these weak points, we address a novel nano-technology, '**one molecule imaging with quantum dot**' for the future research of septic encephalopathy.

A quantum dot (q-dot) is a nanometer-sized semiconductor particle (2-10 nm diameter). Cadmium selenide (CdSe) and cadmium telluride (CdTe) are well-utilized for the nano-materials of q-dot. When q-dot is placed in the crystallized structure, its electrical state for the fluorescence emission is discretized (Reed MA et al, 1988). As a result, only the fluorescence with a specific wavelength is amplified. Immunohistochemical studies using q-dot have a high signal to noise ratio and few photobleaching(Chan WC, Nie S, 1998). Although normal q-dots are hydrophobic, it can be changed their property to hydrophilic in order to apply to living organism. Jin T et. al (2008) develop a water-soluble glutathione-coated Q-dots. They successfully detect q-dot signals in the lymph node in the mouse (Fig. 7). In addition, q-dot is available to track the molecules expressed in the brain. Intraperitoneally-injected q-dots can be found in the brain (Kato S et al, 2010; Yeh TK et al, 2011). Hence, q-dot is a hopeful nano-material to track a molecule associated with sepsis. Then, how do we track the molecules associated with septic encephalopathy with q-dots?

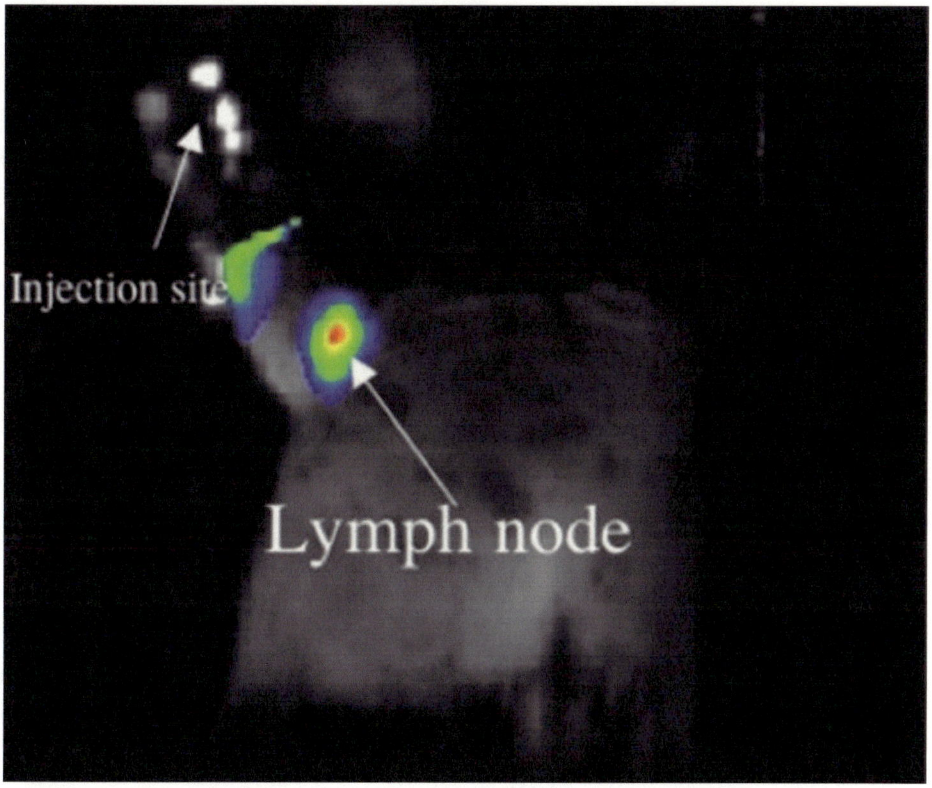

Fig. 7. Lymph node imaging by near infra-red q-dot (from Jin T. (2008))

Near infrared spectroscopy (NIRS) uses near infra-red region (800-2500nm) of light. Since the light in near infra -red range can pass through the skull, reach to the surface of the brain and coincide with the fast event-related responses in human recorded by electroencephalograms (Medvedev AV et al, 2010), it has been used to track cerebral hemodynamics (Gratton E et al, 2005) and human brain activity(Perrey S, 2008). On the other hand, trials to apply q-dots to the molecules associated with pathological states are performed in neurosurgery (Taghva A et al, 2010) and brain tumor (Popescu MA & Toms SA, 2006). Therefore, if labeling of brain with q-dot which emits the fluorescence light in the near infra-red region becomes successful, we can track the molecules associated with septic encephalopathy in higher temporal resolution in the future studies.

6. Conclusion

Septic encephalopathy is associated with many kinds of inflammatory cytokines, receptors, chemicals such as interleukin family, toll-like receptor, tumor necrosis factor, high mobility group box. Since these inflammatory molecules induce systemic inflammatory response in the whole body and affect the brain function after blood brain barrier disruption, they occurs neurological symptoms such as vasogenic edema, aberrant synaptic transmission and plasticity. In addition, the weakness of vagus nerve after septic encephalopathy is related to the pathophysiology. Although the molecular mechanisms for sepsis are explained, medical intervention for patients of septic encephalopathy in intensive care unit is largely limited to symptomatic treatment. The reason is that spatial and temporal dynamics of the functional molecular patterns in various organs for the cause of septic symptoms are still not fully described. For the future medical treatment of septic encephalopathy, we address the two possibilities. First, to find the spatial and temporal dynamics of molecules, q-dots labeled with molecules for septic encephalopathy are recorded with both of near infra-red spectroscopy and functional magnetic resonance imaging. Second, to alleviate the symptoms, it may be effective to stimulate the vagus nerve with non-invasive method, since vagus nerve stimulation can reduce the excess inflammatory cytokine release by mechanisms of nicotinic acetylcholine receptor activation, which inhibits apoptotic and necrotic pathway of cells and tissues after sepsis. These novel approaches will progress the intervention for the sepsis and its encephalopathy in the future studies.

7. Acknowledgement

This work is supported by cooperation of Trauma and Acute Critical Care Center, Osaka University Hospital and Units for Liveable Cities, Kyoto University, JAPAN

8. References

Boland C, Collet V, Laterre E, Lecuivre C, Wittebole X & Laterre PF (2011) Electrical vagus nerve stimulation and nicotine effects in peritonitis-induced acute lung injury in rats. *Inflammation*, Vol. 34, No. 1, pp. 29-35, ISSN 0360-3997

Bolton CF, Young GB & Zochodne DW (1993) The neurological complications of sepsis. *Ann Neurol*, Vol. 33, No. 1, pp. 94-100, ISSN 0364-5134

Bone RC, Balk RA, Cerra FB, Dellinger RP, Fein AM, Knaus WA, Schein RM & Sibbald WJ (1992) Definitions for sepsis and organ failure and guidelines for the use of innovative therapies in sepsis. The ACCP/SCCM Consensus Conference Committee. American College of Chest Physicians/Society of Critical Care Medicine. *Chest*, Vol. 101, No. 6, pp. 1644-1655, ISSN 0012-3692

Bozza FA, Garteiser P, Oliveira MF, Doblas S, Cranford R, Saunders D, Jones I, Towner RA & Castro-Faria-Neto HC (2010) Sepsis-associated encephalopathy: a magnetic resonance imaging and spectroscopy study. *J Cereb Blood Flow Metab*, Vol. 30, No. 2, pp. 440-448, ISSN 0271-678X

Casanova E, Fehsenfeld S, Mantamadiotis T, Lemberger T, Greiner E, Stewart A F & Schutz G (2001) A CamKIIalpha iCre BAC allows brain-specific gene inactivation *Genesis*, Vol. 31, No. 1, pp. 37-42, ISSN 1846-1920

Chan WC & Nie S (1998) Quantum dot bioconjugates for ultrasensitive nonisotopic detection. *Science*, Vol. 281, No. 5385, pp. 2016-2018, ISSN 0036-8075

Clark IA, Alleva LM & Vissel B (2010) The roles of TNF in brain dysfunction and disease. *Pharmacol Ther*, Vol. 128, No. 3, pp. 519-548, ISSN 0163-7258

Coogan A & O'Connor JJ (1997) Inhibition of NMDA receptor-mediated synaptic transmission in the rat dentate gyrus in vitro by IL-1 beta. *Neuroreport*, Vol. 8, No. 9-10, pp. 2107-2110, ISSN 0959-4965

Dellinger RP, Levy MM, Carlet JM, Bion J, Parker MM, Jaeschke R, Reinhart K, Angus DC, Brun-Buisson C, Beale R, Calandra T, Dhainaut JF, Gerlach H, Harvey M, Marini JJ, Marshall J, Ranieri M, Ramsay G, Sevransky J, Thompson BT, Townsend S, Vender JS, Zimmerman JL & Vincent JL (2008) Surviving Sepsis Campaign: international guidelines for management of severe sepsis and septic shock: 2008. *Crit Care Med*, Vol. 36, No. 1, pp. 296-327, ISSN 0090-3493

Eisner F, Jacob P, Frick JS, Feilitzsch M, Geisel J, Mueller MH, Kuper MA, Raybould HE, Konigsrainer I & Glatzle J (2011) Immunonutrition with long-chain fatty acids prevents activation of macrophages in the gut wall. *J Gastrointest Surg*, Vol. 15, No. 5, pp. 853-859, ISSN 1091-255x

El-Mas MM, Fan M & Abdel-Rahman AA (2011) Upregulation of cardiac NOS due to endotoxemia and vagal overactivity contributes to the hypotensive effect of chronic ethanol in female rats. *Eur J Pharmacol*, Vol. 650, No. 1, pp. 317-323, ISSN 0014-2999

Flierl MA, Stahel PF, Rittirsch D, Huber-Lang M, Niederbichler AD, Hoesel LM, Touban BM, Morgan SJ, Smith WR, Ward PA & Ipaktchi K (2009) Inhibition of complement C5a prevents breakdown of the blood-brain barrier and pituitary dysfunction in experimental sepsis. *Crit Care*, Vol. 13, No.1, pp. R12, ISSN 1364-8535

Freund H, Atamian S, Holroyde J & Fischer JE (1979) Plasma amino acids as predictors of the severity and outcome of sepsis. *Ann Surg*, Vol. 190, No. 5, pp. 571-576, ISSN 0003-4932

Freund HR, Muggia-Sullam M, LaFrance R, Holroyde J & Fischer JE (1986) Regional brain amino acid and neurotransmitter derangements during abdominal sepsis and septic encephalopathy in the rat. The effect of amino acid infusions. *Arch Surg*, Vol. 121, No. 2, pp. 209-216, ISSN 0004-0010

Freund HR, Ryan JA Jr & Fischer JE (1978) Amino acid derangements in patients with sepsis: treatment with branched chain amino acid rich infusions. *Ann Surg*, Vol. 188, No. 3, pp. 423-430, ISSN 0004-0010

Gratton E, Toronov V, Wolf U, Wolf M & Webb A (2005) Measurement of brain activity by near-infrared light. *J Biomed Opt*, Vol. 10, No. 1, pp. 11008, ISSN 1083-3668

Harrison C (2010) Sepsis: calming the cytokine storm. *Nat Rev Drug Discov*, Vol. 9, No. 5, pp. 360-361, ISSN 1474-1776

Hotchkiss RS & Nicholson DW (2006) Apoptosis and caspases regulate death and inflammation in sepsis. *Nat Rev Immunol*, Vol. 6, No. 11, pp. 813-822, ISSN 1474-1733

Huang J, Wang Y, Jiang D, Zhou J & Huang X (2010) The sympathetic-vagal balance against endotoxemia. *J Neural Transm*, Vol. 117, No. 6, pp. 729-735, ISSN 0300-9564

Huston JM, Ochani M, Rosas-Ballina M, Liao H, Ochani K, Pavlov VA, Gallowitsch-Puerta M, Ashok M, Czura CJ, Foxwell B, Tracey KJ & Ulloa L (2006) Splenectomy inactivates the cholinergic antiinflammatory pathway during lethal endotoxemia and polymicrobial sepsis. *J Exp Med*, Vol. 203, No.7, pp. 1623-1628, ISSN 0022-1007

Imamura Y, Wang H, Matsumoto N, Muroya T, Shimazaki J, Ogura H & Shimazu T (2011) Interleukin-1beta causes long-term potentiation deficiency in a mouse model of septic encephalopathy. *Neuroscience*, Vol. 187, pp. 63-69, ISSN 0306-4522

Jin T, Fujii F, Komai Y, Seki J, Seiyama A & Yoshioka Y (2008) Preparation and characterization of highly fluorescent, glutathione-coated near infrared quantum dots for in vivo fluorescence imaging. *Int J Mol Sci*, Vol. 9, No. 10, pp. 2044-2061, ISSN 1422-0067

Kafa IM, Ari I & Kurt MA (2007) The peri-microvascular edema in hippocampal CA1 area in a rat model of sepsis. *Neuropathology*, Vol. 27, No. 3, pp. 213-220, ISSN 0919-6544

Kato S, Itoh K, Yaoi T, Tozawa T, Yoshikawa Y, Yasui H, Kanamura N, Hoshino A, Manabe N, Yamamoto K & Fushiki S (2010) Organ distribution of quantum dots after intraperitoneal administration, with special reference to area-specific distribution in the brain. *Nanotechnology*, Vol. 21, No. 33, pp. 335103, ISSN 0957-4484

Katsuki H, Nakai S, Hirai Y, Akaji K, Kiso Y & Satoh M (1990) Interleukin-1 beta inhibits long-term potentiation in the CA3 region of mouse hippocampal slices. *Eur J Pharmacol*, Vol. 181, No. 3, pp. 323-326, ISSN 0014-2999

Kim KD, Zhao J, Auh S, Yang X, Du P, Tang H & Fu YX (2007) Adaptive immune cells temper initial innate responses. *Nat Med*, Vo. 13, No. 10, pp. 1248-1252, ISSN 1078-8956

Lai AY, Swayze RD, El-Husseini A & Song C (2006) Interleukin-1 beta modulates AMPA receptor expression and phosphorylation in hippocampal neurons. *J Neuroimmunol*, Vol. 175, No. 1-2, pp. 97-106, ISSN 0165-5728

Medvedev AV, Kainerstorfer JM, Borisov SV, Gandjbakhche AH & Vanmeter J (2010) "Seeing" electroencephalogram through the skull: imaging prefrontal cortex with fast optical signal. *J Biomed Opt*, Vol. 15, No. 6, pp. 061702, ISSN 1083-3668

Nauwynck M & Huyghens L (1998) Neurological complications in critically ill patients; septic encephalopathy, critical illness polyneuropathy. *Acta Clin Belg*, Vol. 53, No. 2, pp. 92-97

Papadopoulos MC, Lamb FJ, Moss RF, Davies DC, Tighe D & Bennett ED (1999) Faecal peritonitis causes oedema and neuronal injury in pig cerebral cortex. *Clin Sci (Lond)*, Vol. 96, No. 5, pp. 461-466, ISSN 0143-5221

Perrey S (2008) Non-invasive NIR spectroscopy of human brain function during exercise. *Methods*, Vol. 45, No. 4, pp. 289-299, ISSN 1046-2023

Pfister D, Schmidt B, Smielewski P, Siegemund M, Strebel SP, Ruegg S, Marsch SC, Pargger H & Steiner LA (2008) Intracranial pressure in patients with sepsis. *Acta Neurochir Suppl*, Vol. 102, pp. 71-75, ISSN 0065-1419

Popescu MA & Toms SA (2006) In vivo optical imaging using quantum dots for the management of brain tumors. *Expert Rev Mol Diagn*, Vol. 6, No. 6, pp. 879-890, ISSN 1473-7159

Reed MA, Randall JN, Aggarwal RJ, Matyi RJ, Moore TM & Wetsel AE (1988) Observation of discrete electronic states in a zero-dimensional semiconductor nanostructure. *Phys Rev Lett*, Vol. 60, No.6, pp. 535-537, ISSN 0031-9007

Rittirsch D, Flierl MA & Ward PA (2008) Harmful molecular mechanisms in sepsis. *Nat Rev Immunol*, Vol. 8, No. 10, pp. 776-787, ISSN 1474-1733

Rosas-Ballina M, Ochani M, Parrish WR, Ochani K, Harris YT, Huston JM, Chavan S & Tracey KJ (2008) Splenic nerve is required for cholinergic antiinflammatory pathway control of TNF in endotoxemia. *Proc Natl Acad Sci U S A*, Vol. 105, No. 31, pp. 11008-11013, ISSN 1091-6490

Ross FM, Allan SM, Rothwell NJ & Verkhratsky A (2003) A dual role for interleukin-1 in LTP in mouse hippocampal slices. *J Neuroimmunol*, Vol. 144, No. 1-2, pp. 61-67, ISSN 0165-5728

Serantes R, Arnalich F, Figueroa M, Salinas M, Andres-Mateos E, Codoceo R, Renart J, Matute C, Cavada C, Cuadrado A & Montiel C (2006) Interleukin-1beta enhances GABAA receptor cell-surface expression by a phosphatidylinositol 3-kinase/Akt pathway: relevance to sepsis-associated encephalopathy. *J Biol Chem*, Vol. 281, No.21, pp. 14632-14643, ISSN 0021-9258

Sharshar T, Annane D, de la Grandmaison GL, Brouland JP, Hopkinson NS & Francoise G (2004) The neuropathology of septic shock. *Brain Pathol*, Vol. 14, No. 1, pp. 21-33, ISSN 1015-6305

Sprung CL, Peduzzi PN, Shatney CH, Schein RM, Wilson MF, Sheagren JN & Hinshaw LB (1990) Impact of encephalopathy on mortality in the sepsis syndrome. The Veterans Administration Systemic Sepsis Cooperative Study Group. *Crit Care Med*, Vol. 18, No. 8, pp. 801-806, ISSN 0090-3493

Streck EL, Comim CM, Barichello T & Quevedo J (2008) The septic brain. *Neurochem Res*, Vol. 33, No. 11, pp. 2171-2177, ISSN 0364-3190

Taghva A, Khalessi AA, Kim PE, Liu CY & Apuzzo ML (2010) From atom to brain: applications of molecular imaging to neurosurgery. *World Neurosurg*, Vol. 73, No. 5, pp. 477-485, ISSN 1878-8750

Tracey KJ (2002) The inflammatory reflex. *Nature*, Vol. 420, No. 6917, pp. 853-859, ISSN 0028-0836

Tracey KJ (2009) Reflex control of immunity. *Nat Rev Immunol*, Vol. 9, No. 6, pp. 418-428, ISSN 1474-1733

Tsao J (2010) Ultrafast imaging: principles, pitfalls, solutions, and applications. *J Magn Reson Imaging*, Vol. 32, No. 2, pp. 252-266, ISSN 1053-1807

Vida G, Pena G, Deitch EA & Ulloa L (2011) alpha7-cholinergic receptor mediates vagal induction of splenic norepinephrine. *J Immunol*, Vol. 186, No. 7, pp. 4340-4346, ISSN 0022-1767

Wang H, Liao H, Ochani M, Justiniani M, Lin X, Yang L, Al-Abed Y, Wang H, Metz C, Miller EJ, Tracey KJ & Ulloa L (2004) Cholinergic agonists inhibit HMGB1 release and improve survival in experimental sepsis. *Nat Med*, Vol. 10, No. 11, pp. 1216-1221, ISSN 1078-8956

Wang H, Yu M, Ochani M, Amella CA, Tanovic M, Susarla S, Li JH, Wang H, Yang H, Ulloa L, Al-Abed Y, Czura CJ & Tracey KJ (2003) Nicotinic acetylcholine receptor alpha7 subunit is an essential regulator of inflammation. *Nature*, Vo. 421, No. 6921, pp. 384-388, ISSN 0028-0836

Ward PA (2010) Role of C5 activation products in sepsis. *ScientificWorldJournal*, Vol. 10, pp. 2395-2402

Wu JY, Xiaoying Huang & Chuan Zhang (2008) Propagating waves of activity in the neocortex: what they are, what they do. *Neuroscientist*, Vol. 14, No. 5, pp. 487-502, ISSN 1073-8584

Yeh TK, Wu JP, Chang LW, Tsai MH, Chang WH, Tsai HT, Yang CS & Lin P (2011) Comparative tissue distributions of cadmium chloride and cadmium-based quantum dot 705 in mice: Safety implications and applications. *Nanotoxicology*, Vol. 5, No. 1, pp. 91-97, ISSN 1743-5390

Zhao X, Kuja-Panula J, Rouhiainen A, Chen YC, Panula P & Rauvala H (2011) High mobility group box-1 (HMGB1; amphoterin) is required for zebrafish brain development. *J Biol Chem*, Vol. 286, No. 26, pp. 23200-23213, ISSN 0021-9258

8

The Neurochemical Anatomy of Trigeminal Primary Afferent Neurons

Nikolai E. Lazarov
Medical University-Sofia, Bulgaria

1. Introduction

Somatic sensations of the head and orofacial region are transmitted by trigeminal primary afferent neurons, a group of neural-crest derived sensory neurons. Most of their cell bodies are located outside the central nervous system, residing in the trigeminal ganglion (TG) but some of them lie centrally within the brainstem, in the mesencephalic trigeminal nucleus (MTN).

The TG represents a cranial analog of the dorsal root ganglia in the peripheral nervous system (Darian-Smith, 1973). TG neurons have a unique morphology and are classified as pseudounipolar (Krastev, 2009). Their centripetal processes, usually called trigeminal primary afferents, carry somatosensory information from mechanoreceptors, thermoreceptors and nociceptors in the face, the oral and nasal cavities, and through the portio major of the trigeminal nerve reach their main target neurons in the trigeminal sensory nuclei (Fig. 1), where they establish synaptic contacts with their perikarya (for reviews, see Darian-Smith, 1973; Dubner et al., 1978; Kruger & Young, 1981).

Mesencephalic trigeminal neurons are considered centrally displaced ganglion cells but in spite of their curious central location they maintain some characteristics of neural crest cell derivates. The great majority of MTN cells are large pseudounipolar neurons which provide the innervation of the masticatory muscle spindles and periodontal ligament pressoreceptors. Their central branches enter the trigeminal motor nucleus and several other brainstem nuclei around it (Fig. 1), where they make excitatory synaptic connections with jaw-closing motor or premotor (last-order interneurons) neurons, respectively (see Capra & Dessem, 1992 for a review). Unlike the TG cells however, MTN neurons receive synaptic inputs that potentially modify their output (reviewed in Lazarov, 2000). MTN neurons are also remarkable insofar as they, without an exception, constitute one distinct functional class of trigeminal sensory neurons, i.e. proprioceptive neurons (Jerge, 1963; Cody et al., 1972). Due to their ectopic location within the brain, in addition to this classical function, some mesencephalic trigeminal neurons may act as interneurons capable of integrating peripheral and central information prior to reaching the trigeminal motor nucleus (Kolta et al., 1995). The functional segregation between peripheral and central primary afferent neurons is a further striking feature of the mammalian trigeminal sensory system (reviewed in Waite, 2004).

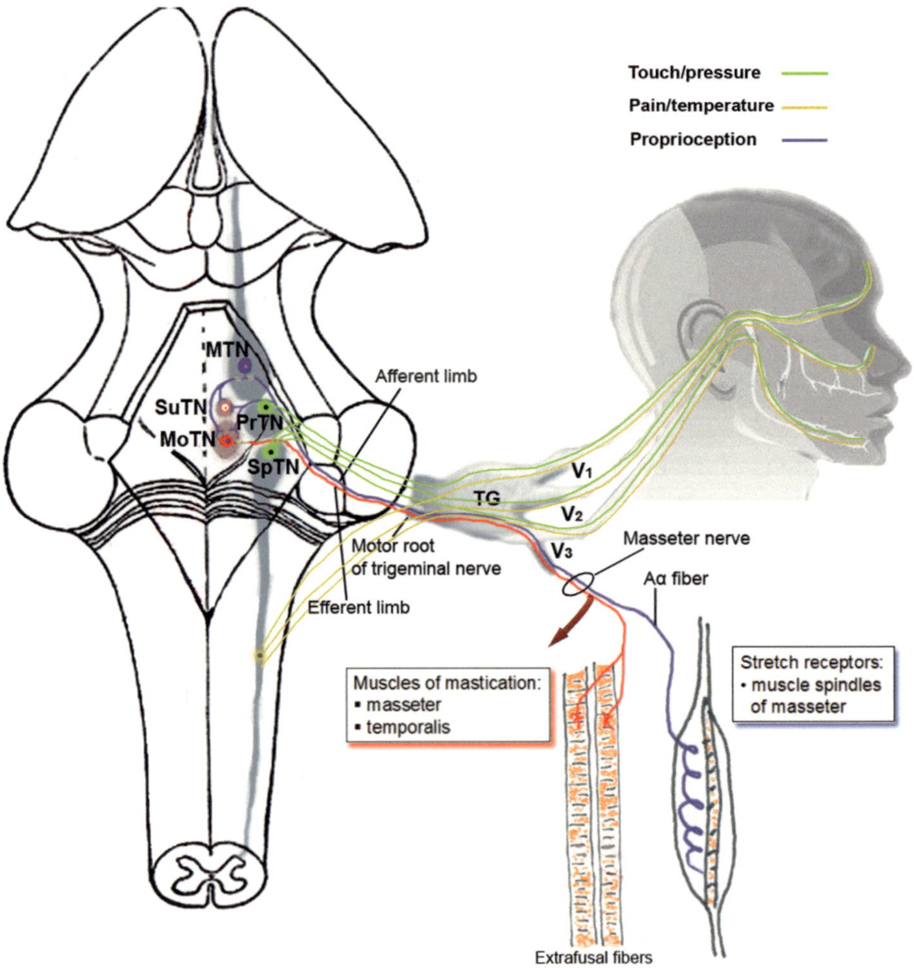

Fig. 1. Schematic illustration of the trigeminal pathways for orofacial somatic sensation. Tactile (touch and pressure) sensibility of the face and mouth is relayed through the large diameter Aβ axons of the trigeminal ganglion (TG) neurons to the principal sensory trigeminal nucleus (PrTN) and rostral part (subnucleus oralis and interpolaris) of the spinal trigeminal nucleus (SpTN), while pain and thermal sensations from the orofacial structures are conveyed by the thin Aδ and C trigeminal primary afferents to the subnucleus caudalis of the SpTN. Proprioceptive sensation from the face and oral cavity is transmitted directly or through premotor neurons in the supratrigeminal nucleus (SuTN) to the motor trigeminal nucleus (MoTN) via the central processes of primary afferent neurons whose pseudounipolar cell bodies are mainly located in the mesencephalic trigeminal nucleus (MTN). The efferent limb (depicted in red) of the reflex arc producing jaw closure (jaw jerk or masseteric reflex) is formed by the axons of trigeminal motoneurons traveling through the motor root of the trigeminal nerve to the muscles of mastication. V_1, V_2, V_3, ophthalmic, maxillary and mandibular divisions of the trigeminal nerve, respectively.

A commonly held hypothesis in neurobiology is that neuronal morphology frequently mirrors chemical neuroanatomy and also neurons in different functional pathways, within which they lie, can be characterized by their neurochemical profiles. In this respect, the various neuronal populations that constitute the TG and MTN can be identified not only on the basis of their morphological characteristics and electrophysiological properties but also by their neurochemical content. This issue is of key importance since the transmitter content of different neuronal populations often correlates well with their target projections. It is assumed that trigeminal primary afferent neurons exhibit pathway-specific patterns of neurochemical expression, a concept that has been called chemical coding (Costa et al., 1986). It has also been proposed that the differently fated embryonic migration, synaptogenesis, and peripheral and central target field innervation could affect the individual neurochemical phenotype of TG and MTN neurons. Trigeminal primary afferent neurons utilize a wide variety of chemical neuromessengers for synaptic transmission and possess the ability to produce relevant adaptive changes in their neurochemical phenotype in response to environmental cues (for recent reviews, see Lazarov, 2002, 2007).

This chapter therefore focuses on the chemical neuroanatomy of the TG and MTN neuronal populations under normal conditions, the role and relationship of neurotransmitters and their corresponding receptors in relaying orofacial sensations and also refers to the interactions with other atypical neuromessengers and neurotrophic factors. We have also surveyed the chemical plasticity of developing and mature TG and MTN neurons to gain insight into their structural and functional properties in an altered neurochemical balance, with special reference to trigeminal nerve degeneration and regeneration, and clinical implications.

2. Neurotransmitters and their known receptors in trigeminal primary afferent neurons

Using immunohistochemistry and *in situ* hybridization histochemistry we have identified distinct neuronal, partly chemically coded, subpopulations in the intact TG and MTN. Our findings suggest that trigeminal primary afferent neurons are chemically heterogeneous and appear to use various chemical neuromediator candidates for synaptic transmitters. These include classical and peptide transmitters, calcium-binding proteins as neuronal markers and other neuroactive molecules (Table 1). In addition, we have demonstrated that TG and MTN neurons receive inputs from different groups of neurons that contain multiple transmitter substances. Indeed, both the TG and MTN receive catecholaminergic, nitrergic and peptidergic innervation in the form of perineuronal arborizations encircling in a basket-like manner the perikarya of large unstained neurons. It is assumed that the pericellular baskets can function as a key communication medium between immunopositive projections and immunonegative neuronal somata in the orofacial somatosensory information processing. Last but not least, it is now well established that the cell bodies of TG and MTN neurons are richly endowed with postsynaptic receptors for a huge array of neurotransmitters and neuroactive substances.

2.1 Classical transmitters

In recent years, a variety of 'classical' transmitter substances and their receptors have been associated with subsets of trigeminal primary afferent neurons. Among them are amino acids (both excitatory and inhibitory) and monoamines. On the other hand, our studies

Neuroactive substance	Trigeminal ganglion	Mesencephalic trigeminal nucleus	Effect of activation
Neurotransmitters and their known receptors			
Glutamate (GLU)	+	+IC, F/T	Membrane depolarization: fast and/or slow excitation
AMPA receptors	-	+IC	Postsynaptic rapid excitation
KA receptors	+	+IC	Presynaptic modulation of transmitter release
NMDA receptors	-	+IC	Presynaptic auto- or postsynaptic heteroreceptors
metabotropic receptors	mGluR5	mGluR1α, mGluR2/3	Heteroreceptors and/or autoreceptors: neuronal excitability and transmission regulation
Aspartate	+	±IC, F/T	Membrane depolarization
Gamma aminobutyric acid (GABA)	+	±IC, F/T	Membrane hyperpolarization: inhibition Membrane depolarization: excitation
$GABA_A$ receptor	+ (γ1, γ2 subunits)	+IC	Postsynaptic fast inhibition
$GABA_B$ receptor	+ ($GABA_{B2}$ subunit)	+IC	Presynaptic regulation of K^+, Ca^{2+}channels: long-term inhibition of synaptic transmission Postsynaptic facilitation of ATP, SER and DA release
Glycine	-	-	
Dopamine (DA)	-	+F/T	Membrane hyperpolarization
D_1 receptor	-	+IC	Masseter muscle proprioceptive processing
D_2 receptor	+	+P	Periodontal ligament proprioceptive processing
Serotonin (SER)	-	+F/T	Membrane depolarization: modulation of sodium currents
5-HT_{1B} receptor	+	ND	

Neuroactive substance	Trigeminal ganglion	Mesencephalic trigeminal nucleus	Effect of activation
5-HT_{1D} receptor	+	ND	
5-HT_{1F} receptor	+	ND	
5-HT_{2} receptor	ND	+IC	Intracellular transduction pathways activation
5-HT_{3} receptor	ND	+IC	Postsynaptic slow excitation
5-HT_{7} receptor	+	ND	
Histamine (HIS)	ND	+F/T	Membrane depolarization
H_1 receptor	+	+IC	Postsynaptic excitation
H_3 receptor	-	+P	Presynaptic inhibition
Adenosine 5'-triphosphate (ATP)	ND	+F/T	Membrane depolarization Facilitation of neuronal discharge
P2X_2 receptor	+	+	Postsynaptic fast excitation
P2X_3 receptor	-	+	Presynaptic modulation of neurotransmitter release
P2X_4 receptor	+	+	
P2X_5 receptor	+	+	
P2X_6 receptor	+	+	
P2Y receptor	-	-	
Nitric oxide (NO)	+	+IC	Membrane depolarization: promotion of intracellular cGMP synthesis;
Carbon monoxide (CO) Neuropeptides and their known receptors	+	+	tonic background stimulation
Substance P (SP)	+	-	Neuromodulation
SP receptor	-	-	Neuromodulation
SOM ss2(b) receptor	-	+	
Neuropeptide Y (NPY)	+	-	
NPY Y_1 receptor	+	-	
NPY Y_2 receptor	+	-	
NPY Y_5 receptor	-	+	
Enkephalin (ENK)	+	-	Neuromodulation
Preprodynorphin	+	ND	
μ-opioid receptor	+	-	
δ-opioid receptor	+	-	
κ-opioid receptor	+	-	
Orexin (hypocretin) A	-	+F/T	Neuromodulation
Orexin receptor-1	ND	+	Induction of calcium currents

Neuroactive substance	Trigeminal ganglion	Mesencephalic trigeminal nucleus	Effect of activation
Orexin (hypocretin) B	-	+F/T	Neuromodulation
Orexin receptor-2	ND	+	Induction of calcium currents
Calcium-binding proteins			
Parvalbumin (PV)	+	+IC	Intracellular Ca buffering Selective marker for orofacial proprioceptors
Calbindin D-28 (CB)	+	+IC	Selective neuronal marker
Calretinin (CR)	+	+IC	NA
S-100	+	-	Selective glial marker
Neurocalcin	+	-	
Osteocalcin	+	+IC	Selective marker
Osteopontin	+	+IC	Selective marker
Peptide 19	+	+IC	Selective marker
Nerotrophic factors and their receptors			
Pan-neurotrophin receptor $P75^{NTR}$	+	+IC	Increase in mature neuronal excitability
Nerve growth factor (NGF)	+	+IC,F	Trophic support
TrkA	+	+IC	NA
Brain derived neurotrophin factor (BDNF)	+	+IC	Trophic support Neuronal phenotype maintenance
Neurotrophin 4-5 (NT-4/5)	+	-	NA
TrkB	+	+IC	Neuronal survival
Neurotrophin 3 (NT-3)	+	+IC	Trophic support Modulation of neuronal electric activity
TrkC	+	+IC	Neuronal survival
Glial cell line-derived neurotrophic factor (GDNF)			Trophic support
GFRalpha-1 receptor	+	+IC	NA
Ret receptor	+	+IC	NA

IC, intracellular; F/T, fibers and/or terminals; ND, no data; NA, not analyzed; P, pontine portion of MTN

Table 1. Overview of the established and putative neuromessengers, specific markers, neurotrophic factors and their known receptors and major functions in orofacial somatosensory signaling under normal conditions

clearly show that other classical neurotransmitters, such as acetylcholine, and purines like adenosine 5'-triphosphate (ATP) and its metabolite adenosine are not present in TG and MTN neurons.

2.1.1 Amino acids

There are three major amino acid neurotransmitters in the nervous system: glutamic acid (L-glutamate), gamma-amino butyric acid (GABA) and glycine. Glutamate (Glu) is considered a promising excitatory transmitter of the trigeminal primary afferent neurons in rats and cats. It is stored in both the large and small TG cells (Wanaka et al., 1987; Azérad et al., 1992; Stoyanova et al., 1998), and, in addition, all five known kainate (KA) ionotropic receptor subtypes are expressed in a majority of them, occasionally combined with metabotropic mGluR5 subunits (Sahara et al., 1997). Experimental results indicate that the metabotropic Glu receptors play an important role in the somatic sensation of TG neurons together with the ionotropic ones (Araki et al., 1993). Functional contribution of peripherally localized Glu receptors in acute and chronic pain processing is amply documented (Carlton, 2001) and further discussed in Section 5. Similarly, most mammalian MTN neurons contain glutaminase, a major enzyme involved in the biosynthesis of Glu (Kaneko et al., 1989; Turman & Chandler, 1994b) and receive glutamatergic synaptic input (Chandler, 1989; Copray et al., 1990). Further, recent research has revealed that vesicular glutamate transporter 1 is expressed in the cell bodies as well as both in the central axon terminals and peripheral sensory endings of MTN neurons in newborn and adult rats (Pang et al., 2006). Finally, all ionotropic receptor subtypes, AMPA (Mineff et al., 1998; Pelkey & Marshall, 1998; Petralia & Wenthold, 1992; Turman et al., 2000), KA and NMDA (Pelkey & Marshall, 1998; Petralia et al., 1994a,b,c; Turman et al., 2002) and some metabotropic subtypes, mGluR1α, mGluR5 and mGluR2/3 (Turman et al., 2001) have been localized on mesencephalic trigeminal neurons. Iontophoretic studies have also suggested that monosynaptic transmission between jaw-closing primary afferents and jaw-closing motoneurons is mediated primarily by non-NMDA receptors (Chandler, 1989), whereas both NMDA and non-NMDA receptors have been involved in the transmission from premotoneurons to jaw-opening motoneurons (Katakura & Chandler, 1990). The identification of mGluR subunits in mesencephalic trigeminal neurons which receive, as already noted, axosomatic input and/or synthesize mGluRs in the soma and then translocate the proteins to central terminals suggests that these, along with NMDA but not AMPA receptors, may function as either auto- or heteroreceptors in central MTN terminals (Turman et al., 2001).

GABA and glycine are both known to participate in the control of masticatory rhythms (Chandler et al., 1985). The presence of glycine, however, has been reported neither in TG nor in MTN neurons (Copray et al., 1990; Lazarov, 2002). On the other hand, GABA is localized in a substantial number of TG cells in rats (Szabat et al., 1992) and cats (Stoyanova et al., 1998). In addition, TG cells express two distinct GABA receptors, ionotropic $GABA_A$ γ1 and γ2 subunits, mostly co-localized in the same neuron (Kondo et al., 1994), and metabotropic $GABA_{B2}$ (Durkin et al., 1999). Our experiments have also pointed out that a subpopulation of smaller MTN cells, presumably interneurons, which are apposed to large mesencephalic trigeminal neurons, may be of a GABAergic nature (Lazarov & Chouchkov,

1995b; Lazarov, 2000, 2002). Besides, molecular biological studies have shown that pseudounipolar MTN neurons respond to GABA and accordingly express $GABA_A$ receptor α2, β2 and γ2 subunit mRNAs (Hayar et al., 1997; Ishii & Kang, 2002), and $GABA_{B1}$ (Margeta-Mitrovic et al., 1999) and $GABA_{B2}$ (Li et al., 2001) receptor proteins. In line with this evidence, several research groups have consequently reported GABAergic innervation of the MTN in rats (Copray et al., 1990; Ginestal & Matute, 1993), guinea pigs (Turman & Chandler, 1994a), rabbits (Kolta et al., 1991a,b) and cats (Lazarov & Chouchkov, 1995b; Lazarov, 2000, 2002). Ultrastructural and confocal laser-scanning studies have additionally revealed the existence of GABAergic synapses upon the cell bodies of MTN neurons in the rat (Chen et al., 2001). Taken together, these results suggest that excitability of jaw muscle spindle afferents is presynaptically controlled by interneurons containing GABA and these play an important role in modulating the jaw-jerk reflex.

Our findings now permit definitive conclusions that both TG and MTN neurons contain a stable concentration of Glu and GABA as possible transmitters. It still remains to clarify the possible synaptic relationships between Glu- and GABA-immunoreactive profiles in the TG and MTN, and their related functional implications. We have observed that both amino acid neurotransmitters are present in separate subpopulations of trigeminal neurons, e.g. most large neurons are glutamatergic while certain small neurons are GABAergic (Lazarov, 2002). Thus, it seems likely that excitatory amino acid(s) may be the transmitter(s) of large myelinated non-nociceptive primary afferents whereas GABA is probably the mediator of smaller trigeminal neurons, as suggested by Salt & Hill (1983).

2.1.2 Monoamines

Out of the six different types of monoamines, catecholamines [dopamine (DA), noradrenaline (NA) and adrenaline (A)] are the most important group. The earliest evidence for the catecholaminergic innervation of the TG sprang from the works of Santini (1966) and Lukás et al. (1970). In these initial studies by using immunocytochemistry with antiserum against tyrosine hydroxylase (TH), the rate-limiting enzyme of catecholamine synthesis, the immunostained neurons within the ganglion were proposed to be DAergic. Applying an antibody against the DA molecule itself, it is now inferred that TH-containing neurons in the TG do not synthesize DA but they are enveloped by DAergic pericellular arborizations (Kummer et al., 1990). A similar pattern has been observed for NA within the ganglion: TG cells are immunonegative to the NA-synthesizing enzyme, dopamine-β-hydroxylase (Katz et al., 1983) but receive dense NAergic innervation from postganglionic sympathetic neurons (Kummer et al., 1990). Hence, immunohistochemical evidence has suggested that TG neurons do not utilize catecholamines as possible transmitters but are under the influence of catecholaminergic afferent fibers of presumable sympathetic origin. Clinical observations imply that primary afferent neurons whose cell bodies reside in the TG express receptors for DA of the D_2 subtype, although these receptors do not function as autoreceptors but rather have a role in pain syndromes involving the head and the neck (Peterfreund et al., 1995).

In the same way, none of the MTN neurons in rats (Copray et al., 1990; Liem et al., 1997), cats (Lazarov & Chouchkov, 1995b) and humans (Usunoff et al., 1997) exhibits immunoreactivity for DA or NA but their perikarya are closely surrounded by fine DAergic and NAergic baskets originating from the A9 and A10 cell groups, the substantia nigra and ventral tegmental area, and the neighboring locus coeruleus, respectively. Our immunohistochemical and *in situ* hybridization experiments have further shown that MTN neurons express the two principal subtypes of DA receptors, though they are unequally distributed within the nucleus: as in muscle spindle afferents, D_1 receptors are found throughout the MTN of the rat, whereas D_2 receptors and periodontal afferent neurons are confined to the caudal part of the nucleus (Lazarov & Pilgrim, 1997). This suggests that the two types of primary afferents may be modulated differentially by DA. The DA input to the MTN may modulate neuronal excitability, rates of transmitter synthesis, transport and release, as well as the number of pre- and postsynaptic receptors (Liem et al., 1997).

In addition to the catecholaminergic input, the TG and MTN are under the influence of another monoaminergic system, namely the serotoninergic system, one of the oldest amine systems in the brain. Indeed, several immunohistochemical studies have revealed the serotoninergic supply of the mammalian TG and MTN. In fact, we have found that the TG lacks intrinsic serotonin (SER)-containing cells but a plexus of varicose nerve fibers of extraganglionic origin covers the immunonegative neurons in a basket-like manner (Chouchkov et al., 1988). Likewise, SER is present neither in the cell bodies nor in neuronal processes of MTN neurons (Lazarov & Chouchkov, 1995a). However, SERergic axonal varicosities reaching the MTN from the mesopontine and medullary raphe nuclei form a pericellular basket-like network around immunonegative mesencephalic trigeminal neurons (Tashiro et al., 1989). Electron microscopic studies show direct synaptic contacts between SER-containing terminals and MTN perikarya in rats (Copray et al., 1991; Liem et al., 1993; Liem & Copray, 1996; Li et al., 2000), cats (Lazarov & Chouchkov, 1995a) and rabbits (Kolta et al., 1993). Out of the large group of the serotonin receptors, also known as 5-hydroxytryptamine receptors or 5-HT receptors, the presence of high affinity 5-HT_{1B} and 5-HT_{1D} receptors is demonstrated at protein and mRNA levels in TG neurons of the rat (Bruinvels et al., 1992; Wotherspoon & Priestley, 2000), guinea pig (Bonaventure et al., 1998) and human (Longmore et al., 1997). The mRNA encoding the 5-HT_7 receptor is also found to be expressed in the human TG (Terrón et al., 2001). At the same time, in the rat MTN an abundant number of the 5-HT_2 (Cornea-Hébert et al., 1999), 5-HT_3 (Morales et al., 1998) and 5-HT_4 receptor (Lazarov, 2007) have been established. SER has been hypothesized to be involved in trigeminal pain (Moskowitz et al., 1979) and SER antagonists have important clinical implications for antimigraine drug development (discussed later in Section 5). Recent data indicate that SER plays a significant role in the control of oral-motor activity as well (Li et al., 2000) and various oral-motor disorders, either drug induced or occurring as a consequence of injury, might result from altered modulation of sodium channels by SER (Tanaka & Chandler, 2006).

As in the case of catecholamines, both peripheral and central trigeminal primary afferent neurons do not contain histamine in their cell bodies but MTN neuronal perikarya receive a direct histaminergic input by hypothalamic descending fibers (Inagaki et al., 1987). In particular, neuronal somata throughout the whole rostrocaudal length of the nucleus are encircled by histaminergic fibers and their terminals, many of the latter forming axo-somatic synapses on them. Our laboratory has provided immunohistochemical evidence for the presence of two distinct histamine receptor subtypes, H_1 and H_3, in the rat MTN, albeit in different neuronal subpopulations (Lazarov & Gratzl, 2006). Overlapping with muscle spindle afferents, histamine H_1 receptors are scattered throughout the full extent of the MTN, whereas H_3 receptors and periodontal afferent neurons are restricted to its caudal region. Since H_1 receptors are excitatory, histamine may act in this way on MTN neurons via the axo-somatic synapses, as suggested by Inagaki et al. (1987). Conversely, the H_3 receptors do not function only as autoreceptors but also as heteroreceptors, modulating MTN neuronal activity and release of other neurotransmitters from them. Therefore, it seems that the majority of MTN neurons respond to central histamine via the activation of H_1 and inhibition of H_3 receptors, thus participating in the control of feeding behavior.

The purine nucleosides adenosine and ATP can function as neurotransmitters or neuromodulators in both the CNS and PNS by signaling through specific receptors termed adenosine (also known as P1) and P2 receptors, respectively. Our attempts fail to identify purines in the TG and MTN neurons, though the latter are innervated by adenosine deaminase-containing projections from the hypothalamus (Nagy et al., 1986). Inasmuch as their terminals contacting MTN perikarya also express immunoreactivity to histamine, it seems that the two substances may coexist there, as noted by Yamamoto et al. (1988). In the TG, an abundant expression of the adenosine A1 receptor protein (Schindler et al., 2001) and the six P2X receptor subtypes (Xiang et al., 1998; Dunn et al., 2001) has been shown in a large number of small nociceptive neurons, which may be suggestive of a role of these receptors in analgesia. The existence of excitatory adenosine $A2_A$ receptors (Rosin et al., 1998) and $P2X_2$, $P2X_3$, $P2X_4$, $P2X_5$ and $P2X_6$ purinoceptors (Khakh et al., 1997; Patel et al., 2001; Lazarov, 2007) has been shown in populations of large proprioceptive mesencephalic trigeminal neurons. P2X receptors, which are ATP-gated cation channels, have been shown to be responsible for mediating both fast excitatory responses in central and peripheral neurons and the presynaptic modulation of neurotransmitter release (reviewed by Ralevic & Burnstock, 1998). It is likely that certain ionotropic P2X purinoceptors may be involved in the processing of proprioceptive information, thus suggesting a potentially important physiological role of ATP at sites where it is released extracellularly (Khakh et al., 1997).

2.2 Neuropeptides

Neuropeptides are a heterogeneous group of several hundred biologically active peptides, present in neurons of both the mammalian CNS and PNS, and involved in the transmission of signals as pure neuromediators or neuromodulators. In general, a large number of putative peptide transmitters have been identified in neurons and/or neuronal processes in the TG, but none of them has been found in mammalian MTN neuronal somata under normal conditions (see reviews by Lazarov, 1994, 2002, 2007). In particular, two subpopulations of primary afferent neurons, containing neuroactive peptides are distinguished in the TG: a number of substance P (SP)-, neurokinin A (NKA)-, calcitonin gene-related peptide (CGRP)-, cholecystokinin (CCK)-, somatostatin (SOM)-, vasoactive intestinal polypeptide (VIP)- and galanin (GAL)-immunoreactive ganglion cells with small- and medium-sized somata, and relatively fewer in number larger-sized neuropeptide Y (NPY)- and peptide 19 (PEP 19)-immunoreactive trigeminal neurons. It is noteworthy that SP, CGRP, SOM and GAL are found in small-diameter TG cells with conduction velocities in the C-fiber range, PEP 19 and NPY are usually expressed in the large ones, and opioid peptides, CCK, VIP and pituitary adenylate cyclase activating polypeptide (PACAP) are observed in both small and large trigeminal neurons (Kummer & Heym, 1986; Weihe, 1990). Our previous studies have also revealed that although devoid of synaptic contacts, TG neurons express an array of peptide receptors for SP, CGRP, CCK, opioid peptides and NPY (see Lazarov, 2002, and references therein). The occurrence of peptidergic arborizations of extrinsic origin around the perikarya of some TG neurons suggests that these are under the influence of multiple biologically active peptides.

Several lines of physiological evidence indicate that SP and CGRP have excitatory effects and depolarize TG neurons (Otsuka & Konishi, 1976; Spigelman & Puil, 1991) while SOM and opioids appear to be inhibitory in nature (Randic & Miletic, 1978). Considering the important functional segregation of TG cells into large (mostly mechanoreceptive) and small (mainly nociceptive) neurons, it is not surprising that the neuropeptides SP and CGRP have been associated with the transmission of nociceptive impulses. However, small-diameter primary afferent neurons not only transmit noxious messages to central neurons but are also active in the periphery in mediating axon-reflex mechanisms and an inflammation response (Couture & Cuello, 1984; Foreman, 1987). Therefore, it is more reasonable to consider the role of SP and CGRP both in the transmission of sensory information from the periphery and in the peripheral effector functions such as neurogenic vasodilatation (McCarthy & Lawson, 1989, 1990), thus implicating them into the pathophysiology of migraine. Moreover, SOM can interact with SP causing inhibition of its release and consequent neurogenic vasodilatation (Brodin et al., 1981). Several lines of evidence indicate that sensory opioids could act synergistically with SP to induce histamine release (Foreman, 1987) and GAL may have an inhibitory effect on the nociceptive transmission (see Xu et al., 1990, and references therein). Therefore, all these peptides play a co-transmitter role and may have significant functions in disease mechanisms associated with head pain in humans (for a recent review, see Edvinsson & Uddman, 2005).

In view of the presence of a large number of neuropeptides in the TG cells, their absence in the morphologically homologous MTN neurons is rather surprising. Obviously, the absence of a peptide in two distinct populations of trigeminal primary afferent neurons indicates that different peptides subserve diverse sensory modalities, at least under normal conditions. In extension of previous inferences, we are confident that there exists a complex coexistent relationship between the chemoanatomical constellation of trigeminal primary afferent neurons and sensory modality transmission (Lazarov, 2002). Notwithstanding that intact mesencephalic trigeminal neurons do not express neuropeptides in their perikarya they are largely influenced by various synaptic inputs. Relevant to the dense peptidergic innervation of the nucleus, receptors for certain peptides have been localized on MTN neuronal somata (reviewed in Lazarov, 2002, 2007). According to Copray et al. (1990) it is likely that the synaptic input on MTN cells only affects the neuronal activity expressed at the central and peripheral terminals, in a more indirect mode and after a longer interval. The authors claim that this points to the presence and involvement of receptor systems that are not directly linked to ion channels but to a much slower secondary-messenger-induced biochemical effector cascade. As argued in the Introduction section, MTN neurons may operate under some circumstances like traditional "integrate and fire" neurons in addition to typically sensory neurons, which generally do not receive synaptic contacts at their somata and do not discharge repetitively (Del Negro & Chandler, 1997).

2.3 Gaseous neuromessengers

In addition to the classical and peptide transmitters, several second messenger systems may be involved in orofacial signal processing. During the last decade the free radical gases nitric oxide (NO) and carbon monoxide (CO) have been found to function as putative messenger molecules both in central and peripheral trigeminal primary afferent neurons. Indeed, recent research in animals and humans has shown that the neurons in the MTN, along with TG cells, contain heme oxygenase, the CO-synthesizing enzyme (Uddman et al., 2004; Fan et al., 2008). The enzyme responsible for the synthesis of NO, nitric oxide synthase (NOS), and its histochemical marker, NADPH-diaphorase are expressed both in TG and MTN neurons in rats (Stoyanova & Lazarov, 2005), rabbits (Kolesar et al., 2006) and cats (Lazarov & Dandov, 1998) as well. The nerve cell bodies containing NOS are predominantly of small to medium size and they also express SP and CGRP (Edvinsson et al., 1998). Moreover, all these studies demonstrate that large unstained trigeminal neurons are innervated by nitrergic fibers and that NO increases the excitability and modifies other electrophysiological properties of these cells. Rather than acting via traditional receptors on the postsynaptic membrane, NO exerts its effect by diffusion into the adjacent neurons to activate soluble guanylyl cyclase, leading to an increase in intracellular cGMP. Furthermore, NO possibly produces an increase in MTN neuronal electrotonic coupling and therefore is involved in the synchronization of their activity too. Finally, there is functional evidence to support the involvement of NO in the development and maintenance of inflammation and pain (Yun et al., 1996). It has been suggested that as in other regions, both gaseous messengers possibly interact in a complex, dynamic way in the orofacial sensory processing where CO, being a more stable gas, may be responsible for basal activity and provide tonic background stimulation, whereas surges of NO transiently amplify or deliver phasic signaling (Fan et al., 2008).

2.4 Calcium-binding proteins

The calcium-binding proteins (CaBPs) represent one of the physiological systems for maintaining calcium ion intracellular homeostasis (reviewed in Baimbridge et al., 1992). In the last two decades they have received increased attention due to their implementation as specific markers for large-sized primary afferent subpopulations and their involvement in many calcium-dependent phenomena in the nervous system both under normal and abnormal conditions (Anderssen et al., 1993). Neuron-specific CaBPs, parvalbumin (PV), calbindin D-28k (CB) and calretinin (CR), are observed to be expressed predominantly in the large-sized TG and MTN neurons (Ichikawa et al., 1994; Lazarov et al., 1998), a subpopulation with inward calcium current. Interestingly, a typical glial cell-specific protein, S-100, is also localized, mostly co-expressed with CB, in TG neurons of epibranchial placode origin (Ichikawa et al., 1997). In addition, immunoreactivity to neurocalcin, a newly identified member of the neuronal CaBP family, has been shown in large or medium in size TG cells (Iino et al., 1998). Two additional newly discovered bone matrix CaBPs, osteocalcin and osteopontin, have recently been co-localized with PV in the cell bodies of both TG and

MTN neurons (Ichikawa et al., 1999; 2000). Data from ongoing experiments have provided compelling evidence that CaBPs might function as intracellular calcium transporters or as a buffering system for cell protection during neuronal activity in normal circumstances. They may also affect calcium-dependent neuronal properties such as excitability, release of neurotransmitters and resistance to excitotoxicity in mammals (see Baimbridge et al., 1992). Additionally to intracellular roles, S-100 may be involved in the neurotrophic functions of trigeminal primary afferent neurons.

3. Neurotrophic factors and neurotrophin receptors

Neurotrophic factors or neurotrophins are a family of structurally and functionally related polypeptides that promote neuronal differentiation, survival and neurochemical plasticity during development by signaling via both a low-affinity p75 receptor and high-affinity transmembrane receptors belonging to the Trk proto-oncogene family. It has been proposed that neurotrophins and their receptors play an essential role in long-term neural trophics and trophic mechanisms during adult life, and may also regulate phenotypic expression. Recent advances in neuroscience have shown that in addition to their trophic support actions, neurotrophins share many functional properties with classical neurotransmitters as well and may function as neuromodulators in neuronal signaling.

In fact, the concepts of neurotrophin-dependent survival, neurotrophin switching and neurotrophin co-operativity have largely arisen from works on the trigeminal system (Davies, 1997). Indeed, it is now well documented that developing trigeminal afferent neurons respond to all four known neurotropic factors, albeit in different capacities. Specifically, the localization of the nerve growth factor (NGF), brain-derived neurotrophin factor (BDNF), neurotrophin-3 (NT-3) and NT-4/5 has been demonstrated in discrete neuronal subsets of the human TG at an age ranging from 23 weeks of gestation to adulthood (Quartu et al., 1997). In early development, embryonic TG neurons depend for their survival on the action of the BDNF, NT-3 or NT-4/5 but not on NGF (Buchmann & Davies, 1993). Accordingly, within the developing TG neurotrophin receptor expression is high around the time of target innervation (Ernfors et al., 1992) and, moreover, two or more Trk receptor isoforms are co-expressed in embryonic rat TG neurons (Moshnyakov et al., 1996). Similarly, MTN neurons display modality specific neurotrophin dependence in their development (Davies, 1997). For instance, during the earliest stages of neurogenesis the developing MTN neurons are transiently supported by BDNF and NT-3, but not by NGF (Copray & Liem, 1993; Davies et al., 1987). Recent work on the human MTN also suggests an active role for the glial cell line-derived neurotrophic factor and possibly other cognate ligands in the trophism from prenatal life to adulthood of the cells subserving the proprioceptive sensory transmission (Quartu et al., 2006). Studies on the neurotrophin receptor expression indicate the presence of p75 (Henry et al., 1993) and all the Trk receptor types within the adult (Yamuy et al., 2000) and developing MTN (Williams et al., 1995). Besides, most MTN neurons express multiple Trk isoforms (Jacobs & Miller, 1999). These results conclusively support the notion that MTN neurons are sensitive to the direct effects of more than one neurotrophin. Recent studies provide some of the initial evidence that the neurotrophin requirements of trigeminal primary afferent neurons are related to a specific sensory modality. For example, the high-affinity NGF receptor, TrkA, is considered a marker for peptide-containing nociceptors. Interestingly, Trk receptors appear to be co-expressed with SP and CGRP in a population of small trigeminal primary afferent neurons (Quartu et al., 1996).

4. Trigeminal response to injury and neurochemical plasticity of trigeminal primary afferent neurons

Research on putative neuromessengers in the trigeminal sensory system has reached another peak of interest over the last decade since it was shown that primary afferent neurons possess the ability to make adaptive changes in their transmitter phenotype in response to environmental cues (Table 2). It is now well known that injury to the peripheral trigeminal nerve results in nerve cell degeneration and that peripheral nerve damage evokes dynamic alterations in the levels of expressions of neurotrophins, neuropeptides and their receptors in the projection areas of injured axons, a phenomenon called chemical plasticity (Hökfelt et al., 1994). Indeed, after axotomy of the inferior alveolar nerve, there is a marked reduction in the total SP and CGRP expression in TG neurons (Elcock et al., 2001) and their release is largely enhanced by peripheral inflammation (Neubert et al., 2000). Conversely, the NPY and VIP levels are dramatically increased in axotomized TG neurons (Sasaki et al., 1994; Fristad et al., 1998). It is generally presumed that neuropeptides repressed after axotomy participate normally in sensory transmission while those induced may function as neurotrophic factors involved in the response to injury and in axonal regeneration (Nielsch & Keen, 1989). The axonal signals induced in response to nerve injury activate several signaling pathways of genes in the neuronal cell bodies that may lead to two opposing outcomes: cell death or regenerative response. In effect, peripheral nerve injury causes the surviving neurons to shift their activity away from normal maintenance and neurotransmission toward a regenerative state (Navarro, 2009). It is thought that changes in gene expression after axonal injury are due to a blockage of NGF retrograde axonal flow from the periphery to the cell body. This may explain why both high (TrkA) and low (p75) affinity neurotrophin receptor transcripts in the TG neurons increase after tooth injury (Wheeler et al., 1998)

As it can be inferred from Table 2, axotomy-induced alterations in the expression of neuroactive substances in MTN neurons include a long-lasting decrease (down-regulation) in the content of CaBPs, up-regulation of NO and some neurotrophins, and a *de novo* synthesis of certain neuropeptides, such as GAL, NPY and CGRP (see Lazarov, 2002, 2007, and references therein). A commonly shared view is that a characteristic of neuropeptides is the plasticity in their expression, reflecting the fact that release has to be compensated by *de novo* synthesis in the neuronal body (Navarro et al., 2007). It may be postulated that the newly synthesized neuropeptides can enhance MTN neuronal survival and neurite regeneration in the adaptive processes following nerve injury. Therefore, a peptide involvement in the proprioceptive function develops mainly in abnormal conditions. Navarro and co-workers (2007) also state that injured neurons respond by up-regulation of neurotrophins, either by autocrine or paracrine sources, and that additional exogenous supply of neurotrophic factors may further enhance the regenerative response of peripherally axotomized neurons. It should be noted that the survival of proprioceptors during the early postnatal period is probably dependent upon BDNF since its application to the proximal stump of the transected masseteric nerve delays the loss of MTN neurons after the cut (Ichikawa et al., 2007). On the other hand, altered levels of CaBPs may be related to adequate cell body response since the sensitivity of damaged neurons to the intracellular

Neuroactive substance	Trigeminal ganglion	Mesencephalic trigeminal nucleus	Effect
	Injury consequence		
Neurotransmitters			
NO	Upregulation	Upregulation	Cell death or defenc
Neuropeptides			
SP	Downregulation		
CGRP	Downregulation	De novo synthesis	Supportive role in
NPY	Upregulation	De novo synthesis	Cell protection
GAL	Upregulation	De novo synthesis	Cell regeneration
PACAP	Upregulation	De novo synthesis Increase in neurotrophin responsiveness	Increase in neurotrophin responsiveness
Calcium-binding proteins			
Parvalbumin (PV)	Downregulation	Downregulation	Cell defence
Calbindin D-28 (CB)	Downregulation	Downregulation	Cell survival
Neurotrophic factors and their receptors			
NGF	Upregulation	Upregulation	Peptide synthesis induction Enhancement membrane Enhancement of membrane potential oscillations
TrkA	Upregulation	Upregulation	Enhanced neuronal survival and maintenance
BDNF	Upregulation	Upregulation	Cell protection

Table 2. Summary of the injury-induced alterations in the expression of neuroactive substances and their effects on mammalian trigeminal primary afferent neurons

calcium concentration is different from that of intact ones. A logical explanation for the reported down-regulation in CaBP expression may be the actual reduction of the MTN cell number following periphery axotomy (Ichikawa et al., 2007). This would be in line with the suggestion that persistently increased levels of NOS in mesencephalic trigeminal neurons may be involved in slowly progressive nerve cell death following nerve damage because they may lead to an augmented vulnerability of the neurons to calcium-mediated neurotoxicity. Alternatively, it is reasonable to speculate that the possible endogenous production of NO might underlie a defense mechanism of the neurons against nerve injury and, thus, improve survival and active regeneration of MTN neurons.

In summary, these findings provide compelling evidence that the content of the neurochemicals in both central and peripheral trigeminal primary afferent neurons is not static and their level may vary in case of marked changes in the environmental conditions, thus implying neuroplasticity as another major attribute of theirs.

5. Clinical relevance

Trigeminal primary afferent neurons have been the focus of intense research also because of their contribution to acute and chronic pain states, and the important role played by trigeminal nociceptive pathways in most clinically significant pain disorders. In response to trigeminal nerve activation, craniofacial pain symptoms can manifest as transient pain conditions as reported with toothaches and headaches, or can transform into more chronic pain conditions such as migraine, temporomandibular joint disorders or trigeminal neuralgia (Durham & Garrett, 2010). Apart from electrical activation, chemical activation of the trigeminal nerve leads to an afferent and efferent release of certain neuropeptides that facilitate peripheral inflammatory responses and causes activation of second-order neurons involved in pain transmission (Buzzi, 2001). Accumulating evidence suggests that CGRP and NO are involved in the underlying pathophysiology of all vascular headaches, the vast majority of which are associated with an inflammatory process. In particular, CGRP, a potent vasodilator and pro-inflammatory agent which is expressed by trigeminal nociceptors, has been identified as a key player in the pathomechanism of migraine headache (McCulloch et al., 1986). Clinical studies have also shown a clear association between the head pain and the release of CGRP, from the trigeminovascular system (for a review, see Edvinsson & Uddman, 2005). For example, during migraine attacks there is a marked increase in the plasma levels of CGRP and the administration of a recently developed CGRP blocker, BIBN4096BS, causes the headache to subside and the neuropeptide levels to normalize (Olesen et al., 2004). On the other hand, the efficacy of SER agonists for migraine therapy is known, and this amine, probably along with CGRP, has been hypothesized to be involved in trigeminal pain (Moskowitz et al., 1979) by activating 5-HT_{1B}, 5-HT_{1D} (Bonaventure et al., 1998; Wotherspoon & Priestly, 2000) and 5-HT_7 (Terrón et al., 2001; see also Classey et al., 2010) receptors. Indeed, the systemic administration of sumatriptan, the most-studied of the serotonergic drugs now collectively known as the triptans, lowers CGRP levels to nearly normal levels coincident with headache relief (Goadsby & Edvinsson, 1991). NO, an inflammatory mediator, is also currently thought of as a key molecule in migraine pain, possibly in concert with CGRP (Thomsen & Olesen, 1996). Results from animal studies have provided evidence for the involvement of NO in sensitation and/or activation of the trigeminovascular system and repressed release of CGRP from trigeminal neurons in response to treatment with NO donors or application of the anti-migraine drug sumatriptan, which has affinity for 5-HT_{1B}, 5-HT_{1D} and 5-HT_{1F} receptors (Bellamy et al., 2006). It seems likely that NO production and neuropeptide release are functionally linked in severe vascular headaches. Conversely, SP, which along with CGRP is the most definitely characterized peptide in the TG, is not released in the cranial blood flow in migraine suggesting that SP does not take part in vascular nociception in man

(Holthusen et al., 1997). It has recently been demonstrated that SP release in the TG is predominantly increased after orofacial inflammation (Neubert et al. 2000) and such a release may play an important role in determining the trigeminal inflammatory alloying concerning the temporomandibular joint disorder (Takeda et al., 2005). The authors point out that NK1 receptor antagonists may be useful as therapeutic agents to prevent the mechanical allodynia. $P2X_3$ receptors may be another therapeutic target for treating temporomandibular joint disorder pain (Shinoda et al., 2005).

Another common clinical concern regarding the trigeminal nerve is trigeminal neuralgia. Evidence for the role of SP and CGRP in trigeminal neuralgia pain is clearly apparent (Stoyanova & Lazarov, 2001). Inhibitory neurotransmitters, such as GABA, are thought to have a role in analgesia and many GABAergic drugs, acting through metabotropic $GABA_B$ receptors, are useful in the treatment of migraine and trigeminal neuralgia. With regard to the latter, a GABA analogue, gabapentin, has been reported to be effective in the management of migraine and trigeminal neuralgia, and also displays anti-nociceptive activity in various animal pain models. In addition, a selective $GABA_B$ receptor agonist, baclofen, has been shown to elicit pain relief and, thus, it might play a therapeutic role in the inhibition of nociceptive hypersensitivity in trigeminal neuralgia (Fromm, 1994).

Clinically relevant is also pain, caused by a central or peripheral nerve lesion which is commonly termed neuropathic pain, and the concomitant neurogenic inflammation. Orofacial neuropathic pain, like anywhere in the body, may occur as a result of tissue damage and the activation of nociceptors, which transmit a noxious stimulus to the brain (Vickers & Cousins, 2000). The abnormal facial pain involves regeneration of damaged nerve fibers and may account for chemical changes in injured neuronal cell bodies. As mentioned above, a variety of neuropeptides, such as SP, CGRP, GAL and NPY, are up-regulated following peripheral axotomy (see Table 2) and craniofacial muscle inflammation (Ambalavanar et al., 2006). Results from studies on animal pain models have suggested that NPY and its receptors are potential targets for treatment of pain, especially neuropathic pain (Silva et al., 2002). The efficacy of opioid receptor agonists in modulation of nociceptive inputs in a wide range of orofacial pain models, including neuropathic pain (Catheline et al., 1998) and inflammatory pain (Ko et al., 1998) is also acknowledged. Given that NGF is responsible for the increased expression of SP and CGRP during neurogenic inflammation (Lundy & Linden, 2004), it is not much surprising that the systemic administration of anti-NGF neutralizing antibodies prevents the up-regulation of neuropeptides in primary afferent neurons innervating the inflamed skin (Woolf et al., 1994). Changes in the injured neurons can also influence the ability of the surrounding glial cells to release neuromodulators such as NO and ATP, thus implicating satellite glial cells in the TG as a determinant of orofacial neuropathic pain. This fits well with the notion that the $P2X_3$ receptor is transiently up-regulated and anterogradely transported in trigeminal primary afferent neurons after neuropathic injury (Eriksson et al., 1998). Purinergic receptors on TG neurons are thus likely to be a legitimate target for therapeutic intervention in neuropathic pain and orofacial inflammation (Ambalavanar et al., 2005). Recent findings further demonstrate that masseter inflammation differentially modulates Glu receptor subunits and that the induced changes in them may contribute to functionally different aspects of craniofacial muscle pain processing under inflammatory conditions (Lee and Ro, 2007).

6. Concluding remarks

Based on the information now available, it has become evident that miscellaneous transmitter candidates are associated with a subset of trigeminal primary afferent neurons and, besides, these are well-innervated by aminergic, peptidergic and nitrergic fibers of a probable extrinsic origin. The data also suggest that some classical neurotransmitters and neuropeptides not only mediate trans-synaptic information coding but can also act as long-term morphogenetic signals and trophic factors. Progressive discovery of the multiplicity of chemical messengers, of coexistent transmitters (or transmitter candidates), their receptors and transducing mechanisms, and of local mechanisms for transmitter release, has reinforced the view that chemical coding in trigeminal primary afferent neurons, either peripherally or centrally, is multiple, heterogeneous, plastically varying and characterized by a wide spectrum of co-existing messenger substances. In line with similar morphological features and trophic factor requirements, as well as diverse central and peripheral targets, and physiological properties, we show that TG and MTN neurons have both similarities and differences in their neurochemical content. On the one hand, the most important similarity relates to the fact that both central and peripheral trigeminal primary afferent neurons express, indeed to a varying degree, classical transmitters and neuronal markers, such as calcium-binding proteins. On the other hand, the most marked spatial difference is the presence of certain neuropeptides in the TG cell bodies and their absence in the MTN neuronal somata under normal conditions. As argued before, we believe that the differently fated embryonic migration, synaptogenesis, and peripheral and central target field innervation can possibly affect the individual neurochemical phenotypes of trigeminal primary afferent neurons.

7. Acknowledgments

I am grateful to all members of my laboratory for their generous help and to many colleagues whose constructive suggestions enriched this chapter. I would also like to thank Dr. Angel Dandov for critical reading and editing of the manuscript.

8. References

Ambalavanar, R., Moritani, M. & Dessem, D. (2005). Trigeminal P2X3 receptor expression differs from dorsal root ganglion and is modulated by deep tissue inflammation. *Pain* Vol. 117, No. 3, 280-291.

Ambalavanar, R., Moritani, M., Moutanni, A., Gangula, P., Yallampalli, C. & Dessem, D. (2006). Deep tissue inflammation upregulates neuropeptides and evokes nociceptive behaviors which are modulated by a neuropeptide antagonist. *Pain* Vol. 120, No. 1-2, 53-68.

Andressen, C., Blümcke, I. & Celio, M.R. (1993). Calcium-binding proteins: selective markers of nerve cells. *Cell Tissue Res* Vol. 271, No. 2, 181-208.

Araki, T., Kenimer, J.G., Nishimune, A., Sugiyama, H., Yoshimura, R. & Kiyama, H. (1993). Identification of the metabotropic glutamate receptor-1 protein in the rat trigeminal ganglion. *Brain Res* Vol. 627, No. 2, 341-344.

Azérad, J., Boucher, Y. & Pollin, B. (1992). Occurrence of glutamate in primary sensory trigeminal neurons innervating the rat dental pulp. *C R Acad Sci Paris III* Vol. 314, No. 10, 469-475.

Baimbridge, K.G., Celio, M.R. & Rogers, J.H. (1992). Calcium-binding proteins in the nervous system. *Trends Neurosci* Vol. 15, No. 8, 303–308.

Bellamy, J., Bowen, E.J., Russo, A.F. & Durham, P.L. (2006). Nitric oxide regulation of calcitonin gene-related peptide gene expression in rat trigeminal ganglia neurons. *Eur J Neurosci* Vol. 23, No. 8, 2057-2066.

Bonaventure, P., Voorn, P., Luyten, W.H. & Leysen, J.E. (1998). 5HT1B and 5HT1D receptor mRNA differential co-localization with peptide mRNA in the guinea pig trigeminal ganglion. *NeuroReport* Vol. 9, No. 4, 641-645.

Brodin, E.B, Gazelius, B., Lundberg, J.M. & Olgart, L. (1981). Substance P in trigeminal nerve endings: occurrence and release. *Acta Physiol Scand* Vol. 111, No. 4, 501-503.

Bruinvels, A.T., Landwehrmeyer, B., Moskowitz, M.A. & Hoyer, D. (1992). Evidence for the presence of 5-HT1B receptor messenger RNA in neurons of the rat trigeminal ganglia. *Eur J Pharmacol* Vol. 227, No. 3, 357-359.

Buchman, V.L. & Davies, A.M. (1993). Different neurotrophins are expressed and act in a developmental sequence to promote the survival of embryonic sensory neurons. *Development* Vol. 118, No. 3, 989-1001.

Buzzi, M.G. (2001). Trigeminal pain pathway: peripheral and central activation as experimental models of migraine. *Funct Neurol* Vol. 16, Suppl. 4, 77-81.

Capra, N.F. & Dessem, D. (1992). Central connections of trigeminal primary afferent neurons: topographical and functional considerations. *Crit Rev Oral Biol Med* Vol. 4, No. 1, 1–52.

Catheline, G., Guilbaud, G. & Kayser, V. (1998). Peripheral component in the enhanced antinociceptive effect of systemic U-69,593, a kappa-opioid receptor agonist in mononeuropathic rats. *Eur J Pharmacol* Vol. 357, No. 2-3, 171-178.

Chandler, S.H. (1989). Evidence for excitatory amino acid transmission between mesencephalic nucleus of V afferents and jaw-closer motoneurons in the guinea pig. *Brain Res* Vol. 477, No. 1-2, 252–264.

Chandler, S.H., Nielsen, S.A. & Goldberg, L.J. (1985). The effects of a glycine antagonist (strychnine) on cortically induced rhythmical jaw movements in the anesthetized guinea pig. *Brain Res* Vol. 325, No. 1-2, 181–186.

Chen, P., Li, J.-L., Li, J.-S. & Mizuno, N. (2001). Glutamic acid decarboxylase-like immunoreactive axon terminals in synaptic contact with mesencephalic trigeminal nucleus neurons in the rat. *Neurosci Lett* Vol. 298, No. 3, 167–170.

Chouchkov, C., Lazarov, N. & Davidoff, M. (1988). Serotonin-like immunoreactivity in the cat trigeminal ganglion. *Histochemistry* Vol. 88, No. 3-6, 637-639.

Classey, J.D., Bartsch, T. & Goadsby, P.J. (2010). Distribution of 5-HT_{1B}, 5-HT_{1D} and 5-HT_{1F} receptor expression in rat trigeminal and dorsal root ganglia neurons: relevance to the selective anti-migraine effect of triptans. *Brain Res* Vol. 1361, 76-85.

Cody, F.W.J., Lee, R.W.H. & Taylor, A. (1972). A functional analysis of the components of the mesencephalic nucleus of the fifth nerve in the cat. *J Physiol (London)* Vol. 226, No. 1, 249–261.

Copray, J.C.V.M. & Liem, R.S.B. (1993). Survival and neurite formation of mesencephalic trigeminal neurones of the rat in vitro. *Arch Oral Biol* Vol. 38, No. 7, 547–557.

Copray, J.C.V.M., Ter Horst, G.J., Liem, R.S.B. & van Willigen, J.D. (1990). Neurotransmitters and neuropeptides within the mesencephalic trigeminal nucleus of the rat: an immunohistochemical analysis. *Neuroscience* Vol. 37, No. 2, 399–411.

Copray, J.C.V.M., Liem, R.S.B., Ter Horst, G.J. & van Willigen, J.D. (1991). Origin, distribution and morphology of serotonergic afferents to the mesencephalic trigeminal nucleus of the rat. *Neurosci Lett* Vol. 121, No. 1-2, 97–101.

Cornea-Hébert, V., Riad, M., Wu, C., Singh, S.K. & Descarries, L. (1999). Cellular and subcellular distribution of the serotonin 5-HT2A receptor in the central nervous system of adult rat. *J Comp Neurol* Vol. 409, No. 2, 187–209.

Costa, M., Furness, J.B. & Gibbins, I.L. (1986). Chemical coding of enteric neurons. *Prog Brain Res* 68, 217–239.

Couture R. & Cuello, A.C. (1984). Studies on the trigeminal antidromic vasodilatation and plasma extravasation in the rat. *J Physiol (London)* Vol. 346, 273-285.

Darian-Smith, I. (1973). The trigeminal system. In: Iggo A. (Ed.), *Handbook of Sensory Physiology, Somatosensory System*, Vol. 2, Springer, Berlin, pp. 271-314.

Davies, A.M. (1997). Studies of neurotrophin biology in the developing trigeminal system. *J Anat* Vol. 191, No. 4, 483-491.

Davies, A.M., Lumsden, A.G.S. & Rohrer, H. (1987). Neural-crest-derived proprioceptive neurons express NGF receptors but are not supported by NGF in culture. *Neuroscience* Vol. 20, No. 1, 37–46.

Del Negro, C.A. & Chandler, S.H., 1997. Physiological and theoretical analysis of K^+ currents controlling discharge in neonatal rat mesencephalic trigeminal neurons. *J Neurophysiol* Vol. 77, No. 2, 537–553.

Dubner, R., Sessle, B. & Storey, A. (1978). The Neural Basis of Oral and Facial Function, Plenum Press, London.

Dunn, P.M., Zhong, Y. & Burnstock, G. (2001). P2X receptors in peripheral neurons. *Prog Neurobiol*, Vol. 65, No. 2, 107–134.

Durham, P.L. & Garrett, F.G. (2010). Development of functional units within trigeminal ganglia correlates with increased expression of proteins involved in neuron-glia interactions. *Neuron Glia Biology* Vol. 6, No. 3, 171-181.

Durkin, M.M., Gunwaldsen, C.A., Borowsky, B., Jones, K.A. & Branchek, T.A. (1999). An in situ hybridization study of the distribution of the GABA(B2) protein mRNA in the rat CNS. *Mol Brain Res* Vol. 71, No. 2, 185-200.

Edvinsson, L. & Uddman, R. (2005). Neurobiology in primary headaches. *Brain Res Rev* Vol. 48, No. 3, 438-456.

Edvinsson, L., Mulder, H., Goadsby, P.J. & Uddman, R. (1998). Calcitonin gene-related peptide and nitric oxide in the trigeminal ganglion: cerebral vasodilatation from trigeminal nerve stimulation involves mainly calcitonin gene-related peptide. *J Auton Nerv Syst* Vol. 70, No. 1-2, 15-22.

Elcock, C., Boissonade, F.M. & Robinson, P.P. (2001). Changes in neuropeptide expression in the trigeminal ganglion following inferior alveolar nerve section in the ferret. *Neuroscience* Vol. 102, No. 3, 655-667.

Eriksson, J., Bongenhielm, U., Kidd, E., Matthews, B. & Fried, K. (1998). Distribution of P2X3 receptors in the rat trigeminal ganglion after inferior alveolar nerve injury. *Neurosci Lett* Vol. 254, No. 1, 37-40.

Ernfors, P., Merlio, J.P. & Persson, H. (1992). Cells expressing mRNA for neurotrophins and their receptors during embryonic rat development. *Eur J Neurosci* Vol. 4, No. 11, 1140-1158.

Fan, W., Dong, W., Leng, S., Li, D., Cheng, S., Li, C., Qu, H. & He, H. (2008). Expression and colocalization of NADPH-diaphorase and heme oxygenase-2 in trigeminal ganglion and mesencephalic trigeminal nucleus of the rat. *J Mol Histol* Vol. 39, No. 4, 427-433.

Foreman, J.C. (1987). Peptides and neurogenic inflammation. *Br Med Bull* Vol. 43, No. 2, 386-400.

Fristad, I., Jacobsen, E.B. & Kvinnsland, I.H. (1998). Coexpression of vasoactive intestinal polypeptide and substance P in reinnervating pulpal nerves and in the trigeminal ganglion neuons after axotomy of the inferior alveolar nerve in the rat. *Arch Oral Biol* Vol. 43, No. 3, 183-189.

Fromm, G.H. (1994). Baclofen as an adjuvant analgesic. *J Pain Symptom Manage* Vol. 9, No. 8, 500-509.

Ginestal, E. & Matute, C. (1993). Gamma-aminobutyric acid-immunoreactive neurons in the rat trigeminal nuclei. *Histochemistry* Vol. 99, No. 1, 49–55.

Goadsby, P.J. & Edvinsson, L. (1991). Sumatriptan reverses the changes in calcitonin gene-related peptide seen in the headache phase of migraine. *Cephalalgia* Vol. 11, Suppl. 11, 3-4.

Hayar, A., Poulter, M.O., Pelkey, K., Feltz, P. & Marshall, K.C. (1997). Mesencephalic trigeminal neuron responses to γ-aminobutyric acid. *Brain Res* Vol. 753, No. 1, 120–127.

Henry, M.A., Westrum, L.E., Bothwell, M. & Johnson, L.R. (1993). Nerve growth factor receptor (p75)-immunoreactivity in the normal adult feline trigeminal system and following retrogasserian rhizotomy. *J Comp Neurol* Vol. 335, No. 3, 425-436.

Hökfelt, T., Zhang, X. & Wiesenfeld-Hallin, Z. (1994). Messenger plasticity in primary sensory neurons following axotomy and its functional implications. *Trends Neurosci* Vol. 17, No. 1, 22–30.

Holthusen, H., Kindgen-Milles, D. & Ding, Z.P. (1997). Substance P is not involved in vascular nociception in humans. *Neuropeptides* Vol. 31, No. 5, 445-448.

Ichikawa, H., Deguchi, T., Nakago, T., Jacobowitz, D.M. & Sugimoto, T. (1994). Parvalbumin, calretinin and carbonic anhydrase in the trigeminal and spinal primary neurons of the rat. *Brain Res* Vol. 655, No. 1-2, 241-245.

Ichikawa, H., Jacobowitz, D.M. & Sugimoto, T. (1997). S100 protein-immunoreactive primary sensory neurons in the trigeminal and dorsal root ganglia of the rat. *Brain Res* Vol. 748, No. 1-2, 253-257.

Ichikawa, H., Itota, T., Torii, Y., Inoue, K. & Sugimoto, T. (1999). Osteocalcin-immunoreactive primary sensory neurons in the rat spinal and trigeminal nervous systems. *Brain Res* Vol. 838, No. 1-2, 205–209.

Ichikawa, H., Itota, T., Nishitani, Y., Torii, Y., Inoue, K. & Sugimoto, T. (2000). Osteopontin-immunoreactive primary sensory neurons in the rat spinal and trigeminal nervous systems. *Brain Res* Vol. 863, No. 1-2, 276–281.

Ichikawa, H., Jin, H.W., Terayama, S., Yamaai, T., Matsuo, S. & Sugimoto, T. (2007). The reduction of proprioceptors in the mesencephalic trigeminal tract nucleus after neonatal masseteric nerve transection; effect of brain-derived neurotrophic factor. *Brain Res* Vol. 1153, 98–102.

Iino, S., Kato, M., Hidaka, H. & Kobayashi, S. (1998). Neurocalcin-immunopositive neurons in the rat sensory ganglia. *Brain Res* Vol. 781, No. 1-2, 236-243.

Inagaki, N., Yamatodani, A., Shinoda, K., Shiotani, Y., Tohyama, M., Watanabe, T. & Wada, H. (1987). The histaminergic innervation of the mesencephalic nucleus of the trigeminal nerve in rat brain: a light and electron microscopical study. *Brain Res* Vol. 418, No. 2, 388–391.

Ishii, H. & Kang, Y. (2002). Molecular basis underlying $GABA_A$ responses in rat mesencephalic trigeminal neurons. *NeuroReport* Vol. 13, No. 17, 2265–2269.

Jacobs, J.S. & Miller, M.W. (1999). Expression of nerve growth factor, p75, and the high affinity neurotrophin receptors in the adult rat trigeminal system: evidence for multiple trophic support systems. *J Neurocytol* Vol. 28, No. 7, 571–595.

Jerge, C.R. (1963). Organization and function of the trigeminal mesencephalic nucleus. *J Neurophysiol* Vol. 26, 379–392.

Kaneko, T., Itoh, K., Shigemoto, R. & Mizuno, N. (1989). Glutaminase-like immunoreactivity in the lower brainstem and cerebellum of the adult rat. *Neuroscience* Vol. 32, No. 1, 79–98.

Katz, D.M., Markey, K.A., Goldstein, M. & Black, I.B. (1983). Expression of catecholaminergic characteristics by primary sensory neurons in the normal adult rat in vivo. *Proc Natl Acad Sci U S A* Vol. 80, No. 11, 3526-3530.

Khakh, B.S., Humphrey, P.P.A. & Henderson, G. (1997). ATP-gated cation channels (P_{2X} purinoceptors) in trigeminal mesencephalic nucleus neurones of the rat. *J Physiol (London)* Vol. 498, No. 3, 709–715.

Ko, M.C., Butelman, E.R. & Woods, J.H. (1998). The role of peripheral mu opioid receptors in the modulation of capsaicin-induced thermal nociception in rhesus monkeys. *J Pharmacol Exp Ther* Vol. 286, No. 1, 150-156.

Kolesar, D., Kolesarova, M., Schreiberova, A., Lackova, M. & Maršala, J., (2006). Distribution of NADPH diaphorase-exhibiting primary afferent neurons in the trigeminal ganglion and mesencephalic trigeminal nucleus of the rabbit. *Cell Mol Neurobiol* Vol. 26, No. 7-8, 1265–1279.

Kolta, A., Dubuc, R., Campistron, G. & Lund, J.P. (1991a). Investigation of possible neurotransmitters responsible for the inhibition of trigeminal primary afferents. *IBRO* Abstr. 3, 86.

Kolta, A., Dubuc, R., Reader, T.A. & Lund, J.P. (1991b). Serotoninergic and GABAergic innervation of the trigeminal mesencephalic and motor nuclei. *Can J Physiol Pharmacol* 69, AXIV.

Kolta, A., Dubuc, R. & Lund, J.P. (1993). An immunocytochemical and autoradiographic investigation of the serotoninergic innervation of trigeminal mesencephalic and motor nuclei in the rabbit. *Neuroscience* Vol. 53, No. 4, 1113–1126.

Kolta, A., Lund, J.P., Westberg, K.G. & Clavelou, P. (1995). Do muscle-spindle afferents act as interneurons during mastication? *Trends Neurosci* Vol. 18, No. 10, 441.

Kondo, E., Kiyama, H., Araki, T., Shida, T., Ueda, Y. & Tohyama, M. (1994). Coexpression of $GABA_A$ receptor gamma 1 and gamma 2 subunits in the rat trigeminal ganglion. *Mol Brain Res* Vol. 21, No. 3-4, 185-200.

Krastev, D. (2009). Trigeminal ganglion - lightmicroscopical presentation of large pseudounipolar neurons. *Comp rend Acad bulg Sci* Vol. 62, No. 11, 1469-1472.

Kruger, L. & Young, R.F. (1981). Specialised features of the trigeminal nerve and its central connections. In: Samii, M., Janeta P.J. (Eds.), *The Cranial Nerves*, Springer, Berlin, pp. 273–301.

Kummer, W., Gibbins, I.L., Stefan, P. & Kapoor, V. (1990). Catecholamines and catecholamine-synthesizing enzymes in guinea-pig sensory ganglia. *Cell Tissue Res* Vol. 261, No. 3, 595-606.

Lazarov, N.E. (1994). Primary trigeminal afferent neuron of the cat. II. Neuropeptide- and serotonin-like immunoreactivity. *J Brain Res* Vol. 35, No. 3, 373-389.

Lazarov, N.E. (2000). The mesencephalic trigeminal nucleus in the cat. *Advances in Anatomy, Embryology and Cell Biology* Vol. 153, Springer, Berlin Heidelberg, pp. 1-103.

Lazarov, N.E. (2002). Comparative analysis of the chemical neuroanatomy of the mammalian trigeminal ganglion and mesencephalic trigeminal nucleus. *Prog Neurobiol* Vol. 66, No. 1, 19-59.

Lazarov, N.E. (2007). Neurobiology of orofacial proprioception. *Brain Res Rev* Vol. 56, No. 2, 362-383.

Lazarov, N.E. & Chouchkov, C.N. (1995a). Serotonin-containing projections to the mesencephalic trigeminal nucleus of the cat. *Anat Rec* Vol. 241, No. 1, 136–142.

Lazarov, N.E. & Chouchkov, C.N. (1995b). Immunocytochemical localization of tyrosine hydroxylase and γ-aminobutyric acid in the mesencephalic trigeminal nucleus of the cat: a light and electron microscopic study. *Anat Rec* Vol. 242, No. 1, 123–131.

Lazarov, N.E. & Dandov, A. (1998). Distribution of NADPH-diaphorase and nitric oxide synthase in the trigeminal ganglion and mesencephalic trigeminal nucleus of the cat: a histochemical and immunohistochemical study. *Acta Anat (Basel)* Vol. 163, No. 4, 191–200.

Lazarov, N.E. & Gratzl, M. (2006). Selective expression of histamine receptors in rat mesencephalic trigeminal neurons. *Neurosci Lett* Vol. 404, No. 1-2, 67–71.

Lazarov, N.E. & Pilgrim, C. (1997). Localization of D_1 and D_2 dopamine receptors in the rat mesencephalic trigeminal nucleus by immunocytochemistry and in situ hybridization. *Neurosci Lett* Vol. 236, No. 2, 83–86.

Lazarov, N.E., Dandov, A., Stoyanova, I. & Chouchkov, C.N., (1998). Calcium-binding proteins in the mesencephalic trigeminal nucleus of the cat. *Arch Physiol Biochem* Vol. 106, No. 5, 370–377.

Lee, J. & Ro, J.Y. (2007). Differential regulation of glutamate receptors in trigeminal ganglia following masseter inflammation. *Neurosci Lett* Vol. 421, No. 2, 91-95.

Li, J.-L., Xiong, K.-H., Li, Y.-Q., Kaneko, T. & Mizuno, N. (2000). Serotonergic innervation of mesencephalic trigeminal nucleus neurons: a light and electron microscopic study in the rat. *Neurosci Res* Vol. 37, No. 2, 127–140.

Li, J.-L., Shigemoto, R., Kulik, A., Chen, P., Nomura, S. Kaneko, T. & Mizuno, N. (2001). Immunocytochemical localization of $GABA_B$ receptors in mesencephalic trigeminal nucleus neurons in the rat. *Neurosci Lett* Vol. 315, No. 1-2, 93–97.

Liem, R.S.B. & Copray, J.C.V.M. (1996). Immunogold localization of serotonin within synaptic terminals in the rat mesencephalic trigeminal nucleus. *Acta Anat (Basel)* Vol. 155, No. 1, 50–56.

Liem, R.S.B., Copray, J.C.V.M. & van Willigen, J.D. (1993). Serotonin-immunoreactive terminals in the mesencephalic trigeminal nucleus of the rat: an electron microscopic immunocytochemical study. *Acta Anat (Basel)* Vol. 148, No. 1, 34–41.

Liem, R.S.B., Copray, J.C.V.M. & Van der Want, J.J.L. (1997). Dopamine-immunoreactivity in the rat mesencephalic trigeminal nucleus: an ultrastructural analysis. *Brain Res* Vol. 755, No. 2, 319-325.

Longmore, J., Shaw, D., Smith, D., Hopkins, R., McAllister, G., Pickard, J.D., Sirinathsinghji, D.J., Butler, A.J. & Hill, R.G. (1997). Differential distribution of 5HT1D- and 5HT1B-immunoreactivity within the human trigemino-cerebrovascular system: implications for the discovery of new antimigraine drugs. *Cephalalgia* Vol. 17, No. 8, 833-842.

Lukás, Z., Czech, S. & Buriánek, P. (1970). Cholinesterase and biogenic monoamines in ganglion semilunare (Gasseri). *Histochemie* Vol. 22, 163-168.

Lundy, F.T. & Linden, G.J. (2004). Neuropeptides and neurogenic mechanisms in oral and periodontal inflammation. *Crit Rev Oral Biol Med* Vol. 15, No. 2, 82-98.

Margeta-Mitrovic, M., Mitrovic, I., Riley, R.C., Jan, L.Y. & Basbaum, A.I. (1999). Immunohistochemical localization of GABA(B) receptors in the rat central nervous system. *J Comp Neurol* Vol. 405, No. 3, 299–321.

McCarthy, P.W. & Lawson, S.N. (1989). Cell type and conduction velocity of rat primary sensory neurons with substance P-like immunoreactivity. *Neuroscience* Vol. 28, No. 3, 745-753.

McCarthy, P.W. & Lawson, S.N. (1990). Cell type and conduction velocity of rat primary sensory neurons with calcitonin gene-related peptide-like immunoreactivity. *Neuroscience* Vol. 34, No. 3, 623-632.

McCulloch, J., Uddman, R., Kingman, T.A. & Edvinsson, L. (1986). Calcitonin gene-related peptide: functional role in cerebrovascular regulation. *Proc Natl Acad Sci U S A* Vol. 83, No. 15, 5731-5735.

Mineff, E.M., Popratiloff, A., Usunoff, K.G. & Marani, E. (1998). Immunocytochemical localization of the AMPA receptor subunits in the mesencephalic trigeminal nucleus of the rat. *Arch Physiol Biochem* Vol. 106, No. 3, 203–209.

Morales, M., Battenberg, E. & Bloom, F.E. (1998). Distribution of neurons expressing immunoreactivity for the 5HT3 receptor subtype in the rat brain and spinal cord. *J Comp Neurol* Vol. 402, No. 3, 385–401.

Moshnyakov, M., Arumäe, U. & Saarma, M. (1996). mRNAS for one, two or three members of trk receptor family are expressed in single rat trigeminal ganglion neurons. *Mol Brain Res* Vol. 43, No. 1-2, 141-148.

Moskowitz, M.A., Reinhard, J.F. Jr., Romero, J., Melamed, E. & Pettibone, D.J. (1979). Neurotransmitters and the fifth cranial nerve: is there a relation to the headache phase of migraine? *Lancet* Vol. 2, No. 8148, 883-885.

Nagy, J.I., Buss, M. & Daddona, P.E. (1986). On the innervation of trigeminal mesencephalic primary afferent neurons by adenosine deaminase-containing projections from the hypothalamus in the rat. *Neuroscience* Vol. 17, No. 1, 141–156.

Navarro, X. (2009). Neural plasticity after peripheral nerve injury and regeneration. *Int Rev Neurobiol* Vol. 87, 483–505.

Navarro, X., Vivó, M. & Valero-Cabré, A. (2007). Neural plasticity after peripheral nerve injury and regeneration. *Prog Neurobiol* Vol. 82, No. 4, 163–201.

Neubert, J.K., Maidment, N.T., Matsuka, Y., Adelson, D.W., Kruger, L. & Spigelman, I. (2000). Inflammation-induced changes in primary afferent-evoked release of substance P within trigeminal ganglia in vivo. *Brain Res* Vol. 871, No. 2, 181-191.

Nielsch, U. & Keen, P. (1989). Reciprocal regulation of tachykinin and vasoactive intestinal peptide-gene expression in rat sensory neurons following cut and crush injury. *Brain Res* Vol. 481, No. 1, 25–30.

Olesen, J., Diener, H.C., Husstedt, I.W., Goadsby, P.J., Hall, D., Meier, U., Pollentier, S. & Lesko, L.M. (2004). Calcitonin gene-related peptide receptor antagonist BIBN 4096 BS for the acute treatment of migraine. *N Engl J Med* Vol. 350, No. 11, 1104-1110.

Otsuka, M. & Konishi, S. (1976). Substance P and excitatory transmitter of primary sensory neurons. *Cold Spring Harb Symp Quant Biol* Vol. 40, 135-143.

Pang, Y.W., Li, J.-L., Nakamura, K., Wu, S.X., Kaneko, T. & Mizuno, N. (2006). Expression of vesicular glutamate transporter 1 immunoreactivity in peripheral and central endings of trigeminal mesencephalic nucleus neurons in the rat. *J Comp Neurol* Vol. 498, No. 1, 129–141.

Patel, M.K., Khakh, B.S. & Henderson, G. (2001). Properties of native P2X receptors in rat trigeminal mesencephalic nucleus neurones: lack of correlation with known, heterologously expressed P2X receptors. *Neuropharmacology* Vol. 40, No. 1, 96–105.

Pelkey, K.A. & Marshall, K.C. (1998). Actions of excitatory amino acids on mesencephalic trigeminal neurons. *Can J Physiol Pharmacol* Vol. 76, No. 9, 900–908.

Peterfreund, R.A., Kosofsky, B.E. & Fink, J.S. (1995). Cellular localization of dopamine D2 receptor messenger RNA in the rat trigeminal ganglion. *Anesth Analg* Vol. 81, No. 6, 1181-1185.

Petralia, R.S. & Wenthold, R.J. (1992). Light and electron immunocytochemical localization of AMPA-selective glutamate receptors in the rat brain. *J Comp Neurol* Vol. 318, No. 3, 329–345.

Petralia, R.S., Wang, Y. X. & Wenthold, R.J. (1994a). The NMDA receptor subunits NR2A and NR2B show histological and ultrastructural localization patterns similar to those of NR1. *J Neurosci* Vol. 14, No. 10, 6102–6120.

Petralia, R.S., Wang, Y. X. & Wenthold, R.J. (1994b). Histological and ultrastructural localization of the kainate receptor subunits, KA2 and GluR6/7, in the rat nervous system using selective antipeptide antibodies. *J Comp Neurol* Vol. 349, No. 1, 84–110.

Petralia, R.S., Yokotani, N. & Wenthold, R.J. (1994c). Light and electron microscope distribution of the NMDA receptor subunit NMDAR1 in the rat nervous system using a selective anti-peptide antibody. *J Neurosci* Vol. 14, No. 2, 667–696.

Quartu, M., Setzu, M.D. & Del Fiacco, M. (1996). trk-like immunoreactivity in the human trigeminal ganglion and subnucleus caudalis. *NeuroReport* Vol. 7. No. 5, 1013-1019.

Quartu, M., Geic, M. & Del Fiacco, M. (1997). Neurotrophin-like immunoreactivity in the human trigeminal ganglion. *NeuroReport* Vol. 8, No. 16, 3611-3617.

Quartu, M., Serra, M.P., Mascia, F., Boi, M., Lai, M.L., Spano, A. & Del Fiacco, M. (2006). GDNF family ligand receptor components Ret and GFRalpha-1 in the human trigeminal ganglion and sensory nuclei. *Brain Res Bull* Vol. 69, No. 4, 393–403.

Ralevic, V. & Burnstock, G. (1998). Receptors for purines and pyrimidines. *Pharmacol Rev* Vol. 50, No. 3, 413–492.

Randić, M. & Miletić, V. (1978). Depressant actions of methionine-enkephalin and somatostatin in cat dorsal horn neurones activated by noxious stimuli. *Brain Res* Vol. 152, No. 1, 196-202.
Rosin, D.L., Robeva, A., Woodard, R.I., Guyenet, P.G. & Linden, J. (1998). Immunohistochemical localization of adenosine A_{2A} receptors in the rat central nervous system. *J Comp Neurol* 401, No. 2, 163–186.
Sahara, Y., Noro, N., Iida, Y., Soma, K. & Nakamura, Y. (1997). Glutamate receptor subunits GluR5 and KA-2 are coexpressed in rat trigeminal ganglion neurons. *J Neurosci* Vol. 17, No. 17, 6611-6620.
Salt, T.E. & Hill, R.G. (1983). Neurotransmitter candidates of somatosensory primary afferent fibres. *Neuroscience* Vol. 10, No. 4, 1083-1103.
Santini, M. (1966). Adrenergic fibres in the feline Gasserian ganglion. *Life Sci* Vol. 5, 283-287.
Sasaki, Y., Wakisaka, S. & Kurisu, K. (1994). Effects of peripheral axotomy of the inferior alveolar nerve on the levels of neuropeptide Y in rat trigeminal primary afferent neurons. *Brain Res* Vol. 664, No. 1-2, 108-114.
Schindler, M., Harris, C.A., Hayes, B., Papotti, M. & Humphrey, PP. (2001). Immunohistochemical localization of adenosine A1 receptors in human brain regions. *Neurosci Lett* Vol. 297, No. 3, 211-215.
Shinoda, M., Ozaki, N., Asai, H., Nagamine, K. & Sugiura, Y. (2005). Changes in P2X3 receptor expression in the trigeminal ganglion following monoarthritis of the temporomandibular joint in rats. *Pain* Vol. 116, No. 1-2, 42-51.
Silva, A.P., Cavadas, C. & Grouzmann, E. (2002). Neuropeptide Y and its receptors as potential therapeutic drug targets. *Clin Chim Acta* Vol. 326, No. 1-2, 3-25.
Spigelman, I. & Puil, E. (1991). Substance P actions on sensory neurons. *Ann N Y Acad Sci* Vol. 632, 220-228.
Stoyanova, I. & Lazarov, N. (2001). Role of calcitonin gene-related peptide (CGRP) and substance P (SP) in migraine pain and trigeminal neuralgia. *Pro Otology* Vol. 1, No. 1, 33-35.
Stoyanova, I.I. & Lazarov, N.E., (2005). Localization of nitric oxide synthase in rat trigeminal primary afferent neurons using NADPH-diaphorase histochemistry. *J Mol Histol* Vol. 36, No. 3, 187–193.
Stoyanova, I., Dandov, A., Lazarov, N. & Chouchkov, C. (1998). GABA- and glutamate-immunoreactivity in sensory ganglia of cat: a quantitative analysis. *Arch Physiol Biochem* Vol. 106, No. 5, 362-369.
Szabat, E., Soinila, S., Häppölä, O., Linnala, A. & Virtanen, I. (1992). A new monoclonal antibody against the GABA-protein conjugate shows immunoreactivity in sensory neurons of the rat. *Neuroscience* Vol. 47, No. 2, 409-420.
Takeda, M., Tanimoto, T., Nasu, M., Ikeda, M., Kadoi, J. & Matsumoto, S. (2005). Activation of NK1 receptor of trigeminal root ganglion via substance P paracrine mechanism contributes to the mechanical allodynia in the temporomandibular joint inflammation in rats. *Pain* Vol. 116, No. 3, 375-385.
Tanaka, S. & Chandler, S.H. (2006). Serotonergic modulation of persistent sodium currents and membrane excitability via cyclic AMP-protein kinase A cascade in mesencephalic V neurons. *J Neurosci Res* Vol. 83, No. 7, 1362–1372.
Tashiro, T., Satoda, T., Matsushima, R. & Mizuno, N. (1989). Enkephalin-, substance P- and serotonin-like immunoreactive axonal varicosities in close apposition to perikarya

of mesencephalic trigeminal nucleus neurons in the cat. *Brain Res* Vol. 494, No. 1, 162–167.

Terrón, J.A., Bouchelet, I. & Hamel, E. (2001). 5-HT7 receptor mRNA expression in human trigeminal ganglia. *Neurosci Lett* Vol. 302, No. 1, 9-12.

Thomsen, L.L. & Olesen, J. (1996). The role of nitric oxide in migraine pain. In: Sandler, M., Ferrari, M., Harnett, S. (Eds.), *Migraine Pharmacology and Genetics*. Chapman & Hall, London, pp. 154-166.

Turman, J.E. & Chandler, S.H. (1994a). Immunohistochemical evidence for GABA and glycine-containing trigeminal premotoneurons in the guinea pig. *Synapse* Vol. 18, No. 1, 7–20.

Turman, Jr., J.E. & Chandler, S.H. (1994b). Immunohistochemical localization of glutamate and glutaminase in guinea pig trigeminal premotoneurons. *Brain Res* Vol. 634, No. 1, 49–61.

Uddman, R., Tajti, J., Sundler, F. & Cardell, L.O. (2004). The presence of heme-oxygenase and biliverdin reductase in human cranial ganglia indicates a role for carbon monoxide in neural transmission. *Neuro Endocrinol Lett* Vol. 25, No. 6, 423-428.

Usunoff, K.G., Marani, E. & Schoen, J.H.R. (1997). The trigeminal system in man. *Advances in Anatomy, Embryology and Cell Biology* Vol. 136, Springer, Berlin Heidelberg, pp. 1-126.

Vickers, E.R. & Cousins, M.J. (2000). Neuropathic orofacial pain. Part 1 - Prevalence and pathophysiology. *Aust Endod J* Vol. 26, No. 1, 19-26.

Wanaka, A., Shiotani, Y., Kiyama, H., Matsuyama, T., Kamada, T., Shiosaka, S. & Tohyama, M. (1987). Glutamate-like immunoreactive structures in primary sensory neurons in the rat detected by a specific antiserum against glutamate. *Exp Brain Res* Vol. 65, No. 3, 691-694.

Waite, P.M.E. (2004). Trigeminal sensory system. In: Paxinos G. (Ed.), *The Rat Nervous System*. 3rd ed., Academic Press, San Diego, pp. 1093–1124.

Weihe, E. (1990). Neuropeptides in primary sensory neurons. In: Zenker, W., Neuhuber, W. (Eds.), *The Primary Afferent Neuron—A Survey of Recent Morpho-Functional Aspects*. Plenum Press, New York, pp. 127-159.

Wheeler, E.F., Naftel, J.P., Pan, M., von Bartheld, C.S. & Byers, M.R. (1998). Neurotrophin receptor expression is induced in a subpopulation of trigeminal neurons that label by retrograde transport of NGF or fluoro-gold following tooth injury. *Mol Brain Res* Vol. 61, No. 1-2, 23-38.

Williams, R., Bäckström, A., Kullander, K., Hallböök, F. & Ebendal, T. (1995). Developmentally regulated expression of mRNA for neurotrophin high-affinity (trk) receptors within chick trigeminal sensory neurons. *Eur J Neurosci* Vol. 7, No. 1, 116-128.

Woolf, C.J., Safieh-Garabedian, B., Ma, Q.P., Crilly, P. & Winter, J. (1994). Nerve growth factor contributes to the generation of inflammatory sensory hypersensitivity. *Neuroscience* Vol. 62, No. 2, 327-331.

Wotherspoon, G. & Priestley, J.V. (2000). Expression of the 5-HT1B receptor by subtypes of rat trigeminal ganglion cells. *Neuroscience* Vol. 95, No. 2, 465-471.

Xiang, Z., Bo, X. & Burnstock, G. (1998). Localization of ATP-gated P2X receptor immunoreactivity in rat sensory and sympathetic ganglia. *Neurosci Lett* Vol. 256, No. 2, 105-108.

Yamamoto, T., Shiosaka, S., Daddona, P.E. & Nagy, J.I. (1988). Further observations on the relationship between adenosine deaminase-containing axons and trigeminal mesencephalic neurons: an electron microscopic, immunohistochemical and anterograde tracing study. *Neuroscience* Vol. 26, No. 2, 669–680.

Yamuy, J., Sampogna, S. & Chase, M.H. (2000). Neurotrophin-receptor immunoreactive neurons in mesopontine regions involved in the control of behavioral states. *Brain Res* Vol. 866, No. 1-2, 1–14.

Yun, H.Y., Dawson, V.L. & Dawson, T.M. (1996). Neurobiology of nitric oxide. *Crit Rev Neurobiol* Vol. 10, No. 3-4, 291-316.

9

β-Endorphin and Alcoholism

Sarah M. Barry[1] and Judith E. Grisel[2]
[1]*Department of Neurosciences, The Medical University of South Carolina, Charleston, SC,*
[2]*Neuroscience Program, Department of Psychology, Furman University, Greenville, SC, USA*

1. Introduction

Extensive research over several decades indicates a strong relationship between alcohol use disorders and anxiety. Stress and anxiety are implicated in both the initiation of alcohol consumption and the maintenance of heavy drinking (Kushner et al., 1990; Pohorecky, 1981). For instance, anxiety disorders reliably precede the onset of alcoholism (Hettema et al., 2003) and over 35% of patients diagnosed with generalized anxiety disorder have engaged in self-medication with alcohol, defined as "drinking more than usual" in response to a stressor (Bolton et al., 2006). Stressors have also been linked to relapse in abstinent adults (Adinoff et al., 2005; Brown et al., 1995). Moreover, there is strong support suggesting that stress and alcohol abuse co-present so frequently as a result of common genetic factors in stress response systems. Genetically inherited variations in the hypothalamic-pituitary-adrenal (HPA) axis have been implicated in vulnerability to initial alcohol abuse, sustained alcohol addiction, and relapse (Crabbe et al., 2006; Kreek & Koob, 1998; Shaham et al., 2003). This paper will discuss the putative contribution of b-endorphin to the negatively reinforcing effects of alcohol.

2. The hypothalamo-pituitary-adrenocortical axis and β-endorphin

Although a thorough understanding of this nebulous concept is lacking, stress has been operationally defined as activation of the hypothalamo-pituitary-adrenocortical (HPA) axis in response to both physical and psychological stressors (for example, Pacak and Palkovits, 2001; Uhart and Wand 2009). The stress response is coordinated by neuronal activation of the paraventricular nucleus in the hypothalamus leading to the release of corticotrophin-releasing hormone (CRH) into the hypothalamic-hypophyseal portal. CRH reaches receptors on the anterior pituitary and initiates the synthesis of ACTH from its precursor, proopiomelanocortin (POMC). ACTH is released into the bloodstream where it influences the adrenal glands, initiating production and release of cortisol into the blood (corticosterone in rodents). Cortisol plays a fundamental role in the systemic reaction that characterizes physiological stress, though high levels of cortisol act in a negative feedback loop, inhibiting further CRH and ACTH synthesis in the brain.

Like stress, alcohol also leads to CRH release from the hypothalamus, initiating activation of this system (Hsu et al., 1998; see Gianoulakis, 2009; Uhart & Wand, 2009 for reviews). Indeed, the physiological effects of alcohol are in part mediated by the HPA axis and dependent upon neuronal activation of the paraventricular nucleus, and the subsequent release of CRH, ACTH and, eventually, adrenal activation (Lee et al., 2004).

Related to these endocrine changes, endogenous opioids are also synthesized and released in response to both the experience of stress and alcohol consumption (Keith et al, 1986; Sarkar & Minami, 1990; Schedlowski et al, 1995; Thiagarajan, 1989). Opioids are primarily known for their analgesic properties, but they are highly implicated in the physiological rewarding effects of alcohol and other drugs of abuse (Wei & Loh, 1976; Van Ree, 1979; Zalewska-Kaszubska et al., 2006; see Crabbe et al., 2006 for review) as well as a wide array of other behavioral states. One class of endogenous opioids is the endorphins. The primary endorphin is β-endorphin, which is both analgesic and addictive in human and animal studies (Janssen & Arntz, 2011; Wie & Loh, 1976), and contributes to the rewarding and reinforcing properties of alcohol (Grahame 1998; Grisel et al, 1999; Williams et al, 2007).

3. β-endorphin and alcohol

POMC is the precursor to all endorphins, including β-endorphin, which is synthesized in both the hypothalamus and the anterior pituitary. Endorphin producing neurons are located primarily in the arcuate nucleus of the hypothalamus, and project to other areas of the hypothalamus (supraoptic nucleus, paraventricular nucleus, and lateral hypothalamus) as well as to the amygdala, ventral tegmental area (VTA), periaqueductal gray, and bed nucleus of the stria terminalis (King & Hentges, 2011; McGinty & Bloom, 1983). Thus, β-endorphin is well situated to influence reward, stress and pain (see Kreek & Koob, 1998 for review). Moreover, EtOH-initiated dopamine release in the nucleus accumbens (NAC; de Waele & Gianoulakis, 1993; Koob & Le Moal, 1997) is thought to involve endorphin, which hyperpolarizes GABAergic neurons, and thereby disinhibits dopaminergic firing in the VTA (Johnson & North, 1992). Thus, the effects of acute alcohol administration on β-endorphin in the hypothalamus (Gianoulakis, 1990; Sakar et al. 2007) contribute to the positive reinforcing effects of alcohol. Additionally, acute administration of alcohol initiates synthesis and release of β-endorphin into the bloodstream (de Waele & Gianoulakis, 1993; Keith et al., 1986).

The relationship between β-endorphin and alcohol suggests at least two fundamental ways by which this peptide may be contributing to alcoholism. The first may underlie the heritable liability to develop an alcohol use disorder while the second comes into play as β-endorphin synthesis is down-regulated following chronic exposure.

4. β-endorphin and acute alcohol exposure

Individual variation in β-endorphin levels, as determined by heritable factors, predisposes individual differences in reinforcing properties of alcohol. Low β-endorphin may mediate enhanced reward either through more salient negative reinforcement or positive reinforcement from the drug. For example, the 'opioid deficiency hypothesis' builds on the fact that individuals predisposed to alcoholism have low basal levels of β-endorphin and suggests that alcohol administration will ameliorate this deficiency (see Gianoulakis et al., 2006; Herz, 1997, 1998; Zalewska-Kaszubska & Czarnecka, 2004 for reviews).

Gianoulakis et al. (1996) examined the possibility that high risk individuals (as identified by familial history) will have increased sensitivity to EtOH-induced release of endogenous opioids, thus mediating the apparent enhanced reward those at high risk for alcoholism presumably experience with EtOH consumption. Subjects were between twenty and thirty years old and were categorized as either high risk (HR) or low risk (LR) based upon known family history of alcoholism. The results showed an EtOH-dose dependent increase in plasma β-endorphin levels in HR subjects, but not in LR subjects. This finding supports the notion that augmented sensitivity of β-endorphin release to EtOH could increase sensitivity to the positive rewards of EtOH.

Animal studies provided further support for the idea that increased sensitivity to an EtOH-mediated rise in β-endorphin might facilitate acquisition of alcohol drinking. We (Grisel et al. 1999) demonstrated that mice with low levels of β-endorphin self-administer more EtOH than either wild type (C57BL/6J) controls or mice that entirely lack the capacity for β-endorphin production. In these studies we used either homozygous or heterozygous B6.129S2-*Pomc*^{tm1Low}/J mice, commercially available from Jackson Laboratories, in Bar Harbor, ME. The mice with low β-endorphin self-administered more EtOH and exhibited higher alcohol preference than controls, regardless of EtOH dose, while those without any capacity to synthesize the peptide consistently drank the least. This experiment suggests two hypotheses. One is that those with low levels of β-endorphin are more inclined to drink. The other, that β-endorphin contributes to the rewarding effects of EtOH.

In animals, pharmaceutical agents that increase plasma β-endorphin levels have been most effective in attenuating self-administration of EtOH. Treatment of Warsaw High and Low Alcohol Preferring rats with the opioid antagonist naltrexone, stopped the plasma β-endorphin increase after EtOH administration in low-preference rats, and normalized β-endorphin plasma levels in high-preferring rats so that before and after alcohol exposure plasma levels were similar. These results indicate the clinical effectiveness of naltrexone in treatment of alcoholism may in part be due to both normalization of plasma β-endorphin levels and an attenuation of alcohol-rewarding properties (Zalewska-Kaszubska et al., 2006). In the same strains of rats, β-endorphin levels and EtOH intake were examined following treatment with acamprosate, which is approved for relapse prevention in withdrawing alcoholics. Chronic administration of acamprosate decreased voluntary intake of EtOH and increased plasma β-endorphin levels in high-preferring rats. Chronic administration of acamprosate also increased β-endorphin levels in rats in withdrawal from free EtOH access, suggesting that the clinical efficacy of this novel pharmacotherapy may be mediated by opioid effects.

The specific influence of β-endorphin on negatively reinforcing effects of EtOH has been examined in animals. Negative reinforcement occurs as alcohol alleviates an aversive state or condition. We (Grisel et al., 2008) looked at anxious behavior as a function of basal levels of β-endorphin. These studies utilized the Light-Dark Box and Elevated Plus Maze to evaluate anxious behavior in wild-type C57BL/6J (WT), heterozygous (HT) and β-endorphin deficient mice (B6.129S2-*Pomc*^{tm1Low}/J). In these assays, anxious behavior is inversely related to time spent in the open or light areas of the assay apparatuses. In naïve subjects, the amount of time spent in the open arms of the Plus Maze or Light-Dark Box was inversely correlated with the amount of basal β-endorphin. These findings are consistent with the suggestion that β-endorphin release produces a calming and relaxing effect and thus lower levels of β-endorphin result in less regulation of HPA axis stress response (Gianoulakis, 1998; Sarkar et al., 2007). It follows that those with low basal β-endorphin levels, and therefore exaggerated stress responses, would be more inclined to self medicate with drugs of abuse, specifically anxiolytics such as EtOH (Zalewska-Kaszubska and Czarnecka, 2004).

Similar experiments were also conducted following acute exposure to EtOH (Grisel et al., 2008). Here, despite more anxious behavior at baseline, β-endorphin-deficient mice exhibited an exaggerated anxiolytic response after EtOH administration in both the plus maze and light-dark box in comparison to controls. These data may help explain the clinical relationship between this peptide and the propensity for alcoholism by suggesting that individuals with chronic β-endorphin deficiency have an increased sensitivity to the rewarding properties of EtOH, at least in part, because it alleviates their anxiety.

5. Interaction between β-endorphin and sex in acute EtOH exposure

Recent studies suggest that sex differences may play a moderating role in acute EtOH sensitivity differences. It is widely appreciated that females have lower incidence of alcoholism than males (Hunt and Zakhari, 1995), and these differences are theorized to manifest differences in coping response between sexes (Hettema et al., 2003). A burgeoning body of research supports the contention that females are more sensitive to stress than males (see Kleim et al., 2010; Maestripieri et al., 2010; Paris et al., 2010; Pratchett et al., 2010 for recent reviews of the human literature and Bangasser et al., 2010; Mogil et al., 1997; and Palanza 2001 for some basic research findings). For example, females, whose use and abuse of alcohol are increasing dramatically, also appear to be more sensitive to stress-induced changes in EtOH sensitivity (see Greenfield et al., 2010; Hudson & Stamp, 2010; Przybycien-Szymanska et al., 2010; Sartor et al., 2010).

Sex differences in stress sensitivity appear to result, at least in part, from differences in hypothalamic-pituitary-adrenal (HPA) functioning mediated by an interaction between gonadal hormones and β-endorphin (Hudson and Stamp, 2010). In β-endorphin deficient animals, stress response to EtOH becomes increasingly more hormone dependent (Barfield et al., 2010). In addition to main effects of both sex and β-endorphin on measures of stress-induced behavior, the effect of EtOH was most profound in females deficient in endorphin. This triple interaction between peptide, sex and EtOH sensitivity on stress response was evident in females during their sexually-receptive phase, but not at other times in their estrous cycle.

These data suggest a biologic mechanism for sexually-dimorphic coping responses to stress that is β-endorphin dependent. Unfortunately, there is a paucity of basic biomedical research on sex differences (Beery and Zucker, 2010) but these data suggest the need for future studies to examine the role the estrous cycle plays in the interaction between stress response and alcohol to further understand differences between males and females.

6. β-endorphin and chronic alcohol use

Though genetics certainly contribute to the liability toward alcohol use disorders, excessive drinking in virtually anyone will lead to neural adaptations that underlie dependence, and β-endorphin is also implicated in those changes. The hedonic dysregulation model suggests that a decrease in opioid peptide function (along with other adaptations) following chronic alcohol consumption results in dysregulation of opioid-mediated reward transmission. This blunted reward circuitry is expressed phenotypically as a negative affect that exacerbates the potency of negative reinforcement following drug administration or adds increased salience to relapse related cues (Koob 2008).

Indeed, empirical studies in humans have provided an extensive body of evidence supporting opioid dysregulation following chronic alcohol abuse. Chronic alcoholic patients exhibit decreased synthesis and release of β-endorphin as measured by plasma levels (Aguirre et al., 1990; see Zalewska-Kaszubska & Czarnecka, 2004 for review), and HPA axis dysregulation is a primary characteristic of withdrawal (Adinoff et al., 2005). Furthermore, the functional response of the mu-opioid receptor (which has a high affinity for β-endorphin) is impaired after chronic exposure to EtOH (He & Whistler, 2011). It is thus likely that overactivity of the HPA is at least partly a result of low β-endorphin and that this change contributes to chronically higher basal levels of anxiety and stress during withdrawal (Aguirre et al., 1990; Aguirre et al., 1995 Wand, 2001).

Investigations of recovering alcoholics have shown that levels of plasma β-endorphin are inversely correlated with self-rated measures of anxiety during the withdrawal period (Kiefer et al., 2002). Augmented negative reinforcement following alcohol consumption for subjects with low β-endorphin is likely because of its role in inhibiting CRH secretion. High levels of cortisol act as negative feedback for HPA axis stress response, (Buckingham, 1986) implicating β-endorphin in both behavioral allostasis and endocrine allostasis. Thus, it is likely that an alcohol-induced reduction of increased basal anxiety levels is a strong negative reinforcing factor in the maintenance of chronic alcohol dependence (Goldowitz et al., 2006; Kiefer et al., 2002).

Further support for the dysregulation models comes from Aguirre et al. (1995) who examined the possibility of classifying individuals as alcoholics or non-alcoholics based on plasma β-endorphin levels. They were able to identify alcoholics and non-alcoholics over 70% of the time by this measure alone. Even more impressively, they found a negative predictive value of 93.55% such that for every 100 people found to have normal plasma β-endorphin levels, 93 would actually be non-alcoholics. The results of this study supported a previous finding that low β-endorphin levels are significantly more common in clinical cases of alcoholics (Aguirre et al., 1990).

Plasma β-endorphin levels are involved in the withdrawal process. Kiefer et al. (2006) characterized alcoholics in recovery as either high preference or low preference based on individual average EtOH intake before detoxification. Basal β-endorphin levels of high preference individuals were found to be lower in comparison with low preference subjects. Treatment with acamprosate resulted in a significant increase in β-endorphin in high preference subjects but not in low preference subjects. Because acamprosate administration decreases withdrawal symptoms and increases abstinence, the increased β-endorphin levels in only high preference implicates β-endorphin deficiency as a key aspect in EtOH withdrawal. In addition to acamprosate's efficacy in treating alcoholism, it has recently been shown to reduce anxiety (Schwartz et al., 2010).

7. Conclusion

In conclusion, a growing body of research suggests that sub-optimal levels of β-endorphin result in compromised allostasis of the HPA axis, and that the consequent enhanced sensitivity to stressors facilitates high drinking. Sex differences may play a moderating role in the interaction between stress sensitivity, β-endorphin levels and EtOH. In general, individuals with deficient β-endorphin levels are likely to find EtOH more rewarding from both exaggerated positive and negative reinforcement. Chronic EtOH consumption leads to alterations in β-endorphin activity, and these changes are responsible in part for feelings of anxiety during withdrawal and relapse. Thus, especially in stressful situations, alcohol is likely to serve as an alternative coping mechanism with particular potency for those with labile β-endorphin and therefore predisposed to enhanced sensitivity to its anxiolytic effects.

8. Acknowledgements

This publication was made possible by NIH Grant Numbers P20 RR-016461 from the National Center for Research Resources, AA13259 (through the INIA Stress Consortium) and AA13641 from the National Institute on Alcohol Abuse and Alcoholism.

9. References

Adinoff B, Junghanns K, Kiefer F, Krishnan-Sarin S (2005) Suppression of the HPA axis stress-response: Implications for relapse. *Alcohol Clin and Exp Res,* Vol. 29, pp. 1351-1355, 0145-6008.

Aguirre JC, del Arbol JL, Rico J, Raya J, Mirand MT (1995) Classification of alcoholics on the basis of plasma β-endorphin concentration. *Alcohol,* Vol. 12, pp. 531-534, 0741-8329.

Aguirre JC, del Arbol JL, Raya J, Ruiz-Requena ME, Rico IJ (1990) Plasma beta-Endorphin levels in chronic alcoholics. *Alcohol,* Vol. 7, pp. 409-412, 0741-8329.

Bangasser DA, Curtis A, Reyes BA, Bethea TT, Parastatidis I, Ischiropoulos H, Van Bockstaele EJ, Valentino RJ (2010) Sex differences in corticotropin-releasing factor receptor signaling and trafficking: potential role in female vulnerability to stress-related psychopathology. *Mol Psychiatry,* Vol. 9, pp. 896-904, 1476-5578.

Barfield ET, Barry SM, Hodgin HB, Thompson BM, Allen SS, Grisel JE (2010) β-endorphin mediates behavioral despair and the effect of EtOH on the tail suspension test in mice. *Alcohol Clin and Exp Res,* Vol. 34, pp. 1066-1072, 1530-0277.

Becker HC, Lopez MF, Doremus-Fitzwater TL (2011) Effects of stress on alcohol drinking: a review of animal studies. *Psychopharm.* In press, 1432-2072.

Bolton J, Cox B, Clara I, Sareen J (2006) Use of alcohol and drugs to self-medicate anxiety disorders in a nationally representative sample. *The Journal of Nervous and Mental Disease,* Vol. 194, pp. 818-825, 0022-3018.

Brown SA, Vik PW, Patterson TL, Grant I, Schuckit MA (1995) Stress, vulnerability and adult alcohol relapse. *J Stud Alcohol,* Vol. 56, pp. 538-45, 0096-882X.

Buckingham JC (1986) Stimulation and inhibition of corticotrophin releasing factor by beta endorphin. *Neuroendo,* Vol. 42, pp. 148-52, 0028-3835.

Crabbe JC, Phillips TJ, Harris RA, Arends MA, Koob GF (2006) Alcohol-related genes: contributions from studies with genetically engineered mice. *Addiction Biology,* Vol. 11, pp. 195-269, 1355-6215.

De Waele JP, Gianoulakis C (1993) Effects of single and repeated exposure to ethanol on hypothalamic b-endorphin and CRH release by the C57Bl/6 and DBA/2 strains of mice. *Neuroendo,* Vol, 57, pp. 700-709, 0028-3835.

Gianoulakis C (1998) The roles of the hypothalamic-pituitary-adrenal axis and the endogenous opioid system. *Alco Health Res Wor,* 22, pp. 202-210, 0090-838X.

Gianoulakis C (2001) Influence of the endogenous opioid system on high alcohol consumption and genetic predisposition to alcoholism. *J Psychiatry Neurosci,* Vol. 26, pp. 304-318, 1180-4882.

Gianoulakis C (2004) Endogenous opioids and addiction to alcohol and other drugs of abuse. *Curr Top Med Chem,* Vol. 4, pp. 39-50, 1568-0266.

Gianoulakis C, Beliveau D, Angelogianni P, Meaney M, Thavundayil J, Tawar V, Dumas M (1989) Different pituitary beta-endorphin and adrenal cortisol response to ethanol in individuals with high and low risk for future development of alcoholism. *Life Sci,* Vol. 45, pp. 1097-1109, 0024-3205.

Gianoulakis C, De Waele JP, Thanvundayil J (1996) Implication of the endogenous opioid system in excessive ethanol consumption. *Alcohol,* Vol. 13, pp. 19-23, 0741-8329.

Goldowitz D, Matthews DB, Hamre KM, Mittleman G, Chesler EJ, Becker HC, Lopez MF, Jones SR, Mathews TA, Miles MF, Kerns R, Grant KA (2006) Progress in using mouse inbred strain, consomics, and mutants to identify genes related to stress, anxiety, and alcohol phenotypes. *Alcohol Clin Exp Res,* Vol. 30, pp. 1066-1098, 0145-6008.

Grahame NJ, Low MJ, Cunningham CL (1998) Intravenous self-administration of ethanol in the b-endorphin deficient mice. *Alcohol Clin Exp Res,* Vol. 22, pp. 1093-1098, 0145-6008.

Grisel JE, Mogil JS, Grahame NJ, Rubinstein M, Bellknap JK, Crabbe JC, Low MJ (1999) Ethanol oral self-administration is increased in mutant mice with decreased beta endorphin expression. *Brain Res,* Vol. 835, pp. 62-67, 0006-8993.

Grisel JE, Bartels JL, Allen SA, Turgeon VL (2008) Influence of β-endorphin on anxious behavior in mice: interaction with EtOH. *Psychopharmacol,* Vol. 200, pp. 105-115, 0033-3158.

He L, Whistler JL (2011) Chronic ethanol consumption in rats produces opioid antinociceptive tolerance through inhibition of mu opioid receptor endocytosis. *Plos One,* Vol. 6, No. 5, 1932-6203.

Herz A (1998) Opioid reward mechanisms: a key role in drug abuse? *Canadian Journal of Physiology and Pharmacology,* Vol. 76, No. 3, pp. 252-258, 0008-4212.

Herz A (1997) Endogenous opioids systems and alcohol addiction. *Psychopharmacology,* Vol. 129, No. 2, pp. 99-11, 0033-3158.

Hettema JM, Prescott CA, Kendler KS (2003) The effects of anxiety, substance abuse and conduct disorders on risk of major depressive disorder. *Psych Med,* Vol. 33, pp. 1423-1432, 0033-2917.

Hsu DT, Chen FL, Takahashi LK, Kalin NH (1998) Rapid stress-induced elevations in corticotrophin-releasing hormone mRNA in rat central amygdala nucleus and hypothalamic paraventricuar nucleus: An in situ hybridization analysis. *B Res,* Vol. 788, pp. 305-2310, 0006-8993.

Hunt WA, Zakhari S (1995) Stress, Gender, and Alcohol-Seeking Behavior. NIH, Bethesda.

Janssen SA, Arntz A (2001) Real-life stress and opioid mediated analgesia in novice parachute jumpers. *J Psychophysiol,* Vol. 15, pp. 106-113.

Jarjour S, Bai L, Gianoulakis C (2009) Effect of acute ethanol administration on the release of opioid peptides from the midbrain including the ventral tegmental area. *Alcohol Clin and Exp Res,* Vol. 33, pp. 1033-43, 1530-0277.

Johnson SW, North RA (1992) Opioids excite dopamine neurons by hyperpolarization of local interneurons. *The Journal of Neuroscience,* Vol. 12, No. 2, 483-488, 0270-6474.

Keith LD, Crabbe JC, Robertson LM, Kendall JW (1986) Ethanol stimulated endorphin and corticotrophin secretion *in vitro. Brain Res,* Vol. 367, pp. 222-229, 0006-8993.

Kiefer F, Horntrich M, Jahn H, Wiedemann K (2002) Is withdrawal-induced anxiety in alcoholism based on b-endorphin deficiency? *Pyschopharm,* Vol. 162, pp. 433-437, 0033-3158.

Kiefer F, Jahn H, Otte C, Nakovics H, Wiedemann K (2006) Effects of treatment with acamprosate on β-endorphin plasma concentration in humans with high alcohol preference. *Neurosci Let,* Vol. 404, pp. 103-106, 0304-3940.

King CM, Hentges ST. (2011) Relative number and distribution of murine hypothalamic proopiomelanocortin neurons innervating distinct target sites. *PLoS One.* Vol. 6, e25864, 1932-6203.

Kleim B, Wilhelm FH, Glucksman E, Ehlers A (2010) Sex differences in heart rate responses to script-driven imagery soon after trauma and risk of posttraumatic stress disorder. *Psychosom Med,* Vol. 72, No. 9, pp. 917-24, 1534-7796.

Koob GF (2008) Hedonic dysregulation as a driver of drug-seeking behavior. *Drug Discov Today Dis Models,* Vol. 5, No. 4, pp. 207-215, 1740-6757.

Koob GF, Le Moal ML (1997) Drug abuse: hedonic homeostatic dysregulation. *Science,*Vol. 278, pp. 52-58, 0036-8075.

Kreek MJ, Koob GF (1998) Drug dependence: Stress and dysregulation of brain reward pathways. *Drug Alcohol Depend,* Vol. 51, pp. 23-47, 0376-8716.

Kushner MG, Sher KJ, Meitman BD (1990) The relation between alcohol problems and anxiety disorders. *Am J Psychiatry,* Vol. 147, pp. 685-695, 0002-953X.

Lee S, Selvage D, Hansen K, Rivier C (2004) Site of action of acute alcohol administration in stimulating the rat hypothalamic-pituitary-adrenal axis: Comparison between the effect of systemic and intracerebroventricular injection of this drug on pituitary and hypothalamic response. *Endocrin,* Vol. 145, pp. 4470-4479, 0013-7227.

Maestripieri D, Baran NM, Sapienza P, Zingales L (2010) Between- and within-sex variation in hormonal responses to psychological stress in a large sample of college students. *Stress,* Vol. 13, No. 5, pp. 413-24, 1607-8888.

McGinty JF, Bloom FE (1983) Double immunostaining reveals distinctions among opioid peptidergic neurons in the medial basal hypothalamus. *Brain Res,* Vol. 278, No. 1- 2, pp. 145-153, 0006-8993.

Mogil JS, Richards SP, O'Toole LA, Helms ML, Mitchell SR, Kest B, Belknap JK (1997) Identification of a sex-specific quantitative trait locus mediating nonopioid stress-induced analgesia in female mice. *J Neurosci,* Vol. 17, No. 20, pp. 7995-8002, 0270-6474.

Pacak K, Palkovits M (2001) Stressor specificity of the central neuroendocrine responses: Implications for stress-related disorders. *Endocr Rev*, Vol. 22, pp. 502-548, 0163-769X.

Palanza P (2001) Animal models of anxiety and depression: how are females different? *Neurosci Biobehav Rev*, Vol. 25, No. 3, pp. 219-33, 0149-7634.

Paris JJ, Franco C, Sodano R, Freidenberg B, Gordis E, Anderson DA, Forsyth JP, Wulfert E, Frye CA (2010) Sex differences in salivary cortisol in response to acute stressors among healthy participants, in recreational or pathological gamblers, and in those with posttraumatic stress disorder. *Horm Behav*, Vol. 57, No. 1, pp. 35-45, 1095-6867.

Pohorecky LA (1981) The interaction of alcohol and stress. *Neurosci Behav Rev*, Vol. 5, pp. 209-229, 0149-7634.

Pratchett LC, Pelcovitz MR, Yehuda R (2010) Trauma and violence: are women the weaker sex? *Psychiatr Clin North Am*, Vol. 33, No. 2, pp. 465-74, 1558-3147.

Sarkar DK, Kuhn P, Marano J, Chen C, Boyadjieva N (2007) Alcohol exposure during the developmental period induces beta-endorphin neuronal death and causes alteration in the opioid control of stress axis function. *Endocrinology*, Vol. 148, pp. 2828-2834, 0013-7227.

Schedlowski M, Flu̇ge T, Richter S, Tewes U, Schmidt RE, Wagner TO (1995) Beta-endorphin, but not substance-P, is increased by acute stress in humans. *Psychoneuroendocrinology*, Vol. 20, pp. 103-110, 0306-4530.

Shahman Y, Shalev U, Lu L, de Wit H, Stewart J (2003) The reinstatement model of drug relapse: history, methodology and major findings. *Psychopharm*, Vol. 168, pp. 3-20, 0033-3158.

Schwartz TL, Siddiqui UA, Raza S, Costello A. (2010) Acamprosate calcium as augmentation therapy for anxiety disorders. *Ann Pharmacother*. Vol. 44, pp. 1930-1932, 1060-0280.

Sperling RE, Gomes SM, Sypek EI, Carey AN, McLaughlin JP (2010) Endogenous kappa-opioid mediation of stress-induced potentiation of ethanol-conditioned place preference and self-administration. *Psychopharm*, Vol. 210, pp. 199-209, 1432-2072.

Thiagarajan AB, Mefford IN, Eskay RL (1989) Single-dose ethanol administration activates the hypothalamic-pituitary-adrenal axis; exploration of the mechanism of action. *Neuroendocrinology*, Vol. 50, pp. 427-432, 0028-3835.

Uhart M, Wand GS (2009) Stress, alcohol and drug interaction: an update of human research. *Addict Biol*, Vol. 14, No. 1, pp. 43-64, 1369-1600.

Van Ree JM (1979) Reinforcing stimulus properties of drugs. *Neuropharmacology*, Vol. 18, No. 12, pp. 963-9, 0028-3908.

Wand G, McCaul ME, Gotjen D, Reynolds J, Lee S (2001) Confirmation that offspring from families with alcohol-dependent individuals have greater hypothalamic-pituitary-adrenal axis activation induced by naloxone compared with offspring without a family history of alcohol dependence. *Alcohol Clin Exp Res*, Vol. 25, pp. 1134-1139, 0145-6008.

Wei E, Loh H (1976) Physical dependence of opiate-like peptides. *Science*, Vol. 193, pp. 1262-1263, 0036-8075.

Williams SB, Holloway A, Karwan K, Allen SS, Grisel JE (2007) Oral self-administration of Ethanol in transgenic mice lacking β-endorphin. Impulse Online Journal.

Zalewska-Kaszubska J, Czarnecka E (2005) Deficit in β-endorphin peptide and tendency to alcohol abuse. *Peptides*, Vol. 26, pp. 701-705, 0196-9781.

Zalewska-Kaszubska J, Gorska D, Dyr W, Czarneck E (2006) Effect of acute administration of ethanol on beta-endorphin plasma level in ethanol preferring and non-preferring rats chronically treated with naltrexone. *Pharmacology Biochemistry and Behavior*, Vol. 85, pp. 155-159, 0091-3057.

Zalewska-Kaszubska J, Gorska D, Dyr W, Czarnecka E (2008) Effect of chronic acamprosate treatment on voluntary alcohol intake and β-endorphin levels in rats selectively bred for high alcohol preference. *Neurosci Lett*, Vol. 431, pp. 221-5, 0304-3940.

10

The Role of Delta Opioid Receptors in Ethanol Consumption and Seeking: Implications for New Treatments for Alcohol Use Disorders

Carsten K. Nielsen and Selena E. Bartlett
Ernest Gallo Clinic and Research Center,
University of California San Francisco,
USA

1. Introduction

There are few effective medications available for the treatment of alcohol use disorders (AUDs). To date, the opioid antagonist, naltrexone, is the most effective in reducing alcohol consumption in combination with behavioral therapy. Naltrexone has high affinity for the mu opioid peptide receptor (MOP-R) with moderate activity at the delta opioid peptide receptor (DOP-R) and kappa opioid peptide receptor (KOP-R). Preclinical studies suggest that the MOP-R plays a significant role in ethanol-mediated behaviors, however, there is evidence suggesting the DOP-R may be a better therapeutic target for treating AUDs. This chapter will review studies investigating the role of the opioid receptors in ethanol-mediated behaviors with the view of identifying improved therapeutics for the treatment of AUDs.

1.1 Current therapeutics for the treatment of alcohol use disorders

AUDs are a major public health problem; currently the National Institute on Alcohol Abuse and Alcoholism, reports there are 17.6 million people in the United States either abuse alcohol or are alcohol dependent. There have been three medications approved by the U.S. Food and Drug Administration: disulfiram (Antabuse), acamprosate (Campral), and naltrexone (ReVia, Vivitrol) - all of which suffer from limited effectiveness due to side-effects and compliance issues (Bouza et al., 2004; Mark et al., 2003a; Mark et al., 2003b; Pettinati et al., 2000). The aldehyde dehydrogenase blocker, disulfiram has not been very effective for treating AUDs (Johnson, 2008; O'Shea, 2000) primarily because of patient compliance (Johnson, 2008; O'Shea, 2000). Disulfiram is reportedly only clinically effective in patients who were fully compliant with taking their medication and were under supervision (Fuller et al., 1986). Acamprosate has been shown to be effective for alcohol dependence in European trials, but not in U.S. trials, and has a low incidence of side-effects (Anton et al., 2006; Bouza et al., 2004; Whitworth et al., 1996). To date, the opioid antagonist, naltrexone, appears to be the most effective medication for alcohol dependence (Anton et al., 2006; O'Malley et al., 1992; Volpicelli et al., 1992).

1.2 Preclinical studies with naltrexone

Naltrexone has been shown to effectively reduce ethanol consumption and seeking in a large number of studies (Ciccocioppo et al., 2002a; Critcher et al., 1983; Franck et al., 1998; Gardell et al., 1996; Le et al., 1999; Nielsen et al., 2008; Simms et al., 2008; Stromberg et al., 1998a; Walker & Koob, 2008). Furthermore, intramuscular injections of naltrexone reduce intravenous (i.v.) or oral self-administration of ethanol in rhesus monkeys (Altshuler et al., 1980; Williams et al., 2001). Naltrexone reduces ethanol consumption in both low ethanol consuming rats (Stromberg et al., 1998a) and high ethanol consuming rats (Nielsen et al., 2008; Simms et al., 2008). However, the effects of naltrexone on ethanol consumption are non-selective as fat, sucrose and water intake are also reduced (Corwin & Wojnicki, 2009; Nielsen et al., 2008; Rao et al., 2008; Simms et al., 2008; Wong et al., 2009). Also, naltrexone reduces alcohol- and cue-induced reinstatement, but not foot-shock stress-induced reinstatement of ethanol-seeking in rodents (Ciccocioppo et al., 2002a; Le et al., 1999; Liu & Weiss, 2002).

1.3 Clinical studies with naltrexone

A number of clinical studies have reported that naltrexone effectively reduces relapse in a subset of alcohol-dependent humans (Anton et al., 1999; Anton et al., 2006; O'Malley et al., 1992; Volpicelli et al., 1992) and is more effective at reducing heavy drinking (Pettinati et al., 2006). Alcohol-dependent patients that have a polymorphism in the OPRM1 gene encoding the mu opioid peptide receptor (MOP-R) with a mutation at A118G (Asn40Asp) have greater euphoric responses to alcohol, increased pain thresholds, greater susceptibility to AUDs and greater responses treatment with naltrexone (Anton et al., 2008; Bart et al., 2005; Oroszi et al., 2009; Oslin et al., 2003). More recently, the use of naltrexone in an extended-release intra-muscular (i.m.) depot formulation (Vivitrol®) is more effective in patients who are able to abstain from drinking prior to treatment (O'Malley et al., 2007; Pettinati et al., 2009). Taken together, treatment with naltrexone appears to have the most consistent effects on drinking outcomes in subjects with A118G mutation.

1.4 Pharmacological activity of naltrexone in reducing ethanol-mediated behaviors

Naltrexone has the highest affinity for the MOP-R, moderate activity at the delta (DOP-R) and kappa (KOP-R) opioid peptide receptors, but without activity at nociceptin (NOP-R) and the sigma (SIG-R) receptors (Ananthan et al., 1999; Goldstein & Naidu, 1989; Takemori & Portoghese, 1984). There is a large body of evidence that suggests that the MOP-R plays a significant role in ethanol-mediated reward behavior (Becker et al., 2002; Ciccocioppo et al., 2002a; Gardell et al., 1996; Hall et al., 2001; Le et al., 1999; Reid & Hunter, 1984; Roberts et al., 2000) (Table 1). Ethanol has been reported to stimulate the activity of the endogenous opioids which target the MOP-R leading to increased basal dopamine release in the mesolimbic pathway Herz, 1997). Naltrexone's mechanism of action has been proposed to result from inhibition of ethanol-induced activity of endogenous opioid peptides and dopamine release *in vivo* (Benjamin et al., 1993; Gonzales & Weiss, 1998; Zalewska-Kaszubska et al., 2006; Zalewska-Kaszubska et al., 2008). In comparison, the roles of the other opioid subtypes on ethanol-mediated behaviors, such as the DOP-R (Krishnan-Sarin et al., 1995a; Roberts et al., 2001; Stromberg et al., 1998a) and KOP-R (Kovacs et al., 2005; Lindholm et al., 2001; Mitchell et al., 2005) are less well-defined.

2. The role of the Mu Opioid Peptide Receptor (MOP-R) in ethanol consumption and seeking

2.1 Ethanol consumption in MOP-R knockout mice

Mice with a genetic deletion of the MOP-R have reduced levels of ethanol intake and seeking in comparison to wild-type mice with a mixed C57/129sv background (Becker et al., 2002; Hall et al., 2001; Roberts et al., 2001; Roberts et al., 2000) (Table 1). Although one study using purebred C57BL/6 mice failed to show any difference in ethanol intake (van Rijn & Whistler, 2009), the differences in these studies may reflect the varying degrees of ethanol intake in mice with different genetic backgrounds (Yoneyama et al., 2008) and also the models of ethanol consumption employed.

2.2 MOP-R activation and ethanol consumption

The opioid receptor agonist, morphine increases ethanol (3-26%) intake in solutions containing sucrose (Hubbell et al., 1986; Reid & Hunter, 1984) suggesting an involvement of the opioid system in the reinforcing properties of ethanol (Table 1). Furthermore, microinjections of morphine into the rat nucleus accumbens (NAc), a brain region involved in the reinforcement pathway, increases ethanol and food intake (Barson et al., 2009). The selective MOP-R agonist, DAMGO, into the NAc increases intake of saccharin, salt, fat and ethanol (de Wet et al., 2001). Since morphine has the highest affinity for the MOP-R but also activity at KOP-R and DOP-R (Goldstein & Naidu, 1989), this may explain some of the non-selective effects on consummatory behavior. It cannot be ruled out that the effects of morphine on food and ethanol consumption may be related to morphine's rewarding effects (Gaiardi et al., 1991; Shippenberg et al., 2009; Shippenberg et al., 1996). Taken together, this data suggests that the MOP-R plays a more general role in ingestive behaviors.

2.3 MOP-R antagonists and ethanol consumption and seeking

The MOP-R has been proposed to be primarily responsible for the action of naltrexone in reducing ethanol consumption and seeking (Stromberg et al., 1998a). Although naltrexone has consistently been shown to reduce ethanol consumption and seeking, the effects of opioid antagonists with higher selectivity for the MOP-R have been shown to produce mixed results (Ciccocioppo et al., 2002a; Hyytia & Kiianmaa, 2001; Marinelli et al., 2009) (Table 1). The selective MOP-R antagonist, CTOP (D-Pen-Cys-Tyr-D-Trp-Orn-Thr-Pen-Thr-NH2), reduces operant ethanol responding in rats when administered into either the cerebroventricles or into the amygdala, but not when administered into the NAc or ventral tegmental area (VTA) (Hyytia & Kiianmaa, 2001). In rats trained to self-administer ethanol and subsequently extinguished from responding, CTOP had no effect of light/tone cue-induced reinstatement and only short-lasting reductions on context-induced reinstatement of ethanol-seeking (Marinelli et al., 2009). Furthermore, in a model of cue-induced reinstatement using visual and olfactory discriminative stimuli, the MOP-R1-selective antagonist, naloxonazine, reduced reinstatement but also produced some nonselective behavioral suppression (Ciccocioppo et al., 2002a). In the same study, naltrexone selectively inhibited cue-induced reinstatement of ethanol-seeking (Ciccocioppo et al., 2002a). The irreversible MOP-R-selective antagonist, clocinnamox, did not reduce responding for oral ethanol in rhesus monkeys, except when it was co-administered with naltrexone (Williams & Woods, 1998). These studies suggest that naltrexone's ability to reduce ethanol consumption and seeking may be mediated via a non-MOP-R.

3. The role of the Delta Opioid Peptide Receptor (DOP-R) in ethanol consumption and seeking

3.1 Ethanol consumption in DOP-R knockout mice

Studies in mice with a genetic deletion of the DOP-R (C57BL/6 or mixed C57/129sv background) have increased levels of ethanol intake when compared to wild-type mice (Roberts et al., 2001; van Rijn & Whistler, 2009) (Table 1). This suggests that decreased DOP-R activity is associated with high ethanol consumption. This may be related to the increased anxiety levels in DOP-R knockout mice as anxiety-like responses were reversed by the consumption of ethanol in the DOP-R knockout mice (Roberts et al., 2001).

3.2 DOP-R activation and ethanol consumption

Ethanol has been shown to stimulate the activity of the endogenous opioids, β-endorphins and enkephalins, which target the MOP-R and DOP-R, respectively, to increase basal dopamine release in the mesolimbic pathway (Herz, 1997). Activation of the enkephalinergic system and occupation of DOP-Rs has been proposed to be important for the maintenance of high voluntary ethanol intake (Froehlich et al., 1991). The enkephalinase inhibitor, thiorphan, which potentiates the actions of the endogenous opioids for the DOP-R by protecting the enkephalins from degradation, increased ethanol, but not water, intake in alcohol-preferring rats (Froehlich et al., 1991).

Recently, further studies have examined the effects of activation of the DOP-R on ethanol consumption using various DOP-R agonists (Barson et al., 2009; Barson et al., 2010; van Rijn et al., 2010) (Table 1). In support of the earlier studies, systemic administration of the DOP-R agonist, SNC80, in mice and microinjections of the DOP-R agonist, DALA (7-14 nM), into the NAc and hypothalamic paraventricular nucleus (HPN) of rats lead to increased ethanol consumption (Barson et al., 2009; Barson et al., 2010; van Rijn et al., 2010). In mice trained using the 10% ethanol 4 hr limited access paradigm, SNC80 increased ethanol consumption (van Rijn et al., 2010). In rats trained to consume up to 7% ethanol for 12 h each day with incremental increases in the concentration of ethanol every four days, the administration of DALA into the NAc selectively increased ethanol consumption over food and water (Barson et al., 2009). Similarly, the effects of DALA administered into the HPN were selective for ethanol over food and water consumption (Barson et al., 2010). DOP-R agonists have also been shown to reduce ethanol consumption in rats (Margolis et al., 2008) and mice (van Rijn & Whistler, 2009). Systemic administration of the selective DOP-R agonist, TAN67, reduced voluntary ethanol intake in mice using a 4 hr limited ethanol access paradigm (van Rijn & Whistler, 2009). Following administration of the DOP-R agonist, DPDPE (10 mM), into the ventral tegmental area (VTA) of rats using continuous access to 10% ethanol paradigm, ethanol intake was reduced in low but not high ethanol consuming rats (Margolis et al., 2008). It is hypothesized that DOP-Rs in the VTA play a protective role against elevated ethanol consumption (Margolis et al., 2008).

3.3 Ethanol consumption and seeking with DOP-R antagonists

The administration of DOP-R antagonists decreases ethanol consumption and seeking in rats (Franck et al., 1998; Hyytia & Kiianmaa, 2001; June et al., 1999; Krishnan-Sarin et al., 1995b; Marinelli et al., 2009; Nielsen et al., 2011; Nielsen et al., 2008). However, DOP-R antagonists also have been shown to not affect (Ingman et al., 2003; Stromberg et al., 1998a) or increase ethanol intake (Margolis et al., 2008) (Table 1). Factors likely contributing to these disparities include the length of ethanol exposure, the route of drug administration, different types of drinking models that induce low, moderate and high ethanol consumption, the rodent strains used (such as alcohol-preferring rats) and potential different roles of subtypes of the DOP-R on ethanol-mediated behaviors.

Opioid Rece-ptor	Effects on Ethanol Consumption and Seeking ↓ Decreased, ↑ Increased, or No Effect (Reference)						
	Voluntary ethanol consumption			Operant responding for ethanol		Reinstatement of ethanol-seeking	
	Knock -out mice	Antagonists	Agonists	Antagonists	Agonists	Antagonists	Agonists
MOP-R	↓ (1,2,3)	↓ (6,7,8,10,20,18,36,47,48) No Effect (10)	↓ (6) ↑ (18,33) No Effect (22,23)	↓ (9,27,30.32)	-	↓ (11,30) No Effect (28)	↓ (32)
DOP-R	↑ (4,24)	↓ (10,14,15,20,24) ↑ (21) No Effect (7,13)	↓ (21,24) ↑ (22,23,25)	↓ (9, 12)	-	↓ (11,28,29)	-
KOP-R	↓ (5)	↓ (46) ↑ (16)	↓ (19,23) No Effect (22)	↓ (26, 27)	-	No Effect (17)	↑ (17)
NOP-R	↓ (42)	No Effect (33,38)	↑ (35, 45) ↓ (33,34,35,37,38,40,45)	-	↓ (32,37,41) No Effect (37)	-	↓ (32, 34, 39, 41)
SIG-R	-	↓ (44)	-	↓ (43)	↑ (31)	↓ (44)	-

Table 1. The roles of opioid receptors in ethanol consumption and seeking in rats and mice. 1. Roberts et al., 2000; 2. Hall et al., 2001; 3. Becker et al., 2002; 4. Roberts et al., 2001; 5. Kovacs et al., 2005; 6. Critcher et al., 1983; 7. Stromberg et al., 1998a; 8. Gardell et al., 1996; 9. Hyytia & Kiianmaa, 2001; 10. Franck et al., 1998; 11. Ciccocioppo et al., 2002a; 12. June et al., 1999; 13. Ingman et al., 2003; 14. Krishnan-Sarin et al., 1995a; 15. Krishnan-Sarin et al., 1995b; 16. Mitchell et al., 2005; 17. Holter et al., 2000; 18. Reid & Hunter, 1984; 19. Lindholm et al., 2001. 20. Nielsen et al., 2008; 21. Margolis et al., 2008; 22. Barson et al., 2009; 23. Barson et al., 2010; 24. van Rijn & Whistler, 2009; 25. van Rijn et al., 2010; 26. Walker et al., 2011 ; 27. Walker & Koob, 2008; 28. Marinelli et al., 2009; 29. Nielsen et al., 2011; 30. Le et al., 1999; 31. Sabino et al., 2011; 32. Kuzmin et al., 2007; 33. Ciccocioppo et al., 2007; 34. Ciccocioppo et al., 2003; 35. Ciccocioppo et al., 1999; 36. Simms et al., 2008; 37. Economidou et al., 2008; 38. Ciccocioppo et al., 2002b. 39. Martin-Fardon et al., 2000; 40. Cifani et al., 2006 41. Ciccocioppo et al., 2004; 42. Sakoori & Murphy, 2008; 43. Sabino et al., 2009a; 44. Sabino et al., 2009b; 45. Economidou et al., 2006; 46. Sandi et al., 1990.; 47. Stromberg et al., 2002; 48. Stromberg et al., 1998b.

3.4 DOP-R antagonists in high drinking rats

DOP-R antagonists reduce ethanol consumption in high-ethanol consuming or alcohol-preferring strains of rats (Hyytia & Kiianmaa, 2001; Krishnan-Sarin et al., 1995a; Krishnan-Sarin et al., 1995b; Nielsen et al., 2008). In studies using alcohol-preferring (P) rats, the DOP-R antagonists naltrindole, ICI 174864 and naltriben all effectively reduced ethanol consumption using the two-bottle choice 10% ethanol paradigm (Krishnan-Sarin et al., 1995a; Krishnan-Sarin et al., 1995b). Naltrindole given systemically in the maximally effective dose (15 mg/kg) produced a long-lasting reduction in ethanol intake for at least 8 h following a single dose and for at least 28 h following a second dose given 4 h later (Krishnan-Sarin et al., 1995a). Although the effects of naltrindole were selective for ethanol over water intake, naltrindole also suppressed the intake of saccharin solutions either with or without ethanol (Krishnan-Sarin et al., 1995a). In comparison, another study by the same group showed that systemic administration of the DOP-R2-selective antagonist, naltriben, (6 mg/kg in two doses) reduced ethanol consumption but not water consumption (Krishnan-Sarin et al., 1995b). Furthermore, it was shown that naltriben reduced the intake of solutions containing ethanol with saccharin and ethanol with quinine but did not affect the intake of either saccharin or quinine solutions alone. Taken together, this suggests that the suppressive effects of naltriben are selective for ethanol. In high-drinking AA (Alko, Alcohol) rats trained to operantly respond for 10% ethanol, intracerebroventricular (i.c.v.) administration of naltrindole, but not the MOP-R antagonist, CTOP, produced a significant and dose-dependent suppression of responding for ethanol (Hyytia & Kiianmaa, 2001). Furthermore, both naltrindole and CTOP suppressed responding in non-ethanol preferring Wistar rats suggesting that the DOP-R may play a greater role than the MOP-R in suppressing responding in high drinking rats, regardless of strain. This is further supported by other studies using models of low to moderate ethanol or limited access paradigms in which DOP-R antagonists do not reduce ethanol consumption (Ingman et al., 2003; Margolis et al., 2008; Stromberg et al., 1998a).

The recent recharacterization of a rat model of voluntary high ethanol intake using intermittent access to 20% ethanol without the use of any initiation procedures (Simms et al., 2008; Wise, 1973) has led to the investigation of the roles of opioid receptors and effects of opioid ligands in high-ethanol consuming, albeit non-ethanol preferring, rats. Using this model of high ethanol intake, the naltrexone-derived DOP-R antagonist, SoRI-9409, was shown to be threefold more effective and selective in reducing ethanol intake than naltrexone in Long-Evans rats (Nielsen et al., 2008). SoRI-9409 more potently reduced high ethanol intake using the model of intermittent access to 20% ethanol compared to less potent reductions in moderate ethanol intake using a model of continuous access to 10% ethanol. The effects of single doses of SoRI-9409 were long-lasting such that reductions in high ethanol intake were observed after 24 h of access, in comparison to naltrexone which was only effective after short access periods (30 min). The effects of SoRI-9409, unlike naltrexone, were also selective for ethanol such that water intake was not reduced. Furthermore, SoRI-9409 did not reduce sucrose intake at doses that effectively reduced ethanol intake. Using the high drinking model of intermittent access to 20% ethanol, daily systemic administrations of SoRI-9409 to Long Evans rats for 28 days selectively reduced the onset and escalation of ethanol intake and continued to selectively reduce ethanol intake by > 50%

for up to 28 days compared with vehicle-treated rats (Nielsen et al., 2008). When the daily administrations of SoRI-9409 were ceased after 28 days, ethanol consumption was maintained at approximately one-half of the baseline drinking levels of post-vehicle-treated rats, for a further 28 days. Cessation of SoRI-9409 treatment did not result in any significant escalation in ethanol consumption suggesting that multiple administrations of SoRI-9409 produce long-lasting and permanent effects on the modulation of ethanol consumption. This further suggests that inhibition of DOP-Rs directly reduces ethanol intake during the escalation and maintenance of drinking in high-ethanol–consuming rats.

3.5 DOP-R antagonists in models of relapse to ethanol-seeking

A major problem in treating AUDs is the high rate of relapse, which can be triggered by re-exposure to cues or an environment previously associated with alcohol use and also by stress. An effective pharmacological treatment for AUDs would ideally prevent relapse of alcohol-seeking in addition to reducing consumption of ethanol. Naltrexone reduces alcohol- and cue-induced reinstatement, but not foot-shock stress-induced reinstatement of ethanol-seeking in rodents (Ciccocioppo et al., 2002a; Le et al., 1999; Liu & Weiss, 2002). It has been shown that DOP-Rs, rather than MOP-Rs, are important for cue-induced reinstatement of ethanol-seeking, as the DOP-R antagonist, naltrindole, reduces cue-induced reinstatement of ethanol-seeking behavior in rodents more effectively than the MOP-R selective antagonists, naloxonazine or CTOP (Ciccocioppo et al., 2002a; Marinelli et al., 2009). Furthermore, recent studies show that the DOP-R antagonist, SoRI-9409, effectively and dose-dependently reduces yohimbine stress-induced reinstatement of ethanol-seeking in rats (Nielsen et al., 2011). This study further demonstrated that the DOP-R plays a greater role than MOP-R or KOP-R in yohimbine stress-induced reinstatement of ethanol-seeking in rats as TAN67- and Deltorphin II-mediated DOP-R activity, using the $[^{35}S]GTP\gamma S$ coupling assay in midbrain membranes, were increased in membranes of yohimbine-treated ethanol-extinguished rats compared to vehicle-treated rats. Moreover, the increase in DOP-R-mediated $[^{35}S]$ $GTP\gamma S$ stimulation observed in yohimbine-treated ethanol-trained rats was absent in naive (non ethanol-trained) rats, suggesting that a history of ethanol self-administration plays an important role in the regulation of DOP-R signaling. In contrast with DOP-R activity, there were no changes in DAMGO-mediated MOP-R or (–)U50488-mediated KOP-R activity in ethanol-trained rats, further supporting studies showing DOP-Rs rather than MOP-Rs are important for reinstatement of ethanol-seeking (Ciccocioppo et al., 2002a; Marinelli et al., 2009).

3.6 DOP-R subtypes in ethanol consumption and seeking

Although one DOP-R gene has been cloned (Evans et al., 1992; Kieffer et al., 1992), two DOP-R subtypes, DOP-R1 and DOP-R2, have been pharmacologically identified *in vivo* and in binding studies in rodent brain membranes (Buzas et al., 1994; Mattia et al., 1991; Negri et al., 1991; Sofuoglu et al., 1991; Zaki et al., 1996). However, the roles of DOP-R subtypes in ethanol-mediated behaviors are not well defined. Studies in mice suggest DOP-R1 and DOP-R2 may have opposing effects on voluntary ethanol intake (van Rijn & Whistler, 2009) such that the DOP-R1 agonist, TAN67, and the DOP-R2 antagonist, naltriben, both reduce ethanol consumption. These different roles of DOP-R1 and DOP-R2 on ethanol intake are hypothesized as DOP-R1 existing as a MOP-R/DOP-R heterodimer which opposes the actions of DOP-R2, which may exist as a DOP-R homomer (van Rijn & Whistler, 2009). Another recent study showed that DOP-R1 inhibition appears more important than DOP-R2 inhibition in yohimbine stress-induced reinstatement of ethanol-seeking in rats (Nielsen et al., 2011). Using the [^{35}S]GTPγS signaling assay in midbrain membranes prepared from yohimbine-treated rats previously responding for ethanol and subsequently extinguished, there was higher TAN67-mediated DOP-R1 activity (> 700-fold) than deltorphin II-mediated DOP-R2 activity (≥ 4-fold) compared to vehicle-treated rats (Nielsen et al., 2011). Pre-treatment with the DOP-R antagonist, SoRI-9409, in yohimbine-treated rats reduced DOP-R1 activity by 37-fold, but did not change DOP-R2, MOP-R or KOP-R activity. The potent inhibition of TAN67-stimulated DOP-R1 activity in yohimbine-treated rat membranes by SoRI-9409, naltrindole and the DOP-R1 antagonist, 7-Benzylidenenaltrexone (BNTX) (Sofuoglu et al., 1993), further suggests that DOP-R1 inhibition is important for reducing yohimbine-induced ethanol-seeking (Nielsen et al., 2011). As SoRI-9409 effectively reduces ethanol consumption in rats and potently reduces DOP-R1 activity in brain membranes of high-ethanol consuming rats (Nielsen et al., 2008), DOP-R1 inhibition appears to play a role in both reducing reinstatement of ethanol-seeking and voluntary ethanol intake in rats. However, as SoRI-9409 inhibits both deltorphin II-mediated DOP-R2 analgesia and DPDPE-mediated DOP-R1 analgesia in mice (Wells et al., 2001), it appears that the subtypes of the DOP-R have different roles in different behaviors and species.

3.7 The role of the DOP-R in the rewarding effects of ethanol

The DOP-R has been shown to play a role in the reinforcing effects of ethanol (Borg & Taylor, 1997; Froehlich et al., 1998; Froehlich et al., 1991; Shippenberg et al., 2008). Activation of DOP-Rs in the NAc and VTA leads to increased basal dopamine release (Borg & Taylor, 1997; Devine et al., 1993b; Herz, 1997; Vetulani, 2001). Dopamine release in the striatum is stimulated by ethanol, DOP-R agonists and enkephalinase inhibitors (Dourmap et al., 1990; Petit et al., 1986; Spanagel et al., 1990) and ethanol-induced release of dopamine in the striatum is blocked by DOP-R antagonists (Acquas et al., 1993; Widdowson & Holman, 1992). DOP-R agonists increase and DOP-R antagonists decrease, respectively, ethanol-induced place preference in rats (Bie et al., 2009; Matsuzawa et al., 1999a; Matsuzawa et al., 1999b) and DOP-R antagonists can make a nonaversive dose of alcohol aversive (Froehlich et al., 1998). A series of studies demonstrated that the DOP-R plays a role in conditioned place preference (CPP) to ethanol using a model of conditioned fear stress (Matsuzawa et al., 1998; Matsuzawa et al., 1999a; Matsuzawa et al., 1999b). In this model, ethanol produced a significant CPP only in rats that were exposed to an environment previously paired with an electric foot shock (Matsuzawa et al., 1998; Matsuzawa et al., 1999a; Matsuzawa et al., 1999b). Significant CPP to ethanol (300 mg/kg, intraperitoneal (i.p.) in rats was attenuated following systemic administration of the non-selective opioid receptor antagonist naloxone (1-3 mg/kg, subcutaneous (s.c.)), the MOP-R antagonist beta-funaltrexamine (3-10 mg/kg, i.p.), the DOP-R antagonist naltrindole (1-3 mg/kg, s.c.) and the KOP-R agonist, U50488 (0.3-1 mg/kg, s.c.)(Matsuzawa et al., 1998; Matsuzawa et al., 1999a). This is in contrast to enhanced place preference to ethanol following systemic administration of the KOP-R antagonist, nor-binaltorphimine (nor-BNI; 3 mg/kg, i.p.) (Matsuzawa et al., 1999a).

Conversely, when ethanol (75-150 mg/kg) was combined with the MOP-R-preferring agonist, morphine (0.1 mg/kg), or the selective DOP-R agonist, TAN-67 (20 mg/kg, s.c.), at doses below the threshold to produce place preference on their own, there was an enhancement of place preference to ethanol (Matsuzawa et al., 1998; Matsuzawa et al., 1999a). Furthermore, naltrindole (3 mg/kg, s.c.) significantly attenuated the enhancement of the ethanol-induced (75 mg/kg, i.p) place preference produced by TAN67 (20 mg/kg, s.c.) suggesting DOP-R receptors may be involved in the rewarding mechanism of ethanol under psychological stress (Matsuzawa et al., 1999b). The attenuation of CPP to ethanol and increased conditioned taste aversion to ethanol by the DOP-R antagonist, naltrindole (Froehlich et al., 1998; Matsuzawa et al., 1998; Matsuzawa et al., 1999a; Matsuzawa et al., 1999b) may contribute, at least in part, to the reductions in ethanol consumption following administration of DOP-R antagonists (Hyytia & Kiianmaa, 2001; Krishnan-Sarin et al., 1995a; Krishnan-Sarin et al., 1995b; Nielsen et al., 2008). However, whether enhanced CPP to ethanol following treatment with TAN67 would explain the effects of DOP-R agonists on ethanol consumption and seeking is unclear. An increase in the rewarding actions of ethanol by TAN67 may subsequently lead to reduced consumption (van Rijn & Whistler, 2009) as less ethanol may be required to produce ethanol's effects. Conversely, activation of DOP-Rs and the subsequent increased rewarding effects of ethanol may have contributed to further increased levels of ethanol consumption following treatment with DOP-R agonists (Barson et al., 2009; Barson et al., 2010; van Rijn et al., 2010). Collectively, these studies suggest that activation and inhibition of DOP-R activity may modulate ethanol consumption via different mechanisms in the central nervous system.

4. The role of the Kappa Opioid Peptide Receptor (KOP-R) in ethanol consumption and seeking

4.1 Ethanol consumption in KOP-R knockout mice

Mice with a genetic deletion of the KOP-R (mixed C57BL/6-129SvJ background) have reduced levels of ethanol intake in animals consuming 12% ethanol and saccharin using a two-bottle choice paradigm (Kovacs et al., 2005) (Table 1). In contrast to the MOP-R and DOP-R, stimulation of the KOP-R is associated with dysphoria, suppression of reward, induced states of aversion, reduced dopamine release in the NAc, inhibition of dopaminergic neurons in the VTA and promotion of negative reinforcement (Bruijnzeel, 2009; Ebner et al., 2010; Margolis et al., 2003; Shippenberg & Herz, 1986).

4.2 KOP-R activation and ethanol consumption

Systemic administration of the KOP-R agonist, U50488, reduces intake of 10% ethanol using two-bottle choice paradigms (Lindholm et al., 2001; Nestby et al., 1999) (Table 1). Furthermore, administration of the KOP-R agonists, dynorphin1-17 or MR-2266-BS, prior to the first free-choice session following a period of forced ethanol exposure reduced preference for ethanol (Sandi et al., 1988; Sandi et al., 1990). The long-acting benzomorphan opioid compound, bremazocine, which acts as an antagonist at MOP-R and DOP-R and an agonist at KOP-R, was shown to more potently reduce 10% ethanol intake than the non-selective opioid antagonist, naltrexone (Nestby et al., 1999). However, as KOP-R agonists produce aversion, this may lead to reductions in ethanol consumption but this remains to be studied. The KOP-R agonist, U69593, produces conditioned place aversion (CPA) in animals (Shippenberg & Herz, 1986) and KOP-R agonists induce dysphoria in humans (Kumor et al., 1986; Pfeiffer et al., 1986; Rimoy et al., 1994). In contrast, the KOP-R agonist, enadoline (or CI-977), when delivered via mini-osmotic subcutaneous pumps increased 10 and 20% ethanol consumption (Holter et al., 2000). However, in rats responding for ethanol for long periods, the lever pressing for ethanol was either decreased or increased following acute systemic administration of higher or lower doses of enadoline, respectively (Holter et al., 2000). As lever pressing for water was also reduced with enadoline treatment, these reductions in responding for ethanol may have been due to sedative effects of this treatment at higher doses.

4.3 KOP-R antagonists and ethanol consumption and seeking

A number of studies have shown mixed results for the selective KOP-R antagonist, nor-BNI using a variety of models of ethanol consumption and seeking (Table 1). In rats given continuous access to 10% ethanol using the two-bottle choice paradigm, a single systemic injection of nor-BNI induced a long-lasting increase in ethanol consumption, particularly in higher drinking rats without inducing CPP (Mitchell et al., 2005). However, nor-BNI has been shown to increase ethanol-induced place preference in rats (Matsuzawa et al., 1999a). In rhesus monkeys responding for solutions of 1-2% ethanol, nor-BNI reduced responding for ethanol on the day of the systemic injection (Williams & Woods, 1998). nor-BNI has low affinity for the MOP-R at 2 h post-injection time point and high affinity for the KOP-R up to 24 h post-injection (Broadbear et al., 1994; Endoh et al., 1992; Horan et al., 1992) suggesting the reductions in ethanol responding on the day of nor-BNI dosing may be MOP-R mediated. In Wistar rats responding for 10% ethanol, nor-BNI has been shown to be more effective in a rat model of ethanol-dependence, using a 4-week intermittent vapor exposure paradigm, compared to non-ethanol dependent rats (Walker & Koob, 2008). Although i.c.v. administration of nor-BNI given immediately before the testing session reduced responding for ethanol in dependent rats (Walker & Koob, 2008), further studies performed with systemically administered nor-BNI given 24 h before the test session similarly reduced responding in ethanol-dependent rats but not in non-dependent rats (Walker et al., 2011). These studies suggest that the dynorphin/KOP-R systems are dysregulated in dependence and contribute to the increased consumption observed during acute withdrawal in dependent rats. Systemic administration of nalmefene, which has similar affinity for MOP-R but higher affinity for KOP-R and DOP-R, compared to naltrexone (Michel et al., 1985), was found to more effectively reduce responding for ethanol in dependent rats than naltrexone (Walker and Koob, 2008). As nalmefene and naltrexone had similar effects on reducing responding in non-dependent rats, this further supports a specific role of the KOP-R in ethanol-dependence (Walker & Koob, 2008).

5. Nociceptin/Orphanin FQ Receptors (NOP-R) and ethanol consumption and seeking

A number of studies have investigated the role of the nociceptin receptor (NOP-R), also known as the opioid receptor-like 1 receptor (ORL1), using the endogenous ligand for the NOP-R, nociceptin/orphanin FQ. Although nociceptin has structural homology with opioid peptides, it does not bind to MOP-R, DOP-R or KOP-R (Reinscheid et al., 1996;

Reinscheid et al., 1998) and appears to possess anti-opioid functional activity (Mogil et al., 1996a; Mogil et al., 1996b; Mogil & Pasternak, 2001). Opioid antagonists, such as naloxone and naltrexone, are not reported to have activity at the NOP-R (Ciccocioppo et al., 2007; Darland et al., 1998; Henderson & McKnight, 1997), although indirect interactions between NOP-R and the classical opioid receptors have been suggested (Yu et al., 2002). In mice with a genetic deletion of the NOP-R ethanol consumption was reduced and ethanol-induced CPP was increased compared to wild-type mice (Koster et al., 1999; Sakoori & Murphy, 2008). However, activation of the NOP-R, using NOP-R agonists including nociceptin and R0-64-6198, have consistently shown reductions in ethanol intake and ethanol CPP (Ciccocioppo et al., 2003; Ciccocioppo et al., 2007; Ciccocioppo et al., 1999; Ciccocioppo et al., 2002b; Economidou et al., 2006; Kuzmin et al., 2007) . In addition, NOP-R agonists have been shown to increase food intake (Cifani et al., 2006). In contrast, the effects of NOP-R antagonists administered alone to rats have not resulted in altered ethanol consumption and seeking. The results of these studies are summarized in Table 1 and have been previously reviewed (Ciccocioppo et al., 2000; Ciccocioppo et al., 2003).

6. Sigma Receptors and ethanol consumption

Sigma receptors (SIG-R) were originally categorized as members of the opioid receptor family (Quirion et al., 1992) although more recent studies suggested SIG-Rs are unique binding sites including phencyclidine binding sites (Gundlach et al., 1985; Gundlach et al., 1986; Martin et al., 1976; Walker et al., 1990). Furthermore, the opioid antagonist, naltrexone, is not reported to have activity at the SIG-R (Holtzman, 1989; Vaupel, 1983).

The SIG-Rs antagonist, BD1047, reduces ethanol-induced locomotion, ethanol-induced place preference and taste conditioning in Swiss mice (Maurice et al., 2003). Conversely, the SIG-R agonist, PRE-084, increased ethanol CPP without effects on ethanol-induced locomotion (Maurice et al., 2003). A series of studies have shown the SIG-R to play a role in ethanol consumption and seeking in Sardinian alcohol-preferring (sP) rats (Sabino et al., 2011; Sabino et al., 2009a; Sabino et al., 2009b) (Table 1). Administration of the SIG-R antagonists, BD1063 NE-100, selectively reduces ethanol consumption, responding for ethanol and also prevents the increase in ethanol intake after an ethanol-deprivation period in rats (Sabino et al., 2009b). Chronic administration of the SIG-R agonist, DTG, increased responding for ethanol in rats, an effect that was blocked with BD-1063 pretreatment (Sabino et al., 2011). However, DTG treatment also increased responding for saccharin and sucrose (Sabino et al., 2011). Chronic administration of DTG to naive rats resulted in increased mRNA expression of MOP-R and DOP-R, but not KOP-R, in the VTA (Sabino et al., 2011). This increased opioid mRNA expression was suggested to be responsible for the excessive alcohol intake following DTG treatment, in agreement with previous studies reporting the importance of DOP-R activity in maintaining high ethanol intake in alcohol-preferring rats (Froehlich et al., 1991) and the roles of MOP-R and DOP-R activation on VTA-mediated dopamine release (Devine et al., 1993b).

7. Brain-region specific roles of opioid receptors in ethanol consumption and seeking

The mesolimbic dopamine system plays a key role in mediating the reinforcing properties of ethanol and other drugs of abuse (Herz, 1997). Moreover, ethanol reinforcement and high alcohol drinking behavior have been suggested to involve the ethanol-induced activation of endogenous opioid systems (Froehlich et al., 1991). Ethanol may alter opioidergic transmission at different levels, including opioid peptide biosynthesis and release, as well as binding to opioid receptors. Ethanol stimulates the activity of the endogenous opioids for MOP-R (β-endorphins) and DOP-R (enkephalins) leading to an enhanced release of dopamine in the mesolimbic pathway (Herz, 1997). Activation of MOP-R in the VTA leads to dopamine release in the NAc (Leone et al., 1991; Spanagel et al., 1992), however modulation of dopamine terminal activity is also reported to involve DOP-R (Borg & Taylor, 1997; Widdowson & Holman, 1992).

7.1 Brain-region specific activity of DOP-R with ethanol consumption

Studies have shown that ethanol differentially alters opioid receptor binding in brain tissue and neuroblastoma cell lines depending on the conditions of study (Charness et al., 1993; Charness et al., 1986). Rat brain membranes treated with ethanol show inhibited enkephalin and DOP-R binding (Hiller et al., 1981). However, treatment of DOP-R-expressing neuroblastoma x glioma NG108-15 hybrid cells with ethanol (200 mM for 4 days or 25 mM for 2 weeks) results in increased DOP-R gene expression and increases in DOP-R binding sites (Charness et al., 1993; Charness et al., 1986), which was hypothesized to be due to a neuronal adaption to ethanol involving changes in receptor density. The discrepancies in ethanol responses in these studies may be explained by differences in ethanol doses and route of administration, time of exposure to the drug, time elapsed after ethanol administration at the moment the experiment was carried out, and receptor ligand used. A series of studies have demonstrated that an acute injection of ethanol given to rats results in altered DOP-R binding affinity, mRNA expression and release of enkephalins (Mendez et al., 2010; Mendez & Morales-Mulia, 2006; Mendez et al., 2004)(Table 2). The most consistent changes in DOP-R activity following acute ethanol treatment have been increased binding and met-enkephalin release, but not content, in mesocorticolimbic and nigrostriatal pathways (Mendez et al., 2010; Mendez et al., 2004). A number of studies have shown that rats given chronic or long-term access to ethanol have altered DOP-R activity in mesocorticolimbic and nigrostriatal pathways (Table 3). Long-term ethanol exposure in rats has been shown to increase DOP-R binding and supersensitivity of striatal DOP-Rs which has been suggested to be due to decreased endogenous peptide release (Lucchi et al., 1985; Lucchi et al., 1984). In comparison, the effects of long-term ethanol treatment in mice have been less consistent. CF-1 mice given ethanol for 5 days had an intermediate DOP-R binding site compared to a high and a low affinity DOP-R binding site in control mice (Hynes et al., 1983). Higher enkepahlin degrading enzyme activity was detected in the striatum of alcohol preferring C57/BL6 mice compared to the alcohol-avoiding DBA/2 mice (Winkler et al., 1998). However, enkephalin degrading enzyme activity was reduced in the hypothalamus, but not the striatum, following long-term ethanol treatment and ethanol withdrawal (Winkler et al., 1998). Furthermore, a higher density of DOP-Rs was found in the VTA and NAc of C57/BL6 mice compared to DBA/2 mice (Moller et al., 2002).

7.2 Brain region-specific effects on ethanol consumption by DOP-R ligands

The different effects on ethanol consumption by cerebral injections of the DOP-R agonists, DPDPE and DALA, (Barson et al., 2009; Barson et al., 2010; Margolis et al., 2008) suggest that

DOP-Rs in specific brain regions have different roles in ethanol consumption and seeking. This is further supported by the increased ethanol consumption observed following administration of the DOP-R antagonist, TIPP-Ψ, into the VTA (Margolis et al., 2008) compared to reduced responding for ethanol following administration of naltrindole, given either systemically (Krishnan-Sarin et al., 1995a) or microinjected into the cerebroventricles, the NAc and basolateral amygdala (BLA), but not into the VTA (Hyytia & Kiianmaa, 2001). Furthermore, the reductions in ethanol consumption following administration of DOP-R antagonists into the cerebroventricles, the NAc and BLA are consistent with the reductions in ethanol consumption following systemic administration of DOP-R antagonists (Franck et al., 1998; Hyytia & Kiianmaa, 2001; June et al., 1999; Krishnan-Sarin et al., 1995b; Marinelli et al., 2009; Nielsen et al., 2008).

Strain	Model	Assay	Brain tissue	Effect on DOP-R	Reference
Wistar rats	Acute ethanol 2.5 g/kg , i.p.	[3H]DPDPE autoradiography	Substantia nigra, Frontal cortex Prefrontal cortex Nucleus accumbens shell Nucleus accumbens core caudate putamen (anterior-medial) caudate putamen (medial-posterior) caudate putamen (posterior)	Increased Increased Increased Increased Increased Increased Increased Reduced	Mendez et al., 2004
Wistar rats	Acute ethanol 2.5 g/kg, i.p.	Pro-enkephalin mRNA expression by in situ hybridization and densitometry	VTA Prefrontal cortex Nucleus accumbens shell Nucleus accumbens core	Reduced Increased Increased Increased	Mendez & Morales-Mulia, 2006
Wistar rats	Acute ethanol treatment 0.5, 1, 2.5 g/kg i.p.	Microdialaysis/ radioimmunoassay of Met-enkephalin release and content	Nucleus accumbens Caudate Putamen Prefrontal cortex	Increased release Reduced content; Reduced content No change	Mendez et al., 2010

Table 2. Table of DOP-R activity in brain regions following acute ethanol treatment in rats.

8. Preclinical considerations of targeting the DOP-R for the treatment of AUDs

In view of the potential development of opioid-receptor selectively acting compounds for the treatment of AUDs, it is important to consider adverse effects associated with opioid receptor activity. A number of adverse effects have been reported with the use of the non-

Species/strain	Model	Assay	Brain tissue	Effect on DOP-R	Effect on MOP-R	Reference
Sprague-Dawley rats	6.5% ethanol (v/v) for 3 weeks	[3H]DADLE and [3H]dihydromorphine [3H]naloxone binding	Whole minus cerebellum	Increased	Increased	Sommer et al., 2001
Wistar rats	1-6% ethanol for 4 weeks	[3H]H-Tyr-Tic psi[CH2-NH]Phe-Phe-OH and [3H]Ile5,6deltorphin b [3H]Tyr-D-Ala-Gly-MePhe-Gly-ol binding	Striatum Nucleus Accumbens	No change No change	Reduced Reduced	Turchan et al., 1999
Sprague-Dawley rats	1-6.7% ethanol (v/v) for 16 days	[35S]GTPγS binding	Hippocampal Dentate gyrus Hippocampal CA1 Interior colliculus Cerebellum Superior colliculus Medial frontal cortex Caudate nucleus Nucleus accumbens	Reduced Reduced Reduced Reduced No change No change No change No change	Reduced Reduced Reduced No change Reduced No change No change No change	Saland et al., 2004
Sprague-Dawley rats	1-6.7% ethanol (v/v) for 16 days	Immunohistochemical staining	Hippocampal CA1 Hippocampal CA3 Hippocampal Dentate gyrus Cerebral cortex Midbrain colliculi Inferior colliculi Striatum Nucleus accumbens	Increased No change No change No change No change No change No change No change	No change Reduced No change Reduced Reduced Reduced Reduced Reduced	Saland et al., 2005
Sprague-Dawley rats	6% ethanol for 6 weeks	[3H]DADLE [3H]etorphin [3H]met-enkephalin [3H]dihydromorphine binding	Striatum	Increased	Reduced	Lucchi et al., 1985; Lucchi et al., 1984
Sprague-Dawley rats	6% ethanol for 6 weeks	Enkephalin release	Striatum	Reduced	-	Lucchi et al., 1984
Fisher 344 rats	1-5% ethanol for 70 days and 24 h withdrawal	[35S]GTPγS binding	Spinal cord	No change	Reduced	Morley et al., 1985
Sprague-Dawley rats	3 weeks of access to 15% ethanol (forced)	[3H]DADLE, [3H]dihydromorphine binding	Forebrain containing striatum	Increase	No change	Moller et al., 1999

Table 3. Table of DOP-R and MOP-R activity in brain regions following long-term ethanol consumption in rats.

selective opioid antagonists (naloxone, naltrexone and methylnaltrexone) in both preclinical (Brown & Holtzman, 1979; Holtzman, 1979; Yuan et al., 2009a; Yuan et al., 2009b) and clinical studies (Bertino et al., 1991; Spiegel et al., 1987; Sternbach et al., 1982; Yeomans & Gray, 1996; Yeomans & Gray, 1997). In humans, naltrexone has neuropsychiatric side effects including anxiety, chills, dizziness, drowsiness, depression, headache, irritability, nervousness and insomnia (Oncken et al., 2001). Furthermore, gastrointestinal side effects associated with naltrexone treatment include appetite loss, constipation, diarrhea, nausea, vomiting and stomach pain/cramps (Oncken et al., 2001). High doses of naltrexone are also associated with hepatotoxicity (Mitchell et al., 1987). Preclinical testing of compounds utilize a number of animal behavioral models to test for adverse effects including effects on nonselective consummatory behavior (self-administration of sugar solutions, food, fat, water), anxiety (elevated plus maze), pain perception (tail-flick, hotplate, paw pressure, von Frey tests), abuse potential (conditioned place preference/aversion), depression (forced swim, learned helplessness), seizure thresholds, (scored observations of clonic movements and catalepsy-like behaviors), and sedation (rotarod and righting reflex tests). Using both opioid receptor knockout mice and opioid receptor subtypes-selective compounds, the roles of opioid receptors in the development of these adverse effects have been investigated in a number of studies. Compounds with affinity for the DOP-R have been tested for adverse effects using a number of these behavioral methods.

8.1 Selective effects on ethanol and general consummatory behaviors

A pharmacotherapeutic for the treatment of AUDs would ideally have selective activity on alcohol consumption and seeking over general consummatory behaviors such as food and fluid intake. Preclinical studies show that naltrexone reduces fat, sucrose and water consumption (Corwin & Wojnicki, 2009; Nielsen et al., 2008; Rao et al., 2008; Wong et al., 2009). Similarly, preclinical studies have shown reduced food intake and weight loss with the opioid antagonists, naloxone (Brown & Holtzman, 1979; Holtzman, 1979; Yuan et al., 2009a; Yuan et al., 2009b) and methylnaltrexone (Yuan et al., 2009a; Yuan et al., 2009b). Conversely, preclinical studies have shown that the MOP-R agonist, morphine, increases both ethanol and food intake (Barson et al., 2009) and the selective MOP-R agonist, DAMGO, increases intake of saccharin, salt, fat and ethanol (de Wet et al., 2001; Tatsuo et al., 1999). Clinical studies have reported that naltrexone treatment leads to reduced food intake and weight loss (Atkinson et al., 1985; Bertino et al., 1991; Spiegel et al., 1987; Sternbach et al., 1982; Yeomans & Gray, 1996; Yeomans & Gray, 1997), although the effects of naltrexone on the eating behavior of obese subjects have been less consistent with reports of either reductions (Spiegel et al., 1987) or no effects on food intake and body weight (Atkinson, 1987; Atkinson et al., 1985; Maggio et al., 1985; Malcolm et al., 1985). Conversely, studies in humans have found that treatment with an opioid agonist with highest affinity for the MOP-R, such as methadone and butorphanol, results in increased food intake and weight gain (Atkinson, 1987; Levine & Atkinson, 1987). Taken together, these studies suggest that the MOP-R plays a more general role in ingestive behaviors.

Activation of the KOP-R has been suggested to affect taste responses due to a non-selective aversive action which could explain changes in levels of ethanol intake (Kovacs et al., 2005). KOP-R knockout mice have a reduced preference for saccharin solutions and a greater preference for quinine solutions (Kovacs et al., 2005). Unlike ligands with highest activity for the MOP-R (such as naltrexone), KOP-R, NOP-R and SIG-R, the ligands which have selective for DOP-R appear to have greater selectivity for ethanol consumption with reduced activity on general consummatory behavior, such as food, sugar or water consumption (Barson et al., 2009; Barson et al., 2010; Froehlich et al., 1991; Krishnan-Sarin et al., 1995b). Central administration of naltrexone, nor-BNI and β-funaltrexamine, but not naltrindole, reduces intake of sucrose solutions in rats (Beczkowska et al., 1992; Koch et al., 1995). Furthermore, central administration of naltrexone, naloxonazine and nor-BNI, but not naltrindole or the DOP-R agonis DALCE, reduces fat intake in food-deprived rats (Koch & Bodnar, 1994). The enkephalinase inhibitor, thiorphan, increased ethanol, but not water, intake in alcohol-preferring rats (Froehlich et al., 1991). Central administration of the DOP-R agonist, DALA, to rats selectively increased ethanol consumption over food and water in comparison to non-selective actions on ethanol intake by the MOP-R agonists, DAMGO and morphine (Barson et al., 2009; Barson et al., 2010). The naltrexone-derived DOP-R antagonist, SoRI-9409, was shown to be much more effective and selective in reducing ethanol consumption than naltrexone such that, unlike naltrexone, SoRI-9409 did not reduce water intake and did not reduce sucrose intake in doses that effectively reduced ethanol intake (Nielsen et al., 2008). Although one study found that the DOP-R antagonist, naltrindole, reduced ethanol and saccharin, but not water, consumption in rats (Krishnan-Sarin et al., 1995a), further studies by these same researchers showed that the DOP-R antagonist, naltriben, reduced the intake of solutions containing ethanol with saccharin and ethanol with quinine but no effects on the intake of either saccharin or quinine solutions alone (Krishnan-Sarin et al., 1995b). Taken together, these studies suggest that compounds with activity at the DOP-R selectively alter ethanol intake over general consummatory behavior.

8.2 Anxiety and stress

A major problem in treating AUDs is the high rate of relapse which is usually triggered by stress and anxiety (Sinha, 2007; Sinha & Li, 2007). Recent preclinical studies have suggested that potential new pharmacotherapies for AUDs act by reducing anxiety and cravings in alcohol-dependent subjects (George et al., 2008; Heilig et al., 2010). Treatment options to control stress and anxiety disorders include benzodiazepines, which carry the risk of abuse potential, and antidepressants, which demonstrate a relative large interindividual variability in terms of drug response (O'Brien, 2005; Tiwari et al., 2009). Studies investigating the roles of opioid receptors in anxiety and stress indicate that the DOP-R plays a significant role. DOP-R knockout mice have increased anxiety (Filliol et al., 2000). In comparison, rats administered the DOP-R agonist, SNC80 have increased anxiolytic activity, an effect that is reversed by naltrindole (Perrine et al., 2006; Saitoh et al., 2004). Naltrindole was found to have anxiogenic activity when given in higher, but not lower doses (Perrine et al., 2006; Saitoh et al., 2004) although the DOP-R antagonist, SoRI-9409 has neither anxiogenic nor anxiolytic activity (Nielsen et al., 2008). In contrast, β-funaltrexamine and nor-BNI did not produce any anxiogenic or anxiolytic effects, suggesting the MOP-R and KOP-R do not play a role in anxiety states (Saitoh et al., 2004). Following the forced swim test, plasma levels of the stress hormone, corticosterone are the same, in triple opioid receptor knockout (MOP-R, DOP-R, KOP-R) knockout and wild-type mice (Contet et al., 2006). This suggests that opioid receptors are not involved in the hormonal stress response. However, other studies have shown that rats housed in a stressful environment were more sensitive to the sedative effects of the DOP-R agonist, SNC80, compared to stimulant effects by SNC80 in rats that were not stressed (Pohorecky et al., 1999). In contrast, plasma corticosterone levels were increased in rats following acute intracerebral administration of the DOP-R agonists DPDPE and DADLE (Gonzalvez et al., 1991; Iyengar et al., 1987). Increased plasma corticosterone levels were found in rats administered naltrindole but not in rats co-administered naltrindole and SNC80 (Saitoh et al., 2005) or rats administered SoRI-9409 (Nielsen et al., 2008). Furthermore, pre-treatment with SoRI-9409 decreased yohimbine stress-induced reinstatement of ethanol-seeking in rats but did not affect yohimbine-induced increases in plasma corticosterone (Nielsen et al., 2011).

8.3 Abuse potential

An issue with the use of pharmacotherapeutics for the treatment of addiction is the incidence of potential abuse of the therapeutic itself. For example, the MOP-R agonist methadone, which is used to treat heroin addiction, has been reported to be widely abused (Li et al., 2011; Simonsen et al., 2011a; Simonsen et al., 2011b; Tormoehlen et al., 2011). Although the use of "substitution" therapy with opioid agonists has been effective for some patients, it has remained controversial (Gerra et al., 2009; Ling et al., 1994; Rhodes & Grossman, 1997). However, as naltrexone induces aversive side-effects in humans and conditioned place aversion in rats (Mitchell et al., 2009), it does not appear to be rewarding itself. Furthermore, naltrexone attenuates the expression of ethanol place conditioning in mice (Middaugh & Bandy, 2000). MOP-R agonists increase and MOP-R antagonists decrease, respectively, ethanol-induced CPP in rats (Matsuzawa et al., 1998; Matsuzawa et al., 1999a; Matsuzawa et al., 1999b). In comparison, activation of the KOP-R is associated with general aversive activity in rats (Shippenberg & Herz, 1986) and induces dysphoria in humans (Kumor et al., 1986; Pfeiffer et al., 1986; Rimoy et al., 1994). The KOP-R agonist, U50488, attenuates ethanol-induced CPP in rats (Matsuzawa et al., 1999a). KOP-R agonists, therefore, do not appear to be carry the risk of abuse potential. In comparison, KOP-R antagonists, such as nor-BNI do not produce CPP or CPA (Mitchell et al., 2005; Sante et al., 2000) although nor-BNI did increase ethanol-induced CPP in one study (Matsuzawa et al., 1999a).

As described earlier, DOP-R agonists increase and DOP-R antagonists attenuate, respectively, ethanol-induced CPP in rats (Bie et al., 2009; Matsuzawa et al., 1998; Matsuzawa et al., 1999a; Matsuzawa et al., 1999b) and DOP-R antagonists can make a nonaversive dose of alcohol aversive (Froehlich et al., 1998). DOP-R antagonists administered alone do not induce CPP or CPA (Nielsen et al., 2008) suggesting they are not rewarding themselves. The increase in the rewarding actions of ethanol by DOP-R agonists may contribute to the altered levels of ethanol consumption following treatment with DOP-R agonists, as described above (Barson et al., 2009; Barson et al., 2010; Margolis et al., 2008; van Rijn et al., 2010; van Rijn & Whistler, 2009). Furthermore, DOP-R (and MOP-R) agonists have been shown to be rewarding themselves such that DPDPE is self-administered into the VTA of rats (Devine & Wise, 1994; McBride et al., 1999). Activation of DOP-R (and MOP-R) leads to increased basal dopamine release in brain regions involved in the reward pathway

(Borg & Taylor, 1997; Devine et al., 1993a; Devine et al., 1993b; Herz, 1997; Vetulani, 2001). The DOP-R agonists, BW373U86 and SNC80, induce significant CPP in rats, effects of which are reversed by pretreatment with naltrindole given in doses which does not modify preference when given alone (Ehlers et al., 1999). Collectively, as DOP-R antagonists inhibit the actions of ethanol-induced endogenous opioids and subsequent dopamine release, and also reduce the rewarding effects of ethanol without being rewarding themselves, these compounds do not appear to be prone to potential abuse.

8.4 Pain perception

Hyperalgesia has been commonly noted following alcohol withdrawal in alcohol-dependent patients (Dina et al., 2008; Gatch, 2009; Jochum et al., 2010) and so analgesic medications may be prescribed to provide pain relief in the early stages of withdrawal (Gillman & Lichtigfeld, 1990). As naltrexone has been shown to block morphine-mediated analgesia in mice (Yan et al., 2003) and in rats (Nielsen et al., 2008), naltrexone treatment may therefore interfere with pain-relieving medications. Furthermore, as naltrexone can precipitate withdrawal symptoms in opioid-dependent rats (Adams & Holtzman, 1990) and monkeys (Paronis & Bergman, 2011), naltrexone treatment may potentially lead to exacerbation of withdrawal-induced hyperalgesia in alcohol-withdrawn patients. Although opioid receptor agonists with highest affinity for the MOP-R, such as morphine and methadone, have been widely used in the clinic for the treatment of pain (Nissen et al., 2001; Peng et al., 2008), preclinical studies have also demonstrated that KOP-R and DOP-R both play roles in analgesia. The administration of opioid agonists acting at the KOP-R (Leighton et al., 1988; Nielsen et al., 2007; Ross & Smith, 1997; Tiseo et al., 1988) and DOP-R (Kamei et al., 1994; Kamei et al., 1997; Scherrer et al., 2004) produce analgesia and anti-allodynia in rats and mice. Furthermore, co-administration of morphine with a KOP-R or a DOP-R agonist results in enhanced analgesia (Ross et al., 2000; Suzuki et al., 1995). A recent study showed that the DOP-R antagonist, SoRI-9409, does not reduce morphine-mediated tail-flick analgesia compared to the significant reduction in morphine-mediated analgesia by naltrexone (Nielsen et al., 2008). When administered alone, SoRI-9409, did not produce tail-flick analgesia or hyperalgesia (Nielsen et al., 2008) but did produce analgesia in the acetic acid writhing test in mice (Wells et al., 2001). Although DOP-R antagonists attenuate DOP-R agonist-mediated analgesia in mice (Kamei et al., 1995; Tseng et al., 1997), they do not block the analgesic effects of clinically used opioid analgesics (Nielsen et al., 2008).

8.5 Seizure thresholds

Seizures have commonly been observed following alcohol withdrawal in alcohol-dependent patients (Amato et al., 2011; Eyer et al., 2011a; Eyer et al., 2011b; Kim et al., 2011). Treatment options to control alcohol-withdrawal convulsions include carbamazepine, valproate and benzodiazepines (Amato et al., 2011; Eyer et al., 2011a) which all have a number of undesirable side-effects. A number of studies have indicated that activation of the DOP-R is associated with an increased incidence of convulsive activity. The DOP-R agonists, SNC80 and BW373U86, induce convulsions in mice (Broom et al., 2002b; Comer et al., 1993), rats (Broom et al., 2002a) and monkeys (Dykstra et al., 1993; Negus et al., 1994). The BW373U86-induced convulsant activity was reduced by naltrindole, naltriben and 7-benzylidenenaltrexone, suggesting the convulsive activity by BW373U86 is DOP-R-mediated (Broom et al., 2002a; Broom et al., 2002b; Comer et al., 1993), Furthermore, the BW373U86-induced convulsive effects were reduced by naltrexone given in very high doses (10-100 mg/kg), doses of which would presumably block DOP-R (Comer et al., 1993). However, recent studies in the pursuit of the development of DOP-R agonists for the treatment of pain and depression have discovered new DOP-R agonists, such as KNT-127, which are devoid of convulsant activity, while still retaining analgesic and antidepressant activity (Saitoh et al., 2011). However, since inhibition of the DOP-R reduces the incidence of DOP-R agonist-induced convulsive activity, the use of DOP-R antagonists may also provide an additional benefit for alcohol-dependent patients to prevent seizures in the early stages of withdrawal.

9. Conclusions

Although naltrexone has the most consistent effects in reducing alcohol consumption, it only effectively prevents relapse in a subset of alcohol-dependent patients. Preclinical studies suggest that potential new therapeutics that target the DOP-R may offer advantages in the treatment and prevention of relapse compared with agents that have activity for the other opioid receptor subtypes. DOP-R agonists may offer advantages for the relief of ethanol withdrawal-induced anxiety and hyperalgesia. DOP-R antagonists appear to effectively and selectively reduce ethanol consumption and seeking with limited effects on general consummatory behavior. The particular effectiveness of DOP-R antagonists in models of high ethanol consumption and relapse to ethanol-seeking may represent an alternative therapeutic strategy for reducing heavy drinking and relapse to alcohol abuse. Furthermore, DOP-R antagonists do not appear to have any abuse potential, effects on pain perception or inductions of convulsive activity. Taken together, the DOP-R represents a very promising candidate therapeutic target for the treatment of alcohol use disorders.

10. Acknowledgements

This work was supported by funding from the State of California for Medical Research through UCSF (to SEB). CKN was supported in part by the Essel Foundation as a National Alliance for Research on Schizophrenia and Depression Young Investigator. We thank Jeffrey Simms for critically reviewing the manuscript.

11. References

Acquas, E.; Meloni, M. & Di Chiara, G. (1993). Blockade of delta-opioid receptors in the nucleus accumbens prevents ethanol-induced stimulation of dopamine release. *Eur J Pharmacol,*Vol.230, No.2, (Jan 12), pp. 239-241

Adams, J.U. & Holtzman, S.G. (1990). Tolerance and dependence after continuous morphine infusion from osmotic pumps measured by operant responding in rats. *Psychopharmacology,*Vol.100, No.4, 451-458, ISSN 0033-3158

Altshuler, H.L.; Phillips, P.E. & Feinhandler, D.A. (1980). Alteration of ethanol self-administration by naltrexone. *Life Sci,*Vol.26, No.9, (Mar 3), pp. 679-688

Amato, L.; Minozzi, S. & Davoli, M. (2011). Efficacy and safety of pharmacological interventions for the treatment of the Alcohol Withdrawal Syndrome. *Cochrane database of systematic reviews,*Vol., No.6, CD008537, ISSN 1469-493X

Ananthan, S.; Kezar, H.S., 3rd; Carter, R.L.; Saini, S.K.; Rice, K.C.; Wells, J.L.; Davis, P.; Xu, H.; Dersch, C.M.; Bilsky, E.J.; Porreca, F. & Rothman, R.B. (1999). Synthesis, opioid receptor binding, and biological activities of naltrexone-derived pyrido- and pyrimidomorphinans. *J Med Chem,*Vol.42, No.18, (Sep 9), pp. 3527-3538

Anton, R.F.; Moak, D.H.; Waid, L.R.; Latham, P.K.; Malcolm, R.J. & Dias, J.K. (1999). Naltrexone and cognitive behavioral therapy for the treatment of outpatient alcoholics: results of a placebo-controlled trial. *Am J Psychiatry,*Vol.156, No.11, (Nov), pp. 1758-1764

Anton, R.F.; O'Malley, S.S.; Ciraulo, D.A.; Cisler, R.A.; Couper, D.; Donovan, D.M.; Gastfriend, D.R.; Hosking, J.D.; Johnson, B.A.; LoCastro, J.S.; Longabaugh, R.; Mason, B.J.; Mattson, M.E.; Miller, W.R.; Pettinati, H.M.; Randall, C.L.; Swift, R.; Weiss, R.D.; Williams, L.D. & Zweben, A. (2006). Combined pharmacotherapies and behavioral interventions for alcohol dependence: the COMBINE study: a randomized controlled trial. *Jama,*Vol.295, No.17, (May 3), pp. 2003-2017,

Anton, R.F.; Oroszi, G.; O'Malley, S.; Couper, D.; Swift, R.; Pettinati, H. & Goldman, D. (2008). An evaluation of mu-opioid receptor (OPRM1) as a predictor of naltrexone response in the treatment of alcohol dependence: results from the Combined Pharmacotherapies and Behavioral Interventions for Alcohol Dependence (COMBINE) study. *Archives of general psychiatry,*Vol.65, No.2, pp. 135-144, ISSN 1538-3636

Atkinson, R.L. (1987). Opioid regulation of food intake and body weight in humans. *Fed Proc,*Vol.46, No.1, (Jan), pp. 178-182, ISSN 0014-9446

Atkinson, R.L.; Berke, L.K.; Drake, C.R.; Bibbs, M.L.; Williams, F.L. & Kaiser, D.L. (1985). Effects of long-term therapy with naltrexone on body weight in obesity. *Clinical pharmacology and therapeutics,*Vol.38, No.4, (Oct), pp. 419-422, ISSN 0009-9236

Barson, J.R.; Carr, A.J.; Soun, J.E.; Sobhani, N.C.; Leibowitz, S.F. & Hoebel, B.G. (2009). Opioids in the nucleus accumbens stimulate ethanol intake. *Physiol Behav,*Vol.98, No.4, (Oct 19), pp. 453-459

Barson, J.R.; Carr, A.J.; Soun, J.E.; Sobhani, N.C.; Rada, P.; Leibowitz, S.F. & Hoebel, B.G. (2010). Opioids in the hypothalamic paraventricular nucleus stimulate ethanol intake. *Alcohol Clin Exp Res,*Vol.34, No.2, (Feb), pp. 214-222

Bart, G.; Kreek, M.J.; Ott, J.; LaForge, K.S.; Proudnikov, D.; Pollak, L. & Heilig, M. (2005). Increased attributable risk related to a functional mu-opioid receptor gene polymorphism in association with alcohol dependence in central Sweden. *Neuropsychopharmacology: official publication of the American College of Neuropsychopharmacology,*Vol.30, No.2, pp. 417-422, ISSN 0893-133X

Becker, A.; Grecksch, G.; Kraus, J.; Loh, H.H.; Schroeder, H. & Hollt, V. (2002). Rewarding effects of ethanol and cocaine in mu opioid receptor-deficient mice. *Naunyn Schmiedebergs Arch Pharmacol,*Vol.365, No.4, (Apr), pp. 296-302

Beczkowska, I.W.; Bowen, W.D. & Bodnar, R.J. (1992). Central opioid receptor subtype antagonists differentially alter sucrose and deprivation-induced water intake in rats. *Brain research,*Vol.589, No.2, (Sep 4), pp. 291-301, ISSN 0006-8993

Benjamin, D.; Grant, E.R. & Pohorecky, L.A. (1993). Naltrexone reverses ethanol-induced dopamine release in the nucleus accumbens in awake, freely moving rats. *Brain research,*Vol.621, No.1, (Sep 3), pp. 137-140, ISSN 0006-8993

Bertino, M.; Beauchamp, G.K. & Engelman, K. (1991). Naltrexone, an opioid blocker, alters taste perception and nutrient intake in humans. *Am J Physiol,*Vol.261, No.1 Pt 2, (Jul), pp. R59-63, ISSN 0002-9513

Bie, B.; Zhu, W. & Pan, Z.Z. (2009). Ethanol-induced delta-opioid receptor modulation of glutamate synaptic transmission and conditioned place preference in central amygdala. *Neuroscience,*Vol.160, No.2, (May 5), pp. 348-358

Borg, P.J. & Taylor, D.A. (1997). Involvement of mu- and delta-opioid receptors in the effects of systemic and locally perfused morphine on extracellular levels of dopamine, DOPAC and HVA in the nucleus accumbens of the halothane-anaesthetized rat. *Naunyn Schmiedebergs Arch Pharmacol,*Vol.355, No.5, (May), pp. 582-588

Bouza, C.; Angeles, M.; Munoz, A. & Amate, J.M. (2004). Efficacy and safety of naltrexone and acamprosate in the treatment of alcohol dependence: a systematic review. *Addiction,*Vol.99, No.7, (Jul), pp. 811-828

Broadbear, J.H.; Negus, S.S.; Butelman, E.R.; de Costa, B.R. & Woods, J.H. (1994). Differential effects of systemically administered nor-binaltorphimine (nor-BNI) on kappa-opioid agonists in the mouse writhing assay. *Psychopharmacology,*Vol.115, No.3, (Jul), pp. 311-319, ISSN 0033-3158

Broom, D.C.; Jutkiewicz, E.M.; Folk, J.E.; Traynor, J.R.; Rice, K.C. & Woods, J.H. (2002a). Convulsant activity of a non-peptidic delta-opioid receptor agonist is not required for its antidepressant-like effects in Sprague-Dawley rats.

Broom, D.C.; Nitsche, J.F.; Pintar, J.E.; Rice, K.C.; Woods, J.H. & Traynor, J.R. (2002b). Comparison of receptor mechanisms and efficacy requirements for delta-agonist-induced convulsive activity and antinociception in mice. *The Journal of pharmacology and experimental therapeutics,*Vol.303, No.2, (Nov), pp. 723-729, ISSN 0022-3565

Brown, D.R. & Holtzman, S.G. (1979). Suppression of deprivation-induced food and water intake in rats and mice by naloxone. *Pharmacology, biochemistry, and behavior,*Vol.11, No.5, (Nov), pp. 567-573, ISSN 0091-3057

Bruijnzeel, A.W. (2009). kappa-Opioid receptor signaling and brain reward function. *Brain Res Rev,*Vol.62, No.1, (Dec 11), pp. 127-146, ISSN 1872-6321

Buzas, B.; Izenwasser, S.; Portoghese, P.S. & Cox, B.M. (1994). Evidence for delta opioid receptor subtypes regulating adenylyl cyclase activity in rat brain. *Life Sci,*Vol.54, No.7, PL101-106

Charness, M.E.; Hu, G.; Edwards, R.H. & Querimit, L.A. (1993). Ethanol increases delta-opioid receptor gene expression in neuronal cell lines. *Mol Pharmacol,*Vol.44, No.6, (Dec), pp. 1119-1127

Charness, M.E.; Querimit, L.A. & Diamond, I. (1986). Ethanol increases the expression of functional delta-opioid receptors in neuroblastoma x glioma NG108-15 hybrid cells. *J Biol Chem,*Vol.261, No.7, (Mar 5), pp. 3164-3169, ISSN 0021-9258

Ciccocioppo, R.; Angeletti, S.; Panocka, I. & Massi, M. (2000). Nociceptin/orphanin FQ and drugs of abuse. *Peptides,*Vol.21, No.7, (Jul), pp. 1071-1080

Ciccocioppo, R.; Economidou, D.; Fedeli, A. & Massi, M. (2003). The nociceptin/orphanin FQ/NOP receptor system as a target for treatment of alcohol abuse: a review of recent work in alcohol-preferring rats. *Physiol Behav,*Vol.79, No.1, (Jun), pp. 121-128

Ciccocioppo, R.; Economidou, D.; Fedeli, A.; Angeletti, S.; Weiss, F.; Heilig, M. & Massi, M. (2004). Attenuation of ethanol self-administration and of conditioned reinstatement of alcohol-seeking behaviour by the antiopioid peptide nociceptin/orphanin FQ in alcohol-preferring rats. *Psychopharmacology (Berl),*Vol.172, No.2, (Mar), pp. 170-178

Ciccocioppo, R.; Economidou, D.; Rimondini, R.; Sommer, W.; Massi, M. & Heilig, M. (2007). Buprenorphine reduces alcohol drinking through activation of the nociceptin/orphanin FQ-NOP receptor system. *Biol Psychiatry,*Vol.61, No.1, (Jan 1), pp. 4-12

Ciccocioppo, R.; Martin-Fardon, R. & Weiss, F. (2002a). Effect of selective blockade of mu(1) or delta opioid receptors on reinstatement of alcohol-seeking behavior by drug-associated stimuli in rats. *Neuropsychopharmacology,*Vol.27, No.3, (Sep), pp. 391-399

Ciccocioppo, R.; Panocka, I.; Polidori, C.; Regoli, D. & Massi, M. (1999). Effect of nociceptin on alcohol intake in alcohol-preferring rats. *Psychopharmacology (Berl),*Vol.141, No.2, (Jan), pp. 220-224

Ciccocioppo, R.; Polidori, C.; Antonelli, L.; Salvadori, S.; Guerrini, R. & Massi, M. (2002b). Pharmacological characterization of the nociceptin receptor which mediates reduction of alcohol drinking in rats. *Peptides,*Vol.23, No.1, (Jan), pp. 117-125,

Cifani, C.; Guerrini, R.; Massi, M. & Polidori, C. (2006). Chronic intracerebroventricular infusion of nociceptin/orphanin FQ increases food and ethanol intake in alcohol-preferring rats. *Peptides,*Vol.27, No.11, (Nov), pp. 2803-2810, ISSN 0196-9781

Comer, S.D.; Hoenicke, E.M.; Sable, A.I.; McNutt, R.W.; Chang, K.J.; De Costa, B.R.; Mosberg, H.I. & Woods, J.H. (1993). Convulsive effects of systemic administration of the delta opioid agonist BW373U86 in mice. *The Journal of pharmacology and experimental therapeutics,*Vol.267, No.2, (Nov), pp. 888-895, ISSN 0022-3565

Contet, C.; Gaveriaux-Ruff, C.; Matifas, A.; Caradec, C.; Champy, M.F. & Kieffer, B.L. (2006). Dissociation of analgesic and hormonal responses to forced swim stress using opioid receptor knockout mice. *Neuropsychopharmacology,*Vol.31, No.8, (Aug), pp. 1733-1744

Corwin, R.L. & Wojnicki, F.H. (2009). Baclofen, raclopride, and naltrexone differentially affect intake of fat and sucrose under limited access conditions. *Behavioural pharmacology,*Vol.20, No.5-6, (Sep), pp. 537-548, ISSN 1473-5849

Critcher, E.C.; Lin, C.I.; Patel, J. & Myers, R.D. (1983). Attenuation of alcohol drinking in tetrahydroisoquinoline-treated rats by morphine and naltrexone. *Pharmacol Biochem Behav,*Vol.18, No.2, (Feb), pp. 225-229

Darland, T.; Heinricher, M.M. & Grandy, D.K. (1998). Orphanin FQ/nociceptin: a role in pain and analgesia, but so much more. *Trends Neurosci,*Vol.21, No.5, (May), pp. 215-221, ISSN 0166-2236

de Wet, J.; Lichtigfeld, F.J. & Gillman, M.A. (2001). Psychotropic analgesic nitrous oxide (PAN) for hyperactivity. *Aust N Z J Psychiatry,*Vol.35, No.4, (Aug), pp. 543-544, ISSN 0004-8674

Devine, D.P. & Wise, R.A. (1994). Self-administration of morphine, DAMGO, and DPDPE into the ventral tegmental area of rats. *The Journal of neuroscience : the official journal of the Society for Neuroscience,*Vol.14, No.4, (Apr), pp. 1978-1984, ISSN 0270-6474

Devine, D.P.; Leone, P.; Carlezon, W.A., Jr. & Wise, R.A. (1993a). Ventral mesencephalic delta opioid receptors are involved in modulation of basal mesolimbic dopamine neurotransmission: an anatomical localization study. *Brain research,*Vol.622, No.1-2, (Sep 17), pp. 348-352, ISSN 0006-8993

Devine, D.P.; Leone, P.; Pocock, D. & Wise, R.A. (1993b). Differential involvement of ventral tegmental mu, delta and kappa opioid receptors in modulation of basal mesolimbic dopamine release: in vivo microdialysis studies. *J Pharmacol Exp Ther,*Vol.266, No.3, (Sep), pp. 1236-1246

Dina, O.A.; Khasar, S.G.; Alessandri-Haber, N.; Green, P.G.; Messing, R.O. & Levine, J.D. (2008). Alcohol-induced stress in painful alcoholic neuropathy. *The European journal of neuroscience,* Vol.27, No.1, (Jan), pp. 83-92, ISSN 1460-9568

Dourmap, N.; Michael-Titus, A. & Costentin, J. (1990). Local enkephalins tonically modulate dopamine release in the striatum: a microdialysis study. *Brain Res,* Vol.524, No.1, (Jul 30), pp. 153-155

Dykstra, L.A.; Schoenbaum, G.M.; Yarbrough, J.; McNutt, R. & Chang, K.J. (1993). A novel delta opioid agonist, BW373U86, in squirrel monkeys responding under a schedule of shock titration. *The Journal of pharmacology and experimental therapeutics,* Vol.267, No.2, (Nov), pp. 875-882, ISSN 0022-3565

Ebner, S.R.; Roitman, M.F.; Potter, D.N.; Rachlin, A.B. & Chartoff, E.H. (2010). Depressive-like effects of the kappa opioid receptor agonist salvinorin A are associated with decreased phasic dopamine release in the nucleus accumbens. *Psychopharmacology,* Vol.210, No.2, (Jun), pp. 241-252, ISSN 1432-2072

Economidou, D.; Fedeli, A.; Fardon, R.M.; Weiss, F.; Massi, M. & Ciccocioppo, R. (2006). Effect of novel nociceptin/orphanin FQ-NOP receptor ligands on ethanol drinking in alcohol-preferring msP rats. *Peptides,* Vol.27, No.12, (Dec), pp. 3299-3306

Economidou, D.; Hansson, A.C.; Weiss, F.; Terasmaa, A.; Sommer, W.H.; Cippitelli, A.; Fedeli, A.; Martin-Fardon, R.; Massi, M.; Ciccocioppo, R. & Heilig, M. (2008). Dysregulation of nociceptin/orphanin FQ activity in the amygdala is linked to excessive alcohol drinking in the rat. *Biol Psychiatry,* Vol.64, No.3, (Aug 1), pp. 211-218

Ehlers, C.L.; Somes, C.; Lumeng, L. & Li, T.K. (1999). Electrophysiological response to neuropeptide Y (NPY): in alcohol-naive preferring and non-preferring rats. *Pharmacology, biochemistry, and behavior,* Vol.63, No.2, (Jun), pp. 291-299, ISSN 0091-3057

Endoh, T.; Matsuura, H.; Tanaka, C. & Nagase, H. (1992). Nor-binaltorphimine: a potent and selective kappa-opioid receptor antagonist with long-lasting activity in vivo. *Arch Int Pharmacodyn Ther,* Vol.316, (Mar-Apr), pp. 30-42, ISSN 0301-4533

Evans, C.J.; Keith, D.E., Jr.; Morrison, H.; Magendzo, K. & Edwards, R.H. (1992). Cloning of a delta opioid receptor by functional expression. *Science,* Vol.258, No.5090, (Dec 18), pp. 1952-1955

Eyer, F.; Schreckenberg, M.; Hecht, D.; Adorjan, K.; Schuster, T.; Felgenhauer, N.; Pfab, R.; Strubel, T. & Zilker, T. (2011a). Carbamazepine and valproate as adjuncts in the treatment of alcohol withdrawal syndrome: a retrospective cohort study. *Alcohol Alcohol Suppl,* Vol.46, No.2, (Mar-Apr), pp. 177-184, ISSN 1464-3502

Eyer, F.; Schuster, T.; Felgenhauer, N.; Pfab, R.; Strubel, T.; Saugel, B. & Zilker, T. (2011b). Risk assessment of moderate to severe alcohol withdrawal--predictors for seizures and delirium tremens in the course of withdrawal. *Alcohol Alcohol Suppl,* Vol.46, No.4, (Jul-Aug), pp. 427-433, ISSN 1464-3502

Filliol, D.; Ghozland, S.; Chluba, J.; Martin, M.; Matthes, H.W.; Simonin, F.; Befort, K.; Gaveriaux-Ruff, C.; Dierich, A.; LeMeur, M.; Valverde, O.; Maldonado, R. & Kieffer, B.L. (2000). Mice deficient for delta- and mu-opioid receptors exhibit opposing alterations of emotional responses. *Nat Genet,* Vol.25, No.2, (Jun), pp. 195-200

Franck, J.; Lindholm, S. & Raaschou, P. (1998). Modulation of volitional ethanol intake in the rat by central delta-opioid receptors. *Alcohol Clin Exp Res,* Vol.22, No.6, (Sep), pp. 1185-1189

Froehlich, J.C.; Badia-Elder, N.E.; Zink, R.W.; McCullough, D.E. & Portoghese, P.S. (1998). Contribution of the opioid system to alcohol aversion and alcohol drinking behavior. *J Pharmacol Exp Ther,*Vol.287, No.1, (Oct), pp. 284-292

Froehlich, J.C.; Zweifel, M.; Harts, J.; Lumeng, L. & Li, T.K. (1991). Importance of delta opioid receptors in maintaining high alcohol drinking. *Psychopharmacology (Berl),*Vol.103, No.4, 467-472

Fuller, R.K.; Branchey, L.; Brightwell, D.R.; Derman, R.M.; Emrick, C.D.; Iber, F.L.; James, K.E.; Lacoursiere, R.B.; Lee, K.K.; Lowenstam, I. & et al. (1986). Disulfiram treatment of alcoholism. A Veterans Administration cooperative study. *Jama,*Vol.256, No.11, (Sep 19), pp. 1449-1455

Gaiardi, M.; Bartoletti, M.; Bacchi, A.; Gubellini, C.; Costa, M. & Babbini, M. (1991). Role of repeated exposure to morphine in determining its affective properties: place and taste conditioning studies in rats. *Psychopharmacology,*Vol.103, No.2, 183-186, ISSN 0033-3158

Gardell, L.R.; Hubbell, C.L. & Reid, L.D. (1996). Naltrexone persistently reduces rats' intake of a palatable alcoholic beverage. *Alcohol Clin Exp Res,*Vol.20, No.3, (May), pp. 584-588

Gatch, M.B. (2009). Ethanol withdrawal and hyperalgesia. *Current drug abuse reviews,*Vol.2, No.1, (Jan), pp. 41-50, ISSN 1874-4745

George, D.T.; Gilman, J.; Hersh, J.; Thorsell, A.; Herion, D.; Geyer, C.; Peng, X.; Kielbasa, W.; Rawlings, R.; Brandt, J.E.; Gehlert, D.R.; Tauscher, J.T.; Hunt, S.P.; Hommer, D. & Heilig, M. (2008). Neurokinin 1 receptor antagonism as a possible therapy for alcoholism. *Science,*Vol.319, No.5869, (Mar 14), pp. 1536-1539, ISSN 1095-9203

Gerra, G.; Maremmani, I.; Capovani, B.; Somaini, L.; Berterame, S.; Tomas-Rossello, J.; Saenz, E.; Busse, A. & Kleber, H. (2009). Long-acting opioid-agonists in the treatment of heroin addiction: why should we call them "substitution"? *Subst Use Misuse,*Vol.44, No.5, 663-671, ISSN 1532-2491

Gillman, M.A. & Lichtigfeld, F.J. (1990). Analgesic nitrous oxide for alcohol withdrawal: a critical appraisal after 10 years' use. *Postgrad Med J,*Vol.66, No.777, (Jul), pp. 543-546, ISSN 0032-5473

Goldstein, A. & Naidu, A. (1989). Multiple opioid receptors: ligand selectivity profiles and binding site signatures. *Mol Pharmacol,*Vol.36, No.2, (Aug), pp. 265-272

Gonzales, R.A. & Weiss, F. (1998). Suppression of ethanol-reinforced behavior by naltrexone is associated with attenuation of the ethanol-induced increase in dialysate dopamine levels in the nucleus accumbens. *The Journal of neuroscience : the official journal of the Society for Neuroscience,*Vol.18, No.24, (Dec 15), pp. 10663-10671, ISSN 0270-6474

Gonzalvez, M.L.; Milanes, M.V. & Vargas, M.L. (1991). Effects of acute and chronic administration of mu- and delta-opioid agonists on the hypothalamic-pituitary-adrenocortical (HPA) axis in the rat. *Eur J Pharmacol,*Vol.200, No.1, (Jul 23), pp. 155-158

Gundlach, A.L.; Largent, B.L. & Snyder, S.H. (1985). Phencyclidine and sigma opiate receptors in brain: biochemical and autoradiographical differentiation. *European journal of pharmacology,*Vol.113, No.3, (Jul 31), pp. 465-466, ISSN 0014-2999

Gundlach, A.L.; Largent, B.L. & Snyder, S.H. (1986). Autoradiographic localization of sigma receptor binding sites in guinea pig and rat central nervous system with (+)3H-3-(3-hydroxyphenyl)-N-(1-propyl)piperidine. *The Journal of neuroscience : the official journal of the Society for Neuroscience,*Vol.6, No.6, (Jun), pp. 1757-1770, ISSN 0270-6474

Hall, F.S.; Sora, I. & Uhl, G.R. (2001). Ethanol consumption and reward are decreased in mu-opiate receptor knockout mice. *Psychopharmacology (Berl)*,Vol.154, No.1, (Feb), pp. 43-49

Heilig, M.; Thorsell, A.; Sommer, W.H.; Hansson, A.C.; Ramchandani, V.A.; George, D.T.; Hommer, D. & Barr, C.S. (2010). Translating the neuroscience of alcoholism into clinical treatments: from blocking the buzz to curing the blues. *Neurosci Biobehav Rev*,Vol.35, No.2, (Nov), pp. 334-344, ISSN 1873-7528

Henderson, G. & McKnight, A.T. (1997). The orphan opioid receptor and its endogenous ligand--nociceptin/orphanin FQ. *Trends Pharmacol Sci*,Vol.18, No.8, (Aug), pp. 293-300, ISSN 0165-6147

Herz, A. (1997). Endogenous opioid systems and alcohol addiction. *Psychopharmacology (Berl)*,Vol.129, No.2, (Jan), pp. 99-111,

Hiller, J.M.; Angel, L.M. & Simon, E.J. (1981). Multiple opiate receptors: alcohol selectively inhibits binding to delta receptors. *Science*,Vol.214, No.4519, (Oct 23), pp. 468-469, ISSN 0036-8075

Holter, S.M.; Henniger, M.S.; Lipkowski, A.W. & Spanagel, R. (2000). Kappa-opioid receptors and relapse-like drinking in long-term ethanol-experienced rats. *Psychopharmacology (Berl)*,Vol.153, No.1, (Dec), pp. 93-102,

Holtzman, S.G. (1979). Suppression of appetitive behavior in the rat by naloxone: lack of effect of prior morphine dependence. *Life sciences*,Vol.24, No.3, (Jan 15), pp. 219-226, ISSN 0024-3205

Holtzman, S.G. (1989). Opioid- and phencyclidine-like discriminative effects of ditolylguanidine, a selective sigma ligand. *The Journal of pharmacology and experimental therapeutics*,Vol.248, No.3, (Mar), pp. 1054-1062, ISSN 0022-3565

Horan, P.; Taylor, J.; Yamamura, H.I. & Porreca, F. (1992). Extremely long-lasting antagonistic actions of nor-binaltorphimine (nor-BNI) in the mouse tail-flick test. *The Journal of pharmacology and experimental therapeutics*,Vol.260, No.3, (Mar), pp. 1237-1243, ISSN 0022-3565

Hubbell, C.L.; Czirr, S.A.; Hunter, G.A.; Beaman, C.M.; LeCann, N.C. & Reid, L.D. (1986). Consumption of ethanol solution is potentiated by morphine and attenuated by naloxone persistently across repeated daily administrations. *Alcohol*,Vol.3, No.1, (Jan-Feb), pp. 39-54, ISSN 0741-8329

Hynes, M.D.; Lochner, M.A.; Bemis, K.G. & Hymson, D.L. (1983). Chronic ethanol alters the receptor binding characteristics of the delta opioid receptor ligand, D-Ala2-D-Leu5 enkephalin in mouse brain. *Life sciences*,Vol.33, No.23, (Dec 5), pp. 2331-2337, ISSN 0024-3205

Hyytia, P. & Kiianmaa, K. (2001). Suppression of ethanol responding by centrally administered CTOP and naltrindole in AA and Wistar rats. *Alcohol Clin Exp Res*,Vol.25, No.1, (Jan), pp. 25-33

Ingman, K.; Salvadori, S.; Lazarus, L.; Korpi, E.R. & Honkanen, A. (2003). Selective delta-opioid receptor antagonist N,N(CH3)2-Dmt-Tic-OH does not reduce ethanol intake in alcohol-preferring AA rats. *Addict Biol*,Vol.8, No.2, (Jun), pp. 173-179

Iyengar, S.; Kim, H.S. & Wood, P.L. (1987). Mu-, delta-, kappa- and epsilon-opioid receptor modulation of the hypothalamic-pituitary-adrenocortical (HPA) axis: subchronic tolerance studies of endogenous opioid peptides. *Brain Res*,Vol.435, No.1-2, (Dec 1), pp. 220-226

Jochum, T.; Boettger, M.K.; Burkhardt, C.; Juckel, G. & Bar, K.J. (2010). Increased pain sensitivity in alcohol withdrawal syndrome. *European journal of pain,*Vol.14, No.7, (Aug), pp. 713-718, ISSN 1532-2149

Johnson, B.A. (2008). Update on neuropharmacological treatments for alcoholism: scientific basis and clinical findings. *Biochem Pharmacol,*Vol.75, No.1, (Jan 1), pp. 34-56

June, H.L.; McCane, S.R.; Zink, R.W.; Portoghese, P.S.; Li, T.K. & Froehlich, J.C. (1999). The delta 2-opioid receptor antagonist naltriben reduces motivated responding for ethanol. *Psychopharmacology (Berl),*Vol.147, No.1, (Nov), pp. 81-89,

Kamei, J.; Iwamoto, Y.; Misawa, M.; Nagase, H. & Kasuya, Y. (1994). Streptozotocin-induced diabetes selectively enhances antinociception mediated by delta 1- but not delta 2-opioid receptors. *Life Sci,*Vol.55, No.6, PL121-126

Kamei, J.; Kawai, K.; Mizusuna, A.; Saitoh, A.; Morita, K.; Narita, M.; Tseng, L.F. & Nagase, H. (1997). Supraspinal delta 1-opioid receptor-mediated antinociceptive properties of (-)-TAN-67 in diabetic mice. *Eur J Pharmacol,*Vol.322, No.1, (Mar 12), pp. 27-30

Kamei, J.; Saitoh, A.; Ohsawa, M.; Suzuki, T.; Misawa, M.; Nagase, H. & Kasuya, Y. (1995). Antinociceptive effects of the selective non-peptidic delta-opioid receptor agonist TAN-67 in diabetic mice. *European journal of pharmacology,*Vol.276, No.1-2, (Mar 24), pp. 131-135, ISSN 0014-2999

Kieffer, B.L.; Befort, K.; Gaveriaux-Ruff, C. & Hirth, C.G. (1992). The delta-opioid receptor: isolation of a cDNA by expression cloning and pharmacological characterization. *Proc Natl Acad Sci U S A,*Vol.89, No.24, (Dec 15), pp. 12048-12052,

Kim, J.H.; Karpyak, V.M.; Biernacka, J.M.; Nam, H.W.; Lee, M.R.; Preuss, U.W.; Zill, P.; Yoon, G.; Colby, C.; Mrazek, D.A. & Choi, D.S. (2011). Functional role of the polymorphic 647 T/C variant of ENT1 (SLC29A1) and its association with alcohol withdrawal seizures. *PLoS One,*Vol.6, No.1, e16331, ISSN 1932-6203

Koch, J.E. & Bodnar, R.J. (1994). Selective alterations in macronutrient intake of food-deprived or glucoprivic rats by centrally-administered opioid receptor subtype antagonists in rats. *Brain research,*Vol.657, No.1-2, (Sep 19), pp. 191-201, ISSN 0006-8993

Koch, J.E.; Glass, M.J.; Cooper, M.L. & Bodnar, R.J. (1995). Alterations in deprivation, glucoprivic and sucrose intake following general, mu and kappa opioid antagonists in the hypothalamic paraventricular nucleus of rats. *Neuroscience,*Vol.66, No.4, (Jun), pp. 951-957, ISSN 0306-4522

Koster, A.; Montkowski, A.; Schulz, S.; Stube, E.M.; Knaudt, K.; Jenck, F.; Moreau, J.L.; Nothacker, H.P.; Civelli, O. & Reinscheid, R.K. (1999). Targeted disruption of the orphanin FQ/nociceptin gene increases stress susceptibility and impairs stress adaptation in mice. *Proc Natl Acad Sci U S A,*Vol.96, No.18, (Aug 31), pp. 10444-10449

Kovacs, K.M.; Szakall, I.; O'Brien, D.; Wang, R.; Vinod, K.Y.; Saito, M.; Simonin, F.; Kieffer, B.L. & Vadasz, C. (2005). Decreased oral self-administration of alcohol in kappa-opioid receptor knock-out mice. *Alcohol Clin Exp Res,*Vol.29, No.5, (May), pp. 730-738

Krishnan-Sarin, S.; Jing, S.L.; Kurtz, D.L.; Zweifel, M.; Portoghese, P.S.; Li, T.K. & Froehlich, J.C. (1995a). The delta opioid receptor antagonist naltrindole attenuates both alcohol and saccharin intake in rats selectively bred for alcohol preference. *Psychopharmacology (Berl),*Vol.120, No.2, (Jul), pp. 177-185

Krishnan-Sarin, S.; Portoghese, P.S.; Li, T.K. & Froehlich, J.C. (1995b). The delta 2-opioid receptor antagonist naltriben selectively attenuates alcohol intake in rats bred for alcohol preference. *Pharmacol Biochem Behav,*Vol.52, No.1, (Sep), pp. 153-159

Kumor, K.M.; Haertzen, C.A.; Johnson, R.E.; Kocher, T. & Jasinski, D. (1986). Human psychopharmacology of ketocyclazocine as compared with cyclazocine, morphine and placebo. *The Journal of pharmacology and experimental therapeutics*,Vol.238, No.3, (Sep), pp. 960-968, ISSN 0022-3565

Kuzmin, A.; Kreek, M.J.; Bakalkin, G. & Liljequist, S. (2007). The nociceptin/orphanin FQ receptor agonist Ro 64-6198 reduces alcohol self-administration and prevents relapse-like alcohol drinking. *Neuropsychopharmacology*,Vol.32, No.4, (Apr), pp. 902-910

Le, A.D.; Poulos, C.X.; Harding, S.; Watchus, J.; Juzytsch, W. & Shaham, Y. (1999). Effects of naltrexone and fluoxetine on alcohol self-administration and reinstatement of alcohol seeking induced by priming injections of alcohol and exposure to stress. *Neuropsychopharmacology*,Vol.21, No.3, (Sep), pp. 435-444

Leighton, G.E.; Rodriguez, R.E.; Hill, R.G. & Hughes, J. (1988). kappa-Opioid agonists produce antinociception after i.v. and i.c.v. but not intrathecal administration in the rat. *British journal of pharmacology*,Vol.93, No.3, (Mar), pp. 553-560, ISSN 0007-1188

Leone, P.; Pocock, D. & Wise, R.A. (1991). Morphine-dopamine interaction: ventral tegmental morphine increases nucleus accumbens dopamine release. *Pharmacol Biochem Behav*,Vol.39, No.2, (Jun), pp. 469-472

Levine, A.S. & Atkinson, R.L. (1987). Opioids in the regulation of food intake and energy expenditure. *Fed Proc*,Vol.46, No.1, (Jan), pp. 159-162, ISSN 0014-9446

Li, L.; Zhang, X.; Levine, B.; Li, G.; Zielke, H.R. & Fowler, D.R. (2011). Trends and pattern of drug abuse deaths in Maryland teenagers. *J Forensic Sci*,Vol.56, No.4, (Jul), pp. 1029-1033, ISSN 1556-4029

Lindholm, S.; Werme, M.; Brene, S. & Franck, J. (2001). The selective kappa-opioid receptor agonist U50,488H attenuates voluntary ethanol intake in the rat. *Behav Brain Res*,Vol.120, No.2, (May), pp. 137-146

Ling, W.; Rawson, R.A. & Compton, M.A. (1994). Substitution pharmacotherapies for opioid addiction: from methadone to LAAM and buprenorphine. *J Psychoactive Drugs*,Vol.26, No.2, (Apr-Jun), pp. 119-128, ISSN 0279-1072

Liu, X. & Weiss, F. (2002). Additive effect of stress and drug cues on reinstatement of ethanol seeking: exacerbation by history of dependence and role of concurrent activation of corticotropin-releasing factor and opioid mechanisms. *J Neurosci*,Vol.22, No.18, (Sep 15), pp. 7856-7861

Lucchi, L.; Rius, R.A.; Govoni, S. & Trabucchi, M. (1985). Chronic ethanol induces changes in opiate receptor function and in met-enkephalin release. *Alcohol*,Vol.2, No.2, (Mar-Apr), pp. 193-195

Lucchi, L.; Rius, R.A.; Uzumaki, H.; Govoni, S. & Trabucchi, M. (1984). Chronic ethanol changes opiate receptor function in rat striatum. *Brain Res*,Vol.293, No.2, (Feb 20), pp. 368-371,

Maggio, C.A.; Presta, E.; Bracco, E.F.; Vasselli, J.R.; Kissileff, H.R.; Pfohl, D.N. & Hashim, S.A. (1985). Naltrexone and human eating behavior: a dose-ranging inpatient trial in moderately obese men. *Brain Res Bull*,Vol.14, No.6, (Jun), pp. 657-661, ISSN 0361-9230

Malcolm, R.; O'Neil, P.M.; Sexauer, J.D.; Riddle, F.E.; Currey, H.S. & Counts, C. (1985). A controlled trial of naltrexone in obese humans. *Int J Obes*,Vol.9, No.5, 347-353, ISSN 0307-0565

Margolis, E.B.; Fields, H.L.; Hjelmstad, G.O. & Mitchell, J.M. (2008). Delta-opioid receptor expression in the ventral tegmental area protects against elevated alcohol consumption. *J Neurosci*,Vol.28, No.48, (Nov 26), pp. 12672-12681

Margolis, E.B.; Hjelmstad, G.O.; Bonci, A. & Fields, H.L. (2003). Kappa-opioid agonists directly inhibit midbrain dopaminergic neurons. *The Journal of neuroscience : the official journal of the Society for Neuroscience,*Vol.23, No.31, (Nov 5), pp. 9981-9986, ISSN 1529-2401

Marinelli, P.W.; Funk, D.; Harding, S.; Li, Z.; Juzytsch, W. & Le, A.D. (2009). Roles of opioid receptor subtypes in mediating alcohol-seeking induced by discrete cues and context. *Eur J Neurosci,*Vol.30, No.4, (Aug), pp. 671-678

Mark, T.L.; Kranzler, H.R. & Song, X. (2003b). Understanding US addiction physicians' low rate of naltrexone prescription. *Drug Alcohol Depend,*Vol.71, No.3, (Sep 10), pp. 219-228

Mark, T.L.; Kranzler, H.R.; Poole, V.H.; Hagen, C.A.; McLeod, C. & Crosse, S. (2003a). Barriers to the use of medications to treat alcoholism. *Am J Addict,*Vol.12, No.4, (Jul-Sep), pp. 281-294

Martin, W.R.; Eades, C.G.; Thompson, J.A.; Huppler, R.E. & Gilbert, P.E. (1976). The effects of morphine- and nalorphine- like drugs in the nondependent and morphine-dependent chronic spinal dog. *The Journal of pharmacology and experimental therapeutics,*Vol.197, No.3, (Jun), pp. 517-532, ISSN 0022-3565

Martin-Fardon, R.; Ciccocioppo, R.; Massi, M. & Weiss, F. (2000). Nociceptin prevents stress-induced ethanol- but not cocaine-seeking behavior in rats. *Neuroreport,*Vol.11, No.9, (Jun 26), pp. 1939-1943

Matsuzawa, S.; Suzuki, T.; Misawa, M. & Nagase, H. (1998). Involvement of mu- and delta-opioid receptors in the ethanol-associated place preference in rats exposed to foot shock stress. *Brain Res,*Vol.803, No.1-2, (Aug 24), pp. 169-177,

Matsuzawa, S.; Suzuki, T.; Misawa, M. & Nagase, H. (1999a). Different roles of mu-, delta- and kappa-opioid receptors in ethanol-associated place preference in rats exposed to conditioned fear stress. *Eur J Pharmacol,*Vol.368, No.1, (Feb 26), pp. 9-16

Matsuzawa, S.; Suzuki, T.; Misawa, M. & Nagase, H. (1999b). Roles of 5-HT3 and opioid receptors in the ethanol-induced place preference in rats exposed to conditioned fear stress. *Life Sci,*Vol.64, No.21, PL241-249

Mattia, A.; Vanderah, T.; Mosberg, H.I. & Porreca, F. (1991). Lack of antinociceptive cross-tolerance between [D-Pen2, D-Pen5]enkephalin and [D-Ala2]deltorphin II in mice: evidence for delta receptor subtypes. *J Pharmacol Exp Ther,*Vol.258, No.2, (Aug), pp. 583-587

Maurice, T.; Casalino, M.; Lacroix, M. & Romieu, P. (2003). Involvement of the sigma 1 receptor in the motivational effects of ethanol in mice. *Pharmacology, biochemistry, and behavior,*Vol.74, No.4, (Mar), pp. 869-876, ISSN 0091-3057

McBride, W.J.; Murphy, J.M. & Ikemoto, S. (1999). Localization of brain reinforcement mechanisms: intracranial self-administration and intracranial place-conditioning studies. *Behavioural brain research,*Vol.101, No.2, (Jun), pp. 129-152, ISSN 0166-4328

Mendez, M. & Morales-Mulia, M. (2006). Ethanol exposure differentially alters pro-enkephalin mRNA expression in regions of the mesocorticolimbic system. *Psychopharmacology (Berl),*Vol.189, No.1, (Nov), pp. 117-124,

Mendez, M.; Barbosa-Luna, I.G.; Perez-Luna, J.M.; Cupo, A. & Oikawa, J. (2010). Effects of acute ethanol administration on methionine-enkephalin expression and release in regions of the rat brain. *Neuropeptides,*Vol.44, No.5, (Oct), pp. 413-420, ISSN 1532-2785

Mendez, M.; Morales-Mulia, M. & Leriche, M. (2004). [3H]DPDPE binding to delta opioid receptors in the rat mesocorticolimbic and nigrostriatal pathways is transiently increased by acute ethanol administration. *Brain Res,*Vol.1028, No.2, (Dec 3), pp. 180-190

Middaugh, L.D. & Bandy, A.L. (2000). Naltrexone effects on ethanol consumption and response to ethanol conditioned cues in C57BL/6 mice. *Psychopharmacology,*Vol.151, No.4, (Sep), pp. 321-327, ISSN 0033-3158

Mitchell, J.E.; Morley, J.E.; Levine, A.S.; Hatsukami, D.; Gannon, M. & Pfohl, D. (1987). High-dose naltrexone therapy and dietary counseling for obesity. *Biological psychiatry,*Vol.22, No.1, (Jan), pp. 35-42, ISSN 0006-3223

Mitchell, J.M.; Bergren, L.J.; Chen, K.S.; Rowbotham, M.C. & Fields, H.L. (2009). Naltrexone aversion and treatment efficacy are greatest in humans and rats that actively consume high levels of alcohol. *Neurobiol Dis,*Vol.33, No.1, (Jan), pp. 72-80, ISSN 1095-953X

Mitchell, J.M.; Liang, M.T. & Fields, H.L. (2005). A single injection of the kappa opioid antagonist norbinaltorphimine increases ethanol consumption in rats. *Psychopharmacology (Berl),*Vol.182, No.3, (Nov), pp. 384-392

Mogil, J.S. & Pasternak, G.W. (2001). The molecular and behavioral pharmacology of the orphanin FQ/nociceptin peptide and receptor family. *Pharmacol Rev,*Vol.53, No.3, (Sep), pp. 381-415, ISSN 0031-6997

Mogil, J.S.; Grisel, J.E.; Reinscheid, R.K.; Civelli, O.; Belknap, J.K. & Grandy, D.K. (1996a). Orphanin FQ is a functional anti-opioid peptide. *Neuroscience,*Vol.75, No.2, (Nov), pp. 333-337, ISSN 0306-4522

Mogil, J.S.; Grisel, J.E.; Zhangs, G.; Belknap, J.K. & Grandy, D.K. (1996b). Functional antagonism of mu-, delta- and kappa-opioid antinociception by orphanin FQ. *Neuroscience letters,*Vol.214, No.2-3, (Aug 23), pp. 131-134, ISSN 0304-3940

Moller, C.; Sommer, W.; Thorsell, A. & Heilig, M. (1999). Anxiogenic-like action of galanin after intra-amygdala administration in the rat. *Neuropsychopharmacology : official publication of the American College of Neuropsychopharmacology,*Vol.21, No.4, (Oct), pp. 507-512, ISSN 0893-133X

Moller, C.; Sommer, W.; Thorsell, A.; Rimondini, R. & Heilig, M. (2002). Anxiogenic-like action of centrally administered glucagon-like peptide-1 in a punished drinking test. *Progress in neuro-psychopharmacology & biological psychiatry,*Vol.26, No.1, (Jan), pp. 119-122, ISSN 0278-5846

Morley, J.E.; Gosnell, B.A.; Krahn, D.D.; Mitchell, J.E. & Levine, A.S. (1985). Neuropeptidergic regulation of feeding. *Psychopharmacol Bull,*Vol.21, No.3, 400-405, ISSN 0048-5764

Negri, L.; Potenza, R.L.; Corsi, R. & Melchiorri, P. (1991). Evidence for two subtypes of delta opioid receptors in rat brain. *Eur J Pharmacol,*Vol.196, No.3, (Apr 24), pp. 335-336

Negus, S.S.; Butelman, E.R.; Chang, K.J.; DeCosta, B.; Winger, G. & Woods, J.H. (1994). Behavioral effects of the systemically active delta opioid agonist BW373U86 in rhesus monkeys. *The Journal of pharmacology and experimental therapeutics,*Vol.270, No.3, (Sep), pp. 1025-1034, ISSN 0022-3565

Nestby, P.; Schoffelmeer, A.N.; Homberg, J.R.; Wardeh, G.; De Vries, T.J.; Mulder, A.H. & Vanderschuren, L.J. (1999). Bremazocine reduces unrestricted free-choice ethanol self-administration in rats without affecting sucrose preference. *Psychopharmacology,*Vol.142, No.3, (Mar), pp. 309-317, ISSN 0033-3158

Nielsen, C.K.; Ross, F.B.; Lotfipour, S.; Saini, K.S.; Edwards, S.R. & Smith, M.T. (2007). Oxycodone and morphine have distinctly different pharmacological profiles:

radioligand binding and behavioural studies in two rat models of neuropathic pain. *Pain,*Vol.132, No.3, (Dec 5), pp. 289-300, ISSN 1872-6623

Nielsen, C.K.; Simms, J.A.; Bito-Onon, J.J.; Li, R.; Ananthan, S. & Bartlett, S.E. (2011). The delta opioid receptor antagonist, SoRI-9409, decreases yohimbine stress-induced reinstatement of ethanol-seeking. *Addict Biol,*Vol., (Feb 11),

Nielsen, C.K.; Simms, J.A.; Pierson, H.B.; Li, R.; Saini, S.K.; Ananthan, S. & Bartlett, S.E. (2008). A novel delta opioid receptor antagonist, SoRI-9409, produces a selective and long-lasting decrease in ethanol consumption in heavy-drinking rats. *Biol Psychiatry,*Vol.64, No.11, (Dec 1), pp. 974-981

Nissen, L.M.; Tett, S.E.; Cramond, T.; Williams, B. & Smith, M.T. (2001). Opioid analgesic prescribing and use - an audit of analgesic prescribing by general practitioners and The Multidisciplinary Pain Centre at Royal Brisbane Hospital. *Br J Clin Pharmacol,*Vol.52, No.6, (Dec), pp. 693-698, ISSN 0306-5251

O'Brien C, P. (2005). Benzodiazepine use, abuse, and dependence. *J Clin Psychiatry,*Vol.66 Suppl 2, 28-33, ISSN 0160-6689

O'Malley, S.S.; Garbutt, J.C.; Gastfriend, D.R.; Dong, Q. & Kranzler, H.R. (2007). Efficacy of extended-release naltrexone in alcohol-dependent patients who are abstinent before treatment. *J Clin Psychopharmacol,*Vol.27, No.5, (Oct), pp. 507-512,

O'Malley, S.S.; Jaffe, A.J.; Chang, G.; Schottenfeld, R.S.; Meyer, R.E. & Rounsaville, B. (1992). Naltrexone and coping skills therapy for alcohol dependence. A controlled study. *Arch Gen Psychiatry,*Vol.49, No.11, (Nov), pp. 881-887,

Oncken, C.; Van Kirk, J. & Kranzler, H.R. (2001). Adverse effects of oral naltrexone: analysis of data from two clinical trials. *Psychopharmacology,*Vol.154, No.4, (Apr), pp. 397-402, ISSN 0033-3158

Oroszi, G.; Anton, R.F.; O'Malley, S.; Swift, R.; Pettinati, H.; Couper, D.; Yuan, Q. & Goldman, D. (2009). OPRM1 Asn40Asp predicts response to naltrexone treatment: a haplotype-based approach. *Alcoholism, clinical and experimental research,*Vol.33, No.3, pp. 383-393, ISSN 1530-0277

O'Shea, B. (2000). Disulfiram revisited. *Hosp Med,*Vol.61, No.12, (Dec), pp. 849-851

Oslin, D.W.; Berrettini, W.; Kranzler, H.R.; Pettinati, H.; Gelernter, J.; Volpicelli, J.R. & O'Brien, C.P. (2003). A functional polymorphism of the mu-opioid receptor gene is associated with naltrexone response in alcohol-dependent patients. *Neuropsychopharmacology: official publication of the American College of Neuropsychopharmacology,* Vol.28, No.8, pp. 1546-1552, ISSN 0893-133X

Paronis, C.A. & Bergman, J. (2011). Buprenorphine and opioid antagonism, tolerance, and naltrexone-precipitated withdrawal. *The Journal of pharmacology and experimental therapeutics,*Vol.336, No.2, (Feb), pp. 488-495, ISSN 1521-0103

Peng, P.; Tumber, P.; Stafford, M.; Gourlay, D.; Wong, P.; Galonski, M.; Evans, D. & Gordon, A. (2008). Experience of methadone therapy in 100 consecutive chronic pain patients in a multidisciplinary pain center. *Pain Med,*Vol.9, No.7, (Oct), pp. 786-794, ISSN 1526-4637

Perrine, S.A.; Hoshaw, B.A. & Unterwald, E.M. (2006). Delta opioid receptor ligands modulate anxiety-like behaviors in the rat. *Br J Pharmacol,*Vol.147, No.8, (Apr), pp. 864-872

Petit, F.; Hamon, M.; Fournie-Zaluski, M.C.; Roques, B.P. & Glowinski, J. (1986). Further evidence for a role of delta-opiate receptors in the presynaptic regulation of newly synthesized dopamine release. *Eur J Pharmacol,*Vol.126, No.1-2, (Jul 15), pp. 1-9

Pettinati, H.M.; Gastfriend, D.R.; Dong, Q.; Kranzler, H.R. & O'Malley, S.S. (2009). Effect of extended-release naltrexone (XR-NTX) on quality of life in alcohol-dependent patients. *Alcohol Clin Exp Res,*Vol.33, No.2, (Feb), pp. 350-356,

Pettinati, H.M.; O'Brien, C.P.; Rabinowitz, A.R.; Wortman, S.P.; Oslin, D.W.; Kampman, K.M. & Dackis, C.A. (2006). The status of naltrexone in the treatment of alcohol dependence: specific effects on heavy drinking. *J Clin Psychopharmacol,*Vol.26, No.6, (Dec), pp. 610-625,

Pettinati, H.M.; Volpicelli, J.R.; Pierce, J.D., Jr. & O'Brien, C.P. (2000). Improving naltrexone response: an intervention for medical practitioners to enhance medication compliance in alcohol dependent patients. *J Addict Dis,*Vol.19, No.1, 71-83,

Pfeiffer, A.; Brantl, V.; Herz, A. & Emrich, H.M. (1986). Psychotomimesis mediated by kappa opiate receptors. *Science,*Vol.233, No.4765, (Aug 15), pp. 774-776, ISSN 0036-8075 *pharmacology,*Vol.12, No.5, (Sep), pp. 325-333, ISSN 0955-8810

Pohorecky, L.A.; Skiandos, A.; Zhang, X.; Rice, K.C. & Benjamin, D. (1999). Effect of chronic social stress on delta-opioid receptor function in the rat. *J Pharmacol Exp Ther,*Vol.290, No.1, (Jul), pp. 196-206, *Psychopharmacology,*Vol.164, No.1, (Oct), pp. 42-48, ISSN 0033-3158

Quirion, R.; Bowen, W.D.; Itzhak, Y.; Junien, J.L.; Musacchio, J.M.; Rothman, R.B.; Su, T.P.; Tam, S.W. & Taylor, D.P. (1992). A proposal for the classification of sigma binding sites. *Trends Pharmacol Sci,*Vol.13, No.3, (Mar), pp. 85-86, ISSN 0165-6147

Rao, R.E.; Wojnicki, F.H.; Coupland, J.; Ghosh, S. & Corwin, R.L. (2008). Baclofen, raclopride, and naltrexone differentially reduce solid fat emulsion intake under limited access conditions. *Pharmacology, biochemistry, and behavior,*Vol.89, No.4, (Jun), pp. 581-590, ISSN 0091-3057

Reid, L.D. & Hunter, G.A. (1984). Morphine and naloxone modulate intake of ethanol. *Alcohol,*Vol.1, No.1, (Jan-Feb), pp. 33-37,

Reinscheid, R.K.; Ardati, A.; Monsma, F.J., Jr. & Civelli, O. (1996). Structure-activity relationship studies on the novel neuropeptide orphanin FQ. *J Biol Chem,*Vol.271, No.24, (Jun 14), pp. 14163-14168, ISSN 0021-9258

Reinscheid, R.K.; Higelin, J.; Henningsen, R.A.; Monsma, F.J., Jr. & Civelli, O. (1998). Structures that delineate orphanin FQ and dynorphin A pharmacological selectivities. *J Biol Chem,*Vol.273, No.3, (Jan 16), pp. 1490-1495, ISSN 0021-9258

Rhodes, D.J. & Grossman, S.A. (1997). Hydromorphone polymer implant. A potential alternative to methadone maintenance. *J Subst Abuse Treat,*Vol.14, No.6, (Nov-Dec), pp. 535-542, ISSN 0740-5472

Rimoy, G.H.; Wright, D.M.; Bhaskar, N.K. & Rubin, P.C. (1994). The cardiovascular and central nervous system effects in the human of U-62066E. A selective opioid receptor agonist. *Eur J Clin Pharmacol,*Vol.46, No.3, 203-207, ISSN 0031-6970

Roberts, A.J.; Gold, L.H.; Polis, I.; McDonald, J.S.; Filliol, D.; Kieffer, B.L. & Koob, G.F. (2001). Increased ethanol self-administration in delta-opioid receptor knockout mice. *Alcohol Clin Exp Res,*Vol.25, No.9, (Sep), pp. 1249-1256

Roberts, A.J.; McDonald, J.S.; Heyser, C.J.; Kieffer, B.L.; Matthes, H.W.; Koob, G.F. & Gold, L.H. (2000). mu-Opioid receptor knockout mice do not self-administer alcohol. *J Pharmacol Exp Ther,*Vol.293, No.3, (Jun), pp. 1002-1008

Ross, F.B. & Smith, M.T. (1997). The intrinsic antinociceptive effects of oxycodone appear to be kappa-opioid receptor mediated. *Pain,*Vol.73, No.2, (Nov), pp. 151-157, ISSN 0304-3959

Ross, F.B.; Wallis, S.C. & Smith, M.T. (2000). Co-administration of sub-antinociceptive doses of oxycodone and morphine produces marked antinociceptive synergy with reduced CNS side-effects in rats. *Pain,*Vol.84, No.2-3, (Feb), pp. 421-428, ISSN 0304-3959

Sabino, V.; Cottone, P.; Blasio, A.; Iyer, M.R.; Steardo, L.; Rice, K.C.; Conti, B.; Koob, G.F. & Zorrilla, E.P. (2011). Activation of sigma-Receptors Induces Binge-like Drinking in Sardinian Alcohol-Preferring Rats. *Neuropsychopharmacology,*Vol., (Feb 23)

Sabino, V.; Cottone, P.; Zhao, Y.; Iyer, M.R.; Steardo, L., Jr.; Steardo, L.; Rice, K.C.; Conti, B.; Koob, G.F. & Zorrilla, E.P. (2009a). The sigma-receptor antagonist BD-1063 decreases ethanol intake and reinforcement in animal models of excessive drinking. *Neuropsychopharmacology,*Vol.34, No.6, (May), pp. 1482-1493

Sabino, V.; Cottone, P.; Zhao, Y.; Steardo, L.; Koob, G.F. & Zorrilla, E.P. (2009b). Selective reduction of alcohol drinking in Sardinian alcohol-preferring rats by a sigma-1 receptor antagonist. *Psychopharmacology (Berl),*Vol.205, No.2, (Aug), pp. 327-335

Saitoh, A.; Kimura, Y.; Suzuki, T.; Kawai, K.; Nagase, H. & Kamei, J. (2004). Potential anxiolytic and antidepressant-like activities of SNC80, a selective delta-opioid agonist, in behavioral models in rodents. *J Pharmacol Sci,*Vol.95, No.3, (Jul), pp. 374-380

Saitoh, A.; Sugiyama, A.; Nemoto, T.; Fujii, H.; Wada, K.; Oka, J.; Nagase, H. & Yamada, M. (2011). The novel delta opioid receptor agonist KNT-127 produces antidepressant-like and antinociceptive effects in mice without producing convulsions. *Behavioural brain research,*Vol.223, No.2, (Oct 1), pp. 271-279, ISSN 1872-7549

Saitoh, A.; Yoshikawa, Y.; Onodera, K. & Kamei, J. (2005). Role of delta-opioid receptor subtypes in anxiety-related behaviors in the elevated plus-maze in rats. *Psychopharmacology (Berl),*Vol.182, No.3, (Nov), pp. 327-334

Sakoori, K. & Murphy, N.P. (2008). Endogenous nociceptin (orphanin FQ) suppresses basal hedonic state and acute reward responses to methamphetamine and ethanol, but facilitates chronic responses. *Neuropsychopharmacology,*Vol.33, No.4, (Mar), pp. 877-891

Saland, L.C.; Abeyta, A.; Frausto, S.; Raymond-Stintz, M.; Hastings, C.M.; Carta, M.; Valenzuela, C.F. & Savage, D.D. (2004). Chronic ethanol consumption reduces delta-and mu-opioid receptor-stimulated G-protein coupling in rat brain. *Alcohol Clin Exp Res,*Vol.28, No.1, (Jan), pp. 98-104

Saland, L.C.; Hastings, C.M.; Abeyta, A. & Chavez, J.B. (2005). Chronic ethanol modulates delta and mu-opioid receptor expression in rat CNS: immunohistochemical analysis with quantitiative confocal microscopy. *Neurosci Lett,*Vol.381, No.1-2, (Jun 10-17), pp. 163-168

Sandi, C.; Borrell, J. & Guaza, C. (1988). Involvement of kappa type opioids on ethanol drinking. *Life Sci,*Vol.42, No.10, 1067-1075

Sandi, C.; Borrell, J. & Guaza, C. (1990). Effects of the kappa opioid receptor antagonist MR-2266-BS on the acquisition of ethanol preference. *Life Sci,*Vol.46, No.16, 1119-1129

Sante, A.B.; Nobre, M.J. & Brandao, M.L. (2000). Place aversion induced by blockade of mu or activation of kappa opioid receptors in the dorsal periaqueductal gray matter. *Behavioural pharmacology,*Vol.11, No.7-8, (Nov), pp. 583-589, ISSN 0955-8810

Scherrer, G.; Befort, K.; Contet, C.; Becker, J.; Matifas, A. & Kieffer, B.L. (2004). The delta agonists DPDPE and deltorphin II recruit predominantly mu receptors to produce thermal analgesia: a parallel study of mu, delta and combinatorial opioid receptor knockout mice. *The European journal of neuroscience,*Vol.19, No.8, (Apr), pp. 2239-2248, ISSN 0953-816X

Shippenberg, T.S. & Herz, A. (1986). Differential effects of mu and kappa opioid systems on motivational processes. *NIDA research monograph,*Vol.75, 563-566, ISSN 1046-9516

Shippenberg, T.S.; Chefer, V.I. & Thompson, A.C. (2009). Delta-opioid receptor antagonists prevent sensitization to the conditioned rewarding effects of morphine. *Biol Psychiatry,*Vol.65, No.2, (Jan 15), pp. 169-174

Shippenberg, T.S.; Heidbreder, C. & Lefevour, A. (1996). Sensitization to the conditioned rewarding effects of morphine: pharmacology and temporal characteristics. *European journal of pharmacology,*Vol.299, No.1-3, (Mar 28), pp. 33-39, ISSN 0014-2999

Shippenberg, T.S.; LeFevour, A. & Chefer, V.I. (2008). Targeting endogenous mu- and delta-opioid receptor systems for the treatment of drug addiction. *CNS Neurol Disord Drug Targets,*Vol.7, No.5, (Nov), pp. 442-453

Simms, J.A.; Steensland, P.; Medina, B.; Abernathy, K.E.; Chandler, L.J.; Wise, R. & Bartlett, S.E. (2008). Intermittent access to 20% ethanol induces high ethanol consumption in Long-Evans and Wistar rats. *Alcohol Clin Exp Res,*Vol.32, No.10, (Oct), pp. 1816-1823

Simonsen, K.W.; Hansen, C.A.; Rollmann, D.; Kringsholm, B.; Muller, I.B.; Johansen, S.S. & Linnet, K. (2011a). Drug-related death in Denmark in 2007. *Dan Med Bull,*Vol.58, No.8, (Aug), pp. A4307, ISSN 1603-9629

Simonsen, K.W.; Normann, P.T.; Ceder, G.; Vuori, E.; Thordardottir, S.; Thelander, G.; Hansen, A.C.; Teige, B. & Rollmann, D. (2011b). Fatal poisoning in drug addicts in the Nordic countries in 2007. *Forensic Sci Int,*Vol.207, No.1-3, (Apr 15), pp. 170-176, ISSN 1872-6283

Sinha, R. & Li, C.S. (2007). Imaging stress- and cue-induced drug and alcohol craving: association with relapse and clinical implications. *Drug Alcohol Rev,*Vol.26, No.1, (Jan), pp. 25-31, ISSN 0959-5236

Sinha, R. (2007). The role of stress in addiction relapse. *Current psychiatry reports,*Vol.9, No.5, (Oct), pp. 388-395, ISSN 1523-3812

Sofuoglu, M.; Portoghese, P.S. & Takemori, A.E. (1991). Differential antagonism of delta opioid agonists by naltrindole and its benzofuran analog (NTB) in mice: evidence for delta opioid receptor subtypes. *The Journal of pharmacology and experimental therapeutics,*Vol.257, No.2, (May), pp. 676-680, ISSN 0022-3565

Sofuoglu, M.; Portoghese, P.S. & Takemori, A.E. (1993). 7-Benzylidenenaltrexone (BNTX): a selective delta 1 opioid receptor antagonist in the mouse spinal cord. *Life Sci,*Vol.52, No.8, 769-775

Sommer, W.; Moller, C.; Wiklund, L.; Thorsell, A.; Rimondini, R.; Nissbrandt, H. & Heilig, M. (2001). Local 5,7-dihydroxytryptamine lesions of rat amygdala: release of punished drinking, unaffected plus-maze behavior and ethanol consumption. *Neuropsychopharmacology : official publication of the American College of Neuropsychopharmacology,*Vol.24, No.4, (Apr), pp. 430-440, ISSN 0893-133X

Spanagel, R.; Herz, A. & Shippenberg, T.S. (1990). The effects of opioid peptides on dopamine release in the nucleus accumbens: an in vivo microdialysis study. *J Neurochem,*Vol.55, No.5, (Nov), pp. 1734-1740

Spanagel, R.; Herz, A. & Shippenberg, T.S. (1992). Opposing tonically active endogenous opioid systems modulate the mesolimbic dopaminergic pathway. *Proc Natl Acad Sci U S A,*Vol.89, No.6, (Mar 15), pp. 2046-2050

Spiegel, T.A.; Stunkard, A.J.; Shrager, E.E.; O'Brien, C.P.; Morrison, M.F. & Stellar, E. (1987). Effect of naltrexone on food intake, hunger, and satiety in obese men. *Physiology & behavior,*Vol.40, No.2, 135-141, ISSN 0031-9384

Sternbach, H.A.; Annitto, W.; Pottash, A.L. & Gold, M.S. (1982). Anorexic effects of naltrexone in man. *Lancet,*Vol.1, No.8268, (Feb 13), pp. 388-389, ISSN 0140-6736

Stromberg, M.F.; Casale, M.; Volpicelli, L.; Volpicelli, J.R. & O'Brien, C.P. (1998a). A comparison of the effects of the opioid antagonists naltrexone, naltrindole, and beta-funaltrexamine on ethanol consumption in the rat. *Alcohol,*Vol.15, No.4, (May), pp. 281-289

Stromberg, M.F.; Sengpiel, T.; Mackler, S.A.; Volpicelli, J.R.; O'Brien, C.P. & Vogel, W.H. (2002). Effect of naltrexone on oral consumption of concurrently available ethanol and cocaine in the rat. *Alcohol,*Vol.28, No.3, (Nov), pp. 169-179,

Stromberg, M.F.; Volpicelli, J.R. & O'Brien, C.P. (1998b). Effects of naltrexone administered repeatedly across 30 or 60 days on ethanol consumption using a limited access procedure in the rat. *Alcohol Clin Exp Res,*Vol.22, No.9, (Dec), pp. 2186-2191

Suzuki, T.; Tsuji, M.; Mori, T.; Misawa, M.; Endoh, T. & Nagase, H. (1995). Effects of a highly selective nonpeptide delta opioid receptor agonist, TAN-67, on morphine-induced antinociception in mice. *Life sciences,*Vol.57, No.2, 155-168, ISSN 0024-3205

Takemori, A.E. & Portoghese, P.S. (1984). Comparative antagonism by naltrexone and naloxone of mu, kappa, and delta agonists. *European journal of pharmacology,*Vol.104, No.1-2, (Sep 3), pp. 101-104, ISSN 0014-2999

Tatsuo, M.A.; Salgado, J.V.; Yokoro, C.M.; Duarte, I.D. & Francischi, J.N. (1999). Midazolam-induced hyperalgesia in rats: modulation via GABA(A) receptors at supraspinal level. *European journal of pharmacology,*Vol.370, No.1, (Apr 1), pp. 9-15, ISSN 0014-2999

Tiseo, P.J.; Geller, E.B. & Adler, M.W. (1988). Antinociceptive action of intracerebroventricularly administered dynorphin and other opioid peptides in the rat. *The Journal of pharmacology and experimental therapeutics,*Vol.246, No.2, (Aug), pp. 449-453, ISSN 0022-3565

Tiwari, A.K.; Souza, R.P. & Muller, D.J. (2009). Pharmacogenetics of anxiolytic drugs. *J Neural Transm,*Vol.116, No.6, (Jun), pp. 667-677, ISSN 1435-1463

Tormoehlen, L.M.; Mowry, J.B.; Bodle, J.D. & Rusyniak, D.E. (2011). Increased adolescent opioid use and complications reported to a poison control center following the 2000 JCAHO pain initiative. *Clin Toxicol (Phila),*Vol.49, No.6, (Jul), pp. 492-498, ISSN 1556-9519

Tseng, L.F.; Narita, M.; Mizoguchi, H.; Kawai, K.; Mizusuna, A.; Kamei, J.; Suzuki, T. & Nagase, H. (1997). Delta-1 opioid receptor-mediated antinociceptive properties of a nonpeptidic delta opioid receptor agonist, (-)TAN-67, in the mouse spinal cord. *The Journal of pharmacology and experimental therapeutics,*Vol.280, No.2, (Feb), pp. 600-605, ISSN 0022-3565

Turchan, J.; Przewlocka, B.; Toth, G.; Lason, W.; Borsodi, A. & Przewlocki, R. (1999). The effect of repeated administration of morphine, cocaine and ethanol on mu and delta opioid receptor density in the nucleus accumbens and striatum of the rat. *Neuroscience,*Vol.91, No.3, 971-977

van Rijn, R.M. & Whistler, J.L. (2009). The delta(1) opioid receptor is a heterodimer that opposes the actions of the delta(2) receptor on alcohol intake. *Biol Psychiatry,*Vol.66, No.8, (Oct 15), pp. 777-784

van Rijn, R.M.; Brissett, D.I. & Whistler, J.L. (2010). Dual efficacy of delta opioid receptor-selective ligands for ethanol drinking and anxiety. *J Pharmacol Exp Ther,*Vol.335, No.1, (Oct), pp. 133-139

Vaupel, D.B. (1983). Naltrexone fails to antagonize the sigma effects of PCP and SKF 10,047 in the dog. *European journal of pharmacology,*Vol.92, No.3-4, (Sep 2), pp. 269-274, ISSN 0014-2999

Vetulani, J. (2001). Drug addiction. Part II. Neurobiology of addiction. *Pol J Pharmacol,*Vol.53, No.4, (Jul-Aug), pp. 303-317,

Volpicelli, J.R.; Alterman, A.I.; Hayashida, M. & O'Brien, C.P. (1992). Naltrexone in the treatment of alcohol dependence. *Arch Gen Psychiatry,*Vol.49, No.11, (Nov), pp. 876-880

Walker, B.M. & Koob, G.F. (2008). Pharmacological evidence for a motivational role of kappa-opioid systems in ethanol dependence. *Neuropsychopharmacology,*Vol.33, No.3, (Feb), pp. 643-652

Walker, B.M.; Zorrilla, E.P. & Koob, G.F. (2011). Systemic kappa-opioid receptor antagonism by nor-binaltorphimine reduces dependence-induced excessive alcohol self-administration in rats. *Addict Biol,*Vol.16, No.1, (Jan), pp. 116-119,

Walker, J.M.; Bowen, W.D.; Walker, F.O.; Matsumoto, R.R.; De Costa, B. & Rice, K.C. (1990). Sigma receptors: biology and function. *Pharmacol Rev,*Vol.42, No.4, (Dec), pp. 355-402, ISSN 0031-6997

Wells, J.L.; Bartlett, J.L.; Ananthan, S. & Bilsky, E.J. (2001). In vivo pharmacological characterization of SoRI 9409, a nonpeptidic opioid mu-agonist/delta-antagonist that produces limited antinociceptive tolerance and attenuates morphine physical dependence. *J Pharmacol Exp Ther,*Vol.297, No.2, (May), pp. 597-605

Whitworth, A.B.; Fischer, F.; Lesch, O.M.; Nimmerrichter, A.; Oberbauer, H.; Platz, T.; Potgieter, A.; Walter, H. & Fleischhacker, W.W. (1996). Comparison of acamprosate and placebo in long-term treatment of alcohol dependence. *Lancet,*Vol.347, No.9013, (May 25), pp. 1438-1442

Widdowson, P.S. & Holman, R.B. (1992). Ethanol-induced increase in endogenous dopamine release may involve endogenous opiates. *J Neurochem,*Vol.59, No.1, (Jul), pp. 157-163

Williams, K.L. & Woods, J.H. (1998). Oral ethanol-reinforced responding in rhesus monkeys: effects of opioid antagonists selective for the mu-, kappa-, or delta-receptor. *Alcoholism, clinical and experimental research,*Vol.22, No.8, (Nov), pp. 1634-1639, ISSN 0145-6008

Williams, K.L.; Kane, E.C. & Woods, J.H. (2001). Interaction of morphine and naltrexone on oral ethanol self-administration in rhesus monkeys. *Behavioural*

Winkler, A.; Buzas, B.; Siems, W.E.; Heder, G. & Cox, B.M. (1998). Effect of ethanol drinking on the gene expression of opioid receptors, enkephalinase, and angiotensin-converting enzyme in two inbred mice strains. *Alcohol Clin Exp Res,*Vol.22, No.6, (Sep), pp. 1262-1271

Wise, R.A. (1973). Voluntary ethanol intake in rats following exposure to ethanol on various schedules. *Psychopharmacologia,*Vol.29, No.3, 203-210

Wong, K.J.; Wojnicki, F.H. & Corwin, R.L. (2009). Baclofen, raclopride, and naltrexone differentially affect intake of fat/sucrose mixtures under limited access conditions. *Pharmacology, biochemistry, and behavior,*Vol.92, No.3, (May), pp. 528-536, ISSN 1873-5177

Yan, L.D.; Gong, Z.H.; Yao, X.J. & Qin, B.Y. (2003). [Comparison of the antagonistic effects of 6 beta-naltrexol and naltrexone against morphine analgesia]. *Yao Xue Xue Bao,*Vol.38, No.8, (Aug), pp. 578-581, ISSN 0513-4870

Yeomans, M.R. & Gray, R.W. (1996). Selective effects of naltrexone on food pleasantness and intake. *Physiology & behavior,*Vol.60, No.2, (Aug), pp. 439-446, ISSN 0031-9384

Yeomans, M.R. & Gray, R.W. (1997). Effects of naltrexone on food intake and changes in subjective appetite during eating: evidence for opioid involvement in the appetizer effect. *Physiology & behavior,*Vol.62, No.1, (Jul), pp. 15-21, ISSN 0031-9384

Yoneyama, N.; Crabbe, J.C.; Ford, M.M.; Murillo, A. & Finn, D.A. (2008). Voluntary ethanol consumption in 22 inbred mouse strains. *Alcohol,*Vol.42, No.3, (May), pp. 149-160, ISSN 0741-8329

Yu, L.C.; Lu, J.T.; Huang, Y.H.; Meuser, T.; Pietruck, C.; Gabriel, A.; Grond, S. & Pierce Palmer, P. (2002). Involvement of endogenous opioid systems in nociceptin-induced spinal antinociception in rats. *Brain research,*Vol.945, No.1, (Jul 26), pp. 88-96, ISSN 0006-8993

Yuan, C.S.; Sun, S.; Attele, A.; Wang, C.Z.; Tong, R. & Israel, R.J. (2009a). Methylnaltrexone potentiates body weight and fat reduction with leptin. *J Opioid Manag,*Vol.5, No.6, (Nov-Dec), pp. 373-378, ISSN 1551-7489

Yuan, C.S.; Wang, C.Z.; Attele, A. & Zhang, L. (2009b). Methylnaltrexone reduced body weight gain in ob/ob mice. *J Opioid Manag,*Vol.5, No.4, (Jul-Aug), pp. 213-218, ISSN 1551-7489

Zaki, P.A.; Bilsky, E.J.; Vanderah, T.W.; Lai, J.; Evans, C.J. & Porreca, F. (1996). Opioid receptor types and subtypes: the delta receptor as a model. *Annu Rev Pharmacol Toxicol,*Vol.36, 379-401

Zalewska-Kaszubska, J.; Gorska, D.; Dyr, W. & Czarnecka, E. (2006). Effect of acute administration of ethanol on beta-endorphin plasma level in ethanol preferring and non-preferring rats chronically treated with naltrexone. *Pharmacology, biochemistry, and behavior,*Vol.85, No.1, (Sep), pp. 155-159, ISSN 0091-3057

Zalewska-Kaszubska, J.; Gorska, D.; Dyr, W. & Czarnecka, E. (2008). Voluntary alcohol consumption and plasma beta-endorphin levels in alcohol-preferring rats chronically treated with naltrexone. *Physiology & behavior,*Vol.93, No.4-5, (Mar 18), pp. 1005-1010, ISSN 0031-9384

11

Normal and Physio-Pathological Striatal Dopamine Homeostasis

Vincent Leviel[1,2,3], Alain Gobert[1], Valérie Olivier[1],
Christine Dentresangle[2], Wadad Hassoun[2] and Kwamivi Dzahini[3]
[1]CNRS, IAF, 91198 Gif sur Yvette,
[2]CNRS, UMR 5542, Lyon
[3]INSERM, U846, SBRI, Bron,
France

1. Introduction

The neurotransmitter Dopamine (DA) exerts a dual function in the striatum (STR), the latter comprising the caudate and putamen nuclei, the main structures in the central nervous system from which it is released. During the last 50 years, numerous studies have highlighted the role of DA in sensory/motor loops. Along with a phasic function exerted in synaptic or close apposition structures, a modulatory role for extracellular DA has also been demonstrated based on the slow and tonic extracellular diffusion of the amine. This duality is probably supported by a metabolic polymorphism, particularly of the release mechanism. The present chapter focuses on works carried out *in vivo* over the last two decades on the control of DA homeostasis in the STR during normal and pathological conditions. It is now generally accepted that the level of extracellular DA is not simply the consequence of dribbling from the synapse after phasic (firing-dependent) overflow but is maintained through tonic, largely non-synaptic, regulatory processes.

The duality of DA release *in vivo* will first be described. An example of an experimental situation allowing this situation to be characterized will be given, followed by a brief overview of the relevant literature from the last three decades.

The tonic regulatory process remains incompletely understood and still requires thorough analysis. In recent years, *in vivo* and *in vitro* studies have led to the development of theoretical models based on the concept of the reversion of the well-known uptake mechanism involving the DA transporter protein (DAT). In particular conditions, DAT could be involved in the control of the extracellular DA concentration through its ability to perform what is called reverse DA transport (DA-RT). Psychotropes from the amphetamine family are known to induce the release of DA through this mechanism, but the physiological involvement of DA-RT has rarely been adressed.

A large number of regulatory processes have been described concerning tonic DA release. Only two aspects of these regulatory processes will be considered here. Specific experiments devoted to showing the role of DA synthesis and extracellular calcium ions will be described and discussed.

The two first paragraphs will be devoted to the duality of normal DA neurotransmission. It is however crucial to understand how the two different mechanisms of release (tonic and phasic) could maintain their equilibrium in pathological situations. Numerous animal models of neurodegeneration have been created. To date, only situations mimicking the early phases of parkinsonian neurodegeneration have been used to explore this equilibrium. Original results will also be presented here. These will provide new information on the regulatory modulation of the tonic and phasic release occurring during the initial pre-symptomatic compensatory phases of Parkinson's disease.

2. The dual DA release process

The extracellular DA concentration in the caudate nucleus could be relevant to something other than the electrical activity of dopaminergic cells. Increased DA release was even observed in the STR under experimental conditions that decreased cell firing in the substantia nigra (SNc, Romo et al., 1986). Since the first proposal by Raiteri et al. (1977) that DA could be released by a calcium-independent and carrier-mediated process, numerous authors have claimed that the firing-dependent release of DA does not explain all the reported alterations in the extracellular DA concentration and that an additional release mechanism must exist (Liang and Rutledge, 1982; Parker and Cubeddu, 1986; Vizi and Labos, 1991). In 1991, A. Grace gathered relevant data and proposed the presence of two modes of release of the amine in the STR (Fig 1), one 'phasic', taking place within the millisecond range, and controlled by The firing running on DA axons, and a 'tonic' mode, taking place over minutes or hours and mainly dependent on various direct influences on the DA terminals including that of Glutamate (GLU). Using differential pulse amperometry (DPA) simultaneously associated with local superfusion and HPLC detection we observed this dual release of DA in response to axonal stimulation and the application of GLU agonists (Fig. 2; Olivier et al., 1995).

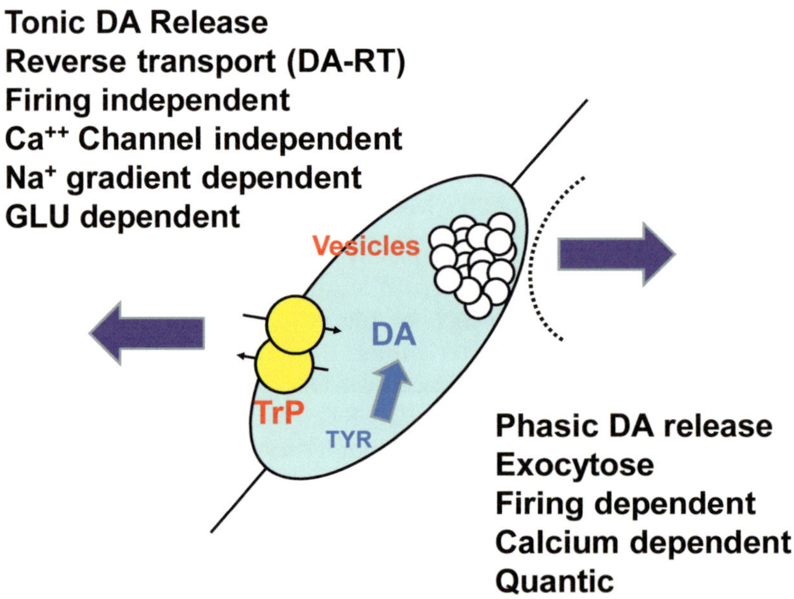

Fig. 1. The dual release of DA through vesicles exocytose or DA transport (TrP).

2.1 Spontaneous and evoked DA release

Dual release can be demonstrated by the simultaneous use of two probes. DPA uses a carbon fiber electrode to detect the DA released following stimulation of the DA axons in the Medial Forebrain Bundle (MFB) in the lateral hypothalamus. Every 4 minutes, a 20-second stimulation-train pulse produces a large increase in the amperometric signal in the STR that is strictly restricted to the stimulation period (Fig. 2, Olivier et al., 1995). The amplitude of the peaks that occur is roughly constant over time. As discussed elsewhere by Gonon (1988) and Suaud-Chagny et al. (1992), the increase in the oxidation current under these conditions is likely to be mainly due to the DA released, despite the fact that some of this increase could be due to dihydroxyphenyl acetic acid (DOPAC), the first DA metabolite. Simulation of the MFB alters the differential oxidation current but is ineffective in terms of the amount of regional extracellular basal DA measured through a cannula close to the probe used for DPA. The DA collected through the superfusion system originates from a region considerably larger than the carbon fiber. The carbon fiber is only sensitive to events occurring in the range of μm from its suface whereas the superfusing probe collects diffusing molecules from within several hundreds of microns. Differences also arise from the duration of the measurements. Stimulation of the MFB only lasts for a short period of the collection time (here 0.08%). Given this short period of time, any increase in the release of the amine remains undetectable in the superfusing fluid. The superfusing methods are particularly useful for detecting 'regional' fluctuations whereas voltammetry reports local events.

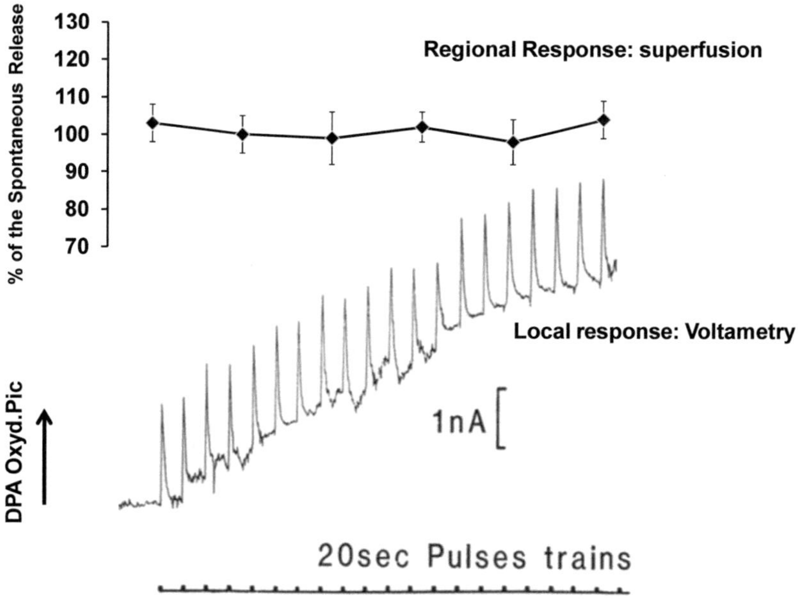

Fig. 2. The effect of MFB stimulation on tonic (up) and phasic down DA release

Superfusion in the presence of cadmium ions:

To block the voltage-dependent calcium channel, 100 μM cadmium was added to the artificial LCR supplying the cannula. This treatment blocks the stimulation-evoked release of DA detected using DPA (Fig. 3). The same effect can be obtained using 1 mM cobalt (not shown) in place of cadmium and remains unchanged in the presence of 0.5 μM GBR12909, a DAT inhibitor. Surprisingly, in the presence of cadmium or cobalt the amount of DA detected in the superfusing fluid greatly increased during the first 40 minutes of application (Fig. 3). Over this period of time, the DA collected fell below control values. When 0.5 μM GBR12909 was simultaneously added with cadmium, no further increase in the amount of DA was detected in the superfusing fluid.

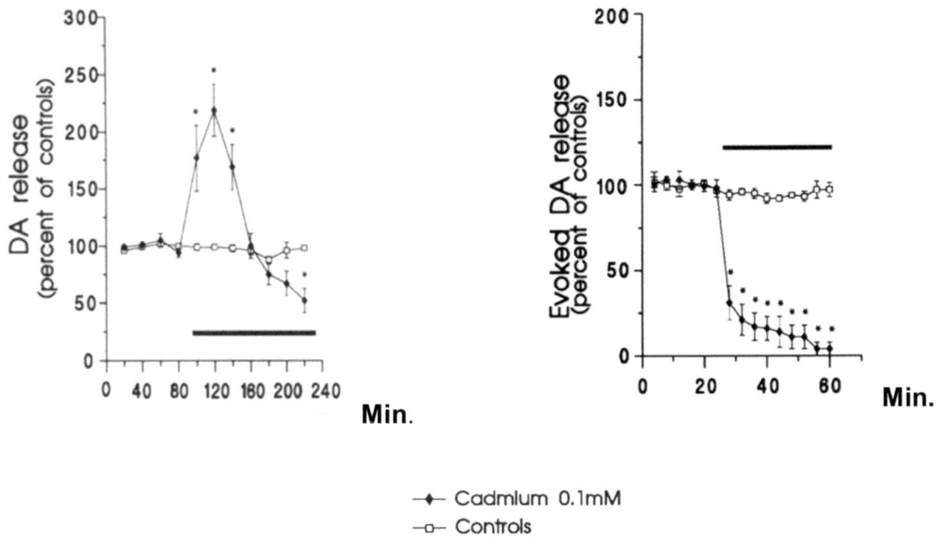

Fig. 3. Blockade of calcium channels via local application of cadmium

Local superfusion with GLU agonists:

Addition of the GLU agonists NMDA (1 mM) and kainate (0.1 mM) to the superfusing fluid increased the amount of DA collected through the push-pull cannula and reduced the amperometric signal evoked by MFB stimulations (Fig. 4). The reduction in the amperometric signal was not counteracted by the presence of 0.5 μM GBR12909. In contrast the increase in the spontaneous release measured through the cannula in response to NMDA or Kainate application completely disappeared.

2.2 From quantal release to reverse transport, the duality of DA release

These experimental observations constitute the most simple and direct evidence of the presence of a double mechanism of release of DA from the DA terminals in the STR. A large set of complementary data will now be briefly reviewed.

Can DA homeostasis be regulated by the firing-evoked synaptic release of DA?

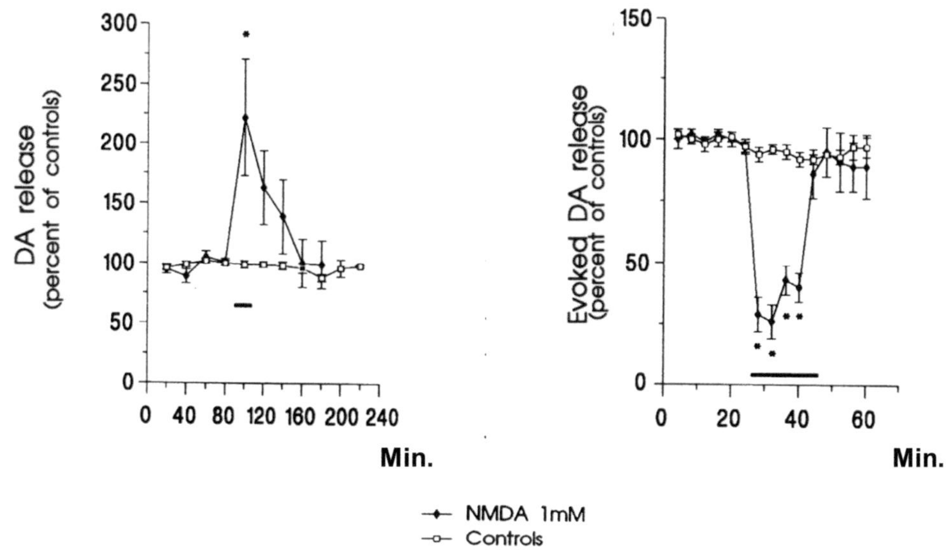

Fig. 4. The dual effect of GLU receptor blockade

The first evidence that regional extracellular DA and synaptic DA are not governed by the same mechanism is derived from the fact that although they should vary in parallel, that is clearly not the case. Many observations based on voltammetry have confirmed the ability of DA axons transiting through the MFB to carry an electrical potential, since an increase in extracellular DA can occur in response to electrical stimulations of the MFB (see above, Ewing and Wightman, 1984; Ewing et al., 1983; Gonon and Buda, 1985; Kuhr et al., 1986; Stamford et al., 1986). The voltammetric approach can only be used in a very restricted region of the space due to the size of the probes used. When using methods suitable for larger regions (micro-dialysis, push-pull cannula systems), it became clear that to alter DA levels in the STR, stimulation of the DA afferents required axonal recruitment and stimulation frequencies outside the physiological range (Grace, 1991; Olivier et al., 1995). Indeed, more than 60–70% of DA varicosities were found to be asynaptic, and DA synapses represent only about 1.8–7% of all striatal synapses (Decarries and Mechawar, 2000). Even if DA cell firing can elicit DA release in the STR for a brief period of time, the synaptic DA released may not be the only contributor to extracellular DA levels and would not be expected to be responsible for homeostatic DA control in the STR (Grace, 1991; Levi and Raiteri, 1993; Olivier, 1995). DA concentration is probably only partially monitored by nigral DA firing cells and DA homeostasis is unlikely to be controlled by spill-over of the amine from synaptic events.

Using DAT to re-visit DA release: DA-RT

It has been known for many years that exocytosis is not the only outward process of the neurotransmitter exchange between neurons and the extracellular space (Stein, 1967). Regarding monoamines, several models in the peripheral nervous system have been proposed that are generally based on exchange diffusion (Bogdanski and Brodie, 1969; Paton 1973a, 1973b). Concerning the release of DA in the central nervous system, DAT was thought to be partly involved in DA release by some authors (Marchi et al., 1985; Olivier et al., 1995; Raiteri et al., 1979) and the mechanism of this carrier-mediated release came from observations on psychostimulants and amphetamine-like substances (Butcher et al., 1988; Fisher and Cho, 1979; Leviel, 2001; Levi and Raiteri, 1993; Nash and Brodkin, 1991). In this process, transmitter molecules are transported outside the cell, most likely via an exchange-diffusion process. This mode of transfer has been extensively studied and various mathematical models have been proposed over the course of the last four decades (Chubb et al., 1972; Stein, 1990, for a review; Thoenen et al., 1969; Wheeler et al., 1993; Ziance and Rutledge, 1972).

During the 1980s, several studies were devoted to the regulatory mechanism of DA release in the STR and the substantia nigra pars reticulate (SNr). Particular attention was given to the control of striatal release, which is known to be regulated by GLU. It appeared that, in addition to a spike-mediated DA efflux, GLU-induced amine overflow could occur independently of any sodium or calcium transfer. This would mean that some of the extracellular DA, the NMDA-mediated DA that is released, is not dependent on the firing of DA neurons (Carter et al., 1988; Cheramy et al., 1986; Giorguieff et al., 1977; Jhamandas and Marien, 1987). The NMDA-mediated release of DA even remained unchanged when the nigrostriatal pathway was blocked with lesions or tetrodotoxin (Keefe et al., 1992, 1993). Recently, using voltammetry associated with electrochemical detection, the same type of observation was again reported (Borland and Michael, 2004). Such observations had already led Anthony Grace to propose, at the beginning of the 1990s, that DA could be released in the STR following two different types of mechanism (Grace, 1991): first, the firing-dependent exocytosis of quantal amounts of amine previously stored in specific pools, and, simultaneously, NMDA-mediated release.

More recently, Falkenburger et al. (2001) confirmed the existence of DA-RT in slices from rat SNc. This explained at least part of the dendritic release of DA. The presence of the somato-dendritic release of DA from the nigrostriatal cells has been known for many years (Cheramy et al., 1981) but the mechanism of this release was, and remains, an open question. As in the experiment conducted by Olivier and co-workers, the demonstration was based on the use of DAT inhibitors (GBR 12909, GBR 12935) that were able to block the GLU-induced release of DA. In a more recent study (Opazo et al., 2010), the voltammetric current corresponding to outward moving DA was increased by adding 1-Aminocyclopentane-trans 1,3 dicarboxylic acid (*trans* ACPD), an activator of the GLU group I mGLUR, to rat nigral slices. This confirmed the role of GLU in this type of DA release. It was also demonstrated that protein kinase C (PKC) activation produced a robust increase in external DA levels that was reversibly inhibited by GBR 12935, a well-known DAT inhibitor. These observations confirmed the identities of the two DA releasing processes. These observations were also made *in vitro* in an engineered neuroblastoma cell line (SH-SY5Y cells) stably expressing DAT (Opazo et al., 2010).

The two release processes act simultaneously in both the SNc and the dSTR. As mentioned above, and given the various morphologies of DA neurons (Arluison et al., 1978; Gauthier et al., 1999; Gerfen et al., 1987; Prensa et al., 2000), the possibility that some types of DA neurons could be specialized in one or the other of the release modes cannot be excluded. For instance, it is noteworthy that mesencephalic DA neurons from the ventral tegmental area poorly express DAT (Blanchard et al., 1994; Ciliax et al., 1999; Mengual and Pickel, 2004; Nirenberg et al., 1996; Sesack et al., 1998). The dual release function of DA neurons may not be equally distributed throughout the whole population of DA cells. The term 'volume transmission', developed in the 1980s (Agnati et al., 1986) and recently used to characterize DA neurotransmission, does not refer to a mode of release but rather to a mode of extracellular transmission. The terms 'phasic release' and 'tonic release' most frequently refer to the pattern of discharge of the DA axons (regular or bursting). The most appropriate terms that have emerged to date to qualify the present types of neurotransmitter release are 'quantal' for the firing-dependent process and 'reverse transport' (DA-RT) or 'lateral release' for the carrier-mediated mechanism. We also use the term 'lateral release' to refer to the non-synaptic localization of this mechanism, due to the extra-synaptic position of the DA transporter. In this case, 'axial release' could refer to synaptic transmission.

3. Regulatory mechanisms

It has already been shown that the extracellular level of calcium (Ca^{++}) ions has an important influence on neurotransmitter release (Katz and Miledi, 1970; Augustine et al., 1987; Smith and Augustine, 1988; Mulkey and Zucker, 1991) and on enzyme activities (Kapatos and Zigmond, 1982; El Mestikawy et al., 1983; Haycock, 1993). Since transient increases in Ca^{++} within nerve terminals are spatially restricted (Lipscombe et al., 1988; Meldolesi et al., 1988; Miller, 1991) it may be hypothesized that Ca^{++} independently affects multiple processes within the different ultrastructural compartments of the nerve terminal. The metabolism and release of DA in the STR constitute an appropriate experimental model with which to investigate the potentially distinct effects of Ca^{++}. In the dopaminergic neurons DA synthesis depends on the activity of tyrosine hydroxylase (TH), the rate-limiting enzyme in its synthetic pathway (Levitt et al., 1965). This enzyme is activated by phosphorylation under the control of various protein kinases, including two Ca^{++}-dependent ones, the Ca^{++}-phospholipid-dependent protein kinases (PKC) and the Ca^{++}-calmodulin-dependent protein kinase (PKII) (El Mestikawy et al., 1983; Albert et al., 1984; Zigmond et al., 1989; Haycock, 1993).

Below we will present further data about the dual control exerted by Ca^{++} ions on DA synthesis and on DA-releasing processes. The apparent challenge between synthesis and release in the effects of Ca^{++} is coming from the fact that DA-RT acts on cytoplasmic DA , unlike exocytosis, which affects a previously vesicularysed stored pool of DA. It can thus be hypothesizd that DA-RT should be more sensitive to those treatments affecting synthesis.

3.1 Synthesis, calcium ions and DA release – Experimental report

We describe here the only method known to evaluate DA synthesis and release simultaneously *in vivo* in anesthetized rats. The method is based on the measurement of the specific activity (DA_{sa}) of the DA released during continuous superfusion of the tissue with the tritiated DA precursor, [^{3}H]tyrosine. It was previously observed that the neosynthesized amine is released preferentially to an oldly stored pool. Taking advantage of this metabolic specificity, it can be postulated that: 1) increased DA_{sa} during higher levels of release reflects enhanced synthesis and 2) decreased DA_{sa} associated with increased levels of release reveals the involvement of stored amine (vesicular) and suggests reduced or insufficient synthesis. The DOPAC efflux is also considered to be a robust index of DA synthesis (Zetterström et al., 1988; Leviel et al., 1989). In other words, any treatment reducing synthesis should reduce cytoplasmic DA_{sa} and the DOPAC efflux. In contrast, any treatment activating synthesis should elevate DA_{sa} and the DOPAC efflux.

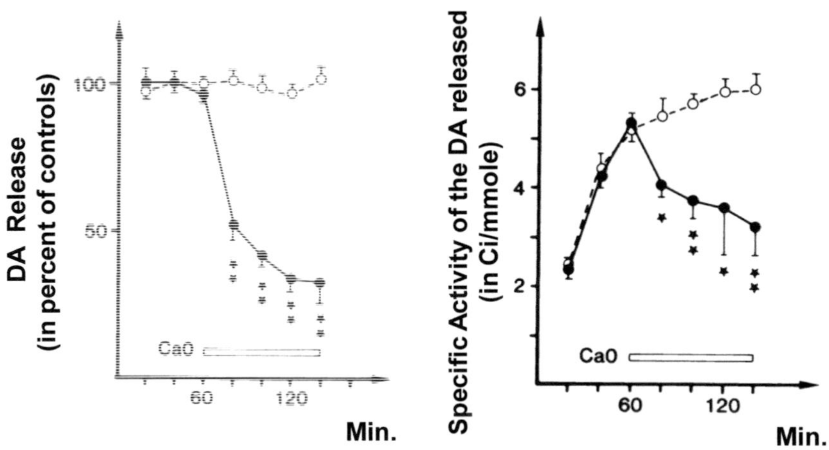

Fig. 5. Superfusion with CSF from which Ca^{++} was omitted

Superfusion with calcium-free medium and α-methyl para-tyrosine (α-mpt)

We already know that local superfusion with the calcium channel blockers cadmium and cobalt enhances regional DA release and blocks firing-induced exocytosis. Removing Ca^{++} ions from the superfusing medium (Ca0) led to a sharp decrease in DA release, stabilizing at around 30% of the basal value after about 80 min. This effect was accompanied by a lowering of the specific activity of DA_{sa} and of [³H]DOPAC (Fig. 5). The addition of α-mpt, a TH inhibitor, did not modify the effect of Ca0 treatment: the DA collected in each 20-minute fraction also stabilized at around 30% of the spontaneous values (Fig. 6). These two effects were thus not additive, and the lowering of the DA_{sa} produced by superfusion with Ca0 was of the same amplitude as that observed in the α-mpt treatment. This observation strongly suggests that the main effect of Ca0 could be the inhibition of DA synthesis (Olivier et al., 1999).

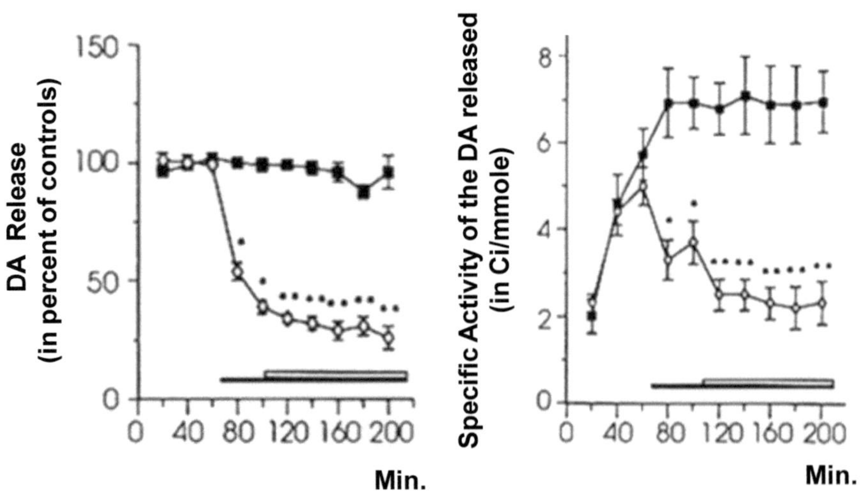

Fig. 6. The inhibition of DA synthesis during superfusion in the absence of Ca^{++}

Superfusion with calcium ionophore (A23187): The forced entry of calcium

Adding the Ca^{++} ionophore A23187 (1 µmol/l) to the superfusing fluid for 20 min had no effect on the spontaneous release of DA or DAsa (Fig. 7). However, an increase in DOPAC (25%) was associated with a 50% increase in the [³H]DOPAC concentration.

It is possible to evaluate the effect of the calcium ionophore A23187 on DA synthesis *'in vivo'*. A high dose of amphetamine can be superfused to produce the maximum overflow of the intraterminal DA. Thus 1 hour after administering 20 min of 1 mmol/l amphetamine, the total intraterminal DA had increased, particularly the DA_{sa} (Olivier et al., 1999). This demonstrates a large increase in synthesis during this period of time.

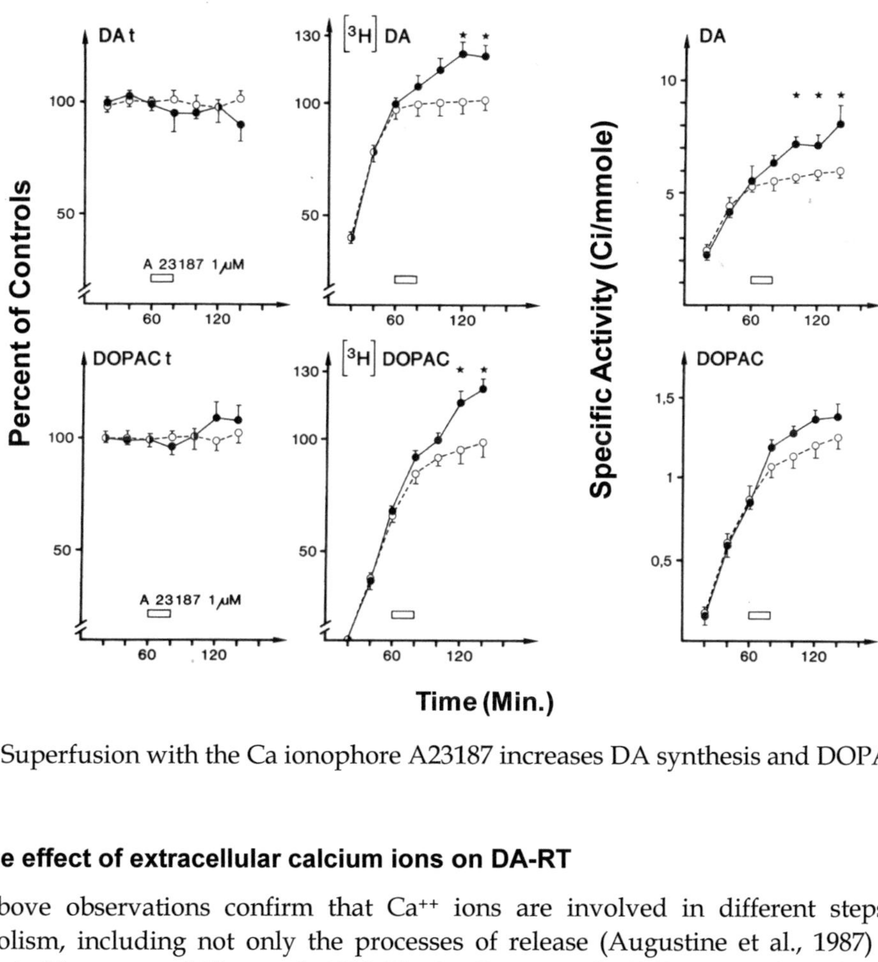

Fig. 7. Superfusion with the Ca ionophore A23187 increases DA synthesis and DOPAC efflux

3.2 The effect of extracellular calcium ions on DA-RT

The above observations confirm that Ca^{++} ions are involved in different steps of DA metabolism, including not only the processes of release (Augustine et al., 1987) but also synthesis (Kapatos and Zigmond, 1982; El Mestikawy et al., 1983; Haycock et al., 1984). We have not directly measured the enzymatic activity of TH, but alterations in synthesis were revealed by the dynamic variations in DA_{sa} and the [³H]DOPAC efflux. Indeed the DA_{sa} can be used as an index of DA synthesis (Herdon et al., 1985) since the newly synthesized DA has a higher specific activity than the stored amine (Leviel et al., 1989). [³H]DOPAC might also be considered as a good index of amine synthesis according to many authors (Herdon et al., 1985; Soares-Da-Silva, 1987; Zetterström et al., 1988; Leviel et al., 1989; Soares-Da-Silva and Garrett, 1990a, 1990b), who have proposed that extracellular DOPAC originates from an unreleased and recently synthesized pool of dopamine.

Ca^{++} ions in the regulation of DA synthesis:

Removal of Ca^{++} from the superfusing fluid induced a large decrease in DA_{sa} and in [^{3}H]DOPAC efflux, suggesting reduced DA synthesis. Futhermore the addition of a TH inhibitor, namely α-mpt, to a Ca^{++}-free superfusing fluid did not further decrease the DA_{sa} or the [^{3}H]DOPAC, suggesting that the activity of TH is already maximally inhibited by Ca^{++} removal. TH activity could be inhibited by a rise in DA feedback inhibition resulting from the lowering of Ca^{++}-dependent exocytosis (Leslie et al., 1985; Zucker and Lando, 1986; Westerink et al., 1988). However, the intracellular accumulation of DA should result in increased DOPAC efflux, which was not observed. Conversely, the reduced DA_{sa} revealed that even to maintain a low rate of DA release, stored amine (with a low specific activity) has to be involved, showing that in the absence of extracellular calcium ions, DA synthesis is unable to sustain the lower DA release (30% of the control value).

Superfusion without Ca^{++} in the CSF appears to be able to reduce synthesis. Forced Ca^{++} entry could have the opposite effect. Indeed a low dose of the Ca^{++} ionophore A23187 (1 µmol/l) slightly increased [^{3}H]DA and [^{3}H]DOPAC efflux, suggesting an increase in DA synthesis (Fig. 7). Such activation of synthesis was confirmed by the potentiation of the amphetamine-induced [^{3}H]DA release that followed pretreatment with A23187 1 µmol/l (Olivier et al., 1999).

This set of simple data is consistent with the concept that moderate Ca^{++} entry is positively coupled with DA synthesis and that its absence from the extracellular medium is negatively coupled with DA synthesis (Kapatos and Zigmond, 1982; El Mestikawy et al., 1983; Haycock et al., 1984).

Ca^{++} ions in the regulation of DA-RT:

Surprisingly, *in vivo* blockade of the Ca^{++} ion channel with Cd^{++} ions activates DA-RT from the DA terminals, an effect that was inhibited by further application of GBR 12909, a DAT inhibitor. The mechanism by which Cd^{++} affects DA-RT is not clear. For a long time, reversal of the Na^+ gradient was proposed to reverse DA transport (Roth et al., 1976; Amejddki-Chab et al., 1992; Levi and Raiteri, 1993; Okada et al., 1990). It was also proposed by Olivier et al. (1999) that Cd^{++} indirectly alters DA-RT via Na^+/K^+ ATPase activity, a hypothesis also proposed for the action of AMPh (Khoshbouei et al., 2003; Pal et al., 1993).

After applying a Ca^{++} ionophore, A23187, DA synthesis increased. With the classical model used for DA-RT of an exchange diffusion process, it is clear that the cytosolic DA constitutes the direct substrate for internal DAT-sites, regardless of its affinity. Thus, from these experiments, and despite the fact that DA-RT can be considered as being firing-independent, many observations during the last decade have confirmed indirect calcium action on DA-RT (Fog et al., 2006; Gnegy et al., 2004; Kantor et al., 2001; Page et al., 2004).

Numerous reports highlight the role of Ca^{++} in the amphetamine-dependent DA-RT. The Ca^{++} chelator BAPTA-AM reduced amphetamine-induced DA efflux as measured by amperometry. A particularly interesting observation was that superfusion of rat striatal slices with 50 µM BAPTA-AM suppressed the amphetamine-induced release of endogenous

DA. However, the same treatment had no effect on basal DA in the absence of AMPh. These studies demonstrated that AMPh-induced and DAT-mediated currents producing substrate efflux require internal Ca^{++} release from intracellular stores and that amphetamine can stimulate dopamine efflux by regulating cytoplasmic Ca^{++} levels (Gnegy et al., 2004). It has also been shown that Ca^{++}/calmodulin-dependent protein kinase-II (CaMKII) plays a key role in the amphetamine-mediated efflux of DA in heterologous cells and dopaminergic neurons. CaMKII binds to the distal C terminus of DAT and co-localizes with DAT in dopaminergic neurons. The distal serines of the N terminus of DAT were phosphorylated by CaMKII *in vitro* and the mutation of these serines eliminated the stimulatory effects of CaMKIIa. A mutation of the DAT C terminus, impairing CaMKIIa binding, also impaired AMPh-induced DA efflux. Thus, it was suggested that the binding of CaMKIIa to the DAT C terminus facilitates phosphorylation of the DAT N terminus, which is responsible for the AMPh-induced dopamine efflux (Fog et al., 2006).

A non-amphetaminic effect of CaMKII was also reported. Pseudo-phosphorylation of the hDAT N-terminal serines (S/D mutation), which appear to be phosphorylated by CaMKII, is largely able to evoke the reverse transport of DA even in unclamped cells, i.e. at resting membrane potential. This showed that activation of this enzymatic system (DAT) constitutes a mechanism of release by itself, even in the absence of amphetamine or any exogenous trigger. CaMKII is the most abundant kinase in the brain and could play a role in the regulation of various neurotransmitters (Colbran et al., 2003; Griffith, 2004). It is well known that local increases in Ca^{++} concentration and the CaMKII complex interact with the transduction of several neuronal signals, whether from DA neurotransmitters or not. Numerous proteins, such as the NR2B subunit of the NMDA receptor, could be involved in tonic release processes. It was recently proposed that tonic hyperactivity of the GLU afferents to the dopaminergic striatal terminals could maintain tonic-activated DA overflow in the rat STR following a 6-OHDA lesion of the SNc (Dzahini et al., 2010), and mechanisms such as those presently known to be evoked could be responsible for the effects observed. The same type of tonic hyperactivity could also be present in the mesencephalic region of the SNc. Sustained hypertonic GLU neurotransmission is often observed and reported in experimental and natural situations of neuro-degeneration, and could maintain secondary amine overflow without immediate consequences, but cause insidious degeneration.

The main finding of recent reports about the regulatory processes of the DAT protein is the complete dissociation between inward (uptake) and outward (release) efflux. Untill recently DAT was considered to be an exchange diffusion system with a stoichiometric equilibrium linking the two functions. It is now clear that this concept should be revisited and that the inward regulatory processes differ from the release mechanism.

In summary, three steps in DA metabolism occur to determine the extracellular DA concentration: synthesis, exocytosis and reverse transport (fig.8). Directly or indirectly, Ca^{++} ions modulate each of these. Thus carrier-mediated release (DA-RT) appears to be indirectly and negatively coupled with calcium entry, whereas synthesis and exocytosis are directly and positively coupled with Ca^{++} entry.

3.3 Intraterminal DA metabolism: From synthesis to release

The observations presented here and the numerous reports about DA synthesis, storage and release have enabled the proposal of a general model of the striatal DA terminal in physiological conditions (Leviel et al., 1989). As mentioned above, components of this model may be attributed to different DA neurons. In the model presented in Fig. 8, a central pool of cytosolic DA constitutes the central point of the functional organization. Three input and four output routes are then described. The major way of supplying this central pool is via DA synthesis. A secondary supply mechanism could involve the intraterminal egress of DA from the vesicular storage pool. The third input comprises DA uptake transport.

The first and major output of cytoplasmic DA involves the formation of DOPAC by the MAO enzyme. The second use of cytoplasmic DA involves terminal overflow through DA-RT. A small proportion of the synthesized DA is vesicularized in a neosynthesized pool constituting the preferentially releasable compartment of the amine, and is released by exocytosis. Some of this vesicularized amine supplies a storage compartment (old stored DA).

This model takes into account the different mechanisms of DA release and DA metabolism that can be independently regulated. For example, reduced exocytotic release (by the blockade of calcium channels) can be accompanied by increased DA-RT, leading to an increase in extracellular amine. Thus even if the depolarization of DA axons is clearly responsible for exocytotic DA release, the preterminal influences could lead to secondary release that is differentially regulated, producing the paradoxical observations that are often reported (Leviel et al., 1989).

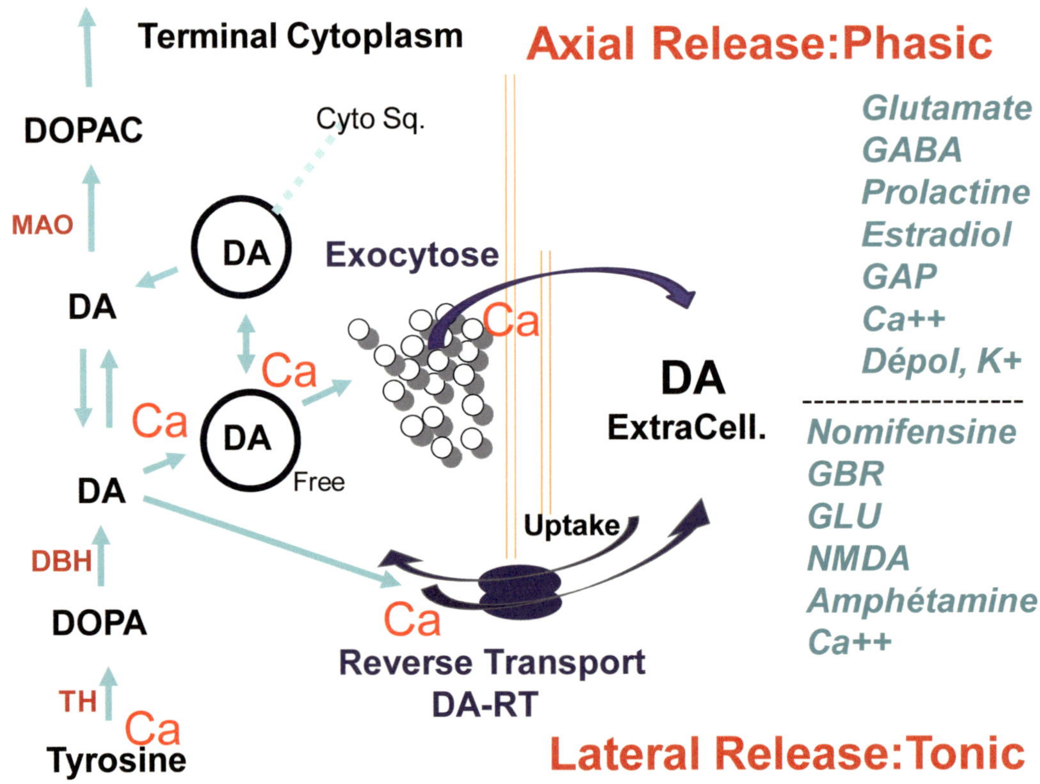

Fig. 8. The four-compartments model of intraterminal DA metabolism including dual release

4. Evolving DA release with DA cell degeneration

4.1 Progressive DA denervation of the STR enhances DA transport in synaptosomal preparations

Why address the consequences of DA cell degeneration? So far we have described the equilibrium between two mechanisms that release DA, but only one of these is likely to be able to maintain DA homeostasis in the extracellular space. For a long time it was thought that the progressive degeneration of the DA cells of the SN, such as observed in Parkinson'disease (PD), is accompanied by the preservation of the DA concentration in the STR, a region that is innervated by DA axons. Basic observations have ascertained that DA metabolism is activated in spared dopaminergic terminals of the partially denervated STR. Both increased DA synthesis and reduced storage capacity were recurrently reported (see Zigmond et al., 1990 for a review). This was considered to be the possible cause of the unmodified (or even sometimes increased) extracellular DA level in this region (Stackowiak et al., 1987; Altar and Marien, 1989; Espino et al., 1995; Dentresangle et al., 2001; Dzahini et al., 2010). Nevertheless, no changes in either the firing pattern or the efficacy of release were observed in nigral DA cells following a moderate partial lesion (Hollerman and Grace, 1990; Dentresangle et al., 2001). On the contrary, spared DA neurons were described as hypoactive and pre-apoptotic (Pasinetti et al., 1989). This adaptation is unlikely to be the result of the electrical hyperactivity of the surviving nigral DA cells.

Extracellular DA is taken up into dopaminergic terminals. In partially lesioned rats, the long-term reduction of this DA uptake may allow more diffusion in tissues (Snyder et al., 1990; van Horn et al., 1992; Gerhardt et al., 1996). This hypothesis is reinforced by the fact that the depolarization of cells bearing the DA transporter reduces their ability to take up extracellular amine (Roth et al., 1976; Zahniser et al., 1998). GLU neurotransmission could be involved in this process. Indeed GLU is responsible for tonic membrane depolarization in CP (Wilson et al., 1995) and GLU neurotransmission is known to be hyperactive following a partial lesion (Lindefors and Ungerstedt, 1990; Samuel *et al.*, 1990; Iwasaki *et al.*, 1992; Wullner *et al.*, 1994).

Reduced DA uptake due to a reduced number of DA terminals is however unable to account for the maintained dopaminergic function as the extracellular DA concentration should also be correlated with a reduction in the number of release sites. No changes in the number of uptake sites *per neuron* were reported and the binding of the transporter ligands was even considered to be a good index of the terminal depopulation (Maloteaux et al., 1988; van Horne et al., 1992). Thus normal or increased levels of extracellular DA, associated with a reduced number of dopaminergic terminals, imply an increased release/uptake ratio *per terminal*. GLU neurotransmission in the STR may mediate this increase. GLU was reported to increase DA synthesis (Desce et al., 1992; Fillenz, 1993; Castro et al., 1996), to activate DA release (Giorguieff et al., 1977; Cheramy et al., 1986; Leviel et al., 1990; Keefe et al., 1992) and to reduce DA uptake (Lin and Chai, 1998). The mechanism by which basal DA release is altered is however poorly understood. In the absence of any change in DA cell activity, alterations should involve DA-RT. This concept of activation of the DA metabolism through local GLU-dependent activation of DA-RT from the striatal DA terminal in response to the DA cell depopulation is widely debated. The following paragraph addresses this problem by analyzing the results of experiments based on progressive or very partial lesions of the nigrostriatal DA pathway in the rat.

4.2 Experimental observations

To address this issue, partial and progressive destruction of the dopaminergic terminals of the STR was achieved and various biochemical parameters were monitored. The injections were not directly located in the striatal tissue but in the lateral ventricle. Recurrent 6-OHDA injections were administered week after week, locally in the rat STR. In these lesioned rats, metabolic alterations of DA were followed along with the kinetic parameters of the uptake process in synaptosomal preparations. These parameters (apparent Km and Vmax) are correlated with the number of uptake sites determined in binding experiments with a ligand of the DAT carrier protein, GBR12935. The possible role of GLU neurotransmission in these alterations was also investigated.

Neither behavioral disturbance nor loss of weight was observed during treatment. Following successive injections, however, progressive biochemical alterations developed in both the median and lateral part of the STR, ipsilaterally to the injected ventricle.

Control values for tissue DA were 54.9±9.3 ng/mg prot and 45.7±6.9 ng/mg prot for the median and lateral STR respectively. For tissue DOPAC, the control values were 27.19±3.6 ng/mg prot and 26.4±4.11 ng/mg prot in the median and lateral STR respectively. The first changes observed were in tissue DA, which began to decrease after the first two injections, reaching only 23.3 and 29.6% (median and lateral STR respectively) of the values of the sham-injected animals after the 8th injection (Fig. 9). The decrease in tissue DOPAC was

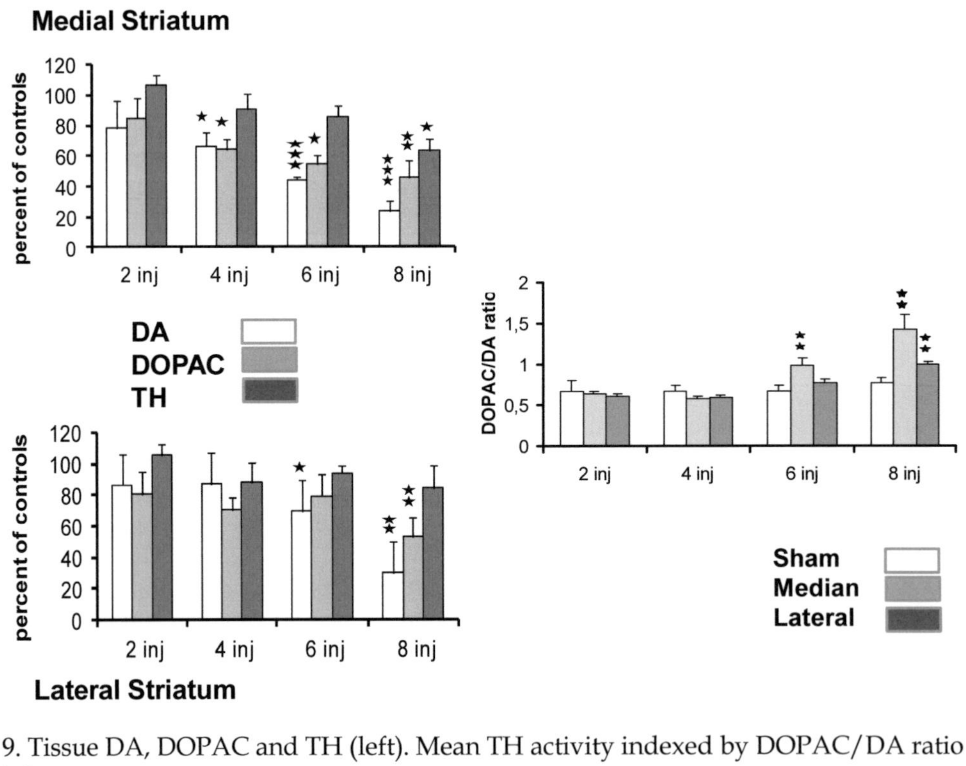

Fig. 9. Tissue DA, DOPAC and TH (left). Mean TH activity indexed by DOPAC/DA ratio (Right).

slower, reaching 45.5 and 52.7% (median and lateral STR respectively) of the controls after the 8th injection. The tissue DOPAC/DA ratio (0.494 in the control rats) increased significantly only after the 6th injection, reaching a value of 1.4 in the median part of the STR after the 8th injection (Fig. 9). The tissue content of TH (Fig. 9) decreased very slowly and the differences compared with control rats (8.94±0.60 UTH in the median STR; 9.24±0.81 UTH in the lateral STR) were only significant after the 8th injection (63 and 84.4% of controls in the median and lateral STR respectively). These alterations were first detected in the medial part of the STR (in the more lesioned part) and 2 weeks later, more laterally. Thus an immediate alteration of tissue DOPAC and DA was observed, followed by a delayed increase in the DOPAC/DA ratio and a late reduction in the amount of TH.

Binding of [^{3}H]GBR12935 was measured in synaptosomes prepared from rats that had been injected for 8 weeks. The B_{max} in the sham-operated group was 3.82 pmole/mg prot. In the lesioned group, B_{max} fell to 2.31 pmole/mg prot (60.4%) but returned to 3.42 pmole/mg prot in lesioned animals treated daily with MK801 (89.5% of sham-operated group). The ability of synaptosomes to load [^{3}H]DA was not greatly affected in lesioned animals. The slopes of the [^{3}H]DA accumulation curves were: 0.101 pmole/mg prot/min for the sham-operated animals, 0.089 pmole/mg prot/min for the lesioned group (88.6% of the sham-operated group, n.s.) and 0.098 pmole/mg prot/min for the lesioned animals treated with MK801 (97.1% of the sham-operated group, n.s.) (Fig. 10). However, the ratio between [^{3}H]DA accumulation and [^{3}H]GBR12935 binding (in pmol/pmol of [^{3}H]GBR12935/min, data not shown) was 0.026 (100%) for the sham-operated animals, 0.038 for the lesioned group (146.5%; $P<0.05$) and 0.028 for the lesioned animals treated with MK801 (108.5% of the sham-operated group, n.s.).

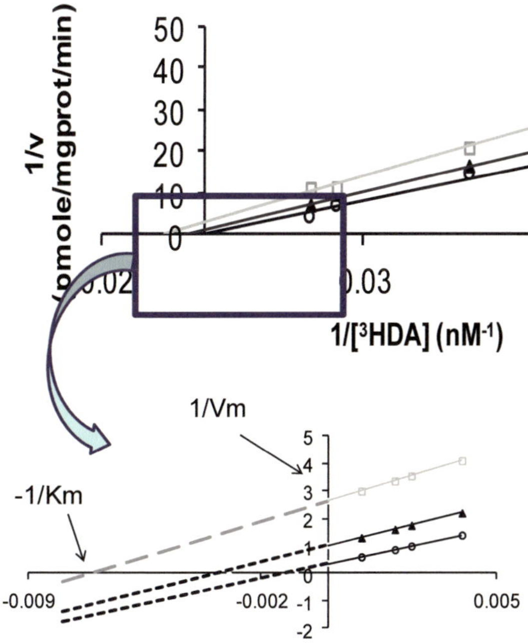

	Vm (Pm/mg/min)	Km (µM)
Lesioned	0.382	013
MK801 Treated	0.824	0.27
Controls	2.967	0.78

Fig. 10. Lineweaver-Burk plot of [^{3}H]DA capture in striatal synaptosomes

The apparent K_m and V_{max} of the [^{3}H]DA transport reaction were calculated by linear regression (Fig. 10). The slopes of the curves obtained for lesioned-only animals and lesioned plus MK801-treated animals were both significantly different from that of sham-operated animals ($P<0.05$). The values of V_{max} were 2.967, 0.382 and 0.824 pmole/mg prot/min respectively for sham-operated, lesioned and lesioned + MK801-injected rats. The K_m values were 0.78, 0.13 and 0.27 μM respectively.

4.3 Nigrostriatal lesion reduces DA uptake but increases DA transport

The reduction in the levels of tissue DA and DOPAC appeared soon after the first injection. The DOPAC/DA ratio, reflecting TH protein activity (Lavielle et al., 1978; Bannon & Roth, 1983; Zetterström et al., 1988; Nissbrandt et al., 1989; Soares da Silva & Garret, 1990), and the amount of TH protein in the tissue remained unchanged during the first 6 weeks. This reduction in intraterminal DA stores that is not associated with changes in DA synthesis is consistent with the observations that we report below of increased basal DA release during the very early phases of denervation (Dentresangle et al., 2001; Dzahini et al., 2010).

After six and eight injections, both the tissue DA and DOPAC continued to decrease and tissue levels of TH protein began to decline. In contrast, the DOPAC/DA ratio increased, confirming a delay in increased DA synthesis. This could be the result of decreased intraterminal DA. TH activity is under the control of cytoplasmic amine levels through an end-product regulatory process (Ames et al., 1978; Mann and Gordon, 1979; Zigmond et al., 1989; Fillenz, 1993). Therefore increased TH activity, which is often reported after partial lesion of the DA pathway (Zigmond et al., 1990) could be, at least in part, a consequence of reduced intraterminal DA pools. The simultaneous reduction in the amount of tissue TH protein may occur in one of two ways: (1) a reduction in the number of DA terminals, or (2) increased protein turnover associated with the increased catalytic activity (Vrana and Roskoski, 1983; Lavergne et al., 1994).

This set of results is consistent with the hypothesis that the preservation of extracellular DA after partial destruction of the nigro-striatal DA pathway is due to activation of basal DA release. However, as already mentioned, this is unlikely to be the result of electrical activation of DA neurons in the SNc. Thus, alterations in DA transport at the level of the DA terminals in the STR are more likely.

The amplitude of the denervation produced by eight injections of the toxin was evaluated initially. The amount of TH protein and the binding of transport sites are considered to be valid indices of DA pathway denervation (van Horne et al., 1992; Maloteau, 1998). In the present experiment, tissue TH protein levels were reduced to 63% of the levels found in controls, and the B_{max} of [^{3}H]GBR12935 was reduced to 60.4% of the value found in sham-operated animals. Thus, about 40% of DA terminals may have degenerated after eight injections of the toxin.

Given this 40% reduction in the number of binding sites in the synaptosomal preparation of lesioned rats, the kinetic parameters of the DA uptake process are apparently paradoxical. First, the global DA uptake was only reduced by 11% (insignificant decrease), and when adjusted according to the number of sites (reduced by 40%), it was actually increased (146% of controls). This observation suggests an increase in the efficiency of the transport process, compensating for the reduction in the population of DA terminals. Second, the V_{max}, which is an index of transport capacity, was only 12% of the value in control rats. This observation shows that a large number of sites, still bound to [^{3}H]GBR12935, had become unable to carry DA. Third, it can be concluded from the low K_m value that the affinity of DA for the carrier protein had increased. These results strongly suggest that moderate DA denervation of the STR results in a reduction in the number of functional DA transporters able to carry DA, but an increase in their affinity, which is responsible in turn for an increased rate of transport. We will see below that a new way to see the structure of the DAT protein could underline this paradoxical data. Indeed DAT is no longer considered as only an uptake processor but rather as a dual actor of the DA transport regulating extracellular DA homeostasis.

5. Presynaptic GLU – Induced activation of DA release in the STR after partial nigral lesion

The behavioral and biochemical recovery, after partial unilateral lesion, of the dopaminergic nigrostriatal path has been reported in various species from rodents to primates (Hefti et al., 1985; McCallum et al., 2006; Boulet et al., 2008; Perez et al., 2008). This recovery is thought to result from normalization of the extracellular dopamine (DA_{ext}) in the STR that was initially reduced by the lesion (Robinson and Whishaw, 1988; Castaneda et al., 1990; Zigmond et al., 1990; Emmi et al., 1996). However, it remains unclear whether this compensation results from overactive nigral neurons, as is proposed to occur after LevoDOPA treatment (Grace, 2008), from direct preterminal influences in the STR (Dentresangle et al., 2001), or from both. A role for GLU in this phenomenon has been proposed given that the GLU tone increases in various regions of the basal ganglia following SNc lesions, including in the STR (Calabresi et al., 1993; Cepeda et al., 2001; Tang et al., 2001), the SNc (Turski et al., 1991; Bezard et al., 1997) and the subthalamic nucleus (Benazzouz et al., 1993; Amalric et al., 1995; Phillips et al., 2006). This was confirmed by the fact that behavioral and biochemical recovery were inhibited by chronic treatment with GLU receptor (GLU_R) antagonists including MK801 (see the preceding paragraph) and 3-[(R)-2-carboxypiperazin-4-yl]-prop-2-enyl-1-phosphonic acid (CPP) (Emmi et al., 1996). The nature of the mechanisms evoked by GLU remains unclear however, because compensatory mechanisms occur very early or following very partial lesions, at a stage at which the spontaneous activity of midbrain DA neurons was not found to be altered (Hollerman and Grace, 1990) and when the impulse/release ratio in the terminal region appeared unchanged (Dentresangle et al., 2001). To complicate the situation, it is now well known that GLU can enhance DA release independently from the spontaneous electrical activity of the midbrain DA neurons (Leviel et al., 1990; Keefe et al., 1992; Olivier et al., 1995, 1999).

5.1 Experimental observations

To understand the functional link between DA and GLU during the compensatory process a very partial and laterally located lesion of the SN was produced in rats using 6-OHDA. Three weeks after this lesion, it was possible to compare the metabolic consequences of a large denervation in the lateral part of the STR with those in a medial region spared by the denervation. Cartography of the tonic extracellular DA and DOPAC concentration was performed using *in vivo* voltammetry. In rats with similar lesions medial and lateral microdialysis approaches allowed us to measure the extracellular GLU concentration. The effect of GLU antagonists (amantadine, memantine and riluzol) on neurotransmission and their neuroprotective action on tonic DA enhancement were also tested.

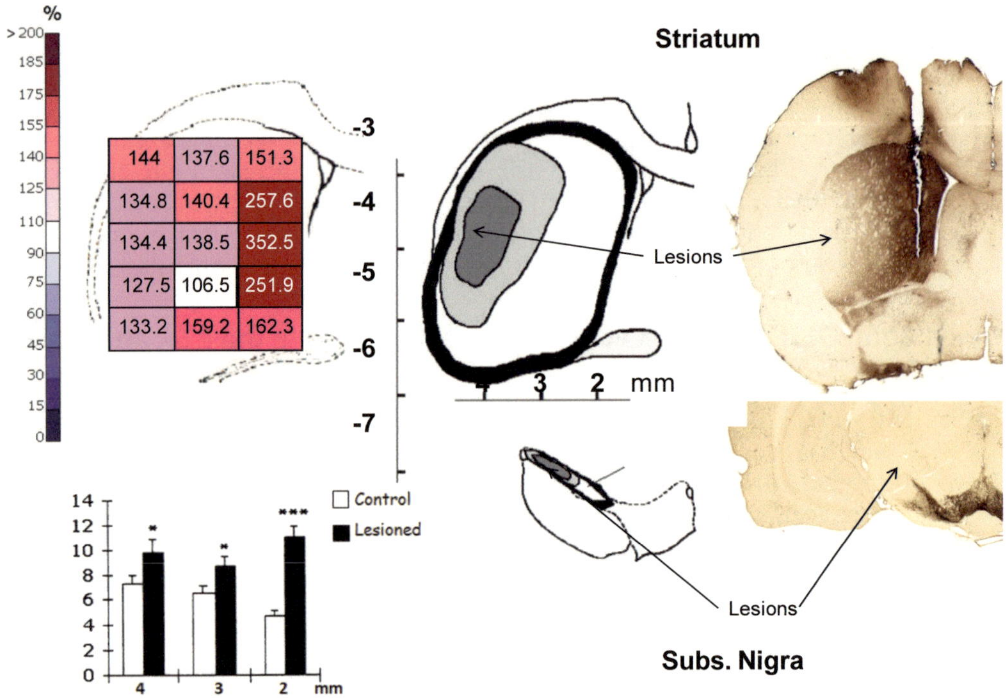

Fig. 11. Lateral lesion of the SN and its consequences for striatal DA denervation and release

Cartography of the STR using voltammetry

The STR was stereotaxically explored in one coronal plane (8.2 mm anterior to the ear axe) to localize biochemical changes *in vivo*. Figure 11 shows the extracellular concentrations of DA expressed in nM and as the ratio (in %) between values obtained in lesioned and control animals in each homologous striatal area for each subregion explored. In the lesioned animals, DA measured in the intact median region (lat. 2) showed a notable increase (352%, $p < 0.001$) in comparison with control values. This effect was less pronounced in the intermediate and lateral striatal areas (lat. 3-4) but was nevertheless present. In the most completely DA-deafferented striatal regions, DA levels did not differ significantly from control values, being only slightly higher. In contrast, the extracellular level of DOPAC decreased enormously (26% of control values; $p < 0.001$) in the lateral part of the STR in comparison with values detected in the homologous striatal region of the control group. In the medial region DOPAC concentrations remained poorly affected (Dzahini et al., 2010).

Effects of partial lesions of the SN and microdialysis results

Voltammetry furnishs excellent stereotaxic localization of biochemical alterations but the use of pargyline to detect DA could produce a bias in the measurements. To better quantify the changes observed with voltammetry, and to extend the measurements to amino acids, the medial spared region was implanted with a microdialysis probe, and superfusates were subjected to HPLC and two analyses, one for catecholamines and the other for amino acids. In sham-operated and untreated rats, the spontaneous extracellular concentrations of DA (7.28±0.36 nM), DOPAC (9.19±1.1 μM), HVA (6.54±0.59 μM), GLU (10.0±0.27 μM), GABA

(0.42±0.06 μM) and ASP (0.47±0.05 μM) were in the range of previously reported values. Importantly, DA was in the nano molar range in the extracellular space whereas metabolites and amino acids were in the micro molar range. Three weeks following the lesion in the lateral part of the SN, an increase in DA was detected in the medial STR (29.2±0.28 nM). Simultaneously an increase in GLU was observed (24.4 ± 0.75 μM). In contrast, the DA metabolites, DOPAC (10.8±0.10 μM) and HVA_{ext} (8.86±0.90 μM), remained unchanged. Likewise, GABA (0.63±0.17 μM) and ASP (0.47±0.05 μM) were not significantly altered.

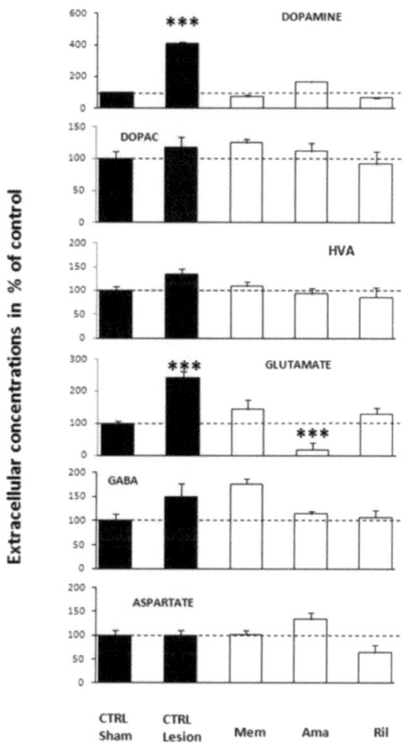

Fig. 12. Tissue DA and amino acid in the striatum 3 weeks following lesioning of the SN using 6-OHDA

Treatment of lesioned rats with GLU antagonists

Treatment with chronic memantine, amantadine or riluzol seemed to counteract the tonic increase in DA induced following the lesion that was observed via voltammetry and confirmed using microdialysis (Fig. 12). Only a moderate increase in DA persisted following chronic amantadine administration (12.4 ± 1.26 nM versus 7.28 ± 0.36 nM in controls). The DA concentration remained at basal levels following treatment with memantine and riluzol (Fig. 12). Acute treatments with the same substances were less efficient at counteracting the increase in DA but the same trends were apparent (15.1 nM, 24.1 nM and 24.4 nM respectively for memantine, amantadine and riluzol versus 29.2 nM in the controls, Dzahini et al., 2010). The GLU antagonists did not interact with the DA metabolites DOPAC and HVA. The results are presented in Fig. 12 as percentages of the values obtained in lesioned rats.

The extracellular GLU concentration increased tonically after the lesion (24.4±0.75 μM versus 10.0+0.27 μM in controls). This effect was counteracted by treatment with either chonic or acute memantine (47.1±2.3 μM and 27.1±1.53 μM respectively). Chronic riluzol also counteracted the lesion-induced increase in GLU after chronic application (21.8±0.68 μM) and acute riluzol drastically reduced GLU (0.7±0.05 μM). GLU was also reduced after both chonic and acute amantadine treatment (1.04±0.4 μM and 0.74±0.26 μM respectively). No alterations in GABA or ASP were detected in response to the treatment of lesioned rats with GLU antagonists. The results obtained after chronic treatments are presented in Fig. 12 as the percentage of values obtained in lesioned rats. The results obtained after acute treatments are presented elsewhere (Dzahini et al., 2010).

Substantially, the lesion produced a large increase in DA and GLU in the medial STR that was not accompanied by noticeable alterations in the two DA metabolites or the other two amino acids that were measured. The three treatments with GLU antagonists seemed to affect DA metabolism in the same way, counteracting the lesion-induced increase in DA. These treatments had differential effects on GLU.

Twenty-one days after the lesion, the denervated part of the STR (lateral) exhibited biochemical responses previously described after high levels of DA cell depopulation: a drastic reduction in DOPAC and an unmodified or slightly increased DA (Zigmond et al., 1984; Altar et al., 1987). In contrast, a large increase in DA (two- to three-fold) and a modest alteration in DOPAC was observed using voltammetry and confirmed using microdialysis in the spared part of the STR (medial). In this case, the levels of DA probably resulted from permanent (tonic) enhancement of the spontaneous release of DA. It has been shown that partial lesions leave the stimulation/release ratio unmodified (Dentresangle et al., 2001). A much larger lesion of the DA cell population seems to be required to alter the spontaneous pattern of discharge of nigral DA cells (Hollerman and Grace, 1990; Harden and Grace, 1995) or stimulation-induced DA release (Stachowiak et al., 1987). These observations strongly suggest that after lateral SN lesion, a global process activates tonic DA release by an indirect mechanism acting presynaptically in the STR.

It has been claimed that recovery of the DA in the STR after partial lesions of the SN could be related to alterations in GLU neurotransmission (Calabresi et al., 2000; Emmi et al., 1996; Kashani et al., 2007). However, the mechanism and the location of this alteration remain unknown. We found that 3 weeks after the lesion, GLU was clearly enhanced in the medial STR. When GLU neurotransmission was pharmacologically interrupted by specific GLU blockers (riluzol, memantine and amantadine), a reduction in extracellular GLU activation was observed, with a simultaneous reduction in the tonic DA increase induced by the nigral lesion.

Amantadine and memantine were proposed to have some neuroprotective effects after discovering the importance of NMDA receptor-mediated excitotoxicity as a factor underlying neurodegeneration in Parkinson's disease (Greenamyre and O'Brien, 1991). Indeed antagonists of NMDA receptors have been shown to inhibit neurodegeneration of the DA system induced by MPP+ and methamphetamine (Sonsalla et al., 1989; Turski et al., 1991). In our case, the effect of the two GLU antagonists was to counteract the increase in GLU and DA induced by the nigral lesion. Several studies have suggested that NMDA-induced DA release could be the main regulatory mechanism of extracellular DA (Bannon et al., 2001; Leviel, 2001; Mortensen and Amara, 2003), and our observations are consistent with the hypothesis of a NMDA-induced mechanism causing stable dopaminergic hypertony. The effects of riluzol strengthen this hypothesis. First proposed to inhibit GLU release (Mantz, 1992), its action has also been attributed to persistent blockade of the sodium current (Del Negro, 2005). In our hands, riluzol reduced the release of GLU in sham-operated animals and counteracted the lesion-induced GLU and DA as well (Dzahini et al., 2010).

6. Conclusions: DA/GLU, a deleterious partnership?

To summarize the present results and referenced data, the most original outcome is that DA release in the STR is not simply a readout of activity in DA neurons that provide a diffuse DA tone in the extracellular space. Rather, DA can be released by at least two different mechanisms with different kinetics, locations and regulatory processes. Based on the data reported here, a working hypothesis can be proposed: that a weak reduction in the DA cell population in the SNc leads to metabolic alterations in the STR that result in further death of DA terminals in this region. The development of this process could follow three major steps (Fig. 13): 1) the activation of diencephalic structures, thalamic or sub-thalamic nuclei that

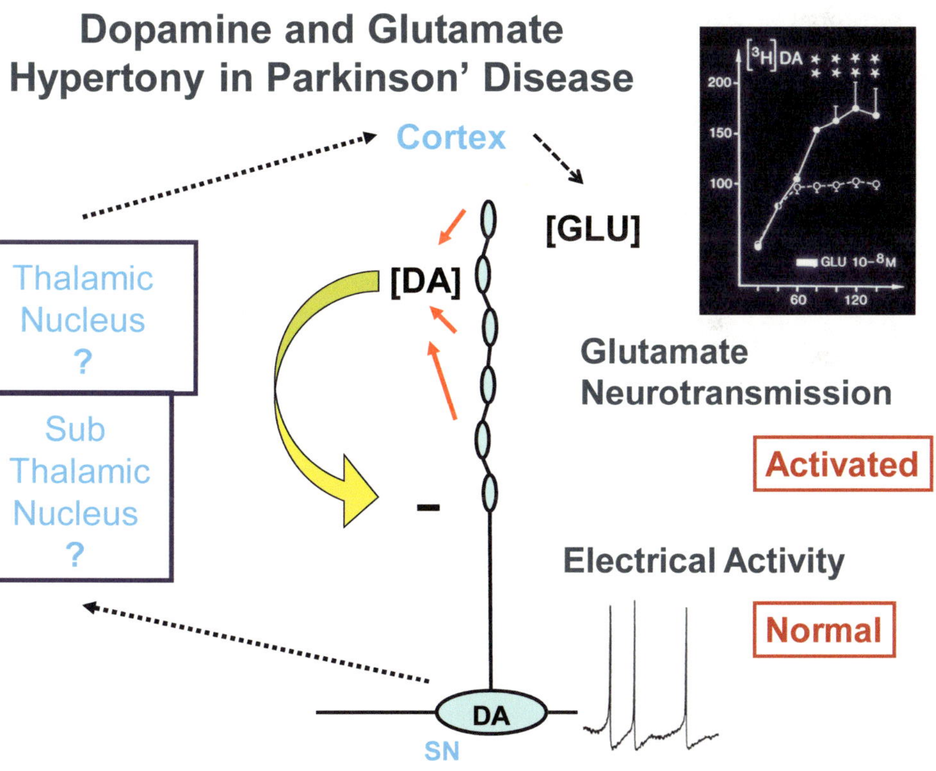

Fig. 13. A working hypothesis of the mechanism involved in the presymptomatic phase of PD

project toward cortical regions; 2) in turn, a tonic increase in some of the corticostriatal pathways that we know to be responsible for different controls of the striatal GABA neurons and DA terminals; 3) indirect activation through GLU afferents to DA terminals of tonic DA release, which initially constitutes autotherapy allowing the behavioral compensation observed in Parkinson's disease. However the toxic effect of DA on the DA terminal (production of H_2O_2 when present in excess) could constitute a secondary pathological agent, maintaining the degenerative process. Each of the three steps mentioned here require further elucidation and demonstration, but a large set of data in each case is consistent with this hypothesis.

DA homeostasis constitutes one of the functions of the DAT via DAT-RT. This is under the control of many regulatory processes including tonic GLU neurotransmission. Experiments regarding the consequences of partial lesions seem to indicate a role for this GLU-dependent regulation in the tonic DA overflow and in maintaining a permanent excess of extracellular DA. It remains to be determined how local GLU can induce the presynaptic and tonic activation of DA release. This could be achieved directly through GLU receptors located on DA terminals or indirectly through heterologous neurotransmission systems such as GABA or ACH.

7. Technical procedures

7.1 Animals

Male Wistar rats (Iffa-Credo France) weighing 250 g were used in the studies reported here. They were maintained and sacrificed in accordance with the European Communities Council Directive (86/609/EEC). The animals were anesthetized with 1.5% isoflurane in pure oxygen in air or were injected with chloral hydrate (400 mg/kg) and spontaneously inspired (Leviel et al., 1989; Olivier et al., 1995). When necessary they were placed in a stereotaxic device. For the short interventions (less than 1 hour), a mixture of ketamine/rompun was used (150/10 mg/Kg). Rectal temperature was maintained at 38 °C. Cardiac and respiratory rhythms were continuously monitored.

7.2 Lesions of the lateral SN

The lateral part of the SN was unilaterally injected with a solution of 6-OHDA (3 µg free base in 1 µl isotonic saline containing 0.2% ascorbic acid, pH 4). The stereotaxic coordinates were, in mm: Ant.: 3.5, Lat.: 2.5 and Ht.: 3.4. The horizontal plane passed through the interaural axis and incisor bar. Unlesioned rats were only submitted to nigral injection of the vehicle (Dentresangle et al., 2001; Dzahini et al., 2010).

7.3 Surgery and procedures for recurrent ventricular injections

Animals were anesthetized with ketamine (150 mg/Kg; Panpharma), maintained in a stereotaxic device and implanted with a cannula (0.71 mm o.d. with a removable mandrel) in the anterior part of the left lateral ventricle. The head of the cannula was sealed with acrylic cement, embedding screws set in the cranial bone. The stereotaxic coordinates were the following (in mm): AP: 0.48; LM: 1; H: 6 from the bregma (following Paxinos and Watson, 1986). Rats were allowed to recover for 2 weeks. In order to inject 6-OHDA (30 min after administering 25 mg/kg imipramine i.p. to protect noradrenergic neurons), the mandrel of the cannula was removed and replaced by an injector connected, through a thin catheter, to a microsyringe. Weekly injections of 10 µl of a solution (0.1% ascorbic acid in 0.9% NaCl) with or without 35 µg of 6-OHDA were given to awake and freely moving animals. Four groups of 12 animals received 2, 4, 6 or 8 weekly injections of the toxin (n=6) or the toxin vehicle only (n=6). A fifth group (n=6) of rats received 8 weekly injections of the toxin and a daily injection of 2 mg/kg MK801 (i.p.).

7.4 Medial Forebrain Bundle (MFB) stimulation

A bipolar electrode was implanted in the medial forebrain bundle (MFB) containing the DA ascending fibers (coordinates: A:5; L:1.3; Ht:2). Every 4 minutes, the MFB was stimulated for 20 seconds by 20 bursts (one per second) of 25 positive square pulses, each lasting 0.5 ms, with a 2 ms interpulse interval (40 Hz theoretical frequency). Each burst was triggered 300 ms after the measurement of DPA (Dentresangle et al., 2001; Dzahini et al., 2010).

7.5 Voltammetric investigations

Difference Normal Pulse Voltammetry (DNPV) and Differential Pulse Amperometry (DPA) were performed using treated carbon fiber electrodes produced as described previously (Olivier et al., 1995; Dentresangle et al., 2001). Their active part was the surface of one pyrolytic carbon fiber (SOFICAR, France), 250 µm long and 8 µm in diameter. A stainless steel tweezer fixed on the interaural bar was used as an auxilliary electrode and the Ag/AgCl reference electrode was a silver wire coated with AgCl. This was maintained in contact with the skull by means of a sponge moistened with Phosphate Buffer Saline (PBS) solution (PBS, pH 7.4). The three electrodes were connected to a pulse voltammetric system (Biopulse, SOLEA Tacussel, France). Carbon-fiber electrodes were electrochemically treated as previously described (Gonon et al., 1984). To calibrate the electrodes, voltammograms were recorded *in vitro* in a standard solution of DOPAC or DA and ascorbic acid in PBS. The values of the oxidation potentials and the amplitude of the peaks were stabilized after 4-5 successive scans (10 to 15 min). Their values were 60 mV for ascorbic acid, 60 mV for DOPAC and 90 mV for DA. It had previously been verified that the amplitude of the oxidation peak for these substances is linearly correlated with their concentrations. The oxidation potentials for DA and DOPAC were however too close to be properly differentiated *in vivo* and DA was three orders of magnitude lower than DOPAC. Thus, for adequate detection of DA, DOPAC formation was inhibited by pretreatment with pargyline (75 mg/kg, i.p.), an inhibitor of monoamine oxidase.

7.6 Superfusion procedures (microdialysis & push-pull cannula)

Animals were submitted to superfusion of the striatum to analyze extracellular DA, DOPA, HVA, GLU, GABA and ASP (Dzahini et al., 2011). They were implanted with a dialysate probe (250 µm in diameter and 4 mm length, cut off 6000 dalton, CMA, Sweden) in the anterior part of the caudate nucleus (Ant.: 8.4 mm; Lat.: 2.5 mm; H.: 6 mm, same stereotaxic references). The cannula was supplied (1 µl/min) with an artificial CSF (in mM, 145 NaCl, 2.7 KCl, 1.0 $MgCl_2$, 1.2 $CaCl_2$, 0.45 NaH_2PO_4, 2.3 Na_2HPO_4, adjusted to pH 7.4).

Push-pull cannulae were used in an experiment devoted to measuring the radioactive form of DA and DOPAC (Leviel et al., 1989, 1990, 1991). The cannulae (1.0 mm outer diameter) were supplied (flow rate: 12.5 µl/min) with an artificial cerebrospinal fluid (CSF) adjusted to pH 7.4 with an O_2-CO_2 (95:5 v/v) mixture. 3,5-[^{3}H]TYR (50 Ci/mmole, Dositek, France) was purified by high performance liquid chromatography (HPLC) on a C_{18} Microbondapak column (Millipore-Waters, France) using H_3PO_4 (1 mmol/l, pH 3) as a mobile phase. [^{3}H]TYR was added to artificial CSF (80 µCi/ml) 1 hour after implantation and superfusates were collected thereafter as successive 20 minute fractions.

7.7 Biochemical analysis

Dialysates collected for measuring catecholamines were protected with 5 µl perchloric acid (0.05 M) and immediately underwent HPLC analysis. Dialysates collected for amino-acid analysis were maintained at -80 °C and kept frozen until analysis.

The catecholamines DA, DOPAC and HVA were measured in the collected fractions by electrochemical detection with the potential of the working electrode maintained at 0.7 V (Antec-Decade) after HPLC separation (column C_{18} Brownlee RP18, 5 µm, 2.1 x 220 mm, maintained at 32 °C; Mobile phase: 50 mM KH_2PO_4, 0.1 mM EDTA-Na_2, 0.28 mM sodium octyl sulfate, 6% methanol, adjusted to pH 4.5; flow rate 0.25 ml/min). Catecholamine peaks were identified based on their retention times (Olivier et al., 1995; Dzahini et al., 2010). Extracellular catecholamine concentrations were estimated by evaluating the peak areas of each substance and their respective external standard (analytical software AZUR, Datalys France). The running time for each determination was 25 min. When superfusion was conducted with 3,5-[^{3}H]TYR added to the CSF, the radioactivity corresponding to each HPLC peak was counted using a continuous flow scintillation detector (Packard-Radiomatic, Flo-One B A250)(Leviel et al., 1989, 1990, 1991).

The concentrations of the amino acids GLU, GABA and ASP in the dialysates were determined after HPLC, via laser-induced fluorescence detection (Dzahini et al., 2010). Briefly, 2 µl of sample or standard was derivatized with naphthalene-2,3-dicarboxaldehyde. The resulting mixture was automatically loaded onto a Symmetry Shield-C_{18} reverse-phase column (100_2.1 mm, 3.5 _m particle size; Waters, Milford, MA), using a refrigerated Triathlon auto injector (Polymer Laboratories, Marseille, France). The mobile phase consisted of 0.04 M NaH_2PO_4, pH6, in a 3–50% acetonitrile gradient. The flow rate was 0.35 ml/min, maintained using two Shimadzu (Kyoto, Japan) LC 10AT pumps. Amino acid peaks were identified based on their retention time. Extracellular amino acid concentrations were estimated by evaluating the peak areas of each amino acid and their respective external standard (analytical software class LC10; Shimadzu). The running time for each determination was 12 min.

7.8 DA and DOPAC tissue concentration

At the end of each experiment, to verify the location of the cannula, the animals were intracardially perfused with a 4% formaldehyde solution, after which the brain was removed, sliced (50 µm) and stained with cresyl violet.

Protein weights were measured using the micro BCA Protein Assay (Pierce, Biorad).

The homogenate (20 µl) was mixed with 20 µl of 0.3 N perchloric acid containing 0.8 mM EDTA, added to an internal standard (3,4-dihydroxybenzylamine) and centrifuged (10,000 g, 10 min). The supernatant of each sample (10 µl) was injected into a C18 reverse-phase microcolumn (Spheri5, RP-18, 220 × 2.1 mm, Browlee labs). The mobile phase consisted of 40 mM KH_2PO_4 (pH 4.5), 0.26 mM octane sulfonic-acid, 15 mg/l EDTA and 11% methanol (vol/vol), and the flow rate was 0.20 ml/min. The liquid chromatography system (TSP) was coupled to an electrochemical detector (Millipore) with a working electrode set at 0.8 V. The concentrations of DA and its metabolites in CP were calculated for each sample (in ng/mg prot). The results were normalized by expressing the changes in DA and DOPAC levels as percentages of the values obtained in control animals (Dentresangle et al., 2001).

7.9 Preparation of synaptosomes

The method for synaptosomal preparation and measurement of [^{3}H]DA uptake was modified from Masserano et al. (1994). Rat brains were rapidly removed and chopped into 1.6-mm-thick slices, in the sagittal plane corresponding to the *anterior commissura*. The median part of the CP, ipsilateral to the injection site, was pooled for all rats of each group and homogenized in 25 ml cold 0.32 M sucrose (10 up and down strokes, at 850 rpm, in a glass-teflon homogenizer). The homogenate was centrifuged at 800 g for 10 min at 4 °C and the pellet was discarded. The supernatant (S1) was kept on ice until it was resuspended for the [^{3}H]DA uptake or [^{3}H]GBR12935 binding protocols.

[^{3}H]DA uptake: The supernatant (S1, 15 ml) was centrifuged (20,000 × g for 10 min at 4 °C), and the resulting pellet (P2) was resuspended in 20 ml of ice-cold incubation buffer (in mM): NaCl, 125; K_2HPO_4, 1.5; $MgSO_4$, 1.5; $CaCl_2$, 1.25; *d*-glucose, 10; HEPES, 25; ascorbic acid, 0.1; pargyline, 1 and EDTA, 0.1, pH 7.4. The buffer was oxygenated with 100% O_2 for 10 min before use. The assays were performed in triplicate with 400 µl of pellet resuspended in 1 ml of incubation buffer. After preincubation of 3 min at 37 °C, the assays were initiated by adding 10 µl of increasing concentrations of [^{3}H]DA (10, 20, 40, 50, 100, 200, 400 nM) for 7 min at 37 °C. Nonspecific values were determined in the presence of Mazindol (1 µM) for 7 min at 4 °C. Assays were terminated by immediate filtration using Whatman GF/B filters soaked in 0.32 M ice-cold sucrose containing 0.05% polyethylenimine. Filters were washed three times with 3 ml of 0.32 M ice-cold sucrose and radioactivity was measured using a Packard TRI-CARB 2100 TR. The apparent K_m and V_{max} of DA uptake were calculated by linear regression of the reciprocal plot ($1/v$ vs. $1/S$). The protein content in the resuspended pellet P2 was measured using the micro BCA kit (Pierce, Biorad).

7.10 [^{3}H]GBR12935 binding

The [^{3}H]GBR12935 binding protocol was modified from Berger et al. (1985). The supernatant (S1, 10 ml) was centrifuged (20,000 g for 10 min at 4 °C), and the resulting pellet (P2) was resuspended in 13 ml of 50 mM ice-cold Tris-HCl buffer, pH 7.7, containing 120 mM NaCl. Assays were performed in triplicate with 500 µl of pellet suspension and 50 mM Tris-HCl buffer, pH 7.7, containing 120 mM NaCl and 0.01% of Bovine Serum Albumin in a final volume of 2 ml. Incubation was initiated by the addition of 100 µl of [^{3}H]GBR12935 (5 µM) for 45 min at 25 °C. Non-specific binding was determined in the presence of 1 µM Mazindol. Filters were washed three times with 4 ml ice-cold Tris-HCl 50 mM buffer pH 7.7 and radioactivity was counted using a Packard TRI-CARB 2100 TR. The protein content in the resuspended pellet P2 was measured using the micro BCA kit (Pierce, Biorad).

7.11 Determination of TH protein content

TH protein content was measured using a semi quantitative immunoblotting technique as previously described by Garcia et al. (1994). Briefly, after centrifugation of the homogenate

(10,000 g, 30 min), 1.5 µl of supernatant was placed onto a nitrocellulose membrane (Bio-rad 162-147, 0.2 µm). Non-specific binding sites were saturated with 50 mM Tris buffer containing 2% bovine serum albumin. The protein was revealed using, in succession, a mouse monoclonal antibody to TH (10 ng/ml; Boehringer Mannheim), a 125I-labeled protein A (S.A: 1.11x 10-9 Bq/mg, 1850 Bq/ml, Amersham) and 3H-hyperfilms (Amersham). The radioimmunochemical labeling was calibrated using a scale of standard TH protein (extracted from adult rat adrenals and diluted in homogenates of cerebellum). One U of TH (UTH) is defined as the mean TH protein content of 10 µg (wet weight) of adult rat adrenal gland. Optical density measurements were converted into UTH/mg tissue by reference to the standards. Each reading provided the surface area (mm^2) of the dot and the TH tissue concentration (UTH/mg tissue). Using the surface area and the TH tissue concentration, the amount of TH (UTH) in the region of interest was calculated and normalized by expressing the amount of TH as a percentage of values in the control rats.

7.12 Immunoprecipitation of TH enzyme

Rats were perfused transcardially with NaCl 9°/°° and PFA 4%. The brain was then removed and stored in PBS buffer containing 0.1% sodium azide pH 7.4 (PBSA). To evaluate the extent of the lesion in the SN and the extent of CPc denervation, TH immuno precipitation was performed on coronally sectioned slices (40–50 µm thickness). Brains were cut on a cryostat (HM440E, Microm); free-floating slices were collected and stored in PBSA. Sections were incubated in 3% H_2O_2 in PBS to block endogenous peroxidase activity and were then incubated overnight with the primary rabbit anti-TH antibody (Chemicon, Temecula, CA; 1/2500) in 10% normal swine serum, TBS, pH 7.4, containing 2% NGS and 0.2%Triton X-100 for 24 h at 4 °C on a platform shaker. After rinsing in PBS 0.1% plus triton X100, sections were incubated with biotinylated swine anti-rabbit secondary antibody for 30 min at room temperature. This was followed by incubation with Strept-ABC-HRP complex (Dako, Glostrup, Denmark). TH immunoreactive neurons were visualized using 3.3-diaminobenzidine (DAB) in N^{2+} 0.5% and H_2O_2. To test the specificity of the staining, control sections were processed in an identical manner but with omission of the primary or secondary antibody. All sections were then washed for 10 min in PBS, mounted on slides, dried, dehydrated in increasing grades of ethanol, cleared in toluene, and mounted with DPX and cover slipped. These sections were scanned and analyzed immediately using Imagemaster Labscan V-3.00 (Pharmacia Biotech, Dzahini et al., 2010).

8. Acknowledgment

The work described here was supported by the Institut National de la Santé et de la Recherché Médicale, le Centre National de la Recherche Scientifique et Rhone Alpes Région.

9. References

Agnati, L. F.;Fuxe, K.;Zoli, M.;Ozini, I.;Toffano, G. & Ferraguti, F. (1986).A correlation analysis of the regional distribution of central enkephalin and beta-endorphin immunoreactive terminals and of opiate receptors in adult and old male rats. Evidence for the existence of two main types of communication in the central nervous system: the volume transmission and the wiring transmission. *Acta Physiol Scand*, Vol.128, No.2, (Oct 1986), pp.(201-207), ISSN 0001-6772

Albert, K. A.;Helmer-Matyjek, E.;Nairn, A. C.;Muller, T. H.;Haycock, J. W.;Greene, L. A.;Goldstein, M. & Greengard, P. (1984).Calcium/phospholipid-dependent protein kinase (protein kinase C) phosphorylates and activates tyrosine hydroxylase. *Proc Natl Acad Sci U S A,* Vol.81, No.24, (Dec 1984), pp.(7713-7717), ISSN 0027-8424

Altar, C. A. & Marien, M. R. (1989).Preservation of dopamine release in the denervated striatum. *Neurosci Lett,* Vol.96, No.3, (Jan 30 1989), pp.(329-334), ISSN 0304-3940

Altar, C. A.;Marien, M. R. & Marshall, J. F. (1987).Time course of adaptations in dopamine biosynthesis, metabolism, and release following nigrostriatal lesions: implications for behavioral recovery from brain injury. *J Neurochem,* Vol.48, No.2, (Feb 1987), pp.(390-399), ISSN 0022-3042

Amalric, M.;Baunez, C. & Nieoullon, A. (1995).Does the blockade of excitatory amino acid transmission in the basal ganglia simply reverse reaction time deficits induced by dopamine inactivation? *Behav Pharmacol,* Vol.6, No.5 And 6, (Aug 1995), pp.(508-519), ISSN 0955-8810

Amejdki-Chab, N.;Benmansour, S.;Costentin, J. & Bonnet, J. J. (1992).Effects of several cations on the neuronal uptake of dopamine and the specific binding of [3H]GBR 12783: attempts to characterize the Na+ dependence of the neuronal transport of dopamine. *J Neurochem,* Vol.59, No.5, (Nov 1992), pp.(1795-1804), ISSN 0022-3042

Ames, M. M.;Lerner, P. & Lovenberg, W. (1978).Tyrosine hydroxylase. Activation by protein phosphorylation and end product inhibition. *J Biol Chem,* Vol.253, No.1, (Jan 10 1978), pp.(27-31), ISSN 0021-9258

Arluison, M.;Agid, Y. & Javoy, F. (1978).Dopaminergic nerve endings in the neostriatum of the rat--2. Radioautographic study following local micro-injections of tritiated dopamine. *Neuroscience,* Vol.3, No.8, 1978), pp.(675-683), ISSN 0306-4522

Augustine, G. J.;Charlton, M. P. & Smith, S. J. (1987).Calcium action in synaptic transmitter release. *Annu Rev Neurosci,* Vol.10, 1987), pp.(633-693), ISSN 0147-006X

Bannon, M. J.;Michelhaugh, S. K.;Wang, J. & Sacchetti, P. (2001).The human dopamine transporter gene: gene organization, transcriptional regulation, and potential involvement in neuropsychiatric disorders. *Eur Neuropsychopharmacol,* Vol.11, No.6, (Dec 2001), pp.(449-455), ISSN 0924-977X

Benazzouz, A.;Gross, C.;Feger, J.;Boraud, T. & Bioulac, B. (1993).Reversal of rigidity and improvement in motor performance by subthalamic high-frequency stimulation in MPTP-treated monkeys. *Eur.J Neurosci.,* Vol.5, No.4, 1993), pp.(389), ISSN

Berger, T. W.;Kaul, S.;Stricker, E. M. & Zigmond, M. J. (1985).Hyperinnervation of the striatum by dorsal raphe afferents after dopamine-depleting brain lesions in neonatal rats. *Brain Res,* Vol.336, No.2, (Jun 17 1985), pp.(354-358), ISSN 0006-8993

Blanchard, V.;Raisman-Vozari, R.;Vyas, S.;Michel, P. P.;Javoy-Agid, F.;Uhl, G. & Agid, Y. (1994).Differential expression of tyrosine hydroxylase and membrane dopamine transporter genes in subpopulations of dopaminergic neurons of the rat mesencephalon. *Brain Res Mol Brain Res,* Vol.22, No.1-4, (Mar 1994), pp.(29-38), ISSN 0169-328X

Bogdanski, D. F. & Brodie, B. B. (1969).The effects of inorganic ions on the storage and uptake of H3-norepinephrine by rat heart slices. *J Pharmacol Exp Ther,* Vol.165, No.2, (Feb 1969), pp.(181-189), ISSN 0022-3565

Borland, L. M. & Michael, A. C. (2004).Voltammetric study of the control of striatal dopamine release by glutamate. *J Neurochem,* Vol.91, No.1, (Oct 2004), pp.(220-229), ISSN 0022-3042

Boulet, S.;Mounayar, S.;Poupard, A.;Bertrand, A.;Jan, C.;Pessiglione, M.;Hirsch, E. C.;Feuerstein, C.;Francois, C.;Feger, J.;Savasta, M. & Tremblay, L. (2008).Behavioral recovery in MPTP-treated monkeys: neurochemical mechanisms studied by intrastriatal microdialysis. *J Neurosci,* Vol.28, No.38, (Sep 17 2008), pp.(9575-9584), ISSN 1529-2401

Butcher, S. P.;Fairbrother, I. S.;Kelly, J. S. & Arbuthnott, G. W. (1988).Amphetamine-induced dopamine release in the rat striatum: an in vivo microdialysis study. *J Neurochem,* Vol.50, No.2, (Feb 1988), pp.(346-355), ISSN 0022-3042

Calabresi, P.;Mercuri, N. B.;Sancesario, G. & Bernardi, G. (1993).Electrophysiology of dopamine-denervated striatal neurons. Implications for Parkinson's disease. *Brain,* Vol.116 (Pt 2), (Apr 1993), pp.(433-452), ISSN 0006-8950

Calabresi, P.;Picconi, B.;Saulle, E.;Centonze, D.;Hainsworth, A. H. & Bernardi, G. (2000).Is pharmacological neuroprotection dependent on reduced glutamate release? *Stroke,* Vol.31, No.3, (Mar 2000), pp.(766-772; discussion 773), ISSN 0039-2499

Carter, C. J.;L'Heureux, R. & Scatton, B. (1988).Differential control by N-methyl-D-aspartate and kainate of striatal dopamine release in vivo: a trans-striatal dialysis study. *J Neurochem,* Vol.51, No.2, (Aug 1988), pp.(462-468), ISSN 0022-3042

Castaneda, E.;Whishaw, I. Q. & Robinson, T. E. (1990).Changes in striatal dopamine neurotransmission assessed with microdialysis following recovery from a bilateral 6-OHDA lesion: variation as a function of lesion size. *J Neurosci,* Vol.10, No.6, (Jun 1990), pp.(1847-1854), ISSN 0270-6474

Castro, S. L.;Sved, A. F. & Zigmond, M. J. (1996).Increased neostriatal tyrosine hydroxylation during stress: role of extracellular dopamine and excitatory amino acids. *J Neurochem,* Vol.66, No.2, (Feb 1996), pp.(824-833), ISSN 0022-3042

Cepeda, C.;Hurst, R. S.;Altemus, K. L.;Flores-Hernandez, J.;Calvert, C. R.;Jokel, E. S.;Grandy, D. K.;Low, M. J.;Rubinstein, M.;Ariano, M. A. & Levine, M. S. (2001).Facilitated glutamatergic transmission in the striatum of D2 dopamine receptor-deficient mice. *J Neurophysiol,* Vol.85, No.2, (Feb 2001), pp.(659-670), ISSN 0022-3077

Cervinski, M. A.;Foster, J. D. & Vaughan, R. A. (2005).Psychoactive substrates stimulate dopamine transporter phosphorylation and down-regulation by cocaine-sensitive and protein kinase C-dependent mechanisms. *J Biol Chem,* Vol.280, No.49, (Dec 9 2005), pp.(40442-40449), ISSN 0021-9258

Cheramy, A.;Leviel, V. & Glowinski, J. (1981).Dendritic release of dopamine in the substantia nigra. *Nature,* Vol.289, No.5798, (Feb 12 1981), pp.(537-542), ISSN 0028-0836

Cheramy, A.;Romo, R.;Godeheu, G.;Baruch, P. & Glowinski, J. (1986).In vivo presynaptic control of dopamine release in the cat caudate nucleus--II. Facilitatory or inhibitory influence of L-glutamate. *Neuroscience,* Vol.19, No.4, (Dec 1986), pp.(1081-1090), ISSN

Chubb, I. W.;De Potter, W. P. & De Schaepdryver, A. F. (1972).Tyramine does not release noradrenaline from splenic nerve by exocytosis. *Naunyn Schmiedebergs Arch Pharmacol,* Vol.274, No.3, 1972), pp.(281-286), ISSN 0028-1298

Ciliax, B. J.;Drash, G. W.;Staley, J. K.;Haber, S.;Mobley, C. J.;Miller, G. W.;Mufson, E. J.;Mash, D. C. & Levey, A. I. (1999).Immunocytochemical localization of the dopamine transporter in human brain. *J Comp Neurol,* Vol.409, No.1, (Jun 21 1999), pp.(38-56), ISSN 0021-9967

Colbran, R. J.;Carmody, L. C.;Bauman, P. A.;Wadzinski, B. E. & Bass, M. A. (2003).Analysis of specific interactions of native protein phosphatase 1 isoforms with targeting subunits. *Methods Enzymol,* Vol.366, 2003), pp.(156-175), ISSN 0076-6879

Del Negro, C. A.;Morgado-Valle, C.;Hayes, J. A.;Mackay, D. D.;Pace, R. W.;Crowder, E. A. & Feldman, J. L. (2005).Sodium and calcium current-mediated pacemaker neurons and respiratory rhythm generation. *J Neurosci,* Vol.25, No.2, (Jan 12 2005), pp.(446-453), ISSN 1529-2401

Dentresangle, C.;Le Cavorsin, M.;Savasta, M. & Leviel, V. (2001).Increased extracellular DA and normal evoked DA release in the rat striatum after a partial lesion of the substantia nigra. *Brain Res,* Vol.893, No.1-2, (Mar 2 2001), pp.(178-185), ISSN 0006-8993

Descarries, L. & Mechawar, N. (2000).Ultrastructural evidence for diffuse transmission by monoamine and acetylcholine neurons of the central nervous system. *Prog Brain Res,* Vol.125, 2000), pp.(27-47), ISSN 0079-6123

Desce, J. M.;Godeheu, G.;Galli, T.;Artaud, F.;Cheramy, A. & Glowinski, J. (1992).L-glutamate-evoked release of dopamine from synaptosomes of the rat striatum: involvement of AMPA and N-methyl-D-aspartate receptors. *Neuroscience,* Vol.47, No.2, 1992), pp.(333-339), ISSN

Dzahini, K.;Dentresangle, C.;Le Cavorsin, M.;Bertrand, A.;Detraz, I.;Savasta, M. & Leviel, V. (2010).Pre-synaptic glutamate-induced activation of DA release in the striatum after partial nigral lesion. *J Neurochem,* Vol.113, No.6, (Jun 2010), pp.(1459-1470), ISSN 1471-4159

Emmi, A.;Rajabi, H. & Stewart, J. (1996).Behavioral and neurochemical recovery from partial 6-hydroxydopamine lesions of the substantia nigra is blocked by daily treatment with glutamate receptor antagonists MK-801 and CPP. *J Neurosci,* Vol.16, No.16, (Aug 15 1996), pp.(5216-5224), ISSN 0270-6474

Espino, A.;Cutillas, B.;Tortosa, A.;Ferrer, I.;Bartrons, R. & Ambrosio, S. (1995).Chronic effects of single intrastriatal injections of 6-hydroxydopamine or 1-methyl-4-phenylpyridinium studied by microdialysis in freely moving rats. *Brain Res,* Vol.695, No.2, (Oct 16 1995), pp.(151-157), ISSN 0006-8993

Ewing, A. G.;Bigelow, J. C. & Wightman, R. M. (1983).Direct in vivo monitoring of dopamine released from two striatal compartments in the rat. *Science,* Vol.221, No.4606, (Jul 8 1983), pp.(169-171), ISSN 0036-8075

Ewing, A. G. & Wightman, R. M. (1984).Monitoring the stimulated release of dopamine with in vivo voltammetry. II: Clearance of released dopamine from extracellular fluid. *J Neurochem,* Vol.43, No.2, (Aug 1984), pp.(570-577), ISSN 0022-3042

Falkenburger, B. H.;Barstow, K. L. & Mintz, I. M. (2001).Dendrodendritic inhibition through reversal of dopamine transport. *Science,* Vol.293, No.5539, (Sep 28 2001), pp.(2465-2470), ISSN 0036-8075

Fillenz, M. (1993).Short-term control of transmitter synthesis in central catecholaminergic neurones. *Prog Biophys Mol Biol,* Vol.60, No.1, 1993), pp.(29-46), ISSN

Fischer, J. F. & Cho, A. K. (1979).Chemical release of dopamine from striatal homogenates: evidence for an exchange diffusion model. *J Pharmacol Exp Ther,* Vol.208, No.2, (Feb 1979), pp.(203-209), ISSN 0022-3565

Fog, J. U.;Khoshbouei, H.;Holy, M.;Owens, W. A.;Vaegter, C. B.;Sen, N.;Nikandrova, Y.;Bowton, E.;McMahon, D. G.;Colbran, R. J.;Daws, L. C.;Sitte, H. H.;Javitch, J. A.;Galli, A. & Gether, U. (2006).Calmodulin kinase II interacts with the dopamine transporter C terminus to regulate amphetamine-induced reverse transport. *Neuron,* Vol.51, No.4, (Aug 17 2006), pp.(417-429), ISSN 0896-6273

Garcia, C.;Marcel, D.;Le Cavorsin, M.;Pujol, J. F. & Weissmann, D. (1994).Phenotypic characteristics of expressed tyrosine hydroxylase protein in the adult rat nucleus tractus solitarius: plasticity revealed by RU24722 treatment. *Neuroscience,* Vol.62, No.4, (Oct 1994), pp.(1201-1205), ISSN 0306-4522

Gauthier, J.;Parent, M.;Levesque, M. & Parent, A. (1999).The axonal arborization of single nigrostriatal neurons in rats. *Brain Res,* Vol.834, No.1-2, (Jul 10 1999), pp.(228-232), ISSN 0006-8993

Gerfen, C. R.;Herkenham, M. & Thibault, J. (1987).The neostriatal mosaic: II. Patch- and matrix-directed mesostriatal dopaminergic and non-dopaminergic systems. *J Neurosci,* Vol.7, No.12, (Dec 1987), pp.(3915-3934), ISSN 0270-6474

Gerhardt, G. A.;Cass, W. A.;Hudson, J.;Henson, M.;Zhang, Z.;Ovadia, A.;Hoffer, B. J. & Gash, D. M. (1996).In vivo electrochemical studies of dopamine overflow and clearance in the striatum of normal and MPTP-treated rhesus monkeys. *J Neurochem,* Vol.66, No.2, (Feb 1996), pp.(579-588), ISSN 0022-3042

Giorguieff, M. F.;Kemel, M. L. & Glowinski, J. (1977).Presynaptic effect of L-glutamic acid on the release of dopamine in rat striatal slices. *Neurosci Lett,* Vol.6, No.1, (Oct 1977), pp.(73-77), ISSN 0304-3940

Gnegy, M. E.;Khoshbouei, H.;Berg, K. A.;Javitch, J. A.;Clarke, W. P.;Zhang, M. & Galli, A. (2004).Intracellular Ca2+ regulates amphetamine-induced dopamine efflux and currents mediated by the human dopamine transporter. *Mol Pharmacol,* Vol.66, No.1, (Jul 2004), pp.(137-143), ISSN 0026-895X

Gonon, F. G. (1988).Nonlinear relationship between impulse flow and dopamine released by rat midbrain dopaminergic neurons as studied by in vivo electrochemistry. *Neuroscience,* Vol.24, No.1, (Jan 1988), pp.(19-28), ISSN 0306-4522

Gonon, F. G. & Buda, M. J. (1985).Regulation of dopamine release by impulse flow and by autoreceptors as studied by in vivo voltammetry in the rat striatum. *Neuroscience,* Vol.14, No.3, (Mar 1985), pp.(765-774), ISSN 0306-4522

Gonon, F. G.;Navarre, F. & Buda, M. J. (1984).In vivo monitoring of dopamine release in the rat brain with differential normal pulse voltammetry. *Anal Chem,* Vol.56, No.3, (Mar 1984), pp.(573-575), ISSN 0003-2700

Grace, A. A. (1991).Phasic versus tonic dopamine release and the modulation of dopamine system responsivity: a hypothesis for the etiology of schizophrenia. *Neuroscience,* Vol.41, No.1, 1991), pp.(1-24), ISSN 0306-4522

Grace, A. A. (2008).Physiology of the normal and dopamine-depleted basal ganglia: insights into levodopa pharmacotherapy. *Mov Disord,* Vol.23 Suppl 3, 2008), pp.(S560-569), ISSN 1531-8257

Greenamyre, J. T. & O'Brien, C. F. (1991).N-methyl-D-aspartate antagonists in the treatment of Parkinson's disease. *Arch Neurol,* Vol.48, No.9, (Sep 1991), pp.(977-981), ISSN 0003-9942

Griffith, L. C. (2004).Regulation of calcium/calmodulin-dependent protein kinase II activation by intramolecular and intermolecular interactions. *J Neurosci,* Vol.24, No.39, (Sep 29 2004), pp.(8394-8398), ISSN 1529-2401

Harden, D. G. & Grace, A. A. (1995).Activation of dopamine cell firing by repeated L-DOPA administration to dopamine-depleted rats: its potential role in mediating the therapeutic response to L-DOPA treatment. *J Neurosci,* Vol.15, No.9, (Sep 1995), pp.(6157-6166), ISSN 0270-6474

Haycock, J. W. (1993).Multiple signaling pathways in bovine chromaffin cells regulate tyrosine hydroxylase phosphorylation at Ser19, Ser31, and Ser40. *Neurochem Res,* Vol.18, No.1, (Jan 1993), pp.(15-26), ISSN 0364-3190

Hefti, F.;Enz, A. & Melamed, E. (1985).Partial lesions of the nigrostriatal pathway in the rat. Acceleration of transmitter synthesis and release of surviving dopaminergic neurones by drugs. *Neuropharmacology,* Vol.24, No.1, (Jan 1985), pp.(19-23), ISSN 0028-3908

Herdon, H.;Strupish, J. & Nahorski, S. R. (1985).Differences between the release of radiolabelled and endogenous dopamine from superfused rat brain slices: effects of depolarizing stimuli, amphetamine and synthesis inhibition. *Brain Res,* Vol.348, No.2, (Dec 2 1985), pp.(309-320), ISSN 0006-8993

Hollerman, J. R. & Grace, A. A. (1990).The effects of dopamine-depleting brain lesions on the electrophysiological activity of rat substantia nigra dopamine neurons. *Brain Res,* Vol.533, No.2, (Nov 19 1990), pp.(203-212), ISSN 0006-8993

Iversen, S. D. & Iversen, L. L. (2007).Dopamine: 50 years in perspective. *Trends Neurosci,* Vol.30, No.5, (May 2007), pp.(188-193), ISSN 0166-2236

Iwasaki, Y.;Ikeda, K.;Shiojima, T. & Kinoshita, M. (1992).Increased plasma concentrations of aspartate, glutamate and glycine in Parkinson's disease. *Neurosci Lett,* Vol.145, No.2, (Oct 12 1992), pp.(175-177), ISSN 0304-3940

Jhamandas, K. & Marien, M. (1987).Glutamate-evoked release of endogenous brain dopamine: inhibition by an excitatory amino acid antagonist and an enkephalin analogue. *Br J Pharmacol,* Vol.90, No.4, (Apr 1987), pp.(641-650), ISSN 0007-1188

Kantor, L.;Hewlett, G. H.;Park, Y. H.;Richardson-Burns, S. M.;Mellon, M. J. & Gnegy, M. E. (2001).Protein kinase C and intracellular calcium are required for amphetamine-mediated dopamine release via the norepinephrine transporter in undifferentiated PC12 cells. *J Pharmacol Exp Ther,* Vol.297, No.3, (Jun 2001), pp.(1016-1024), ISSN 0022-3565

Kapatos, G. & Zigmond, M. J. (1982).Influence of calcium on dopamine synthesis and tyrosine hydroxylase activity in rat striatum. *J Neurochem,* Vol.39, No.2, (Aug 1982), pp.(327-335), ISSN 0022-3042

Kashani, A.;Betancur, C.;Giros, B.;Hirsch, E. & El Mestikawy, S. (2007).Altered expression of vesicular glutamate transporters VGLUT1 and VGLUT2 in Parkinson disease. *Neurobiol Aging,* Vol.28, No.4, (Apr 2007), pp.(568-578), ISSN 1558-1497

Katz, B. & Miledi, R. (1970).Further study of the role of calcium in synaptic transmission. *J Physiol,* Vol.207, No.3, (May 1970), pp.(789-801), ISSN 0022-3751

Keefe, K. A.;Zigmond, M. J. & Abercrombie, E. D. (1992).Extracellular dopamine in striatum: influence of nerve impulse activity in medial forebrain bundle and local glutamatergic input. *Neuroscience,* Vol.47, No.2, 1992), pp.(325-332), ISSN 0306-4522

Keefe, K. A.;Zigmond, M. J. & Abercrombie, E. D. (1993).In vivo regulation of extracellular dopamine in the neostriatum: influence of impulse activity and local excitatory amino acids. *J Neural Transm Gen Sect,* Vol.91, No.2-3, 1993), pp.(223-240), ISSN 0300-9564

Khoshbouei, H.;Wang, H.;Lechleiter, J. D.;Javitch, J. A. & Galli, A. (2003).Amphetamine-induced dopamine efflux. A voltage-sensitive and intracellular Na+-dependent mechanism. *J Biol Chem,* Vol.278, No.14, (Apr 4 2003), pp.(12070-12077), ISSN 0021-9258

Lavergne, A.;Frain, O.;Guibert, B.;Biguet, N. F. & Leviel, V. (1994).Regulation of tyrosine hydroxylase gene expression in mesencephalic dopamine neurons: effect of imipramine treatment. *Neurosci Lett,* Vol.182, No.2, (Dec 5 1994), pp.(167-171), ISSN 0304-3940

Leslie, S. W.;Chandler, L. J.;Barr, E. M. & Farrar, R. P. (1985).Reduced calcium uptake by rat brain mitochondria and synaptosomes in response to aging. *Brain Res,* Vol.329, No.1-2, (Mar 11 1985), pp.(177-183), ISSN 0006-8993

Levi, G. & Raiteri, M. (1993).Carrier-mediated release of neurotransmitters. *Trends Neurosci,* Vol.16, No.10, (Oct 1993), pp.(415-419), ISSN 0166-2236

Leviel, V. (2001).The reverse transport of DA, what physiological significance? *Neurochem Int,* Vol.38, No.2, (Feb 2001), pp.(83-106), ISSN

Leviel, V.;Fayada, C.;Guibert, B.;Chaminade, M.;Machek, G.;Mallet, J. & Biguet, N. F. (1990).Short- and long-term alterations of gene expression in limbic structures by repeated electroconvulsive-induced seizures. *J Neurochem,* Vol.54, No.3, (Mar 1990), pp.(899-904), ISSN 0022-3042

Leviel, V.;Gobert, A. & Guibert, B. (1989).Direct observation of dopamine compartmentation in striatal nerve terminal by 'in vivo' measurement of the specific activity of released dopamine. *Brain Res,* Vol.499, No.2, (Oct 16 1989), pp.(205-213), ISSN

Levitt, M.;Spector, S.;Sjoerdsma, A. & Udenfriend, S. (1965).Elucidation of the Rate-Limiting Step in Norepinephrine Biosynthesis in the Perfused Guinea-Pig Heart. *J Pharmacol Exp Ther,* Vol.148, (Apr 1965), pp.(1-8), ISSN 0022-3565

Liang, N. Y. & Rutledge, C. O. (1982).Evidence for carrier-mediated efflux of dopamine from corpus striatum. *Biochem Pharmacol,* Vol.31, No.15, (Aug 1 1982), pp.(2479-2484), ISSN 0006-2952

Lin, A. M. & Chai, C. Y. (1998).Role of dopamine uptake in NMDA-modulated K(+)-evoked dopamine overflow in rat striatum: an in vivo electrochemical study. *Neurosci Res,* Vol.31, No.3, (Jul 1998), pp.(171-177), ISSN 0168-0102

Lindefors, N. & Ungerstedt, U. (1990).Bilateral regulation of glutamate tissue and extracellular levels in caudate-putamen by midbrain dopamine neurons. *Neurosci Lett,* Vol.115, No.2-3, (Jul 31 1990), pp.(248-252), ISSN 0304-3940

Lipscombe, D.;Madison, D. V.;Poenie, M.;Reuter, H.;Tsien, R. Y. & Tsien, R. W. (1988).Spatial distribution of calcium channels and cytosolic calcium transients in growth cones and cell bodies of sympathetic neurons. *Proc Natl Acad Sci U S A,* Vol.85, No.7, (Apr 1988), pp.(2398-2402), ISSN 0027-8424

Maloteaux, J. M.;Vanisberg, M. A.;Laterre, C.;Javoy-Agid, F.;Agid, Y. & Laduron, P. M. (1988).[3H]GBR 12935 binding to dopamine uptake sites: subcellular localization and reduction in Parkinson's disease and progressive supranuclear palsy. *Eur J Pharmacol,* Vol.156, No.3, (Nov 8 1988), pp.(331-340), ISSN 0014-2999

Mann, S. P. & Bennett, R. C. (1979).The fate of choline in the circulating plasma of the rat. *Experientia,* Vol.35, No.2, (Feb 15 1979), pp.(211-212), ISSN 0014-4754

Mantz, J.;Cheramy, A.;Thierry, A. M.;Glowinski, J. & Desmonts, J. M. (1992).Anesthetic properties of riluzole (54274 RP), a new inhibitor of glutamate neurotransmission. *Anesthesiology,* Vol.76, No.5, (May 1992), pp.(844-848), ISSN 0003-3022

Marchi, M.;Paudice, P.;Bonanno, G. & Raiteri, M. (1985).Presynaptic muscarinic receptor activation enhances striatal dopamine release evoked by depolarization but not that induced by non-depolarizing stimuli. *Neurochem Int,* Vol.7, No.1, 1985), pp.(137-141), ISSN 0197-0186

Masserano, J. M.;Venable, D. & Wyatt, R. J. (1994).Effects of chronic cocaine administration on [3H]dopamine uptake in the nucleus accumbens, striatum and frontal cortex of rats. *J Pharmacol Exp Ther,* Vol.270, No.1, (Jul 1994), pp.(133-141), ISSN 0022-3565

Meldolesi, J.;Volpe, P. & Pozzan, T. (1988).The intracellular distribution of calcium. *Trends Neurosci,* Vol.11, No.10, (Oct 1988), pp.(449-452), ISSN 0166-2236

Mengual, E. & Pickel, V. M. (2004).Regional and subcellular compartmentation of the dopamine transporter and tyrosine hydroxylase in the rat ventral pallidum. *Journal of Comparative Neurology,* Vol.468, No.3, 2004), pp.(395-409), ISSN

Miller, R. J. (1991).The control of neuronal Ca2+ homeostasis. *Prog Neurobiol,* Vol.37, No.3, 1991), pp.(255-285), ISSN 0301-0082

Nash, J. F. & Brodkin, J. (1991). Microdialysis studies on 3,4-methylenedioxymethamphetamine-induced dopamine release: effect of dopamine uptake inhibitors. *J Pharmacol Exp Ther,* Vol.259, No.2, (Nov 1991), pp.(820-825), ISSN 0022-3565

Nirenberg, M. J.;Vaughan, R. A.;Uhl, G. R.;Kuhar, M. J. & Pickel, V. M. (1996).The dopamine transporter is localized to dendritic and axonal plasma membranes of nigrostriatal dopaminergic neurons. *J Neurosci,* Vol.16, No.2, (Jan 15 1996), pp.(436-447), ISSN

Okada, M.;Mine, K. & Fujiwara, M. (1990).The Na(+)-dependent release of endogenous dopamine and noradrenaline from rat brain synaptosomes. *J Pharmacol Exp Ther,* Vol.252, No.3, (Mar 1990), pp.(1283-1288), ISSN 0022-3565

Olivier, V.;Gobert, A.;Guibert, B. & Leviel, V. (1999).The in vivo modulation of dopamine synthesis by calcium ions: influences on the calcium independent release. *Neurochem Int,* Vol.35, No.6, (Dec 1999), pp.(431-438), ISSN 0197-0186

Olivier, V.;Guibert, B. & Leviel, V. (1995).Direct in vivo comparison of two mechanisms releasing dopamine in the rat striatum. *Brain Res,* Vol.695, No.1, (Oct 9 1995), pp.(1-9), ISSN

Opazo, F.;Schulz, J. B. & Falkenburger, B. H. (2010).PKC links Gq-coupled receptors to DAT-mediated dopamine release. *J Neurochem,* Vol.114, No.2, (Jul 2010), pp.(587-596), ISSN 1471-4159

Pal, R.;Nath, R. & Gill, K. D. (1993).Influence of ethanol on cadmium accumulation and its impact on lipid peroxidation and membrane bound functional enzymes (Na+, K(+)-ATPase and acetylcholinesterase) in various regions of adult rat brain. *Neurochem Int,* Vol.23, No.5, (Nov 1993), pp.(451-458), ISSN 0197-0186

Papa, S. M.;Boldry, R. C.;Engber, T. M.;Kask, A. M. & Chase, T. N. (1995).Reversal of levodopa-induced motor fluctuations in experimental parkinsonism by NMDA receptor blockade. *Brain Res,* Vol.701, No.1-2, (Dec 1 1995), pp.(13-18), ISSN 0006-8993

Parker, E. M. & Cubeddu, L. X. (1986).Effects of d-amphetamine and dopamine synthesis inhibitors on dopamine and acetylcholine neurotransmission in the striatum. II. Release in the presence of vesicular transmitter stores. *J Pharmacol Exp Ther,* Vol.237, No.1, (Apr 1986), pp.(193-203), ISSN 0022-3565

Pasinetti, G. M.;Lerner, S. P.;Johnson, S. A.;Morgan, D. G.;Telford, N. A. & Finch, C. E. (1989).Chronic lesions differentially decrease tyrosine hydroxylase messenger RNA in dopaminergic neurons of the substantia nigra. *Brain Res Mol Brain Res,* Vol.5, No.3, (May 1989), pp.(203-209), ISSN 0169-328X

Paton, D. M. (1973).Evidence for carrier-mediated efflux of noradrenaline from the axoplasm of adrenergic nerves in rabbit atria. *J Pharm Pharmacol,* Vol.25, No.3, (Mar 1973), pp.(265-267), ISSN 0022-3573

Paton, D. M. (1973).Mechanism of efflux of noradrenaline from adrenergic nerves in rabbit atria. *Br J Pharmacol,* Vol.49, No.4, (Dec 1973), pp.(614-627), ISSN 0007-1188

Perez, X. A.;Parameswaran, N.;Huang, L. Z.;O'Leary, K. T. & Quik, M. (2008).Pre-synaptic dopaminergic compensation after moderate nigrostriatal damage in non-human primates. *J Neurochem,* Vol.105, No.5, (Jun 2008), pp.(1861-1872), ISSN 1471-4159

Phillips, J. M.;Lam, H. A.;Ackerson, L. C. & Maidment, N. T. (2006).Blockade of mGluR glutamate receptors in the subthalamic nucleus ameliorates motor asymmetry in an animal model of Parkinson's disease. *Eur J Neurosci,* Vol.23, No.1, (Jan 2006), pp.(151-160), ISSN 0953-816X

Prensa, L.;Cossette, M. & Parent, A. (2000).Dopaminergic innervation of human basal ganglia. *J Chem Neuroanat,* Vol.20, No.3-4, (Dec 2000), pp.(207-213), ISSN 0891-0618

Raiteri, M.;Cerrito, F.;Cervoni, A. M. & Levi, G. (1979).Dopamine can be released by two mechanisms differentially affected by the dopamine transport inhibitor nomifensine. *J Pharmacol Exp Ther,* Vol.208, No.2, (Feb 1979), pp.(195-202), ISSN 0022-3565

Raiteri, M.;del Carmine, R. & Bertollini, A. (1977).Effect of desmethylimipramine on the release of (3H)norepinephrine induced by various agents in hypothalamic synaptosomes. *Mol Pharmacol,* Vol.13, No.4, (Jul 1977), pp.(746-758), ISSN 0026-895X

Robinson, T. E. & Whishaw, I. Q. (1988).Normalization of extracellular dopamine in striatum following recovery from a partial unilateral 6-OHDA lesion of the substantia nigra: a microdialysis study in freely moving rats. *Brain Res,* Vol.450, No.1-2, (May 31 1988), pp.(209-224), ISSN 0006-8993

Romo, R.;Cheramy, A.;Godeheu, G. & Glowinski, J. (1986).In vivo presynaptic control of dopamine release in the cat caudate nucleus--III. Further evidence for the implication of corticostriatal glutamatergic neurons. *Neuroscience,* Vol.19, No.4, (Dec 1986), pp.(1091-1099), ISSN 0306-4522

Samuel, D.;Errami, M. & Nieoullon, A. (1990).Localization of N-methyl-D-aspartate receptors in the rat striatum: effects of specific lesions on the [3H]3-(2-carboxypiperazin-4-yl)propyl-1-phosphonic acid binding. *J Neurochem,* Vol.54, No.6, (Jun 1990), pp.(1926-1933), ISSN 0022-3042

Sesack, S. R.;Hawrylak, V. A.;Matus, C.;Guido, M. A. & Levey, A. I. (1998).Dopamine axon varicosities in the prelimbic division of the rat prefrontal cortex exhibit sparse immunoreactivity for the dopamine transporter. *J Neurosci,* Vol.18, No.7, (Apr 1 1998), pp.(2697-2708), ISSN 0270-6474

Snyder, G. L.;Keller, R. W., Jr. & Zigmond, M. J. (1990).Dopamine efflux from striatal slices after intracerebral 6-hydroxydopamine: evidence for compensatory hyperactivity of residual terminals. *J Pharmacol Exp Ther,* Vol.253, No.2, (May 1990), pp.(867-876), ISSN 0022-3565

Soares-da-Silva, P. (1987).Does brain 3,4-dihydroxyphenylacetic acid reflect dopamine release? *J Pharm Pharmacol,* Vol.39, No.2, (Feb 1987), pp.(127-129), ISSN 0022-3573

Sonsalla, P. K.;Nicklas, W. J. & Heikkila, R. E. (1989).Role for excitatory amino acids in methamphetamine-induced nigrostriatal dopaminergic toxicity. *Science,* Vol.243, No.4889, (Jan 20 1989), pp.(398-400), ISSN 0036-8075

Stachowiak, M. K.;Keller, R. W., Jr.;Stricker, E. M. & Zigmond, M. J. (1987).Increased dopamine efflux from striatal slices during development and after nigrostriatal bundle damage. *J Neurosci,* Vol.7, No.6, (Jun 1987), pp.(1648-1654), ISSN 0270-6474

Stein, W. (1967). The movements of molecules across cell membranes, Academic Press, New York, USA

Stein, W.(1990). Channels, carriers and pumps: an introduction to the membrane transport, Academic Press, New York, USA

Suaud Chagn, Y. M. F.;Brun, P.;Buda, M. & Gonon, F. Fast in vivo monitoring of electrically evoked doPamine release by differential pulse amperometry with untreated carbon fibre electrodes. *J Neurosci Methods,* Vol.45, No.3, pp.(183-190), ISSN

Tang, K.;Low, M. J.;Grandy, D. K. & Lovinger, D. M. (2001).Dopamine-dependent synaptic plasticity in striatum during in vivo development. *Proc Natl Acad Sci U S A,* Vol.98, No.3, (Jan 30 2001), pp.(1255-1260), ISSN 0027-8424

Thoenen, H.;Huerlimann, A. & Haefely, W. (1969).Cation dependence of the noradrenaline-releasing action of tyramine. *Eur J Pharmacol,* Vol.6, No.1, (Apr 1969), pp.(29-37), ISSN 0014-2999

Turski, L.;Bressler, K.;Rettig, K. J.;Loschmann, P. A. & Wachtel, H. (1991).Protection of substantia nigra from MPP+ neurotoxicity by N-methyl-D-aspartate antagonists. *Nature,* Vol.349, No.6308, (Jan 31 1991), pp.(414-418), ISSN 0028-0836

van Horne, C.;Hoffer, B. J.;Stromberg, I. & Gerhardt, G. A. (1992).Clearance and diffusion of locally applied dopamine in normal and 6-hydroxydopamine-lesioned rat striatum. *J Pharmacol Exp Ther,* Vol.263, No.3, (Dec 1992), pp.(1285-1292), ISSN 0022-3565

Vizi, E. S. & Labos, E. (1991).Non-synaptic interactions at presynaptic level. *Prog Neurobiol,* Vol.37, No.2, 1991), pp.(145-163), ISSN 0301-0082

Vrana, K. E. & Roskoski, R., Jr. (1983).Tyrosine hydroxylase inactivation following cAMP-dependent phosphorylation activation. *J Neurochem,* Vol.40, No.6, (Jun 1983), pp.(1692-1700), ISSN 0022-3042

Westerink, B. H.;Hofsteede, H. M.;Damsma, G. & de Vries, J. B. (1988).The significance of extracellular calcium for the release of dopamine, acetylcholine and amino acids in conscious rats, evaluated by brain microdialysis. *Naunyn Schmiedebergs Arch Pharmacol,* Vol.337, No.4, (Apr 1988), pp.(373-378), ISSN 0028-1298

Wheeler, D. D.;Edwards, A. M.;Chapman, B. M. & Ondo, J. G. (1993).A model of the sodium dependence of dopamine uptake in rat striatal synaptosomes. *Neurochem Res,* Vol.18, No.8, (Aug 1993), pp.(927-936), ISSN 0364-3190

Wilson, C. J. (1995).Dynamic modification of dendritic cable properties and synaptic transmission by voltage-gated potassium channels. *J Comput Neurosci,* Vol.2, No.2, (Jun 1995), pp.(91-115), ISSN 0929-5313

Wullner, U.;Standaert, D. G.;Testa, C. M.;Landwehrmeyer, G. B.;Catania, M. V.;Penney, J. B., Jr. & Young, A. B. (1994).Glutamate receptor expression in rat striatum: effect of deafferentation. *Brain Res,* Vol.647, No.2, (Jun 6 1994), pp.(209-219), ISSN 0006-8993

Zahniser, N. R.;Gerhardt, G. A.;Hoffman, A. F. & Lupica, C. R. (1998).Voltage-dependency of the dopamine transporter in rat brain. *Adv Pharmacol,* Vol.42, 1998), pp.(195-198), ISSN 1054-3589

Zetterstrom, T.;Sharp, T.;Collin, A. K. & Ungerstedt, U. (1988).In vivo measurement of extracellular dopamine and DOPAC in rat striatum after various dopamine-releasing drugs; implications for the origin of extracellular DOPAC. *Eur J Pharmacol,* Vol.148, No.3, (Apr 13 1988), pp.(327-334), ISSN 0014-2999

Ziance, R. J. & Rutledge, C. O. (1972).A comparison of the effects of fenfluramine and amphetamine on uptake release and catabolism of norepinephrine in rat brain. *J Pharmacol Exp Ther,* Vol.180, No.1, (Jan 1972), pp.(118-126), ISSN 0022-3565

Zigmond, M. J.;Abercrombie, E. D.;Berger, T. W.;Grace, A. A. & Stricker, E. M. (1990).Compensations after lesions of central dopaminergic neurons: some clinical and basic implications. *Trends Neurosci.,* Vol.13, No.7, 1990), pp.(296), ISSN

Zigmond, M. J.;Acheson, A. L.;Stachowiak, M. K. & Stricker, E. M. (1984).Neurochemical compensation after nigrostriatal bundle injury in an animal model of preclinical parkinsonism. *Arch Neurol,* Vol.41, No.8, (Aug 1984), pp.(856-861), ISSN 0003-9942

Zigmond, M. J.;Berger, T. W.;Grace, A. A. & Stricker, E. M. (1989).Compensatory responses to nigrostriatal bundle injury. Studies with 6-hydroxydopamine in an animal model of parkinsonism. *Mol Chem Neuropathol,* Vol.10, No.3, (Jun 1989), pp.(185-200), ISSN 1044-7393

Zucker, R. S. & Lando, L. (1986).Mechanism of transmitter release: voltage hypothesis and calcium hypothesis. *Science,* Vol.231, No.4738, (Feb 7 1986), pp.(574-579), ISSN 0036-8075

12

Activity-Dependent Regulation of the Dopamine Phenotype in the Adult Substantia Nigra: Prospects for Treating Parkinson's Disease

Mal Horne, Kate Lord and Tim Aumann
Florey Neuroscience Institutes,
The University of Melbourne,
Australia

1. Introduction

The motor symptoms of Parkinson's disease (PD) are caused by degeneration of dopamine (DA) neurons in the substantia nigra pars compacta (SNc) and the resulting depletion of DA signaling in their target structure, the dorsal striatum (the nigrostriatal pathway). PD motor symptoms are successfully alleviated by systemic administration of a blood-brain barrier permeable DA precursor (levodopa) or DA receptor agonists (Olanow et al. 2001), however these treatments are marred by side-effects in some patients (Wood 2010), and increasingly unreliable response and shortened duration of effect coupled with the emergence of dyskinesias in most patients (Stocchi et al. 2010, Stocchi & Marconi 2010). These problems probably arise from loss of physiological storage, release and reuptake of nigrostriatal DA and ensuing down-stream changes in post-synaptic signaling, and from increased DA signaling in structures outside the nigrostriatal pathway, especially when D2 agonists are used. Targeted (nigrostriatal) reconstruction of physiological DA signaling, aimed at restoring nigrostriatal DA transmission to at least the level at disease outset, ought to alleviate PD motor symptoms without side-effects. However, attempts to achieve this by replacing SNc DA cells through transplantation or endogenous repair are often hampered by poor acquisition and maintenance of the DA phenotype in the microenvironment of the adult SNc (Brundin et al. 2000, Courtois et al. 2010, Torres et al. 2005, Bauer et al. 2000).

There is evidence that expression of tyrosine hydroxylase (TH, the rate-limiting enzyme in DA synthesis) by adult SNc and midbrain neurons is pliable. TH is down-regulated in cells that survive exposure to neurotoxins [6-hydroxy-dopamine (6-OHDA) or 1-methyl-4-phenyl-1,2,3,6-tetrahydropyridine (MPTP)], and can be up-regulated again, presumably in these same cells, by glial-derived neurotrophic factor (GDNF) (Bjorklund *et al.* 1997, Bowenkamp *et al.* 1996, Gash *et al.* 1996, Sauer & Oertel 1994). There is also a degree of spontaneous recovery in the number of TH immunoreactive (TH+) SNc cells following 6-OHDA, which occurs coincidentally with a decrease in the number of SNc cells that are not immunoreactive against TH (TH-) (Stanic *et al.* 2003), implying acquisition of DA phenotype by extant cells. The DA phenotype of SNc neurons also appears to be regulated in an activity-dependent way. Reduced SNc TH expression following striatal infarct is blocked by intraventricular administration of a $GABA_A$ receptor agonist (Soriano *et al.* 1997, Yamada *et al.* 1996); SNc TH mRNA is elevated followed systemic administration of nicotine or α-7 nicotinic acetylcholine receptor agonists (Serova & Sabban 2002); and we recently reported that the number of SNc TH+ cells in adult mice can be increased or decreased by direct brain infusions of drugs targeting SNc neuronal activity (Aumann *et al.* 2011, Aumann *et al.* 2008). These data are consistent with the possibility that the DA phenotype of adult SNc neurons can be gained or lost in an activity-dependent way.

Understanding how the DA phenotype of neurons in the adult SNc is regulated will highlight strategies and molecular (drug) targets to facilitate DA phenotype acquisition and maintenance by either transplanted or endogenous cells. The aims of the experiments described in this report were to determine whether infusions of drugs that increase the number of SNc DA (TH+) cells in normal mice: (1) increase the number of these cells in a 6-OHDA rodent model of PD; and (2) restore motor deficits.

2. Methods

2.1 Animals

All experimental procedures on animals were approved by the Florey Neuroscience Institutes animal ethics committee and conform to the National Health and Medical Research Council of Australia's published code of practice.

Male C57Bl/6J mice and male Sprague-Dawley rats were used for this study. Throughout the experiments all animals were housed in a climate-controlled (22°C) room on a 12/12hour light/dark cycle with ad libitum access to food (standard rodent chow) and water.

2.2 6-OHDA lesion

Unilateral 6-OHDA lesions were made in the mice and rats when they were 8-weeks old. We aimed for partial (40-60%) loss of SNc DA neurons because another form of compensatory plasticity (i.e. spouting of surviving nigrostriatal projections) in the nigrostriatal system is hampered with lesions >75% (Stanic et al. 2003). Mice were anesthetized with an i.p. injection of 5% chloral-hydrate in sterile phosphate buffered saline, whereas rats were anesthetized with 1-2% isofluorane in air. Their heads were secured in a stereotaxic frame and a midline incision made over the skull. A small (2-3mm diameter) hole was drilled through the skull overlying the left (mice) or right (rats) SNc with a dental burr. In mice, 1.5μg/μl 6-OHDA (Sigma-Aldrich) in distilled H_2O with 0.2mg/ml ascorbic acid was prepared on the morning of the lesions and kept on ice until injected to minimize oxidation. 1.6μl of the 6-OHDA solution was injected slowly (1.0μl/min.) through a 26gauge sterile needle at stereotaxic coordinates: 3.0mm posterior to Bregma, 1.5mm lateral to the midline, 4.0mm deep. In rats, two 1.0μl injections of 2.0μg/μl 6-OHDA in distilled H_2O with 0.2mg/ml ascorbic acid were made through a glass micropipette at stereotaxic coordinates: (1) 3.7mm anterior to Lambda, 1.7mm lateral to the midline, 8.1mm deep; and (2) 3.7mm anterior to Lambda, 2.1mm lateral to the midline, 7.5mm deep. At the completion of each injection the injection needle was left in situ for 2mins. to allow toxin diffusion then the needle was slowly withdrawn to minimize toxin backtracking up the needle track. The skin was sutured and antiseptic applied, an anti-inflammatory [3mg/kg Meloxicam (Metacam®), s.c.] was administered, and the animal was left to recover in a warmed cage.

2.3 Osmotic minipump infusions

Some weeks following the 6-OHDA lesion, when SNc TH+ cell loss was maximal, a cannula [ALZET® (Cupertino, CA, USA) or PlasticsOne® (Roanoke, VA, USA)] was implanted into the midbrain or striatum on the same side as the lesion, through which a drug (or vehicle) was infused continuously via an osmotic pump (ALZET® model #1002 in mice & model #2006 in rats) for a period of time (see Results section for specific timings). To prime the pumps prior to implantation they were filled with drug (or vehicle) and immersed in 37°C sterile saline overnight. The next day animals were anaesthetized and prepared as described above. The cannula was implanted at the following stereotaxic coordinates: (1) For SNc infusions in mice 3.0mm posterior to Bregma, 1.5mm lateral to the midline, 4.0mm deep; (2) For SNc infusions in rats 3.7mm anterior to Lambda, 1.9mm lateral to the midline, 7.8mm deep; (3) For striatal infusions in rats 0.5mm anterior to Bregma, 3.0mm lateral, 3.5mm deep. The cannula was glued to the skull with dental cement and the attached pump was placed in a subcutaneous 'pocket' created in the interscapular region.

In rat experiments the period of drug delivery was extended beyond the lifetime (6 weeks) of the first implanted pump by replacing it with a new filled pump. This was done by anaesthetizing the rat with 1-2% isofluorane in air, making a small incision in the skin overlying the old pump, clamping the vinyl tube closed, removing the old pump (and flow moderator), replacing it with a new primed pump (and new flow moderator), releasing the clamp and suturing the skin. The implanted cannula remained undisturbed throughout this procedure.

2.4 Behavior

The behavioral studies described below were performed on cohorts of animals typically comprising 12 animals, 6 treated with drug and 6 with vehicle. Each behavioral test was performed at the same time of day within each cohort and each animal was studied concurrently. If availability of equipment prevented this, animals were studied consecutively in a different pseudo-randomized order and equipment was thoroughly cleaned with 80% ethanol after each animal to remove any distracting odors.

2.4.1 Rotational response to amphetamine

Animals were injected intraperitonealy with 5mg/kg amphetamine and immediately placed into a cylindrical chamber (17cm diameter by 17cm high for mice & 31cm diameter by 31cm high for rats). In some rat experiments rotational behavior was also assessed for 20mins. prior to amphetamine. The behavior of each animal in its chamber was recorded on videotape for at least 1hour following amphetamine. On days where amphetamine was administered, no other behavioral tests were performed.

Rotational behavior was measured off-line using Ethovision® XT animal tracking software (Noldus Information Technology, Wageningen, Netherlands). One rotation was defined as a cumulative 360° change in heading direction of the animal's centre of mass, with no time limit. If an animal interrupted a turn in one direction with a turn in the other of more than 90°, the cumulative change in the first direction was reset to zero.

2.4.2 Locomotor cells

Locomotion was measured using photo-optic locomotor cells (Truscan Photobeam; Coulbourn Instruments, Allentown, PA, USA), which automatically detect horizontal- (locomotor) and vertical-plane (rearing) movements. Cell dimensions were 42cm wide x 42cm deep x 38cm high. Each rat was placed into a locomotor cell (6 rats at a time) for 30mins. in a quiet room with low-level light.

2.4.3 Cylinder test

Lateralized forelimb movement deficits were assessed using the cylinder test. This test was always performed in conjunction with the locomotor cells - half the cohort was run in the locomotor cells while the other half was run in the cylinder test, then vice verse (in a different pseudo-randomized order each time). Each rat was placed in a clear plastic cylinder (19cm diameter and 26cm high) standing vertically on a bench (1 rat at a time). A video camera recorded behavior for 10mins. in a quiet room with low-level light. Whilst in the cylinder the rats reared up to explore the only route of escape, supporting themselves against the cylinder wall with their left and/or right forelimbs. Two mirrors were positioned behind the cylinder to observe forelimb movements obscured by the rat's body. The number of times each forelimb touched the wall of the cylinder over the 10mins. was counted by an observer without prior knowledge of the treatment received.

2.4.4 Corridor test

Lateralized motor or attention deficits were assessed using the corridor test. No other test was performed on the day of the corridor test. Three days prior to the corridor test, rats were food-deprived by rationing chow at the rate of 2.5g/100g body weight. Two rats were run concurrently (in a different pseudo-randomized order each time). Each rat was placed in a corridor measuring 240cm long by 7cm wide by 21cm high, enclosed at each end but open at the top. Food (chocolate rice-puff cereal) was available *ad libitum* at multiple, evenly spaced points (13cm apart) along the left and right sides of the corridor. A video camera recorded their behavior for 10mins. in a quiet room with low-level light. Whilst in the corridor the rats explored freely along its length including sniffing and eating the cereal at their leisure. The number of times each rat sniffed at or ate cereal on their left and right sides was recorded by an observer without prior knowledge of the treatment received.

2.5 Immunohistochemistry

At the end of the experiment animals were killed with an overdose of anesthetic (sodium pentobarbitone, 100mg/kg, i.p.). Before their heart stopped beating the animals were perfused transcardially with warm (37°C) heparinized (0.1%) 0.1M phosphate buffered saline (PBS) followed by cold (4°C) 4% paraformaldehyde plus 0.2% picric acid in 0.1M phosphate buffer (PB). The brains were removed and placed at 4°C in PBS with 20% sucrose. Once equilibrated with 20% sucrose in PBS, the brains were frozen and 16μm thick coronal sections were cut through the striatum and SNc. Sections were collected directly onto glass slides coated with 0.1% chrome alum and 1% gelatin in distilled H_2O and stored at -80°C until immunohistochemical processing.

For TH immunohistochemistry, mounted sections were post-fixed in 10% neutral buffered formalin (5min.), incubated for 10min. in blocking solution (0.1M PBS, 0.3% Triton X-100 & 3% normal goat serum), then for 72hours at 4°C in rabbit anti-TH primary antibody (1:1500, Chemicon, Temecula, CA, USA) with 0.3% Triton X-100 and 1% normal goat serum in PBS. This was followed by 2hours incubation at room temperature in a biotinylated secondary antibody (1:1000, goat anti-rabbit IgG, Dako, Denmark). Next, sections were incubated for 1hour in 0.02% avidin peroxidase with 0.75% Triton X-100 in PBS at room temperature, then in cobalt- and nickel-intensified diaminobenzidine (DAB) for 20mins., then 3% hydrogen peroxide was added to the DAB solution for a further 2mins. to complete the chromagen reaction. Rinses (3 x 5min. each) in PBS were performed between each step. Sections were counterstained with 1% neutral red for 8min., washed in H_2O, dehydrated in a series of graded ethanol solutions (50-100%) and cleared in X3B before being coverslipped with a polystyrene mounting medium.

For DAT immunohistochemistry the protocol was the same as for TH immunohistochemistry with the following exceptions. Prior to incubation in blocking solution an antigen retrieval step was performed in which the sections were heated in 0.2% citrate buffer (pH 6) and allowed to cool at room temperature for 30min. Sections were incubated in a blocking solution (5% normal goat serum, 0.3% Triton X-100 in 0.1M PBS) for 10min. The primary antibody was mouse anti-DAT (1:3000, Chemicon) and the biotinylated secondary antibody was sheep anti-mouse (1:600, Chemicon). No counterstain was performed.

2.6 Stereology

To estimate the numbers of TH+ and TH- neurons in the SNc following 6-OHDA lesion and drug treatment, a fractionator sampling design was used, as previously described in detail (Parish *et al.* 2001), using a stereology program (Stereo Investigator, MicroBrightField, VT, USA) attached to a microscope. The SNc was delineated at its anatomical boundaries with reference to rodent brain atlases (Franklin & Paxinos 2008, Paxinos & Watson 2007) and based on high cell-packing density, cell morphology, and TH immunoreactivity (Nelson *et al.* 1996). Counts of TH+ and TH- SNc neurons (glia were excluded on the basis of soma diameter <5μm) within a counting frame (45μm x 35μm) were made at regular pre-determined intervals (x=145μm, y=145μm) using a 60x oil-immersion objective lens. The cell nucleus was the counting unit. TH+ cells were immunoreactive against TH and TH- cells were not immunoreactive against TH but counterstained. Every 5th section of the series was analyzed (i.e. 80μm apart) and the volume of the SNc was estimated according to Cavalieri's method (Gundersen *et al.* 1988), which estimates on the basis of area, section thickness and distance between sections. Cells on the treated and contralateral (internal control) sides of each brain were always counted consecutively to ensure consistency of cell classifications. Cell count in the lesioned and treated SNc was expressed as a proportion of cell count in the contralateral internal control SNc in each animal. Cell counts were performed by an experienced SNc stereologist without prior knowledge of the treatment received.

3. Results

3.1 Midbrain infusions of SK channel agonists

3.1.1 1-EBIO in mice

The number of SNc TH+ cells in normal adult mice increased by ~500 following a 2 week infusion of 100μM 1-EBIO (or 30μM riluzole) into midbrain (Aumann et al. 2008, Aumann et al. 2011). To examine whether midbrain 1-EBIO infusion can also increase SNc TH+ cells in a PD model, we repeated this in adult mice with prior depletion of TH+ SNc cells by 6-OHDA.

Eight-week old mice received a single injection of 6-OHDA directly into the left SNc. Two weeks later [when TH+ SNc cell loss is maximal (Aumann et al. 2008)] an infusion cannula was implanted into the left SNc, to allow continuous delivery of vehicle, 100μM 1-EBIO or 200μM 1-EBIO by osmotic pump for a further 2 weeks. The number of TH+ cells in the lesioned then treated SNc [expressed relative to the number of TH+ cells in the contralateral (internal control) SNc] is shown in figure 1. Data from individual mice are represented by the square symbols and the mean of each treatment group by the horizontal line. Note: (1) the relative tightness of the number of TH+ SNc cells in the vehicle-treated group, highlighting the consistency of the effect of our 6-OHDA injections across different mice; (2) the much greater variability in the drug-treated groups, indicating 1-EBIO has a restorative effect in some mice, even at 100μM; and (3) the increasing restorative effect with increasing dose of 1-EBIO. Unfortunately, although there is a net (average) increase in the number of TH+ SNc cells from ~50% (vehicle) to ~80% (200μM 1-EBIO) of the normal number of cells, this difference is not significant ($p=0.068$, one-way ANOVA) due to high variability in the 1-EBIO-treated groups.

We also examined the density of immunoreactivity for the DA transporter (DAT) in the striatum in a cohort of vehicle-treated and 200μM 1-EBIO-treated mice to examine whether 1-EBIO improved striatal DA innervation following 6-OHDA depletion. Although there was a trend for DAT density to be higher in the 1-EBIO-treated group, and specifically in the dorsal striatum, not the ventral striatum, this difference was not statistically significant (data not shown).

3.1.2 Riluzole in mice

Riluzole is approved for the treatment of amyotrophic lateral sclerosis and is reported to affect neuronal excitability through a number of different ion-channels (e.g. voltage-activated Na+, glutamate receptors and SK channels). It activates SK channels at concentrations ≥3μM (Cao et al. 2002, Grunnet et al. 2001) and at 30μM (direct injection) it increases the number of TH+ SNc cells in normal mice (Aumann et al. 2011). We therefore tested its ability to increase the number of TH+ SNc in the PD model. Note that riluzole protects SNc neurons from MPTP and 6-OHDA in animal models of PD (Barneoud et al. 1996, Bezard et al. 1998) but does not provide benefit in PD patients, either early (Jankovic & Hunter 2002) or late (Braz et al. 2004) in disease, or in Parkinson plus disorders (Bensimon et al. 2009). To our knowledge riluzole has not been considered as a neuro-restorative agent in PD, such as we are proposing here (i.e. replenishing SNc DA cells by DA phenotype recruitment). We also note that the doses of riluzole used so far in clinical trials for PD have all been relatively low (around 3μM) rather than the 30μM, which we have shown increases the number of SNc TH+ cells in normal mice (Aumann et al. 2011). Therefore, any restorative benefit of riluzole through DA phenotype recruitment may have been missed.

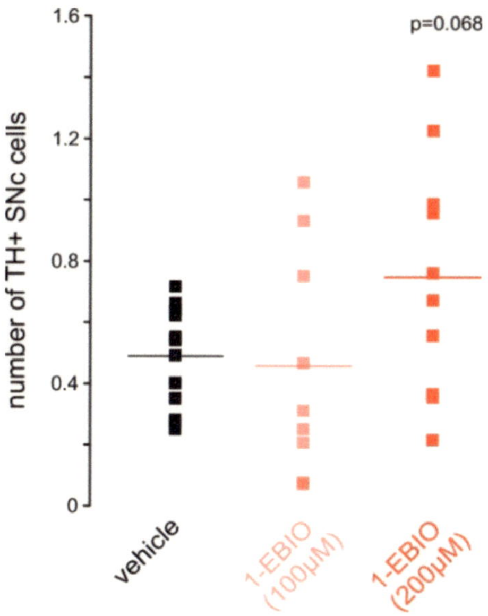

Fig. 1. Effect of the SK channel agonist 1-EBIO on the number of TH+ SNc cells in 6-OHDA-lesioned adult mice. 6-OHDA was injected into the left SNc of 8-week old male C57Bl/6J mice to reduce the number of SNc TH+ cells to ~50% of normal (see vehicle-treated mice, black symbols). Two weeks later a cannula was implanted into the left SNc, through which 1-EBIO or vehicle was infused (from an attached minipump) continuously for a further 2 weeks. The number of TH+ cells in the left and right SNc of each mouse was estimated using unbiased stereology by an observer who was unaware of the treatment received. The data for each mouse (filled squares) are expressed as the ratio of the number of TH+ SNc cells on the lesioned and treated (left) side relative to the internal control (right side). The mean of each treatment group is represented by a horizontal line. Lesion and vehicle-treated mice (n=15, black symbols) have a ~50% reduction, on average, in the number of TH+ SNc cells. Treatment with 100μM 1-EBIO (n=9, pale red symbols) appears to have had a beneficial effect (see text) in some mice, but there was no change on average. Treatment with 200μM 1-EBIO (n=10, red symbols) appears to have had an even stronger beneficial effect in some mice, resulting in an average increase in SNc TH+ cells to ~80% of normal. Note, however, that this increase was not statistically significant (p=0.068, one-way ANOVA).

We tested the neuro-restorative effects of orally administered riluzole on motor symptoms and TH+ SNc cell number in a mouse PD model. Three weeks after 6-OHDA SNc lesion, mice were administered riluzole in their drinking water for 2 weeks. Both 3μM and 30μM riluzole doses were tested. Note these were the projected daily systemic concentrations based on the average daily volume of drinking water consumed and body-weight of each mouse. Every 3 days following the lesion and throughout the treatment period, the rotational behavior of the mice in response to amphetamine (5mg/kg i.p.) was measured (figure 2A & A'). Following 6-OHDA lesion and before treatment began (figure 2A), the relative number of ipsiversive rotations (rotations toward the side of the lesion) increased progressively to reach a maximum by 12 days [p=0.035 (time), two-way ANOVA]. Presumably this reflects gradual depletion of DA in the left striatum caused by progressive degeneration of DA neurons in the left SNc. The relative number of contraversive rotations

(rotations away from the side of the lesion) remained constant throughout this experiment (data not shown). There was no significant difference in rotational behavior amongst the 3 treatment groups in this post-lesion and pre-treatment period [figure 2A, p=0.107 (treatment)], nor was there a treatment by time interaction [figure 2A, p=0.981 (treatment x time)]. Drug (or vehicle) treatment began 18 days following 6-OHDA (figure 2A'). Despite this, the rotational phenotype of the mice in each treatment group remained unchanged throughout the treatment period [figure 2A'; p=0.923 (treatment), p=0.986 (time), p=0.949 (treatment x time), two-way ANOVA]. Thus, riluzole had no effect on 6-OHDA-induced motor dysfunction in this experiment.

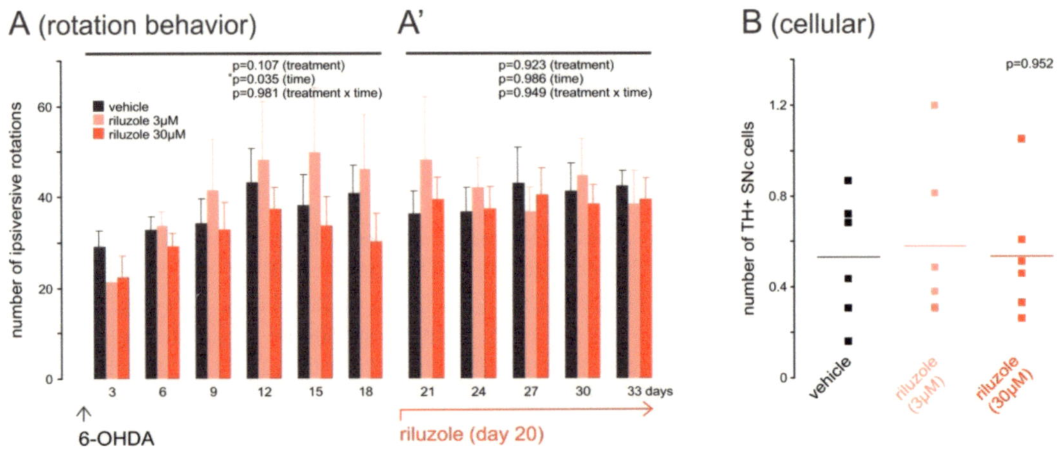

Fig. 2. Effects of the SK channel agonist riluzole on rotational behavior in response to amphetamine and the number of TH+ SNc cells in 6-OHDA-lesioned adult mice. 6-OHDA was injected into the left SNc of 8-week old male C57Bl/6J mice to reduce the number of SNc TH+ cells to ~50% of normal (see vehicle-treated mice, black symbols in B). (A & A') Every 3rd day for the next 18 days the rotational behavior in response to amphetamine was examined. The relative mean ± SE number of ipsiversive rotations performed over a 25 minute interval, beginning 25 minutes following amphetamine injection, is plotted over time for each treatment group. Note, the software used to count rotations was not as accurate as manual counting or other methods (e.g. rotometers); therefore the number of rotations here should not be compared with data collected using these other methods. However, the software consistently counted rotations at different times; therefore any changes in number of rotations accurately reflect behavioral changes. (A) 6-OHDA resulted in progressive increase in the number of ipsiversive rotations over time (p=0.035, two-way ANOVA). No differences in number of contraversive rotations occurred over this same period (data not shown). (A') Over days 20-33, vehicle (black bars), 3μM riluzole (pale red bars), or 30μM riluzole (red bars) was administered to the mice in their drinking water. During this time there was no change in the number of ipsiversive (or contraversive, data not shown) rotations by treatment or by time (two-way ANOVA). (B) At the end of day 33, there were no differences in the number of TH+ cells in the 6-OHDA-lesioned SNc across the three treatment groups (p=0.952, one-way ANOVA). See figure 1 legend for details about how these data are represented.

Following riluzole treatment, we estimated the total number of TH+ SNc cells and measured the density of DAT immunoreactivity in the dorsal striatum in these mice. No differences were found across treatment groups in the number of TH+ SNc cells (figure 2B; $p=0.952$, one-way ANOVA) or the density of DAT immunoreactivity in the dorsal striatum (data not shown).

3.1.3 1-EBIO in rats

We repeated the 200μM 1-EBIO infusion experiment in mice detailed above in unilateral 6-OHDA-lesioned rats, because motor impairments can be more accurately quantified in rats using locomotor cells, the cylinder test, and rotational response to amphetamine. The timecourse of this experiment was longer than the mouse experiment because it takes longer for SNc DA cell degeneration to occur following 6-OHDA, and because we wanted to see whether a treatment period longer than we used in mice (2 weeks) produced any effect.

In summary, there were no effects of 200μM 1-EBIO infusion on motor behavior or number of TH+ SNc cells following 6-OHDA lesion in rats. The rotational behavior in response to amphetamine is plotted against time in figure 3A. This shows that following 6-OHDA, there was a gradual increase in the ratio of ipsiversive:contraversive rotations, as expected, which peaked at 4 weeks. Two weeks later (i.e. 6 weeks following lesion) half the rats were implanted with osmotic pumps infusing 200μM 1-EBIO directly into the lesioned midbrain, and the other half were implanted with osmotic pumps infusing vehicle. Following the onset of drug (or vehicle) treatment, there was a trend (non-significant) for animals receiving 200μM 1-EBIO to show improvement in their rotational response at 9 & 11 weeks (3 & 5 weeks after treatment onset; figure 3A). However, no such trend was apparent at 13 & 15 weeks (7 & 9 weeks after treatment onset; figure 3A). A similar scenario, including a non-significant trend for improvement at 9 & 11 weeks, was also observed in motor behavior during the cylinder test (data not shown).

At the experiment end-point (15 weeks after lesion), the number of SNc TH+ cells was similar in 1-EBIO- and vehicle-infused rats (figure 3B).

3.2 Striatal infusions of quinpirole

While infusion of SK channel agonists (1-EBIO or riluzole) into the normal adult mouse SNc recruited ~500 more TH+ SNc cells (Aumann et al. 2008, Aumann et al. 2011), infusion of the D2 DA receptor agonist quinpirole into the normal adult mouse striatum was far more potent in this respect; recruiting ~3000 new TH+ SNc cells (Aumann et al. 2011). We therefore examined the behavioral and cellular effects of striatal quinpirole infusion in 6-OHDA-lesioned rats.

Four different behaviors were measured before and after unilateral 6-OHDA lesion of the SNc and during treatment (100nM quinpirole or vehicle). These are plotted in figure 4A-D. While there was no obvious effect of lesion or treatment on locomotor and rearing behavior (figure 4A-B), an asymmetry in left/right forelimb use (cylinder test and corridor test) and possibly also left/right side attention (corridor test) was evident following lesion (figure 4C-D). The lesion was made in the right SNc in this experiment, resulting in left forelimb

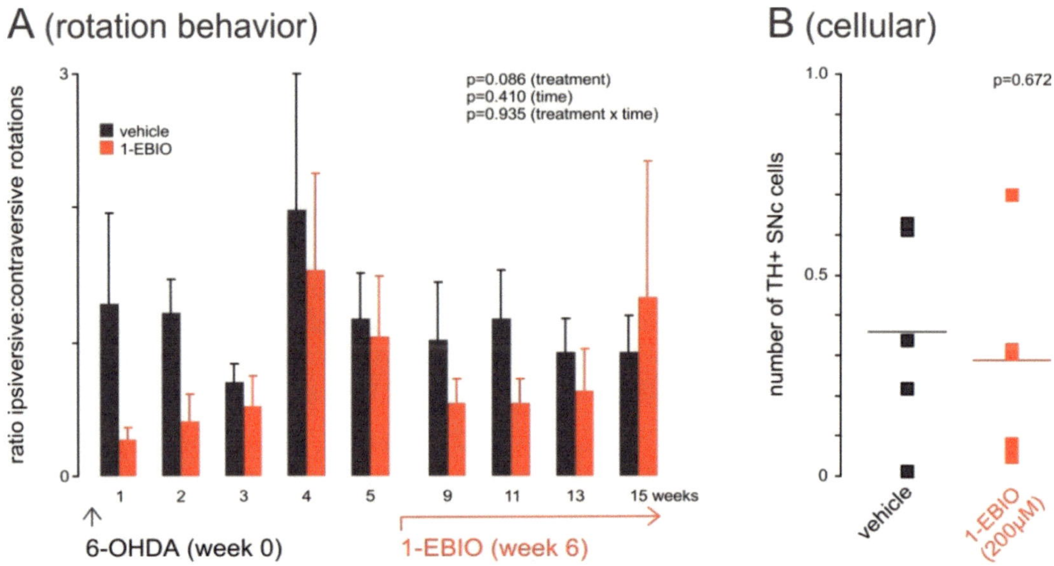

Fig. 3. Effects of the SK channel agonist 1-EBIO (200µM) on rotational behavior in response to amphetamine and the number of TH+ SNc cells in 6-OHDA-lesioned adult rats. (A) 6-OHDA was injected into the right SNc of 8-week old male Sprague-Dawley rats to reduce the number of SNc TH+ cells to ~35% of normal (see vehicle-treated rats, black symbols in B). Over the ensuing 15 weeks the rotational behavior in response to amphetamine was examined. The relative mean ± SE ratio of ipsiversive-to-contraversive rotations performed over a 60 minute interval, beginning immediately following amphetamine injection, is plotted over time for vehicle-treated (black bars) and 1-EBIO-treated (red bars) rats. 6-OHDA resulted in progressive increase in the ratio of ipsiversive:contraversive rotations from weeks 1-5, although this was not evident in the vehicle-treated group and was not statistically significant in either group. At week 6, 200µM 1-EBIO (or vehicle) infusion directly into the right SNc commenced. There was a non-significant trend for 1-EBIO to improve the rotational bias at 9 & 11 weeks, but not at 13 & 15 weeks. There were no effects of treatment or time over the course of this experiment (two-way ANOVA). (B) At the end of week 15, there was no difference in the number of TH+ cells in the 6-OHDA-lesioned SNc between vehicle- (black symbols) and 1-EBIO-infused (red symbols) rats (p=0.672, t-test). See figure 1 legend for details about how these data are represented.

akinesia (and possibly left side attention deficit), evidenced by increases in right:left forelimb use in figure 4C and right:left feeding in figure 4D. There was a degree of normalization of these asymmetries following treatment onset (week 12), however there were no differences in the extent of these normalizations in quinpirole- versus vehicle-infused rats (figure 4C-D).

At the experiment end-point the number of SNc TH+ cells was not different between quinpirole- and vehicle-infused rats (figure 4E).

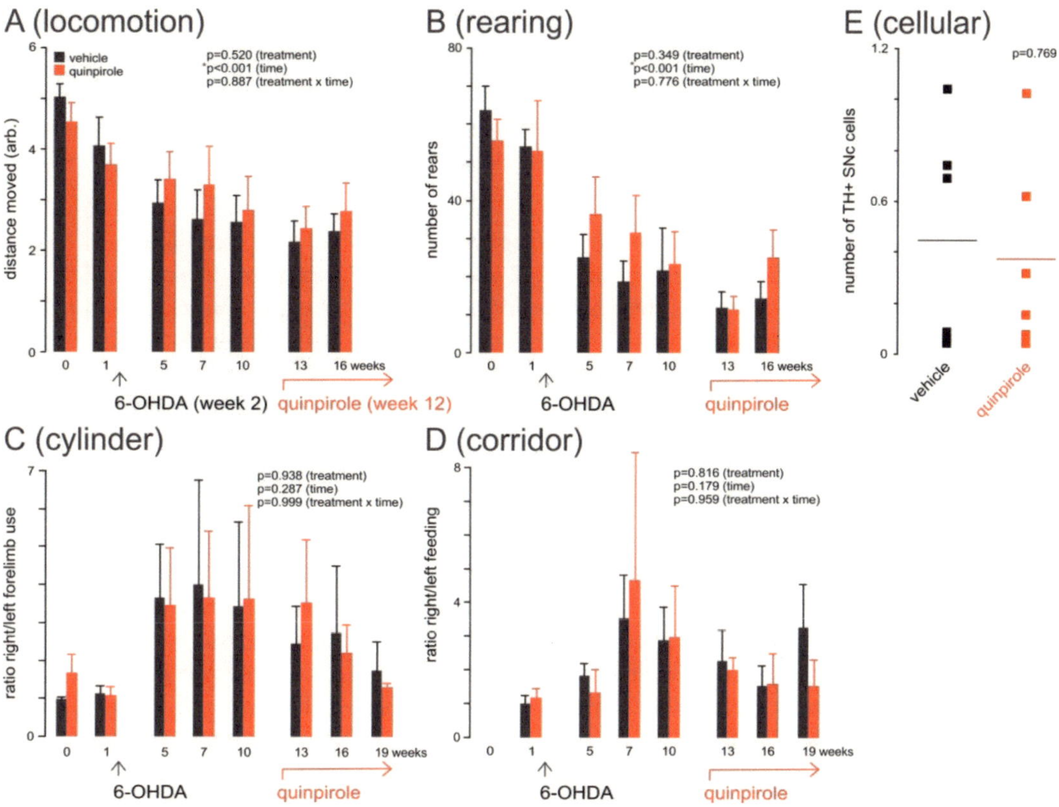

Fig. 4. Effects of the D2 DA receptor agonist quinpirole on motor behavior and the number of TH+ SNc cells in 6-OHDA-lesioned adult rats. (A-D) 6-OHDA was injected into the right SNc of 8-week old male Sprague-Dawley rats to reduce the number of SNc TH+ cells to ~50% of normal (see vehicle-treated rats, black symbols in E). Over the ensuing 19 weeks locomotion (A), rearing (B), right/left forelimb use in the cylinder test (C) and right/left feeding in the corridor test (D) were examined. At week 12, 100nM quinpirole (or vehicle) infusion directly into the right dorsal striatum commenced. The mean ± SE of each of the behavioral measures is plotted over time and treatment (vehicle = black, quinpirole = red). 6-OHDA resulted in an increased ratio of right/left forelimb use in the cylinder test (C) and of right/left side feeding in the corridor test (D). There were no effects on locomotion (A) and rearing (B) beyond the expected habituation over time. Quinpirole had no effect over vehicle on any of the behaviors examined (two-way ANOVAs). (E) At the end of week 19, there was no difference in the number of TH+ cells in the 6-OHDA-lesioned SNc between vehicle- (black symbols) and 1-EBIO-infused (red symbols) rats (p=0.769, t-test). See figure 1 legend for details about how these data are represented.

4. Discussion

These studies were carried out because administration of 1-EBIO, riluzole and quinpirole to normal mice leads to a robust, rapid and reproducible increase in DA cells in the SNc

(Aumann et al. 2011, Aumann et al. 2008). However, these agents failed to alleviate motor deficits and failed to consistently recruit "new" TH+ SNc cells in mice or rats with prior 6-OHDA-induced depletion of SNc DA neurons. The following discussion focuses on caveats of this conclusion, and on what the present experimental outcomes might reveal about the underlying biology. We conclude that these agents warrant further experimentation, perhaps using animal models that more faithfully recapitulate slow nigrostriatal degeneration in PD.

The first caveat is technical and around drug delivery. Given the credible increase in number of SNc TH+ cells brought about by 2-weeks 1-EBIO infusion in some 6-OHDA-lesioned mice (figure 1), we opted for a longer infusion in the rat experiments, expecting cell recruitment would improve. However, the opposite was true. After 9-weeks 1-EBIO infusion in 6-OHDA-lesioned rats, there was no difference in behavior (week 15 in figure 3A) or in the number of SNc TH+ cells (figure 3B), compared with vehicle infusion. However, there was evidence of some behavioral improvement, and presumably nigrostriatal cell recovery, earlier in the course of the 1-EBIO infusion (weeks 9 & 11 in figure 3A). Why then did this potential improvement lapse at weeks 13 & 15? Degradation of the drug is not the explanation because a new pump with a fresh supply of 1-EBIO was introduced at week 12. However, it could have been due to inadvertent and premature termination of drug delivery around week 12. At the experimental endpoint (week 15) it was noted that the majority of pumps were disconnected from their cannula; this was not the case when the pumps were replaced (week 12). Unfortunately we cannot know precisely when this detachment, and therefore cessation of drug infusion, occurred. However, if it was around week 12, it is possible 1-EBIO was having a beneficial effect. Therefore we believe the experiment should be repeated. If future experiments reveal 1-EBIO does facilitate recruitment of new SNc DA neurons and improves motor symptoms in 6-OHDA-lesioned rodents, the present data indicate that these benefits are acutely dependent on the presence of the drug, and therefore continuous drug delivery will be necessary to maintain them.

A second caveat relates to lesion size. In the mouse 1-EBIO experiments (figure 1), lesions were similar in size, evidenced by the relatively tight cluster of data from vehicle-treated mice (black symbols, figure 1). Therefore it is likely that: (1) lesions in the animals receiving 1-EBIO infusion were also of similar size; and (2) 1-EBIO treatment is recruiting new SNc DA neurons in some 6-OHDA lesioned mice. We propose that responsiveness to 1-EBIO may be determined by lesion size, with large 6-OHDA lesions being relatively unresponsive compared to smaller lesions. Our reasoning for this is discussed later. Suffice to point out here that in the 1-EBIO rat experiment (figure 3) [and in the quinpirole rat experiment (figure 4)], lesion size was much more variable than in the 1-EBIO mouse experiments. Moreover, the size of the lesions was ≥ the upper range of mouse lesions [i.e. <40% of TH+ cells remaining, figure 3B (and 4E)] in a significant proportion of rats. Therefore it may be that many of the rats in these experiments were unable to respond to 1-EBIO (or quinpirole) because their lesions were too big (and possibly also too rapid, see discussion below).

A less likely caveat in our opinion is that rats are less able to respond to 1-EBIO or striatal quinpirole than mice. The ability of the rodent SNc to spontaneously compensate following 6-OHDA insult, and in different ways (e.g. recruitment of TH+ SNc cells or sprouting of surviving nigrostriatal axons), is no different in mice versus rats in our experience.

The caveats discussed above are tantalizing and the importance of a positive outcome justifies further experiments that attend to: (1) ensuring drug delivery remains patent; (2) whether continual drug delivery is necessary to maintain the recruited population of DA neurons; (3) whether lesion size (and rate) are confounding factors in the responsiveness to treatment; and (4) whether there are species differences.

We will now turn to discussion of what the present results might reveal about the underlying biology. There is an extensive literature showing that expression of TH in cells is regulated by changes in membrane potential (neuronal activity) and intracellular Ca2+. We recently reported that this is true also in the SNc of normal (i.e. unlesioned) adult mice (Aumann et al. 2011, Aumann et al. 2008). When drugs targeting the activity of SNc neurons are infused into the brain for 2 weeks, both the amount of TH protein/SNc cell and the number of SNc TH+ cells are altered (Aumann et al. 2011, Aumann et al. 2008). Specifically, our data show that when the number of TH+ cells increases, the TH immunoreactivity of each cell decreases, and vice versa. Also, when the number of TH+ cells increases, the number of SNc cells that are not TH immunoreactive (TH-) decreases by the same amount, and vice versa [i.e. the net number of SNc cells (TH+ & TH- combined) does not change]. From a broad perspective these data indicate that TH expression in adult SNc neurons is activity-dependent. More closely they imply a homeostatic mechanism(s) regulating DA neurotransmission in the striatum, but acting at the levels of TH expression and DA phenotype recruitment/loss in SNc. We propose that this homeostatic mechanism(s) operates at two levels. At the level of an individual SNc cell, TH expression is activity- and Ca^{2+}-dependent and is brought about by altered Ca^{2+}-dependent DA gene expression. At the level of nigrostriatal circuitry, striatal DA receptor signaling and feedback circuitry from the striatum to the SNc operates to control the number of SNc DA cells.

The rapid (within 2 weeks) recruitment/loss of the DA phenotype by SNc cells in normal mice (Aumann et al. 2011, Aumann et al. 2008) implies the existence of a population of relatively mature (but not DA) neurons located in and around SNc that can be recruited into and out of the DA population. In other (unpublished) studies we have evidence that significant numbers of new neurons (NeuN+) are generated in the adult mouse midbrain [from Nestin+ (but BrdU-) neural precursor cells], many (~420 over an 8 week period) of which end up in SNc, see also (Shan *et al.* 2006). A very small number of these new midbrain neurons express TH, i.e. demonstrate a capacity to acquire the DA phenotype, but so far these have been observed around the ventral midline and in the ventral tegmental area (VTA), not in SNc. It could be that these newborn NeuN+ but TH- SNc neurons are the same cells in which the DA phenotype can be recruited should appropriate signals arrive. We believe that one of these signals is a change in their electrical activity, such as occurs when 1-EBIO is infused into the midbrain or quinpirole is infused into the striatum.

In this context, it is relevant to consider what might have happened to this putative DA phenotype recruitment when confronted with rapid depletion of SNc DA neurons following direct 6-OHDA injection. Evidence from our laboratory and others (Sauer & Oertel 1994) shows that following 6-OHDA, and in the absence of any further treatment or manipulation, the number of SNc TH+ cells spontaneously recovers toward normal, while at the same time the number of SNc TH- cells declines (Stanic et al. 2003). This suggests DA phenotype recruitment, possibly as part of a process that has directed the homeostasis described above toward repair. The failure of our attempts to facilitate this recruitment using 1-EBIO or quinpirole in the present study might be due to depletion of the population of recruitable cells by this spontaneous recovery. It also indicates the rate of replenishment of the recruitable population (i.e. neurogenesis) is not very high, since not enough were generated within the timeframe of our experiments (4-17 weeks) to significantly impact the TH+ population. This would fit with the consensus in the literature that the rate of adult midbrain neurogenesis is not very high (Shan et al. 2006, Zhao *et al.* 2003) or zero (Aponso *et al.* 2008, Chen *et al.* 2005, Cooper & Isacson 2004, Frielingsdorf *et al.* 2004, Lie *et al.* 2002, Peng *et al.* 2008, Yoshimi *et al.* 2005). This point brings us to another caveat of the present experiments, which is the very rapid depletion of SNc DA neurons by 6-OHDA injection may not be the best PD model in which to study activity-dependent DA phenotype recruitment. Perhaps a model in which the rate of degeneration is much slower, which better mimics the situation in PD, would provide enough time for the recruitable population of cells to be sustained.

5. Conclusion

In summary, our working model is: (1) The nigrostriatal DA pathway is under homeostatic control to maintain a constant level of striatal DA signaling; (2) This is achieved at the level of individual SNc cells via activity- and Ca^{2+}-dependent alterations in DA (TH) gene expression; (3) It is also achieved at the level of D2 DA receptor-mediated striatonigral feedback circuitry (the indirect pathway) leading to changes in the number of SNc DA cells; (4) A population of relatively mature NeuN+ but TH- cells located in and immediately surrounding SNc is available to be rapidly recruited into and out of the DA population; (5) This recruitable population of cells can be rapidly depleted (i.e. recruited into the DA population) in response to perturbations of the system (e.g. altered SNc neuronal activity, nigrostriatal DA signaling, or 6-OHDA), but is only slowly replenished by neurogenesis. The implication of this homeostasis for nigrostriatal DA cell-replacement therapies is that any manipulation designed to increase the number of SNc DA cells is likely to be offset by a homeostatic response. The effects of infusing D2 agonists into the striatum suggest that striatal DA signaling may be a factor. Thus in PD or its models the effect of homeostatic control may be difficult to predict. On the other hand, pharmaceuticals that increase SNc DA cells in normal mice fail to do so in 6-OHDA-lesioned rodents, possibly because the population of recruitable cells is also extensively depleted. Thus, researchers looking to help develop cell-replacement therapies to treat the motor symptoms of PD should consider the effects their interventions might have on nigrostriatal DA homeostasis because: (1) homeostatic responses may be confounding interpretation of the effects of their interventions; and (2) homeostatic responses may need to be addressed also, as part of an overall strategy to increase cell-based nigrostriatal DA transmission.

Future work should therefore aim to better understand these homeostatic responses by: (1) identifying downstream signaling pathways mediating activity- and Ca^{2+}-dependent changes in DA gene expression; (2) identifying mechanisms of SNc DA phenotype recruitment; (3) identifying the phenotype of recruitable cells; (4) characterizing the ontogenesis of newborn SNc neurons; and (5) investigating mechanisms regulating the rate of SNc neurogenesis. Progress in these areas promises to be vital for better treating the motor symptoms of PD, but will also be relevant for other disorders involving dysfunctional midbrain DA signaling (e.g. attention deficit hyperactivity disorder, schizophrenia, drug addiction), and for adult neurogenesis and brain plasticity more generally.

6. Acknowledgements

This study was supported by grants from the National Health & Medical Research Council of Australia, the Bethlehem Griffiths Research Foundation, & the CASS Foundation. The Authors gratefully acknowledge the technical assistance of Doris Tomas, Brett Purcell & Greg Thomas.

7. References

Aponso, P. M., Faull, R. L. and Connor, B. (2008) Increased progenitor cell proliferation and astrogenesis in the partial progressive 6-hydroxydopamine model of Parkinson's disease. *Neuroscience,* 151, 1142-1153.

Aumann, T. D., Egan, K., Lim, J. et al. (2011) Neuronal activity regulates expression of tyrosine hydroxylase in adult mouse substantia nigra pars compacta neurons. *J Neurochem,* 116, 646-658.

Aumann, T. D., Gantois, I., Egan, K., Vais, A., Tomas, D., Drago, J. and Horne, M. K. (2008) SK channel function regulates the dopamine phenotype of neurons in the substantia nigra pars compacta. *Exp Neurol,* 213, 419-430.

Barneoud, P., Mazadier, M., Miquet, J. M., Parmentier, S., Dubedat, P., Doble, A. and Boireau, A. (1996) Neuroprotective effects of riluzole on a model of Parkinson's disease in the rat. *Neuroscience,* 74, 971-983.

Bauer, M., Meyer, M., Grimm, L., Meitinger, T., Zimmer, J., Gasser, T., Ueffing, M. and Widmer, H. R. (2000) Nonviral glial cell-derived neurotrophic factor gene transfer enhances survival of cultured dopaminergic neurons and improves their function after transplantation in a rat model of Parkinson's disease. *Human gene therapy,* 11, 1529-1541.

Bensimon, G., Ludolph, A., Agid, Y., Vidailhet, M., Payan, C. and Leigh, P. N. (2009) Riluzole treatment, survival and diagnostic criteria in Parkinson plus disorders: the NNIPPS study. *Brain,* 132, 156-171.

Bezard, E., Stutzmann, J. M., Imbert, C., Boraud, T., Boireau, A. and Gross, C. E. (1998) Riluzole delayed appearance of parkinsonian motor abnormalities in a chronic MPTP monkey model. *Eur J Pharmacol,* 356, 101-104.

Bjorklund, A., Rosenblad, C., Winkler, C. and Kirik, D. (1997) Studies on neuroprotective and regenerative effects of GDNF in a partial lesion model of Parkinson's disease. *Neurobiology of disease,* 4, 186-200.

Bowenkamp, K. E., David, D., Lapchak, P. L., Henry, M. A., Granholm, A. C., Hoffer, B. J. and Mahalik, T. J. (1996) 6-hydroxydopamine induces the loss of the dopaminergic phenotype in substantia nigra neurons of the rat. A possible mechanism for restoration of the nigrostriatal circuit mediated by glial cell line-derived neurotrophic factor. *Experimental brain research. Experimentelle Hirnforschung. Experimentation cerebrale,* 111, 1-7.

Braz, C. A., Borges, V. and Ferraz, H. B. (2004) Effect of riluzole on dyskinesia and duration of the on state in Parkinson disease patients: a double-blind, placebo-controlled pilot study. *Clin Neuropharmacol,* 27, 25-29.

Brundin, P., Karlsson, J., Emgard, M., Schierle, G. S., Hansson, O., Petersen, A. and Castilho, R. F. (2000) Improving the survival of grafted dopaminergic neurons: a review over current approaches. *Cell transplantation,* 9, 179-195.

Cao, Y. J., Dreixler, J. C., Couey, J. J. and Houamed, K. M. (2002) Modulation of recombinant and native neuronal SK channels by the neuroprotective drug riluzole. *Eur J Pharmacol,* 449, 47-54.

Chen, Y., Ai, Y., Slevin, J. R., Maley, B. E. and Gash, D. M. (2005) Progenitor proliferation in the adult hippocampus and substantia nigra induced by glial cell line-derived neurotrophic factor. *Exp Neurol,* 196, 87-95.

Cooper, O. and Isacson, O. (2004) Intrastriatal transforming growth factor alpha delivery to a model of Parkinson's disease induces proliferation and migration of endogenous adult neural progenitor cells without differentiation into dopaminergic neurons. *J Neurosci,* 24, 8924-8931.

Courtois, E. T., Castillo, C. G., Seiz, E. G., Ramos, M., Bueno, C., Liste, I. and Martinez-Serrano, A. (2010) In vitro and in vivo enhanced generation of human A9 dopamine neurons from neural stem cells by Bcl-XL. *The Journal of biological chemistry,* 285, 9881-9897.

Franklin, K. B. J. and Paxinos, G. (2008) *The mouse brain in stereotaxic coordinates.* Academic Press/Elsevier, New York.

Frielingsdorf, H., Schwarz, K., Brundin, P. and Mohapel, P. (2004) No evidence for new dopaminergic neurons in the adult mammalian substantia nigra. *Proc Natl Acad Sci U S A,* 101, 10177-10182.

Gash, D. M., Zhang, Z., Ovadia, A. et al. (1996) Functional recovery in parkinsonian monkeys treated with GDNF. *Nature,* 380, 252-255.

Grunnet, M., Jespersen, T., Angelo, K., Frokjaer-Jensen, C., Klaerke, D. A., Olesen, S. P. and Jensen, B. S. (2001) Pharmacological modulation of SK3 channels. *Neuropharmacology,* 40, 879-887.

Gundersen, H. J., Bagger, P., Bendtsen, T. F. et al. (1988) The new stereological tools: disector, fractionator, nucleator and point sampled intercepts and their use in pathological research and diagnosis. *APMIS : acta pathologica, microbiologica, et immunologica Scandinavica,* 96, 857-881.

Jankovic, J. and Hunter, C. (2002) A double-blind, placebo-controlled and longitudinal study of riluzole in early Parkinson's disease. *Parkinsonism Relat Disord,* 8, 271-276.

Lie, D. C., Dziewczapolski, G., Willhoite, A. R., Kaspar, B. K., Shults, C. W. and Gage, F. H. (2002) The adult substantia nigra contains progenitor cells with neurogenic potential. *J Neurosci,* 22, 6639-6649.

Nelson, E. L., Liang, C. L., Sinton, C. M. and German, D. C. (1996) Midbrain dopaminergic neurons in the mouse: computer-assisted mapping. *The Journal of comparative neurology,* 369, 361-371.

Olanow, C. W., Watts, R. L. and Koller, W. C. (2001) An algorithm (decision tree) for the management of Parkinson's disease (2001): treatment guidelines. *Neurology,* 56, S1-S88.

Parish, C. L., Finkelstein, D. I., Drago, J., Borrelli, E. and Horne, M. K. (2001) The role of dopamine receptors in regulating the size of axonal arbors. *J Neurosci,* 21, 5147-5157.

Paxinos, G. and Watson, C. (2007) *The rat brain in stereotaxic coordinates.* Elsevier, Amsterdam; Boston.

Peng, J., Xie, L., Jin, K., Greenberg, D. A. and Andersen, J. K. (2008) Fibroblast growth factor 2 enhances striatal and nigral neurogenesis in the acute 1-methyl-4-phenyl-1,2,3,6-tetrahydropyridine model of Parkinson's disease. *Neuroscience,* 153, 664-670.

Sauer, H. and Oertel, W. H. (1994) Progressive degeneration of nigrostriatal dopamine neurons following intrastriatal terminal lesions with 6-hydroxydopamine: a combined retrograde tracing and immunocytochemical study in the rat. *Neuroscience,* 59, 401-415.

Serova, L. and Sabban, E. L. (2002) Involvement of alpha 7 nicotinic acetylcholine receptors in gene expression of dopamine biosynthetic enzymes in rat brain. *The Journal of pharmacology and experimental therapeutics,* 303, 896-903.

Shan, X., Chi, L., Bishop, M., Luo, C., Lien, L., Zhang, Z. and Liu, R. (2006) Enhanced de novo neurogenesis and dopaminergic neurogenesis in the substantia nigra of 1-methyl-4-phenyl-1,2,3,6-tetrahydropyridine-induced Parkinson's disease-like mice. *Stem Cells,* 24, 1280-1287.

Soriano, M. A., Justicia, C., Ferrer, I., Rodriguez-Farre, E. and Planas, A. M. (1997) Striatal infarction in the rat causes a transient reduction of tyrosine hydroxylase immunoreactivity in the ipsilateral substantia nigra. *Neurobiology of disease,* 4, 376-385.

Stanic, D., Finkelstein, D. I., Bourke, D. W., Drago, J. and Horne, M. K. (2003) Timecourse of striatal re-innervation following lesions of dopaminergic SNpc neurons of the rat. *The European journal of neuroscience,* 18, 1175-1188.

Stocchi, F., Jenner, P. and Obeso, J. A. (2010) When do levodopa motor fluctuations first appear in Parkinson's disease? *Eur Neurol,* 63, 257-266.

Stocchi, F. and Marconi, S. (2010) Factors associated with motor fluctuations and dyskinesia in Parkinson disease: potential role of a new melevodopa plus carbidopa formulation (sirio). *Clin Neuropharmacol,* 33, 198-203.

Torres, E. M., Monville, C., Lowenstein, P. R., Castro, M. G. and Dunnett, S. B. (2005) Delivery of sonic hedgehog or glial derived neurotrophic factor to dopamine-rich grafts in a rat model of Parkinson's disease using adenoviral vectors Increased yield of dopamine cells is dependent on embryonic donor age. *Brain research bulletin,* 68, 31-41.

Wood, L. D. (2010) Clinical review and treatment of select adverse effects of dopamine receptor agonists in Parkinson's disease. *Drugs Aging,* 27, 295-310.

Yamada, K., Goto, S., Yoshikawa, M. and Ushio, Y. (1996) Gabaergic transmission and tyrosine hydroxylase expression in the nigral dopaminergic neurons: an in vivo study using a reversible ischemia model of rats. *Neuroscience,* 73, 783-789.

Yoshimi, K., Ren, Y. R., Seki, T. et al. (2005) Possibility for neurogenesis in substantia nigra of parkinsonian brain. *Ann Neurol,* 58, 31-40.

Zhao, M., Momma, S., Delfani, K. et al. (2003) Evidence for neurogenesis in the adult mammalian substantia nigra. *Proc Natl Acad Sci U S A,* 100, 7925-7930.

13

Molecular Mechanisms in Synaptic Plasticity

M. Mayadevi*, G.M. Archana*,
Ramya R. Prabhu* and R.V. Omkumar†
*Molecular Neurobiology Division,
Rajiv Gandhi Centre for Biotechnology, Thycaud, Kerala,
India*

1. Introduction

Brain is a sophisticated information processing and storage system with capabilities unmatched by any manmade computers. Neurons, the primary building blocks of the brain are structurally and functionally specialized to do these functions. The neuronal membrane is equipped with several types of ion channel and ion pump proteins which enable it to conduct nerve impulses in the form of electrochemical signals called action potentials. The highly branched structure of the neuron with dendrites and axons helps in not only transmitting these signals but also in information processing by integrating multiple inputs. Storage of information, on the other hand, happens by permanent changes in the brain consequent to activity that will serve the function of recording information input. This remarkable property of the brain is known as plasticity and brings about changes in the structures and functions of the brain in response to internal and external stimuli. Plasticity can be defined as the ability of neural circuitry to undergo modifications consequent to experience and thereby modify future thought, behaviour and feeling. Neuronal activity can modify the behaviour of neural circuits by one of the three mechanisms : (a) by modifying the strength or efficacy of synaptic transmission at pre-existing synapses, (b) by eliciting the growth of new synaptic connections or the pruning away of existing ones, or (c) by modulating the excitability of individual neurons (Malenka, 2002). It is now reasonably well established that synapses are the primary sites of information storage, enabled by synaptic plasticity.

Synaptic plasticity is the cellular phenomenon by which synapses can undergo permanent changes in their properties consequent to specific patterns of activity. Since synaptic activity represents incoming information into the brain, the consequent permanent changes in synapses are thought to serve as the engram or record of the information. Hence mechanisms underlying synaptic plasticity events have attracted considerable attention as the molecular basis of learning and memory.

Synaptic plasticity was first proposed as a cellular mechanism for memory by Donald Hebb in 1949. According to Hebb's postulate, repeated communication between two neurons via

---

* Equal contribution
† Corresponding Author

synaptic transmission can cause an enhancement in the efficacy of transmission between those neurons, brought about by biochemical changes at the synapses. Accordingly Hebbian conditioning needs both presynaptic and postsynaptic activity for its induction. This was followed by a search for instances where synaptic efficacy is altered. The discovery of Long term potentiation (LTP) by Bliss and Lomo in 1973 (Bliss & Lomo, 1973) was the first demonstration of synaptic plasticity. LTP had all the characteristics necessary for a mechanism responsible for learning and memory and thus gained acceptance as a cellular correlate or cellular model system for learning and memory. Moreover, the cellular system with reduced complexity compared to the animal models was more amenable for interrogations at the molecular level. LTP thus became an essential component of a paradigm in which initial insights on molecular mechanisms are provided by experiments involving LTP which could then be validated in higher animal models.

In addition to the fundamental interest of how learning and memory are performed by brain, the study of synaptic plasticity is also attractive as it could lead to practical applications. The principles governing the workings of the molecular machineries involved in synaptic plasticity could be useful in the design of manmade memory devices. In the case of many CNS disorders, early aberrations at the molecular level are likely to involve synaptic plasticity mechanisms since the initial clinical symptoms very often involve cognitive impairments such as deficits in learning and memory. These mechanisms could be possible targets for early therapeutic intervention, provided they drive further molecular processes leading to the pathology of such diseases. Understanding of the mechanisms of synaptic plasticity would be of great therapeutic value in such instances.

A major challenge in understanding the molecular mechanisms of synaptic plasticity has been the diversity in the underlying mechanisms in different parts of the brain. The current article has reviewed the literature on molecular mechanisms that are involved in the induction and maintenance of different forms synaptic plasticity, mainly LTP and long term depression (LTD) and has attempted to simplify the scenario by extracting general features possessed by these mechanisms. Impairments in synaptic plasticity that could occur in disease conditions have also been touched upon.

2. Synaptic plasticity

The term *Synaptic plasticity* refers to the activity dependent changes in the efficacy of synaptic communication. Donald Hebb in 1949 developed a hypothesis about the mechanism of learning and memory at the neuronal level. Clinical observations enabled investigators to link human memory dysfunction to the hippocampus (Scoville & Milner, 1957; Olds, 1972). These developments stimulated research in the field of synaptic plasticity in the mammalian brain (Blundon, 2008). Synaptic plasticity has been most extensively studied at the Schaffer-collateral pathway (Bliss, 2011) in the hippocampus, the seat of learning and memory, especially declarative memory. In 1973, Bliss and his associates reported that tetanic stimulation of the perforant pathway of presynaptic fibres resulted in high responses at postsynaptic sites on granule cells at the dentate gyrus region, to electric stimulation. The experiments were conducted *in vivo* with anaesthetized rabbits. They called the effect LTP because of the elevation of the postsynaptic potential, which could serve as a cellular substrate for information storage (Bliss & Lomo, 1973).

Several observations from a variety of species indicate that synaptic plasticity and memory are correlative. Behavioural and *in vitro* studies suggest that activity-induced synaptic modulations, such as LTP, play a role in information storage in the brain. This idea has been proposed as the "synaptic plasticity and memory (SPM) hypothesis" (Martin et al., 2000), and has been a major driving force behind the study of synaptic plasticity. Synaptic plasticity includes both short-term changes in the strength or efficacy of neurotransmission as well as longer-term changes in the structure of synapses (Kandel, 2001). Experimental models of changes in synaptic strength or effectiveness in response to repeated electrical stimulation are thought to mimic physiological plasticity at the neuronal level. The efficacy of synaptic transmission could increase as in LTP or it could decrease as in LTD as a result of plasticity. These modifications in synaptic strength, both positive and negative, distributed across millions of connections among neurons, are believed to form the physical and biochemical substrates for learning and memory.

Hippocampal LTP became a favourite model for the study of learning and memory due to the following reasons. First, there is compelling evidence from studies in rodents and higher primates, including humans, that the hippocampus is a critical component of the neural system involved in various forms of long-term memory. Second, several properties of LTP make it an attractive cellular mechanism for information storage. Like memories, LTP can be generated rapidly and is prolonged and strengthened with repetition. It is also input specific in that it is elicited at the synapses activated by afferent activity and not at adjacent synapses on the same postsynaptic cell (Malenka, 2002).

3. Long term potentiation

LTP is an activity-dependent, persistent enhancement of synaptic strength. LTP mainly occurs at glutamatergic synapses and is often measured in terms of the magnitude of excitatory post synaptic potential (EPSP) enhancement at a given time-point after induction. This measurement is influenced by the initial magnitude of potentiation and the decay rate of the potentiation and are independently regulated. Generally longer-lasting forms of plasticity are observed following repetitive or tetanic stimulation of synapses with prolonged (approximately 200-millisecond to 5-second) trains of stimuli applied at high frequencies (10 to 200 Hz).

3.1 Phases of LTP

LTP is formed by a series of distinguishable mechanisms. LTP can be divided into two temporally distinct phases such as early and late phases. Early LTP (E-LTP) lasts for about 1-3 hrs and requires modification of existing proteins and their trafficking at synapses but not *de novo* protein synthesis (Bliss & Collingridge, 1993; Malenka & Bear, 2004). This short lasting form of LTP can be induced by a weak, high frequency tetanus (single train of 100 pulses at 100 Hz). Late LTP (L-LTP) requires the synthesis of RNA, new proteins and protein kinase activity especially cyclic adenosine 3′, 5′-monophosphate (cAMP)-dependent protein kinase or protein kinase A (PKA) (Frey et al., 1993; Huang and Kandel, 1994; Nguyen et al., 1994), which lasts for up to 8-10 hrs *in vitro* and weeks *in vivo*. L-LTP can be induced by repeated strong high frequency stimulation such as multiple trains of 100 pulses at 100 Hz and is necessary for structural modification of synapses (Lu et al., 2007).

3.2 Types of LTP

Even though plasticity events can be distinguished as either LTP or LTD, a huge variation in forms of LTP has also been observed. Several factors contribute to these different types of LTP. LTP varies with the type of molecular pathway involved in its induction as can be seen in the case of LTP in hippocampal CA1 region which is either N-methyl-D-aspartate receptor (NMDAR) dependent or independent. Different regions of brain show different forms of LTP. The age of the organism also contributes to the variation in LTP. LTP in neonatal (<9 postnatal days) rodent hippocampal CA1 region is different from that in mature animals (Yasuda et al., 2003). Based on the pre and postsynaptic activity patterns required for induction, LTP can be classified as Hebbian, Non-Hebbian, anti-Hebbian and neo-Hebbian. Hebbian LTP requires both pre and post synaptic activity at the same time for its induction (Hebb, 1949). Non-Hebbian LTP requires activation of either pre or post synaptic compartment and does not need simultaneous depolarization of pre- and postsynaptic cells; an example of this occurs in the mossy fibre hippocampal pathway. Anti-Hebbian LTP can be formed by a conjunction of presynaptic depolarization and postsynaptic hyperpolarization (Lamsa et al., 2007). This can be induced in several classes of interneurons in strata oriens and pyramidale by high or low frequency stimulation patterns applied to axon collaterals of local pyramidal neurons, as long as the postsynaptic membrane potential is kept negative to the action potential threshold (Kullmann & Lamsa, 2008). In addition to these three forms of LTP, neo-Hebbian LTP has been described recently which is related with the late phase of LTP induced by an NMDAR dependent process (Lisman et al., 2011). This form of LTP not only depends on the two factors of the Hebbian condition (glutamate release and postsynaptic depolarization), but also on a third factor, dopamine release. Dopamine will enhance the protein synthesis within the dendrites of hippocampal neurons (Smith, 2005).

Analyses of LTP decay rates and biochemical mechanisms have revealed three different forms of LTP (LTP-1, 2 and 3) in the hippocampus. LTP-1, induced by a single train of conditioning stimulation, is short lasting (2–3 h *in vitro*) and is dependent on post-translational modifications of existing synaptic proteins. LTP-2, induced by several repetitions of a conditioning train, is an intermediate form of LTP that depends on protein synthesis but not transcription of new mRNA. Finally, LTP-3, induced by multiple, spaced repetitions of conditioning stimulation, is very durable (perhaps even permanent in some cases, e.g. Abraham et al., 2002) and requires gene transcription and translation (Raymond, 2008).

3.3 Properties of LTP

Three key properties of LTP were elucidated in the 1970s and early 1980s. All of these can be explained using NMDA receptor dependent LTP mechanisms.

3.3.1 Input specificity

LTP can be generated only in those synapses which had undergone activation and not in adjacent synapses. But this is not valid for closely located synapses.

3.3.2 Associativity

One of the interesting properties of LTP mechanism is its associativity. If a weak non-LTP inducing stimulation in one afferent is paired with a strong LTP inducing stimulation in another afferent on the same cell, then the weakly stimulated afferent also exhibits LTP (Levy & Steward, 1979). This property is called as associativity. This property makes LTP an attractive mechanism for associating two pieces of information being conveyed by different sets of afferents that synapse on the same postsynaptic cell (Malenka, 2003).

3.3.3 Cooperativity

LTP can also be generated by weaker stimulation of a crucial number of presynaptic fibres to achieve a threshold stimulation to activate a postsynaptic neuron to induce LTP. This property is called cooperativity because different presynaptic fibres are cooperatively eliciting LTP.

3.3.4 Persistence

In addition to the above mentioned three characteristics, persistence can also be included as a fourth characteristic. LTP is persistent, lasting from several minutes to many months as long as the memory persists.

3.4 Molecular mechanisms of LTP

The cellular and molecular mechanisms of LTP induction are comprised of many events such as covalent modification of pre-existing proteins, the activation of cellular programs for gene expression and increased protein synthesis. The regulatory events move from the synapse to the nucleus and then back to the synapse in the course of LTP induction.

LTP induction experiments have mostly been done in hippocampal excitatory synapses. The hippocampus is divided into three distinctive regions composed of three distinctive kinds of cells. The dentate gyrus (DG), which is composed of granule cells and the CA3 and CA1 regions, which are composed of pyramidal cells having different properties. These regions are connected by well defined pathways through which signals traverse the hippocampus. The perforant fibre pathway (pp) from the entorhinal cortex forms excitatory connections with the granule cells of the DG. The granule cells give rise to axons that form the mossy fibre pathway (mf), which connects with the pyramidal cells in area CA3 of the hippocampus. The pyramidal cells of the CA3 region project to the pyramidal cells in CA1 by means of the Schaffer collateral pathway (Fig. 1).

LTP is widely studied in the CA1 region of the hippocampus (Bliss and Collingridge, 1993; Reymann and Frey, 2007). The establishment of LTP in the CA1 region requires both presynaptic activity and large postsynaptic depolarization. The original stimulus protocol used by Bliss and Lomo in the anesthetized rabbit ranged from 10 to 100 Hz (Bliss & Lomo, 1973). Since that time, a variety of LTP induction protocols from different research groups have emerged in the literature. Most involve trains of high-frequency stimulation (tetanization) that are delivered to presynaptic axons. The tetanization typically lasts several seconds and is delivered at frequencies of 25 to 400 Hz.

The induction of LTP requires an influx of calcium into the postsynaptic neuron that can be either through NMDAR dependent or NMDAR-independent mechanisms.

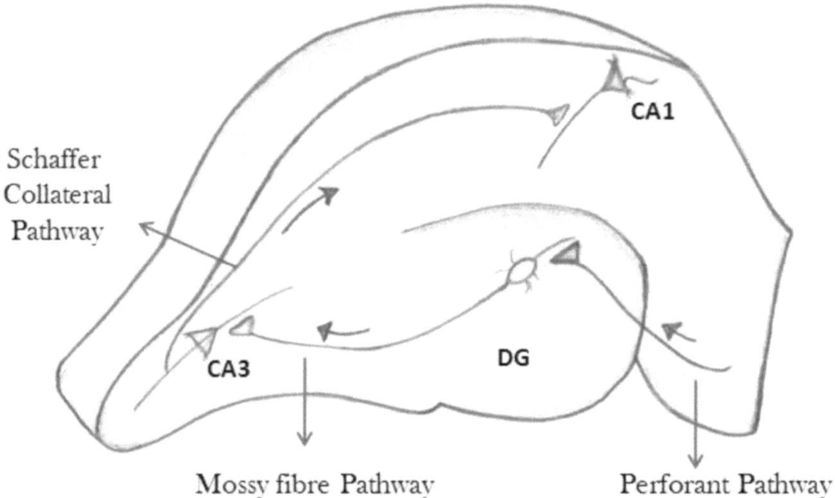

Fig. 1. Hippocampus

3.4.1 NMDAR dependent mechanism (NMDAR-LTP)

The best understood form of LTP is induced by the activation of the NMDAR complex. This subtype of glutamate receptor allows electrical events at the postsynaptic membrane to be transduced into chemical signals which, in turn, are thought to activate both pre and postsynaptic mechanisms to generate a persistent increase in synaptic strength.

Glutamate is a major excitatory neurotransmitter in the brain. During nerve impulse transmission, glutamate will be released into the synapse from the presynaptic terminal. Glutamate receptors present on the postsynaptic membrane are the initial triggers for the ensuing postsynaptic calcium signaling mechanism responsible for the induction of LTP. NMDA, α-amino-3-hydroxy-5-methyl-4-isoxazolepropionic acid (AMPA) and kainate receptors are the ionotropic-glutamate receptors present on the postsynaptic membrane. Among these NMDA and AMPA receptors play an important role in the induction of LTP. NMDARs are formed from hetero-tetrameric assemblies of GluN1 (previously NR1) subunits with GluN2A-D (NR2A-D) and Glu3A/B (NR3A/B). NMDARs require the binding of L-glutamate and the co-agonist glycine, as well as depolarization, to become activated and conduct Na^+, K^+ and Ca^{2+} ions. AMPARs are composed of four subunits, GluA1-4 (previously GluR1-4). The Q/R edited GluA2 subunit is critical for the biophysical properties of AMPARs producing low conductance, non-rectifying, Ca^{2+}-impermeable AMPARs. Postnatally the great majority of AMPARs contain edited GluA2 in excitatory synapses.

Glutamate binding to the AMPA receptor leads to a sodium influx into the postsynaptic compartment. This leads to depolarization causing release of Mg^{2+} block present on the NMDA receptor. The binding of glutamate and the removal of Mg^{2+} block causes NMDA receptor to open and conduct Ca^{2+} and Na^+ into the cell. The influx of Ca^{2+} is essential for LTP induction. With repeated activation of the neuron, sufficient calcium will enter into the postsynaptic compartment and triggers the molecular events needed for the induction of

LTP. This calcium influx activates several important signaling pathways involving different protein kinases and phosphatases. One of the kinases activated by the influx of calcium through NMDARs is Ca^{2+}/calmodulin dependent protein kinase II (CaMKII), which is known as the memory molecule. CaMKII is a Ser/Thr protein kinase, abundant in glutamatergic postsynaptic terminal. The activation of CaMKII by Ca^{2+}/CaM complex leads to the formation of autophosphorylated enzyme at Thr^{286} position, which will make it calcium independent. Thus the Thr^{286} autophosphorylated form of the enzyme will maintain its activity even though Ca^{2+}/CaM complex is removed from its regulatory domain. The autophosphorylation can enhance binding affinity of the enzyme for Ca^{2+}/CaM by a 1000 fold. Studies have shown that Thr^{286} autophosphorylated enzyme is required for the induction of LTP. Upon activation, CaMKII can rapidly translocate to the postsynaptic density (PSD), where postsynaptic receptors such as AMPAR and NMDAR are concentrated. The translocated CaMKII can bind to different subunits of NMDAR such as GluN1, GluN2A and GluN2B, which are the ideal postsynaptic adapters. Of these, GluN2B-CaMKII interaction is well characterized and is essential for the induction and maintenance of LTP (Barria & Malinow, 2005; Lisman et al., 2011). The AMPAR is one of the substrates for CaMKII (as well as for PKC) in the PSD where CaMKII can phosphorylate GluA1 subunit of AMPAR at Ser^{831}. This phosphorylation of GluA1 by CaMKII (Barria et al., 1997b) leads to an increased conductance of homomeric GluA1 channels (Derkach et al., 1999) and is believed to be one of the major contributors to the enhanced efficacy of glutamatergic synapses in CA1 area of hippocampus during LTP (Fig. 2).

LTP can occur either in AMPAR containing synapses or in synapses lacking AMPAR. When a glutamatergic synapse is formed, only NMDAR will be present in the postsynaptic membrane. Such synapses lacking AMPA receptors are called *silent synapses*, where AMPAR gets inserted in the postsynaptic membrane during the activation of nearby synapses. As a consequence of NMDAR activation and the resulting Ca^{2+} influx into the post synaptic dendrite, new AMPARs get inserted into the post synaptic membrane. This *'AMPAfication'* of the synapse makes the transmission stronger (Bear, 2001). Thus enhanced AMPAR activity either by increase in AMPAR abundance in the synapse or by increase in the conductivity of AMPARs is the key postsynaptic mechanism leading to increase in EPSP response seen in LTP. Studies have shown that activated forms of α-CaMKII can enhance the synaptic trafficking of AMPARs. PKA can also participate in *AMPAfication* by phosphorylating GluA1 at Ser^{845} which enhances AMPAR exocytosis (Oh, 2005). AMPAR recruitment mediated by PKA is shown in Fig. 3. Activation of PKA also boosts the activity of CaMKII indirectly by decreasing the competing protein phosphatase activity especially protein phosphatase 1(PP1). PKA inhibits PP1 by activating the inhibitor of PP1 called inhibitor-1(Bryne, 2009).

Several other protein kinases, including protein kinase C (PKC), PKA, the tyrosine kinase Src, and mitogen-activated protein kinase (MAPK), have also been suggested to contribute to LTP (Teyler et al., 1987). The evidence in support of critical roles for these kinases is, however, considerably weaker than that for CaMKII. PKC has been suggested to play a role analogous to that of CaMKII, because PKC inhibitors have been reported to block LTP and increasing postsynaptic PKC activity can enhance synaptic transmission (Hu et al., 1987).

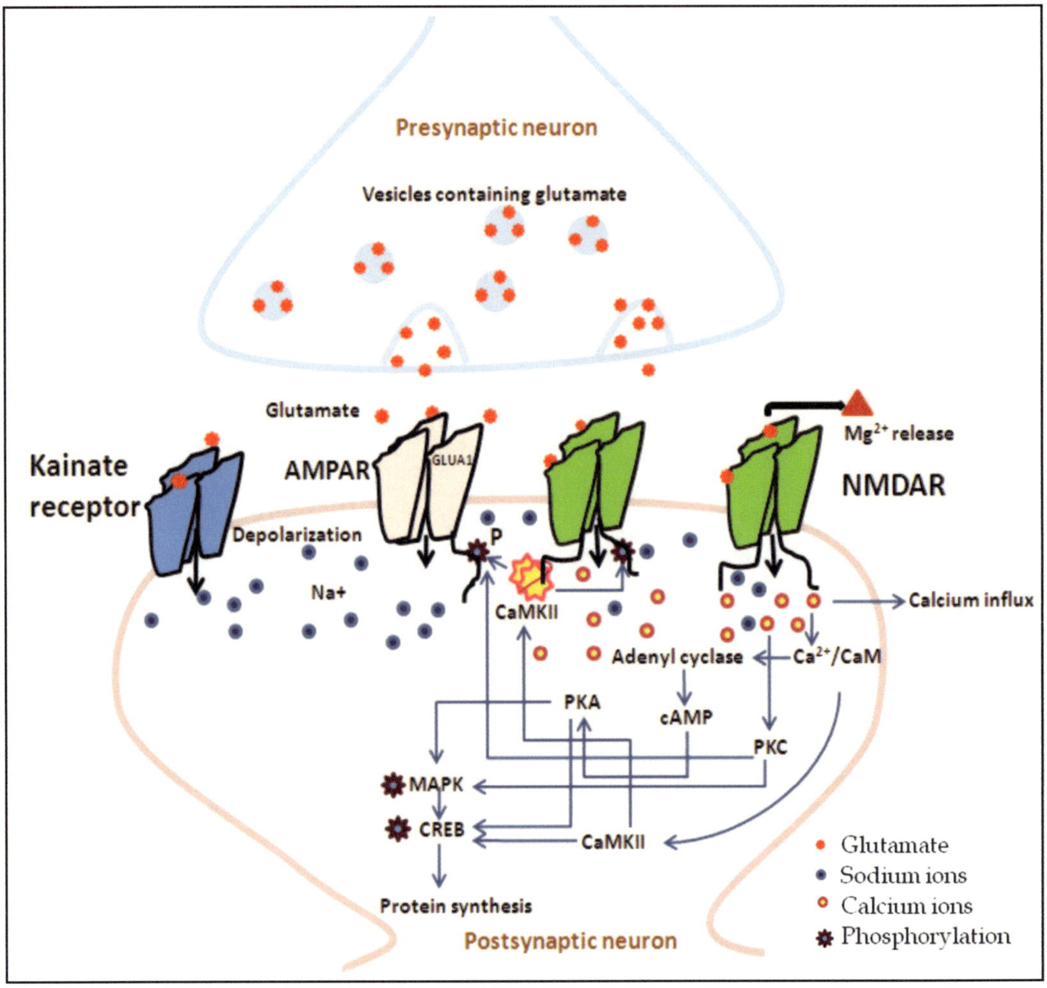

Fig. 2. Molecular mechanisms of NMDAR Dependent LTP.

The calcium influx through NMDAR also activates adenyl cyclase, which generates cAMP in the postsynaptic compartment. This second messenger generated thus triggers a series of downstream signalling mechanisms, which function more in LTP maintenance. The local increase in cAMP levels leads to the activation of PKA by causing the catalytic subunits of this enzyme to dissociate from the regulatory subunits.

The activated PKA can regulate gene expression. PKA can modify transcription by phosphorylating several different transcription factors, one of which is the cAMP response element binding protein (CREB). CREB is a nuclear protein that modulates transcription of genes containing cAMP response elements (CRE) in their promoters (Kandel, 2001). The catalytic subunits of PKA can translocate to nucleus and phosphorylate serine-133 on CREB.

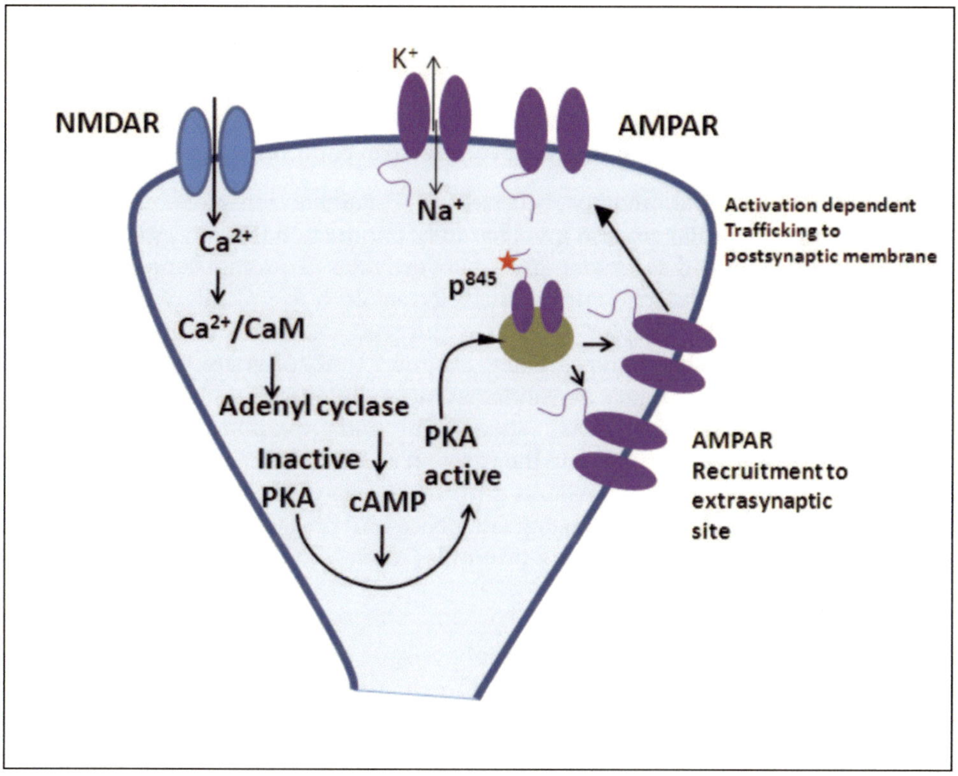

Fig. 3. AMPAR exocytosis regulation by PKA. Ca^{2+} signaling can activate PKA via adenyl cyclase-cAMP pathway. PKA can phosphorylate GluA1 subunit of AMPAR at Ser^{845} and this leads to the recruitment of AMPARs into extrasynaptic site. This extrasynaptic pool of AMPARs can then diffuse to PSD during NMDAR activation.

This phosphorylation can initiate transcription of CRE-associated genes. One protein that is regulated by the CREB family of transcription factors is brain-derived neurotrophic factor (BDNF), a key regulator in the conversion of E-LTP to L-LTP. BDNF can bind to a specific receptor tyrosine kinase, TrkB. This binding results in dimerization and autophosphorylation of the Trk receptors, leading to activation of the tyrosine kinases. Activated receptors in general are capable of triggering a number of signal transduction cascades including the MAPK pathway, the phosphatidylinositol 3-kinase (PI3K) pathway, and the phospholipase C-γ (PLC-γ) pathway. The signals thus generated also can pass on to the nucleus to cause further activation of transcription factors and alterations in gene expression (Lu, 2003).

PKA can also recruit MAPK to the nucleus where it can phosphorylate other kinases and transcription factors (eg: CREB) to activate gene transcription. Extra cellular signal regulated protein kinase (ERK), is a member of the mitogen-activated family of protein kinases, which play a crucial role in L-LTP. ERK activity is required to initiate the local translation of messenger RNAs (mRNAs) that are present at spines into functional proteins. Another function of ERK is its rapid translocation into the nucleus of the neuron where it phosphorylates several regulatory transcription factors. This leads to the transcription of several mRNAs that are transported along dendrites toward the spines and their synapses.

The tyrosine kinases Src and Fyn indirectly affect LTP by modulating NMDAR function. These Src family of tyrosine kinases can alter NMDAR function by phosphorylating GluN2A and 2B subunits, thereby relieving a basal zinc inhibition of the NMDAR. Phosphorylation of GluN2A or 2B thus potentiates the current through NMDAR complex. The increase in calcium concentration thus produced can contribute to the process of LTP.

Recent studies indicate that another subclass of glutamate receptors, the metabotropic glutamate receptors (mGluRs) are also involved in LTP induction (Bashir, 1993). In addition to activating ion channel-linked receptors, glutamate activates G protein-coupled metabotropic receptors which exist in eight different types labeled $mGluR_1$ to $mGluR_8$ which are classified into groups I, II, and III. Receptor types are grouped based on receptor structure and physiological activity. mGluR subtypes 1 and 5 (group I mGluRs) are positively coupled to phospholipase C (PLC), and trigger elevations in intracellular inositol triphosphate (IP3) and diacylglycerol (DAG), followed by mobilization of Ca^{2+} and activation of PKC (Benquet, 2002). Group I mGluRs are known to modulate the function of NMDAR by binding to PDZ proteins near to NMDAR (Yu, 1997). The activation of mGluRs, especially $mGluR_5$ is involved in the induction of large amplitude or long-lasting late phase LTP of AMPAR-mediated transmission induced by strong or repeated stimulation protocols (Anwyl, 2009).

3.4.1.1 Maintenance of LTP

While LTP induction involves enhancement of synaptic efficacy largely by the biochemical events of E-LTP, the long term maintenance of the potentiated state demands for stable and self-sustaining biochemical mechanisms. In the dynamic milieu of the cell where most changes are reversible, stable alterations can be brought about by changes in the size of molecular pools that are dynamically maintained or by establishment of cyclic pathways which can maintain themselves. Increased exocytosis of AMPARs to the synaptic membrane could increase the size of the AMPAR pool in the synapse thereby increasing the response of the synapse. Phosphorylation of AMPARs leads to an increase in the pool of AMPARs with increased conductivity. However sustained maintenance of the larger pools requires adjustments in the kinetics of the pathways that influence these pools. One of the molecules that had been viewed as a candidate for maintenance of the stable state is CaMKII. Theoretical analysis indicates that the pool of CaMKII molecules in the special chemical environment of the PSD acts as a bistable switch. According to this model, the activity level of kinases and phosphatases determine which kind of synaptic plasticity, LTP or LTD is induced. A switch of this kind turns on, when a threshold number of Thr^{286} sites on the kinase are phosphorylated. Thr^{286}-autophosphorylation converts CaMKII to an autonomously active 'on' state. The 'on' state of the switch can last for very long periods, because the kinase acts faster than the PSD phosphatase on Thr^{286} sites (Lisman, 2002). In the early phase of LTP, phospho-CaMKII generated will be more due to the fast activity of the kinase. Activated form of CaMKII can bind to the GluN2B subunit of the NMDAR as described earlier. This binding leads to saturation of CaMKII at very low concentration of ATP and thereby stabilizes the activity of the kinase against variations in the concentrations of ATP at synapses (Pradeep et al., 2009). This binding also leads to reduction in the rates of the phosphorylation and dephosphorylation reactions, resulting in a reduction in the amount of ATP consumed while running the simultaneous kinase and phosphatase reactions. Thereby this biochemical mechanism permits the functioning of the kinase-phosphatase switch in an energy efficient manner (Cheriyan et al., 2011). Activated CaMKII can function in enhancing AMPAR currents and its recruitment. This will contribute to the maintenance of enhanced AMPAR mediated postsynaptic response.

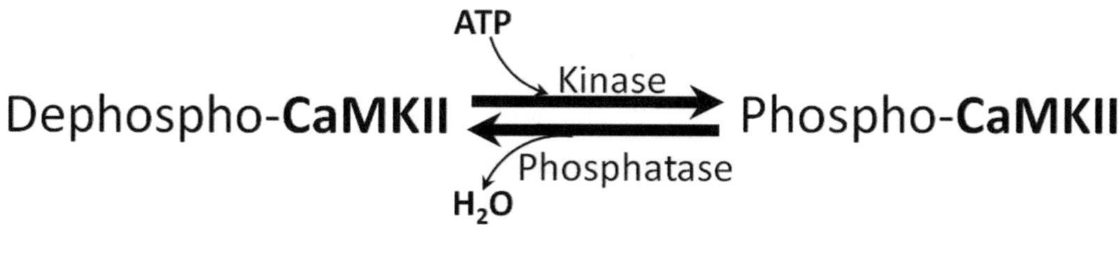

Fig. 4. CaMKII-phosphatase bistable switch model. Continuous interconversion between CaMKII and phospho-CaMKII is catalysed by the kinase activity of Thr^{286} autophosphorylated CaMKII and the phosphatase activity of PP1.

Activated PKA can also contribute to the maintenance of LTP by involving in a self-sustaining mechanism, in addition to its role in promoting AMPAR exocytosis. As described earlier, activated PKA can alter gene expression via cAMP-PKA-CREB pathway. One gene activated by CREB encodes a ubiquitin hydrolase, a component of a specific ubiquitin protease that leads to the regulated proteolysis of the regulatory subunit of PKA. This results in persistent activity of PKA, leading to persistent phosphorylation of PKA substrates such as CREB, MAPK, etc., thereby completing a self-sustaining cycle that can be stably maintained.

3.4.1.2 Synaptic tagging hypothesis

L-LTP requires *de novo* protein synthesis. The long lasting activity changes require nuclear transcription followed by delivery of newly synthesized proteins to the synapse to yield synaptic remodeling. Newly synthesized proteins delivered by non-directed transport from the cell body must be captured locally at the activated synapse in order to function in an input-specific manner (Doyle, 2011). For this, the activated synapse requires a local signal that allows it to capture proteins or mRNAs for protein-synthesis-dependent LTP or LTD. This process has been termed *synaptic tagging*. Based on this proposal, synaptic activity generates a tag, which "captures" the plasticity-related proteins (PRPs) derived outside of synapses (Lu et al., 2011). These findings indicate a tight and extensive dialogue between the synapse and the nucleus in both directions.

3.4.1.3 mRNA transport into the dendrites

mRNA localization to the synapses depends on synaptic activity and the mechanism behind this transport is largely a mystery. This transport mechanism is highly complex and involves multiple mRNA binding proteins. This process can be divided into different stages, (1) the presence of cis-acting localization elements (LEs) or zipcodes generally located in the 3′-untranslated region (3′-UTR) of localized transcripts, (2) the recognition of these signals by trans-acting RNA-binding proteins (RBPs), (3) the assembly of RBPs and their cargo

RNAs into transport ribonucleo-protein particles (RNPs) as a functional complex, (4) the translocation of transport RNPs along the microtubule (MT) cytoskeleton to their final destination at synapses in a translationally repressed state, (5) the anchoring of these particles at or underneath activated synapses in a translationally repressed state and finally (6) the activation of translation of the localized mRNAs (Doyle, 2011).

One of the specific immediately expressed candidate gene is activity-regulated cytoskeleton-associated protein (Arc). Newly synthesized Arc mRNA is targeted rapidly to synapses that have recently undergone specific forms of synaptic activity where it is locally translated. Targeting of *Arc* mRNA depends on NMDAR activity. An increase in Arc expression promotes stable expansion of the F-actin network in dendritic spines, which is believed to underlie morphological enlargement of the synapse and stable LTP (Bramham, 2010).

3.4.1.4 Spine enlargement

Most excitatory synapses in the brain terminate on dendritic spines. Spines are specialized perturbations on dendrites that contain PSD. The PSD includes receptors, channels and signaling molecules that couple synaptic activity with postsynaptic biochemistry. Spines provide a closed compartment that allows rapid changes in the concentrations of signaling molecules, such as calcium, and hereby make efficient responses to inputs possible. Long-term changes in spine morphology could contribute to the modulation of synaptic transmission that occurs in LTP. Shortening or widening the neck of a spine affects calcium influx into the dendrite. Spine enlargement depends on the structure of cytoskeletal filaments. Actin filaments of microfilaments are in close association with PSD. Reorganization of actin filament contributes to the spine enlargement process in LTP. The AMPA class of glutamate receptors has been found to have a stabilizing effect on spine morphology. Rho GTPases and their downstream effectors have an important role in regulating the cytoskeleton, and consequently in regulating spine and dendritic morphology, in response to extracellular stimulation. AMPAR activation by spontaneous glutamate release at synapses is sufficient to maintain dendritic spines (Lamprecht & LeDoux, 2004).

3.4.1.5 Presynaptic mechanisms

Activation of both pre and postsynaptic sites are necessary for the generation of LTP on the basis of Hebbian theory. Neurotransmitter release is one of the presynaptic mechanisms eliciting the induction of LTP. An increase in neuro-transmitter release can be observed together with the postsynaptic mechanisms. This is due to the activation of presynaptic terminals by some factors released by the postsynaptic compartment or cell (Williams et al., 1989). A prominent candidate for such a messenger is arachidonic acid or one of its metabolites, because these compounds can readily cross cell membranes. This can be generated by the degradation of phospholipids by the enzyme phospholipase A_2, a calcium dependent enzyme (Bliss, 1990). Nitric oxide (NO) is another retrograde messenger produced by Ca^{2+}/CaM activated nitric oxide synthase (NOS), which can activate the synthesis of cyclic GMP presynaptic terminal by activating two NO-sensitive guanylyl cyclases (NO-GCs) (NO-GC1 and NO-GC2) leading to increased neurotransmitter release. The physiological consequences of increase in NO/cGMP and the associated cellular mechanisms involved are not well understood.

3.4.2 NMDAR-independent mechanisms

Although a vast majority of studies of NMDAR dependent LTP have been conducted, there are also a few mechanisms that are independent of NMDAR that have been studied. Following section will briefly describe molecular mechanisms of NMDAR independent forms of LTP.

3.4.2.1 200 Hz LTP

NMDAR-independent forms of LTP also can be induced at the Schaffer collateral pathway in CA1. This allows for a comparison of two different types of LTP at the same synapse. NMDAR-independent LTP in CA1 can be elicited by use of four and a half seconds, 200 Hz stimuli separated by five seconds. LTP induced by this stimulation protocol is insensitive to NMDAR selective antagonist such as APV. 200 Hz LTP was shown to be blocked by nifedipine (Grover and Teyler, 1990), a voltage gated calcium channel (VGCC) blocker. This observation led to the conclusion that 200 Hz-LTP stimulation elicits sufficiently large and prolonged membrane depolarization, resulting in the opening of voltage dependent calcium channels, to trigger elevation of postsynaptic calcium sufficient to trigger LTP. It is also reported that L-type Ca^{2+} channel-dependent synaptic plasticity significantly contributes to spatial learning in the behaving mouse (Moosmang et al., 2005).

3.4.2.2 Tetra-Ethyl-Ammonium LTP

NMDAR-independent LTP at the Schaffer collateral pathway in CA1 can also be induced by the bath application of the K^+ channel blocker tetraethylammonium (TEA) (TEA-LTP) (Aniksztejn and Ben-Ari, 1991) and is referred to as LTPk. This nonspecific potassium channel blocker can cause membrane excitability. Like 200 Hz-LTP, TEA-LTP is insensitive to NMDAR antagonists, and is blocked by blockade of voltage sensitive calcium channels. The induction of LTPk is dependent on synaptic activity, as its induction is blocked by AMPAR antagonists. Similar to 200 Hz LTP, the current model for TEA-LTP is that synaptic depolarization via glutamate receptor activation, augmented by the hyperexcitable membrane due to K^+ channel blockade, leads to a relatively large and prolonged membrane depolarization. This leads to the triggering of LTP through postsynaptic calcium influx via the VGCCs.

3.4.2.3 Mossy fiber LTP in CA3

A good model system for studying NMDAR-independent LTP is the mossy fiber inputs into CA3 pyramidal neurons. The mossy fiber synapses are unique, large synapses with unusual presynaptic specializations. The mechanism will be described in later section (3.5.).

3.4.3 Chemical LTP (Chem-LTP)

Early protocols for the induction of LTP in cultures of dissociated hippocampal neurons comprised repetitive high frequency presynaptic stimulation (HFS-LTP) as mentioned above. In some cases this was coupled with postsynaptic depolarization and in others cultures were preincubated with blockers of different channels. High frequency stimulation activates only a small fraction of synapses, making it difficult to detect molecular and cellular changes associated with LTP. Most biochemical analysis and imaging studies require a high proportion of synapses to be potentiated. Therefore, a range of strategies were applied to chemically induce LTP (Chem-LTP). Chem-LTP is an alternative to high frequency stimulation and has the advantage that it can activate all the cells in the culture. One example of Chem-LTP is mentioned below.

3.4.3.1 Forskolin/rolipram-induced LTP

Forskolin/rolipram-induced LTP was predominantly used in slice cultures; it can also be applied for dissociated hippocampal neuronal cultures. This form of chemically induced, highly sensitive plasticity state is based on the increase of intracellular cAMP levels by the application of the adenylyl cyclase activator forskolin (50 μM) and the phosphodiesterase inhibitor rolipram (0.1 μM) in Mg^{2+} and 2-Cl-adenosine free artificial cerebrospinal fluid for 16 min (Otmakhov, 2004). This induction procedure is bypassing the need for synaptic activation, and by raising cAMP concentration directly activates PKA and signaling pathways that underlie synaptic plasticity. However, froskolin/rolipram-LTP still require NMDAR activation and involve the recruitment of CaMKII to dendritic spines (Molnar, 2011).

3.5 LTP in other regions of CNS

Although LTP was first described at the perforant path synapses on the neurons of the DG, subsequently most of the work on the mechanism of LTP is performed on the Schaffer collateral synapses on the CA1 pyramidal neurons.

In the CA1 region, NMDAR-mediated and NMDAR-independent LTP have been described and they are expressed mainly as postsynaptic mechanisms. Presynaptic LTP was also discovered in hippocampus and cerebellum. In hippocampus, presynaptic LTP can be observed in mossy fiber pathway. There is no need for calcium influx in the postsynaptic compartment for eliciting this form of LTP and this is NMDAR-independent. In the induction of presynaptic LTP, presynaptic calcium release is essential. R-type calcium channels are voltage dependent calcium channels that can mediate presynaptic calcium release. This calcium influx can activate several signaling pathways needed for the induction of mossy fiber LTP (MF-LTP). Both pharmacological and genetic analyses indicate that a rise in presynaptic cAMP is a crucial component. The cAMP level is enhanced by the activation of Ca^{2+}/CaM activated adenyl cyclase 1 (AC1) and leads to the activation of PKA. This PKA activation regulates key molecules needed for the enhanced neurotransmitter release (Nicoll, 2005).

3.5.1 Cerebellar LTP

In cerebellum, parallel fibres (PF) of cerebellar granule cells form synapse with Purkinje cells (PC) of Purkinje cell layer (Fig. 5). When the PF is stimulated at 4-8 Hz for 15 s, a presynaptic form of LTP is induced at PF. This shows a similar molecular mechanism as that of the mossy fiber pathway in the hippocampus. A postsynaptically expressed form of LTP was more recently described and is observed as a reversal of PF-LTD. PF–LTP can be induced by repetitive PF stimulation (1 Hz for 5 minutes) without concomitant CF activation and requires a lower calcium transient for its induction than PF-LTD (Vogt & Canepari, 2010). PF-LTP generally depends on the activation of phosphatases such as PP1, PP2A, and PP2B and is independent of activity of kinases such as CaMKII and PKC (Jorntell & Hansel, 2006). In cerebellar PCs, GluR1 expression is weak, and the majority of AMPA receptors consist of

GluR2–GluR3 heteromeric complexes. An activity dependent synaptic delivery of GluR2 has been shown during the induction of LTP in PF-PC synapses. This activity driven process involves NO-mediated binding of *N*-ethylmaleimide sensitive factor (NSF) to GluR2. In PF LTP, GluR2 synaptic delivery is also facilitated by dephosphorylation of GluR2 at Ser^{880}.

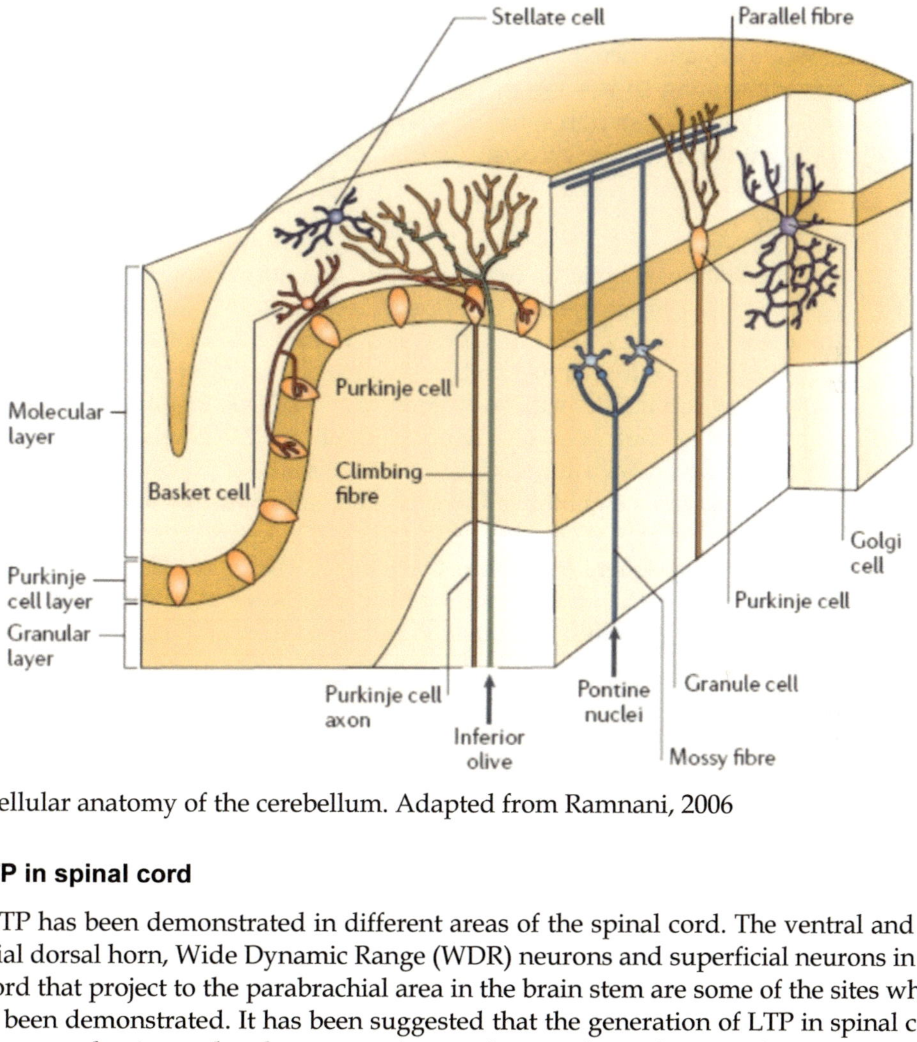

Fig. 5. Cellular anatomy of the cerebellum. Adapted from Ramnani, 2006

3.5.2 LTP in spinal cord

Spinal LTP has been demonstrated in different areas of the spinal cord. The ventral and the superficial dorsal horn, Wide Dynamic Range (WDR) neurons and superficial neurons in the spinal cord that project to the parabrachial area in the brain stem are some of the sites where LTP has been demonstrated. It has been suggested that the generation of LTP in spinal cord may be one mechanism, whereby acute pain may be transformed into a chronic pain state. LTP in superficial spinal dorsal horn involves simultaneous activation of multiple receptors like the NMDAR, the Neurokinin 1 (NK-1) receptor for substance P and mGluRs. This LTP is likely to occur in both the sensory and the affective pain pathways. LTP in deep spinal WDR neurons have a pivotal role in transmission of painful inputs. As with LTP in the superficial spinal cord, activation of the ionotrophic glutamate receptors (AMPA and NMDA subtypes) and the NK1 receptor seems crucial for the induction of LTP in deep WDR neurons (Rygh et al, 2005).

4. Long term depression

LTD is an activity dependent reduction in the efficacy of neuronal synapses. It can generally last for hours or longer. It brings about a long lasting decrease in synaptic strength. LTD can be defined as a long lasting decrease in the synaptic response of neurons to stimulation of their afferents following a long patterned stimulus (Collingrigde et al., 2010). LTD is generally considered as a reversal of LTP as it is understood that if synapses continue to increase in strength, eventually they would reach some level of maximum efficacy which might cause saturation and then they may be unable to encode new information. This would result in neurons coming to a stage of complete inactivity or over activity. LTD is also considered to be the initial step in synaptic elimination (Bastrikova et al., 2008; Beckner et al., 2008) as it is known that those synapses which lose their efficacy are eliminated.

4.1 Types of LTD

LTD can be either homosynaptic or heterosynaptic. Homosynaptic LTD is induced by a conditioning input. It is input specific. It is restricted to the individual synapse which is activated by a low frequency stimulus (LFS) i.e., it happens in the same synapse that receives the induction. It is associative and it correlates with postsynaptic activation of the neuron by an active presynaptic neuron. Homosynaptic LTD is in turn of two types. LTD which follows an LTP is often known as depotentiation. If LTD is observed from base line conditions, with low frequency stimulus, then it is *de novo* LTD. Heterosynaptic LTD refers to depression at synapses neighboring the activated ones but are not directly activated themselves (Abraham et al., 2007). Heterosynaptic LTD occurs at synapses that are not potentiated. It occurs consequent to a non-conditioning input in association with either LTP or LTD. LTD relies on both pre and postsynaptic expression mechanisms although the maintenance mechanism is not fully understood (Bliss and Cooke, 2011).

4.2 LTD in Hippocampus

Unlike LTP, LTD in hippocampus occurs when the postsynaptic cells are weakly depolarized, whereas LTP induction involves strong postsynaptic depolarization. The hippocampal LTD is governed by BCM (Bienenstock Cooper Munro) theory (Bienenstock et al., 1982). It says that the synapses that are active when the postsynaptic cells are weakly polarized undergo LTD. If APs preceed EPSPs, LTD results; i.e., unpaired stimulation causes lower calcium signals and therefore LTD.

In the CA1 region LTD is homosynaptic, and depends on NMDARs and on protein synthesis but in the DG, it is independent of NMDARs and protein synthesis and is found both as heterosynaptic and homosynaptic forms (Kemp and Vaughan, 2007).

The best understood type of LTD is induced in hippocampal area CA1 by LFS via an NMDAR dependent rise in postsynaptic intracellular calcium and the activation of a protein phosphatase cascade which will be discussed hereforth. A brief application of NMDA can also lead to depression, i.e., a form of chem-LTD. LTD is triggered by postsynaptic calcium entry, like LTP, after activation by presynaptic stimulus. The main receptors involved are AMPAR and NMDAR. If the postsynaptic depolarization by AMPAR is weak, it cannot activate NMDARs completely. The partial removal of Mg^{2+} block results in reduced Ca^{2+} entry.

Therefore instead of kinases, phosphatases get activated as they require comparatively lower Ca^{2+} concentrations for activation. The protein phosphatase activated is PP2B or calcineurin. PP2B can in turn activate PP1. PP2B dephosphorylates and inactivates Inhibitor-1. This relieves the inhibition of PP1 by Inhibitor-1 thereby activating it (Mulkey et al., 1993).

In hippocampus, plasticity is mediated by conductance changes of AMPARs which are in turn regulated by phosphorylation. The majority of AMPARs at hippocampal synapses are GluR1/GluR2 and GluR2/GluR3 heteromers. The trafficking of GluR1 plays a dominant role in plasticity. Activated PP1 brings about dephosphorylation of GluR1 at Ser^{845} (Fig. 6) and promotes AMPAR internalization (Lee et al., 2000). Inhibition of PP2B blocks GluR1 internalization and thereby LTD, suggesting the importance of phosphatase activity in LTD (Beattie et al., 2000). Targeting PP1 precisely to synapses upon NMDAR activation is crucial for LTD expression and is facilitated by PP1 binding proteins like spinophilin, neurabin, etc. (Morshita et al., 2001). In hippocampus, AMPARs are stabilized on the membrane by NSF and clathrin adaptor protein AP2, which bind to the NSF binding site on GluR2. During NMDAR-LTD, AP2 replaces NSF and this initiates AMPAR endocytosis. Clathrin mediated endocytosis of AMPARs is triggered by a neuronal calcium sensor known as hippocalcin. Upon activation, hippocalcin translocates to the plasma membrane, where it forms a complex with AP2 and GluR2 and initiates clathrin mediated AMPAR endocytosis. Protein interacting with C-kinase 1 (PICK1) is another protein that binds directly to GluR2 and it can also bind to PKC. PICK1 competes with AMPAR binding protein (ABP) and glutamate receptor interacting protein (GRIP) for binding to C-terminal of GluR2 and promotes internalization. PICK1 also helps in modifying neuronal architecture by interacting with F-actin. PP2B interacts with A-kinase anchor protein-150 (AKAP-150) which in turn interacts with PSD-95. PSD-95 further interacts with NMDAR thereby positioning PP2B near NMDAR (Bhattacharya et al., 2009). This helps in the activation of PP2B by Ca^{2+} influx through NMDARs. Activated PP2B can mediate the NMDAR-induced endocytosis of AMPARs that underlies one major form of LTD. Disruption of the interaction between PSD-95 and AKAP-150 strongly inhibited NMDAR-dependent endocytosis of AMPARs (Bhattacharya et al., 2009). Phosphorylation of Ser^{295} of PSD-95 occurs *in vivo*, and it enhances the ability of PSD-95 to accumulate in the PSD, to recruit surface AMPA receptors, and to strengthen synaptic transmission. During LTD, PSD-95 is dephosphorylated at Ser^{295} facilitating its removal from PSD. This mechanism also plays a role in the NMDAR-dependent endocytosis of AMPAR (Kim et al., 2007).

Although a major form of LTD is mediated by NMDARs, the ultimate direction of change in synaptic efficacy is brought about by changes in AMPAR function (Collingridge et al., 2010). Calcium influx through the NMDAR is central to the induction of both LTP and LTD because intracellular application of calcium chelators, such as BAPTA or EGTA, prevents induction of plasticity. Since induction of LTP and LTD are controlled by the postsynaptic NMDAR, any presynaptic component of expression requires a retrograde messenger that can signal to the presynaptic terminal that coincidence has occurred. Two candidates are nitric oxide (NO) and endocannabinoids (eCB) (Bliss & Cook, 2011). *N*-arachidonylethanolamine (AEA) and 2-arachidonoylglycerol (2-AG) are two major eCBs that activate type I cannabinoid receptors (CB1) receptors on the presynaptic neuron in the brain (Di Marzo et al., 1998). Upon stimulation, eCBs are released from postsynaptic neurons and travel across the synaptic cleft to activate CB1 on presynaptic terminals, resulting in depression of synaptic transmission.

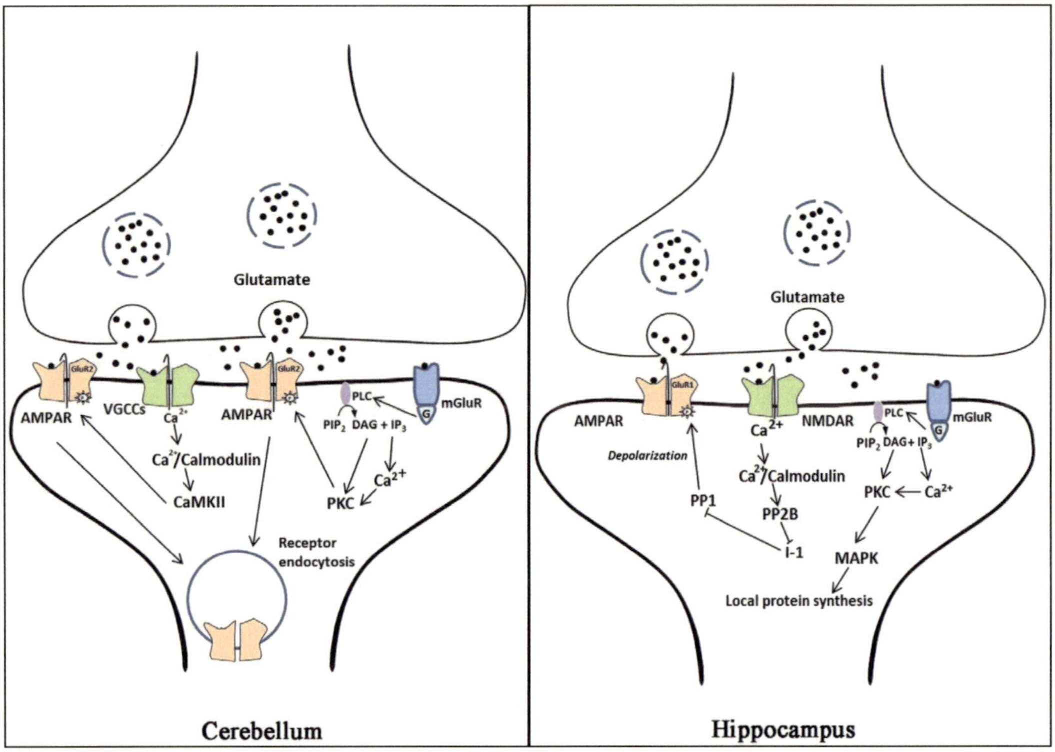

Fig. 6. Mechanisms of LTD induction in hippocampus and cerebellum. Key signaling pathways that lead to LTD in hippocampus and in cerebellum involve AMPAR regulation. Hippocampal LTD involves activation of phosphatases like PP2B and PP1 which dephosphorylate GluR1 resulting in reduced AMPAR conductance, whereas in cerebellum, kinases like CaMKII and PKC are activated resulting in GluR2 phosphorylation and thereby causing AMPAR endocytosis and reduced current.

Of the NMDARs, GluN2B containing NMDARs are supposed to be important for LTD especially in hippocampus as a study using conditional knockout mice showed that the selective ablation of GluN2B subunits in pyramidal neurons in CA1 specifically impairs CA1 NMDAR-LTD. This also results in deficits in several hippocampal dependent learning and memory tasks, providing strong evidence for a key role of this particular from of LTD in memory formation. (Brigman et al., 2010; Collingridge et al., 2010). BDNF is released from glutamatergic neurons in response to high frequency stimulus and is found to have a role in LTP. While BDNF affects synaptic potentiation at hippocampal synapses, proBDNF is involved in LTD. proBDNF, by activating its receptor known as the p75 neurotrophin receptor ($p75^{NTR}$), facilitates hippocampal (LTD). Deletion of $p75^{NTR-/-}$ in mice selectively impaired the NMDAR dependent LTD, without affecting other forms of synaptic plasticity. $p75^{NTR-/-}$ mice also showed a decrease in the expression of GluN2B, an NMDA receptor subunit uniquely involved in LTD. $p75^{NTR-/-}$ mice showed a decrease in the expression of GluN2B in the hippocampus and also a marked reduction in GluN2B-mediated currents at the CA1 synapse. Activation of $p75^{NTR}$ by proBDNF enhanced GluN2B dependent LTD and GluN2B mediated synaptic currents. (Woo et al., 2005).

The events described above depict the importance of GluN2B subunit in LTD. It is also known that CaMKII can phosphorylate GluN2B at Ser^{1303}, both *in vitro* and *in vivo* (Omkumar et al., 1996). This phosphorylation prevents the binding of CaMKII to GluN2B *in vitro* (Strack et al., 2000; O'Leary et al., 2011). Studies from our lab have shown that the phosphorylation status at Ser^{1303} enables GluN2B to distinguish between the Ca^{2+}/CaM activated form and autonomously active Thr^{286}-autophosphorylated form of CaMKII. This highlights the need for a dephosphorylation mechanism at GluN2B-Ser^{1303}. It has been shown that phosphatases in PSD can dephosphorylate GluN2B-Ser^{1303} (Rajeevkumar et al., 2009). Although the physiological role of GluN2B-Ser^{1303} is not known to date, it is likely to be involved in LTD mechanism as phosphatases get activated during induction of LTD.

Another major form of LTD worth mentioning is the one which is dependent on group 1 metabotropic glutamate receptors (mGluR). Chemical LTD is typically induced by activation of mGlu receptors. The most commonly induced chemical LTD is by (*S*)-3, 5-dihydroxyphenylglycine (DHPG), an agonist of mGluR, one which is effective even in the absence of Ca^{2+}. Normally mGluR-LTD is induced in CA1 synapses by a train of LFS consisting of single pulses. The mGluR antagonist α-methyl-4-caboxyphenylglycine (MCPG) blocked depotentiation and *de novo* LTD in CA1 showing the involvement of mGluR in LTD (Bolshakow et al., 1994).

Glutamate binding to mGluR initiates a signaling cascade, involving the breakdown of the membrane lipid PIP2 (Phosphoinositol 4, 5 - bisphosphate) by phospholipase C (PLC) to the important signaling molecules IP3 (Inositol 1, 4, 5 - triphosphate). This also causes release of diacylglycerol (DAG) and calcium mobilization. This leads to the activation of the calcium sensitive kinase, PKC. This enzyme then phosphorylates AMPAR but in such a manner that the conductance is reduced (Bliss et al., 2011). An offshoot is the production of NO, the retrograde messenger. Group I mGluRs (mGluR1/5) activate PLC, leading to Ca^{2+} mobilization, and activation of the ERK–MAPK pathway through which they modulate signals of synapse-to-nucleus communication and triggers protein synthesis. mGluR1 and mGluR2 receptor subtypes mediate *de novo* LTD at cerebellar PF-PC synapses and hippocampal mossy fibre synapses respectively.

mGluRs are the critical regulators of activity-dependent protein synthesis in dendrites. Signaling by mGluR1/5 is critical to synaptic circuitry formation during development and is implicated in LTD (Zukin et al., 2009). mGluR1/5 elicit synapse specific modifications in synaptic strength and spine morphology by stimulating rapid local translation of dendritic mRNAs including *Fmr1*, that encodes fragile X mental retardation protein (FMRP) (Greenough et al., 2001). Expression of mGluR-LTD at Schaffer collateral to CA1 pyramidal cell synapses is mediated by persistent internalization of AMPARs and in adolescent mice requires *de novo* protein synthesis (Huber et al., 2000; Snyder et al., 2001). But mGluR-LTD at cortical synapses (Desai et al., 2006) requires neither local protein synthesis nor FMRP function. mGluR-LTD is also seen in CA1 in neonates and is protein synthesis dependent. (Nosyreva & Huber, 2005).

PICK1 is also required for mGluR-LTD at different synapses. mGluRs are associated with protein tyrosine phosphatases rather than Ser/Thr ones. DHPG, a potent agonist of mGluR, induced LTD that involves tyrosine dephosphorylation of GluA2 and is associated with AMPARs endocytosis (Gladding et al., 2009). DHPG-induced LTD appears not to require extracellular Ca^{2+} (Fitzjohn et al., 2001). It also doesn't require CaMKII. Certain other proteins which are activated by mGluRs are arg 3.1(Arc), striatal-enriched protein tyrosine phosphatase (STEP) and microtubule associated protein 1B which are involved in AMPAR internalization (Collingridge et al., 2010).

4.3 LTD in cerebellum

Cerebellum is involved in motor learning and non-declarative memory. It is required in the adaptation of vestibulo ocular reflex (VOR) movements of the eyes needed to keep the retinal image stable. In the 1980s, Ito and colleagues provided the first experimental evidence for plasticity in the cerebellar cortex.

Of the three layers of cerebellum; the molecular layer, granular layer and the Purkinje layer, the Purkinje cells synapse on deep cerebellar nuclei which are the major output from the cerebellum (Bear et al., 2001). Purkinje cells modify the output. Purkinje cells receive excitatory input from two sources, viz, climbing fibre (CF) and parallel fibre (PF). Each Purkinje cell receives input from one inferior olive cell (which arises from medulla) via CF and this input is very powerful. This generates a very large EPSP that always strongly activates the postsynaptic Purkinje cells. The other input to the Purkinje cells, viz the PF arises from cerebellar granule (CG) cells. The CG cells in turn receive mossy fibres which arise from precerebellar nuclei. Purkinje cells receive synapses from more than one PF. The plasticity at PF-PC synapse is governed by Marr Albus (Marr, 1969; Albus, 1971) theory which explains the mechanism behind motor learning. It says that the plasticity of the PF synapse is effective if it is active at the same time as the CF input to the Purkinje cell. Activating CF results in massive calcium influx. Despite the large calcium influx, paired CF and PF stimulation results in LTD in Purkinje cells (Ito et al., 1982), whereas PF stimulation alone causes LTP (Lev Ram et al., 2002).

CF stimulation results in large input of EPSP. As a result voltage gated sodium channels open causing massive depolarization. This activates VGCCS, facilitating calcium entry. At the same time, the activation of PF results in glutamate release which binds to AMPA receptor and allows sodium ion entry. Altering AMPAR affects synaptic efficacy by changing the channel density. The other receptor activated is mGluR. It activates the release of downstream second messengers such as DAG and results in activation of PKC. αCaMKII is also activated along with PKC (Hansel, 2006). These kinases can phosphorylate the AMPAR. PKC can phosphorylate GluR2, the subunit of AMPAR at Ser^{-880} and this brings about receptor endocytosis (Chung et al., 2003). It is a critical event in the induction of cerebellar LTD (Fig. 6). This phosphorylation disrupts the binding of GluR2 to GRIP1 facilitating binding to PICK1 (Xia et al., 2000). Purkinje cells are enriched with GluR2/GluR3 receptors whereas it is poor in expressing GluR1 subunits. Purkinje cells lack NMDAR and thus LTD is mainly AMPAR mediated. The cerebellar LTD is the type of plasticity where information is stored as a decrease in the effectiveness of synaptic connection.

It is interesting to see that the LTP and LTD induction cascades in hippocampus and cerebellar Purkinje synapses are different and exhibit a mirror image like relationship (Jorntell & Hansel, 2006). As already discussed, LTD in cerebellum, is being brought about by kinases whereas in hippocampus it is brought about by phosphatases.

4.4 LTD induction

LTD can be induced by prolonged periods of LFS by pairing baseline synaptic stimulation with depolarization i.e. normally at a frequency of 10 Hz. LFS of 1 Hz for 15 minutes brings about LTD in CA1 area of hippocampus of anaesthetized rabbit (Bliss & Lomo, 1973). This stimulation is preceded by baseline stimulation at frequencies such as 0.1–0.05 Hz to establish a reference level for basal synaptic transmission. Electrically induced LTD is typically generated by low frequency stimulation (in the range of 1-3 Hz) given for prolonged periods of time (5–15 min) (Braunewell et al., 2001). Coincident EPSPs with action potentials (APs) evokes large calcium signals and leads to LTP whereas unpaired stimulation brings about LTD (Markram et al., 1997). LTD, like LTP possess the characteristics of longevity, input-specificity and associativity. The relative contributions of pre and postsynaptic mechanisms may vary at different times after induction and also across different classes of synapses. In cerebellum, PF-LTD can be induced by paired PF and CF stimulation (Ito et al., 1982), which is typically applied at 1–4 Hz for 5 min.

4.5 Physiological functions of LTD

Elucidating the functional role of LTD *in vivo* has been challenging due to difficulty of inducing it *in vivo* and due to the lack of selective inhibitors for the same (Collingridge et al., 2010). But still some of the physiological functions of LTD are known.

LTD has been implicated in cerebellar motor learning. For example, studies using PKC transgenic mice showed that chronic PKC inhibition restricted to cerebellar PF-PC synapses exhibited compromised LTD and defective adaptation of VOR. But still a causal relationship remains to be demonstatred between PF-PC LTD and motor learning (De Zeeuw et al., 1998). To the contrary, recent studies using knockout mice which target the expression of PF-PC LTD by blocking internalization of AMPARs show that LTD is not necessary for motor learning. The mutant mice lacked PF-PC LTD but had no difficulty in performing motor learning skills like VOR adaptation, eyeblink conditioning, and locomotion learning on the Erasmus Ladder which covers a wide range of cerebellar learning behaviors (Schonewille et al., 2011).

LTD is implicated in hippocampus dependent learning because of its property of depotentiation. Depotentiation in CA1 and DG has been shown when rats explore a novel environment or a familiar environment containing novel objects. Impairment of reversal learning in water maze was found to be associated with severely impaired hippocampal LTD in dopamine transporter knockout mice. LTD is also involved in learning regarding novelty detection. In freely moving rats, LTD is facilitated during exploration of complex environments containing novel objects (Collingridge et al., 2010).

The various molecular mechanisms involved in LTD in brain have been discussed. LTD has been implicated in several physiological processes including learning and memory and also in development of visual system. Future studies will be focused on the aspects of protein synthesis and turnover involved in LTD in detail. Also the mechanisms by which LTD could be induced by neurotransmitters other than glutamate remains to be elucidated. (Collingridge et al., 2010).

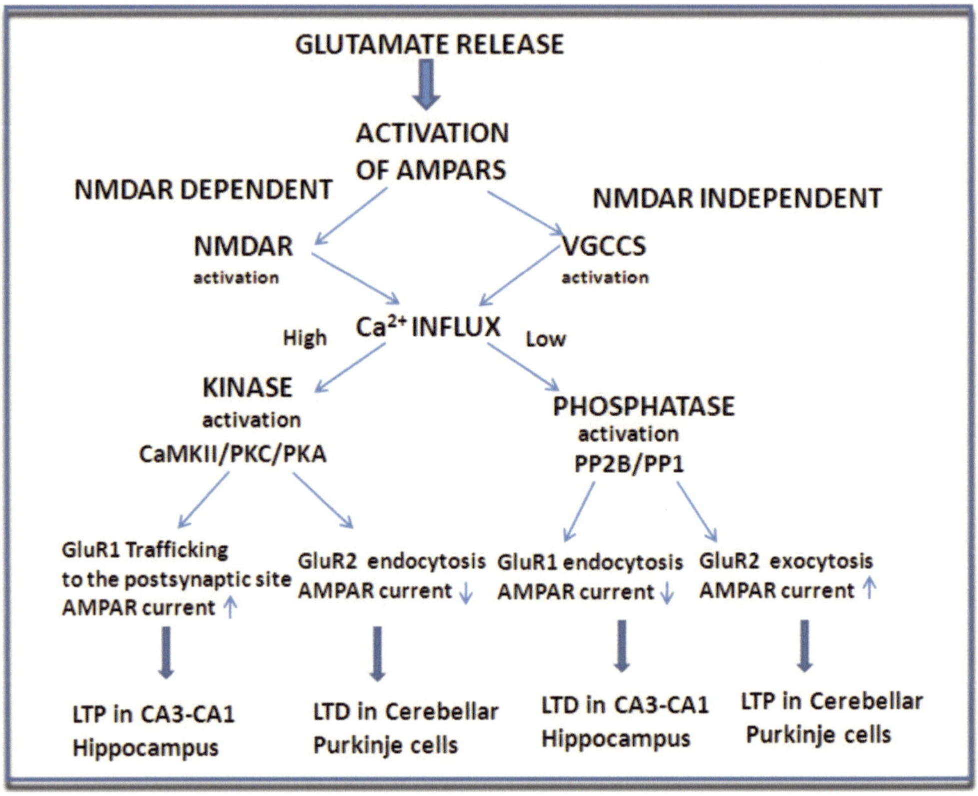

Fig. 7. Scheme of shared post synaptic signaling pathways leading to LTP and LTD

5. Synaptic plasticity and disease

In disease conditions, aberrant synaptic plasticity or any defect in signaling mechanism may cause substantial deficits in different aspects of central nervous system. The role of synaptic plasticity in disease is becoming more evident across a wide range of CNS disorders. Understanding the molecular basis of normal and diseased plasticity will provide a platform to study the molecular basis of many of the diseases and to target drugs on plasticity related molecules to treat many of the CNS disorders. Cognitive deficits are the early symptoms that appear much before the onset of neuritic dystrophy and pathology. Often, it is likely that the immediate consequence of aberrant signaling could be impairment of synaptic plasticity. This would later develop into synaptic and neuronal loss. Thus plasticity related mechanisms could have the advantage of being targets for early therapeutic intervention in CNS disorders.

Among the CNS disorders such as Alzheimer's disease (AD), schizophrenia, epilepsy and in disorders associated with learning disabilities where there are alterations of synaptic plasticity, Alzheimer's disease has been extensively studied.

5.1 Alzheimer's disease

Hippocampus, amygdala, neocortex, anterior thalamus, entrohinal, and transentrohinal cortices are some of the areas affected in Alzheimers disease (Sweatt, 2010). Synapse loss that starts even at early stages of AD, results in a condition where minimum number of synapses are not available for cortical networks and impairment of synaptic plasticity occurs. The neuropathological hallmarks of Alzheimer's disease are the presence of intracellular neurofibrillary tangles (NFT) composed of hyperphosphorylated tau protein and extracellular neuritic plaques composed of amyloid β protein (Aβ) (Montoya, 2011). Aβ is produced by the sequential cleavage of amyloid precursor protein (APP) by β-secretase and γ-secretase (Haass & Selkoe, 1993). 40-residue Aβ (Aβ40) and 42-residue Aβ (Aβ42) are the most common isoforms of Aβ (Xia, 2010). Even before plaques could be observed, significant deficits in synaptic transmission have been detected by electrophysiological recordings from the hippocampus of transgenic mice over expressing APP (Hsia et al., 1999; Mucke et al., 2000). Thus aberrations in synaptic function are the early events followed by the formation of plaques and NFT (Funato et al., 1999; Hartl et al., 2008; Selkoe, 2002; Walsh & Selkoe, 2004, as cited in Proctor et al., 2011).

5.1.1 Disruption of the plasticity of glutamatergic synaptic transmission

The alterations of synaptic plasticity which happens before synaptic loss may be initiating neurodegeneration. The spatial working memory and LTP were normal in young $APP_{695}SWE$ transgenic mice. There was reduction in LTP and deficits in behavioural performance with aged transgenic mice. The deterioration of LTP in dentate gyrus and CA1 and behavioural deficit appear in a correlated manner (Chapman et al., 1999). Aβ concentrations increased with age. Many lines of investigations show that oligomeric forms of Aβ species interfere with synaptic plasticity, inhibit LTP and impairs maintenance of LTP (Barghorn et al., 2005; Klyubin et al., 2008; Shankar et al., 2008; Walsh et al., 2002; Wang et al., 2002; Stephan et al., 2001). Aβ peptide when applied before and during HFS inhibits LTP induction in the dentate medial perforant path and Schaffer colllateral-CA1 pathway (Chen et al., 2000; Chen et al., 2002). The basal synaptic transmission or short-term synaptic plasticity remained intact. Aβ inhibits maintenance phase of L-LTP and also inhibits protein synthesis in the L-LTP phase when applied after HFS. The effects of Aβ on the induction of LTP and on L-LTP are independent of each other, working through multiple mechanisms (Chen et al., 2002). Different forms of LTP affected by Aβ will be reflected as deficits in different phases of memory and also at a concentration of Aβ, below that is required to produce neurotoxicity (Chen et al., 2002).

5.1.2 Molecular events causing disruption of LTP

Aβ was shown to increase intracellular Ca^{2+} concentrations due to potentiation of currents through L-type Ca^{2+} channels (Ueda et al., 1997) and blockade of fast-inactivating K^+ channels that leads to prolonged membrane depolarization and Ca^{2+} influx (Good et al., 1996). Basal synaptic transmission and NMDAR-dependent forms of LTP are impaired in the aging hippocampus (Foster & Norris, 1997), which correlates with deficits in spatial memory (Barnes & McNaughton, 1985; Diana et al., 1995). Aβ induced Ca^{2+} transients activate calcineurin and cause desensitization of NMDAR channels, reducing Ca^{2+} influx through these channels during LTP-inducing stimulus protocol. As a result induction of NMDAR-dependent forms of LTP, E-LTP and also L-LTP are suppressed (Chen et al., 2002). Aβ also inhibited NMDAR mediated EPSCs. Activated calcineurin could impair the mechanisms underlying the components of L-LTP and long-term memory. This could be related to early signs of memory deficits of AD. Under the influence of Aβ oligomers, activation of ERK, MAPK, CaMKII and Akt/PKB were reduced during LTP (Selkoe, 2008; Zeng et al., 2010). In Alzheimer's disease mouse models, erratic regulation of *Arc* expression leads to synaptic dysfunction (Shepherd & Bear, 2011).

NMDAR dependent neocortical plasticity deficits were observed in AD patients (Battaglia et al., 2007). Nanomolar concentrations of Aβ reduced the NMDAR-mediated EPSCs in hippocampal slices (Li et al., 2009; Cerpa et al., 2010, as cited in Hu et al., 2011). In APP transgenic mice, there is lower level of cell surface NMDA receptors. Hence, Aβ peptide may be promoting the endocytosis of NMDA receptors. NMDA receptor endocytosis also requires α-7-nicotinic receptors (nAChRs), PP2B and the STEP tyrosine phosphatase. Autopsy tissues of AD patients show a reduction in the NMDAR subunit levels. PP2B is activated, when Aβ oligomers bind and activate α-7-nicotinic receptors. Tyrosine phosphatase STEP is activated by PP2B-mediated dephosphorylation. Dephosphorylation of Y1472 of GluN2B by the activated STEP removes NMDAR from surface. In both AD transgenic mouse models and in the brains of AD subjects increased levels of STEP were detected (Chin et al., 2005; Kurup et al., 2010, as cited in Proctor et al., 2011). Aβ induced changes in LTP could be due to disruption of plasticity mechanism as a result of NMDAR changes. Postsynaptic protein tyrosine kinase EphB2, a regulator of NMDAR trafficking, is cleaved on binding to Aβ and this promotes the removal of synaptic NMDARs (Cissé et al., 2011). Stimulation of inducible nitric oxide synthase (iNOS), superoxide production and activation of microglia, all by Aβ, may also inhibit NMDAR dependent LTP (Wang et al., 2004). The density of dendritic spines decrease and the active synapses are reduced when exposed to physiological concentration of Aβ. Electrophysiological experiments show that decrease in spine density can be correlated to the loss of excitatory synapses (Selkoe, 2008). Aβ requires the activity of NMDA receptors to bring about morphological changes of the dendrite (Shankar et al., 2007).

An increase in Aβ concentration can decrease AMPA receptor-mediated EPSCs or field EPSPs. Aβ binds to GluA2 containing AMPA receptors and causes the endocytosis of AMPARs in a clathrin-dependent, calcineurin and densin mediated pathway (Liu et al., 2010, as cited in Hu et al., 2011). High concentrations of Aβ also induce phosphorylation of GluA2-Ser^{880} by PKC and subsequent internalization of the receptor. Caspase-3 cleavage of calcineurin facilitates postsynaptic GluA1 dephosphorylation and internalization in the cultured hippocampal neurons from transgenic mouse. This observation was supplemented by hippocampal-dependent contextual fear conditioning (CFC) deficit shown by transgenic AD mouse model and an alteration in basic glutamatergic synaptic transmission and enhanced LTD. The reduced AMPAR-mediated currents are associated with the lower number of AMPAR at the synapse (D'Amelio et al., 2011). The trafficking and anchoring of AMPA and NMDA receptors are disturbed by hyperphosphorylated tau also (Hoover et al., 2010, as cited in Hu et al., 2011).

Aβ is found to be attached to hippocampal neurons and its presence could be seen on dendritic surfaces (Gong et al., 2003). Synapse elimination associated with decrease in size of the synapse can be linked with degradation of the PSD proteinaceous network (Gong & Lippa, 2010). The number and compartmentalization of NMDA and AMPA receptors in PSD are determined by PSD-95, and other scaffolding proteins. PSD-95 and SAP102 are found to be altered in the susceptible regions of AD brain (Gylys et al., 2004; Leuba et al., 2008a, 2008b, as cited in Proctor et al., 2011). The lower levels of NMDA and AMPA receptors can be due to the depletion of PSD-95 from PSD, altering interactions between glutamate receptors and scaffolding proteins. This could possibly be one of the mechanisms leading to the disruption of LTP. AMPA receptors are removed from the synapse by binding to scaffolding protein AKAP-150 and PSD-95 (Bhattacharyya et al., 2009, as cited in Proctor et al., 2011) as seen in LTD. In APP transgenic mouse model loss of AMPARs are seen. The changes in LTP, integrity of spine and reduced NMDAR expression could all be due to the Aβ induced disruption in AMPAR trafficking and expression, as AMPAR regulation is important for NMDAR-dependent LTP (Proctor et al., 2011).

Elevated Aβ blocks neuronal glutamate uptake at synapse, the outcome of which is an increased glutamate at synaptic cleft (Li et al., 2009). This may lead to the activation of extra or perisynaptic NMDAR promoting LTD. The activation of perisynaptic mGluRs may also be involved in the facilitation of LTD by Aβ. The pathway for Aβ induced LTD induction involves an initial synaptic activation of NMDAR by glutamate followed by synaptic NMDAR desensitization, NMDAR and AMPAR internalization, and activation of perisynaptic NMDARs and mGluRs (Hsieh et al., 2006; Li et al., 2009, as cited in Palop and Mucke, 2010). In patients with Alzheimer's disease, glycogen synthase kinase (GSK3β) deregulation due to its increased expression causes reactivation of NMDAR-LTD, which leads to synaptic loss (Collingridge et al., 2010). Hence Aβ induced LTP deficits seem to depend on activation of LTD pathways.

In the dentate gyrus, at medial perforant path synapses on the dentate granule cells, paired-pulse facilitation (PPF) and LTP are impaired in mouse transgenic model of AD (Palop et al., 2007; Harris et al., 2010). Tau reduction eliminates abnormalities in synaptic transmission and plasticity in hippocampal subfields of hAPPJ20 mice (Palop et al., 2007; Harris et al., 2010; Roberson et al., 2011). Phosphorylation of tau by GSK3 modulates the pathway by which Aβ exerts its pathogenic downstream effects on LTP. This is similar to the Aβ mediated neurodegeneration (Tackenberg & Brandt, 2009). The absence of tau prevents the synaptic dysfunction induced by Aβ (Shipton et al., 2011).

5.2 Synaptic plasticity and other diseases

Other diseases conditions where impairments in synaptic plasticity were observed are schizophrenia, Fragile X Syndrome (Lauterborn et al., 2007; Connor et al., 2011, as cited in Kumar, 2011), Parkinson's disease (Bagetta et al., 2010, as cited in Kumar, 2011), Down syndrome (Costa and Grybko, 2005; Siarey et al., 2005, as cited in Kumar, 2011), Rett syndrome (Moretti et al., 2006; Weng et al., 2011, as cited in Kumar, 2011), Huntington's disease (Usdin et al., 1999; Murphy et al., 2000; Lynch et al., 2007, as cited in Kumar, 2011), Niemann-Pick disease type C (Zhou et al., 2011, as cited in Kumar, 2011), Rubinstein-Taybi syndrome (Alarcon et al., 2004, as cited in Kumar, 2011), brain inflammation (Min et al., 2009; Lynch, 2010, as cited in Kumar, 2011), glioma (Wang et al., 2010, as cited in Kumar, 2011) and diabetes (Biessels et al., 1996; Kamal et al., 1999, 2000, 2005; Valastro et al., 2002; Artola et al., 2005; Artola, 2008, as cited in Kumar, 2011).

Schizophrenia is caused by abnormal synaptic regulation. Six genes identified for schizophrenia (Harrison & Weinberger, 2005) encode for proteins involved in synaptic plasticity and its modulation (Stephan, 2006). Neurophysiological studies have reported *in vivo* disturbances of cortical plasticity and excitability in schizophrenia patients. Paired associative stimulation (PAS) induced LTP-like plasticity was disrupted and these plasticity deficits were indicated to be caused by NMDAR abnormalities in schizophrenia patients (Frantseva et al., 2008). Dysfunction of glutamatergic transmission is associated with the pathophysiological state in schizophrenia and this will lead to disturbed plasticity and neurotoxicity (Hasan et al., 2011; Konradi and Heckers, 2003; Paz, 2008).

Hippocampal LTP in CA1 area was greatly reduced in epilepsy. This reduction was associated with altered dendritic morphology and reduced hippocampal non-spatial memory seen in epileptic mouse model (Sgobio et al., 2010). The composition of ionotropic glutamate receptors in the PSD was found to be altered in brain areas where seizure activity is more pronounced (Wyneken et al., 2003). Application of low frequency stimulation to depoteniate the hyperexcitable synapses were found to be effective in epileptic patients (Tergau et al., 1999).

In drug addiction and fear conditioning related to post traumatic stress disorder, normal LTP and learning are responsible for the undesired condition (Mahan and Ressler, 2011). The impairment of hippocampus-dependent memory retrieval under acute stress condition is mediated by hippocampal LTD (Collingridge et al., 2010). In Fragile X syndrome (FXS), FMRP, is mutated and acts as a negative regulator of *Arc* translation. The dysregulated expression of *Arc* may alter plasticity (Shepherd & Bear, 2011).

A plethora of information thus provide concrete evidence that impairment of synaptic plasticity in diseases can contribute to decline in learning and memory.

6. Conclusion

Although a great deal has been learnt regarding the mechanisms that operate during synaptic plasticity, a complete description of the molecular basis of synaptic plasticity that underlies higher brain functions such as learning and memory is yet to be accomplished. While there is strong experimental support for changes in AMPAR activity as a major post synaptic mechanism supporting plasticity at synapses, the role of presynaptic mechanisms is less understood. The diversity in the mechanisms across different brain regions and across different species is a major challenge towards providing a mechanistic explanation of synaptic plasticity. Understanding the deviations in synaptic plasticity mechanisms in diseases may reveal new targets for the early therapeutic intervention in CNS disorders.

7. References

Abraham, W. C., Logan, B., Greenwood, J. M. & Dragunow, M. (2002). Induction and experience-dependent consolidation of stable long-term potentiation lasting months in the hippocampus. *J. Neurosci.,* Vol.22, No.21, pp. 9626-34.

Abraham, W. C., Logan, B., Wolf, A. & Benuskova, L. (2007). "Heterosynaptic" LTD in the Dentate Gyrus of Anesthetized Rat Requires Homosynaptic Activity. *J. Neurophysiol.,* Vol.98, pp. 1048–1051.

Albus, J. S. (1971). A theory of cerebellar function. *Math. Biosci.* Vol.10, pp. 25-61.

Ankisztejn, L. & Ben-Ari, Y. (1991). Novel form of long-term potentiation produced by a K+ channel blocker in the hippocampus. *Nature,* Vol.349, No.6304, pp. 67-9.

Anwyl, R. (2009). Metabotropic glutamate receptor-dependent long-term potentiation. *Neuropharmacology,* Vol.56, No. 4, pp.735-40.

Barghorn, S., Nimmrich, V., Striebinger, A., Krantz, C., Keller, P., Janson, B., Bahr, M., Schmidt, M., Bitner, R. S, Harlan, J., Barlow, E., Ebert, U. & Hillen, H. (2005). Globular amyloid beta-peptide oligomer—a homogenous and stable neuropathological protein in Alzheimer's disease. *J. Neurochem.,* Vol.95, pp834–847.

Barnes, C. A. & McNaughton, B. L. (1985). An age comparison of the rates of acquisition and forgetting spatial information in relation to long-term enhancement of hippocampal synapses. *Behavioral Neuroscience,* Vol.99, pp. 1040–1048.

Barria, A. & Malinow, R. (2005). NMDA receptor subunit composition controls synaptic plasticity by regulating binding to CaMKII. *Neuron,*Vol.48, pp. 289-301.

Barria, A., Muller, D., Derkach, V., Griffith, L. C. & Soderling, T. R. (1997b). Regulatory phosphorylation of AMPA-type glutamate receptors by CaM-KII during long-term potentiation. *Science,* Vol.276, No.5321, pp. 2042-5.

Bashir, Z. I., Jane, D. E., Sunter, D. C., Watkins, J. C. & Collingridge, G. L. (1993). Metabotropic glutamate receptors contribute to the induction of long-term depression in the CA1 region of the hippocampus. *Eur. J. Parmacol.,* Vol.239, No.1-3, pp. 265-6.

Bastrikova, N., Gardner, G. A., Reece, J. M., Jeromin, A. & Dudek, S. M. (2008). Synapse elimination accompanies functional plasticity in hippocampal neurons. *Proc. Natl. Acad. Sci., U S A.,* Vol.105, pp. 3123–3127.

Battaglia, F., Wang, H. Y., Ghilardi, M. F., Gashi, E., Quartarone, A., Friedman, E. & Nixon, R. A. (2007). Cortical plasticity in Alzheimer's disease in humans and rodents. *Biol. Psychiatr.,* Vol.62, pp. 1405–1412, ISSN 0006-3223.

Bear, M. F., Connors, B. W. & Paradiso, M. A. (2001). *Neuroscience Exploring the Brain,* (second edition), Lippincott, Williams and Wilkins, 0-683-30596-4, USA.

Beattie, E. C., Carroll, R. C., Yu, X., Morishita, W., Yasuda, H., von Zastrow, M. & Malenka, R.C. (2000). Regulation of AMPA receptor endocytosis by a signaling mechanism shared with LTD. *Nat. Neurosci.,* Vol.3, pp. 1291–1300.

Becker, N., Wierenga, C. J., Fonseca, R., Bonhoeffer, T. & Nägerl, U. V. (2008). LTD induction causes morphological changes of presynaptic boutons and reduces their contacts with spines. *Neuron,* Vol.60, pp. 590–597.

Bhattacharya, S., Biou, V., Xu, W., Shluter, O. & Malenka, R. C. (2009). A critical role for PSD-95/AKAP interactions in endocytosis of synaptic AMPA receptors. *Nat. Neurosci.,* Vol.12, Issue 2, pp. 172-181.

Bienestock, E. L., Cooper, L. N. & Munro, P. W. (1982). Theory for the development of neuron selectivity: orientation specificity and binocular interaction in visual cortex. *J. Neurosci.,* Vol.2, pp .32-48.

Bliss, T. V. (1990). Long-term potentiation. *Science,* Vol.249, No.4972, pp. 973.

Bliss, T. V. & Cooke, S. F. (2011). Long-term potentiation and long-term depression: a clinical perspective. *Clinics,* Vol.66(S1), pp. 3-17.

Bliss, T. V. & Collingridge, G. L. (1993). A synaptic model of memory: Long-term potentiation in the hippocampus. *Nature,* Vol.361, No.6407, pp. 31-9.

Bliss, T. V. & Lomo, T. (1973). Long-lasting potentiation of synaptic transmission in the dentate area of the anaesthetized rabbit following stimulation of the perforant path. *J. Physiol.,* Vol.232, No.2, pp. 331-56.

Blundon, J. A. & Zakharenko, S. S. (2008). Dissecting the components of long-term potentiation. *Neuroscientist,* Vol.14, No.6, pp. 598-608.

Bolshakow, V. Y & Siegelbaum, S. A. (1994). Postsynaptic induction and presynaptic expression of hippocampal long term depression. *Science,* Vol.264, pp. 1148-1152.

Bramham, C. R., Alme, M. N., Bittins, M., Kuipers, S. D., Nair, R. R., Pai, B., Panja, D., Schubert, M. & Soule, J. (2010). The *Arc* of synaptic memory. *Exp. Brain Res,* Vol.200, pp. 125-140.

Braunewell, K. H. & Manahan-Vaughan, D. (2001). Long-term depression: a cellular basis for learning? *Rev. Neurosci.,* Vol.12, pp. 121–140.

Brigman, J. L., Wright, T., Talani, G., Mulcare, S. P., Jinde, S., Seabold, G. K., Mathu, P., Davis, M. I., Bock, R., Gustin, R. M., Colbran, R. J., Alvarez, V. A., Nakazawa, K., Delpire, E., Lovinger, D. M. & Holmes,A. (2010). Loss of GluN2B-Containing NMDA Receptors in CA1 Hippocampus and Cortex Impairs Long-Term Depression, Reduces Dendritic Spine Density, and Disrupts Learning. *J. Neurosci.,* Vol.30, No.13, pp. 4590–4600.

Bryne, J. H. & Roberts, J. L. (2009). *From Molecules to Networks, An Introduction to Cellular and Molecular Neuroscience,* (Ed.2). Elsevier, ISBN 978-0-12-374132-5, China.

Chapman, P. F., White, G. L., Jones, M. W., Cooper-Blacketer, D., Marshall, V. J., Irizarry, M., Younkin, L., Good, M. A., Bliss, T. V. P. & Hyman, B. T. (1999). Impaired synaptic plasticity and learning in aged amyloid precursor protein transgenic mice. *Nat. Neurosci.,* Vol.l2, pp. 271-276.

Chen, Q. S., Kagan, B. L., Hirakura, Y. & Xie, C. W. (2000). Impairment of hippocampal long-term potentiation by Alzheimer amyloid beta-peptides. *Journal of Neuroscience Research,* Vol.60, pp. 65–72.

Chen, Q. S., Wei, W. Z., Shimahara, T. & Xie, C. W. (2002). Alzheimer amyloid beta peptide inhibits the late phase of long-term potentiation through calcineurin-dependent mechanisms in the hippocampal dentate gyrus. *Neurobiol. Learn. Mem.,* Vol.77, pp. 354 -371.

Cheriyan, J., Kumar, P., Mayadevi, M., Surolia, A. & Omkumar, R. V. (2011). Calcium/calmodulin dependent protein kinase II bound to NMDA receptor 2B subunit exhibits increased ATP affinity and attenuated dephosphorylation. *PLoS One,* Vol.6, e16495.

Chung, H. J., Steinberg, J. P., Huganhir, R. L. & Linden, D. J. (2003). Requirement of AMPA receptor GluR2 phosphorylation for cerebellar long term depression. *Science,* Vol.300, pp. 1751-1755.

Cissé, M., B., Halabisky, J., Harris, N., Devidze, D. B., Dubal, B., Sun, A., Orr, G., Lotz, D. H., Kim & Hamto, P. (2011). Reversing EphB2 depletion rescues cognitive functions in Alzheimer model. *Nature,* Vol.469, pp. 47-52.

Collingridge, G. L., Peineau, S., Howland, J. G. & Wang, Y. T. (2010). Long-term depression in the CNS, *Nature Neurosci.,* Vol.11, pp. 459-473.

Cooke, S. F. & Bliss, T. V. (2006). Plasticity in the human central nervous system. *Brain,* Vol.129, No.Pt 7, pp. 1659-73.

D'Amelio, M., Cavallucci, V., Middei, S., Marchetti, C., Pacioni ,S., Ferri ,A., Diamantini, A., De Zio, D., Carrara, P., Battistini, L, Moreno, S., Bacci, A., Ammassari-Teule, M., Marie, H. & Cecconi, F. (2011). Caspase-3 triggers early synaptic dysfunction in a mouse model of Alzheimer's disease. *Nature Neuroscience*, Vol.14, pp. 69-76.

De Zeeuw, C. I., Hansel, C., Bian, F., Koekkoek, S. K. E., van Alphen, A. M, Linden D. J. & Oberdick, J. (1998). Expression of a Protein Kinase C Inhibitor in Purkinje Cells Blocks Cerebellar LTD and Adaptation of the vestibulo-Ocular Reflex. *Neuron*, Vol.20, pp. 495–508.

Derkach, V., Barria, A. & Soderling, T. R. (1999). Ca^{2+}/calmodulin-kinase II enhances channel conductance of alpha-amino-3-hydroxy-5-methyl-4-isoxazolepropionate type glutamate receptors. *Proc. Natl. Acad. Sci. U S A*, Vol.96, No.6, pp. 3269-74.

Desai, N. S., Casimiro, T. M., Gruber, S. M. & Vanderklish, P. W. (2006). Early postnatal plasticity in neocortex of Fmr1 knockout mice. *J. Neurophysiol.*, Vol.96, pp. 1734–1745.

Di Marzo, V., Melck, D., Bisogno, T. & De Petrocellis, L. (1998). Endocannabinoids: endogenous cannabinoid receptor ligands with neuromodulatory action. *Trends Neurosci.*, Vol.21, pp. 521–528.

Diana, G., Domenici, M. R., Scotti de Carolis, A., Loizzo, A. & Sagratella, S. (1995). Reduced hippocampal CA1 $Ca(^{2+})$-induced long-term potentiation is associated with age-dependent impairment of spatial learning. *Brain Research*, Vol.686, pp. 107–110.

Doyle, M. & Kiebler, M. A. (2011). Mechanisms of dendritic mRNA transport and its role in synaptic tagging. *The EMBO J.*, Vol.30, pp. 3540-3552.

Fitzjohn, S. M., Palmer, M. J., May, J. E. R., Neeson, A., Morris, S. A. C. & Collingridge, G. L. (2001). A characterization of long-term depression induced by metabotropic glutamate receptor activation in the rat hippocampus *in vitro*. *J. Physiol.*, Vol.537.2, pp. 421-430.

Foster, T. C., & Norris, C. M. (1997). Age-associated changes in Ca (2+)-dependent processes: Relation to hippocampal synaptic plasticity. *Hippocampus*, Vol.7, pp. 602–612.

Frey, U., Huang, Y. Y. & Kandel, E. R. (1993). Effects of cAMP simulate a late stage of LTP in hippocampal CA1 neurons. *Science*, Vol.260, No.5114, pp. 1661-4.

Gladding C. M. (2009). Tyrosine dephosphorylation regulates AMPAR internalization in mGluR LTD. *Mol. Cell. Neurosci.*, Vol.40, pp. 267-279.

Good, T. A., Smith, D. O. & Murphy, R. M. (1996). Beta-amyloid peptide blocks the fast-inactivating K+current in rat hippocampal neurons. *Biophysical Journal*, Vol.70, pp. 296–304

Gong, Y., Chang, L., Viola, K. L., Lacor, P. N., Lambert, M. P., Finch, C. E., Krafft, G. A. & Klein, W. L. (2003). Alzheimer's disease-affected brain: presence of oligomeric A beta ligands (ADDLs) suggests a molecular basis for reversible memory loss. *Proc. Natl. Acad. Sci. U S A.*, Vol.100, No.18, pp. 10417–10422.

Gong, Y. & Lippa, C. F. (2010). Review: Disruption of the Postsynaptic Density in Alzheimerâs Disease and Other Neurodegenerative Dementias. *American journal of Alzheimer's disease and other dementias*, Vol.25, pp. 547-555.

Greenough, W. T., Klintsova, A. Y., Irwin, S. A., Galvez, R., Bates, K. E. & Weiler, I. J. (2001). Synaptic regulation of protein synthesis and the fragile X protein. *Proc. Natl. Acad. Sci. U.S.A* Vol.98, pp. 7101–7106.

Haass, C. & Selkoe, D. J. (1993). Cellular processing of beta-amyloid precursor protein and the genesis of amyloid beta-peptide. *Cell.*, Dec 17, Vol.75, No.6, pp.1 039-42.

Hansel C., de Jeu. M., Belmeguenai. A., Houtman S. H., Buitendijk G. H. S, Andreev, D., De Zeeuw, C. I. & Elgersma Y. (2006). αCaMKII is Essential for Cerebellar LTD and motor learning, *Neuron,* Vol.51, pp. 835-843.

Harris, J. A., Devidze, N., Halabisky, B., Lo, I., Thwin, M.T., Yu, G. Q., Bredesen, D. E., Masliah, E. & Mucke, L. (2010). Many neuronal and behavioral impairments in transgenic mouse models of Alzheimer's disease are independent of caspase cleavage of the amyloid precursor protein. *J. Neurosci.*, Vol.30, No.1, pp. 372–381, ISSN 0270-6474.

Harrison, P. J. & Weinberger, D. R . (2005). Schizophrenia genes, gene expression and neuropathology: On the matter of their convergence. *Mol. Psychiatry,* Vol.10, pp. 40–68, ISSN 1359-4184.

Hasan, A., Michael, A., Nitscheb, Reina, N., Schneider-Axmanna, T., Gusea, B., Grubera, O., Falkaia, P. & Wobrocka, T. (2011). Dysfunctional long-term potentiation-like plasticity in schizophrenia revealed by transcranial direct current stimulation. *Behavioural Brain Research,* Vol.224, pp. 15– 22, ISSN 0166-4328.

Hebb, D. (1949). *The organization of behavior,* pp. 319-340.

Hsia, A. Y., Masliah, E., McConlogue, L., Yu, G. Q, Tatsuno, G., Hu, K., Kholodenko, D., Malenka, R. C., Nicoll, R. A. & Mucke L. (1999). Plaque-independent disruption of neural circuits in Alzheimer's disease mouse models, *Proc. Natl. Acad. Sci. U S A.,* Vol.96, No6, pp. 3228–3233.

Hu, G. Y., Hvalby, O., Walaas, S. I., Albert, K. A., Skjeflo, P., Andersen, P. & Greengard, P. (1987). Protein kinase C injection into hippocampal pyramidal cells elicits features of long term potentiation. *Nature,* Vol.328, No 6129, pp. 426-9.

Hu, N. W., Ondrejcak, T. & Rowan, M. J. (2011). Glutamate receptors in preclinical research on Alzheimer's disease: update on recent advances. *Pharmacology Biochemistry and Behavior,* ISSN 0091-3057.

Huang, Y. Y. & Kandel, E. R. (1994). Recruitment of long-lasting and protein kinase a-dependent long-term potentiation in the CA1 region of hippocampus requires repeated tetanization. *Learn. Mem.*, Vol.1, No.1, pp. 74-82.

Huber, K. M., Kayser, M. S. & Bear, M. F. (2000). Role for rapid dendritic protein synthesis in hippocampal mGluR dependent long-term depression. *Science,* Vol.288, pp. 1254–1257.

Ito, M. (1982). Cerebellar control of the vestibule ocular reflex around the flocculus hypothesis. *Annu. Rev. Neurosci.*, Vol.5, pp. 275-296.

Jorntell, H. & Hansel, C. (2006). Synaptic memories upside down: Bidirectional plasticity at cerebellar parallel fiber-purkinje cell synapses. *Neuron,* Vol.52, No.2, pp. 227-38, ISSN 0959-4388.

Kandel, E. R. (2001). The molecular biology of memory storage: A dialogue between genes and synapses. *Science,* Vol.294, No.5544, pp. 1030-8.

Kandel, E. R., Schwartz, J. H. & Jessel, T. M. (2000). Principles of Neural Science. (Ed.4). McGraw-Hill, ISBN 0-8385-7701-6.

Kemp, A. & Manahan-Vaughan, D. (2007). Hippocampal long-term depression: master or minion in declarative memory processes? *TRENDS in Neurosciences,* Vol.30 No.3, pp. 111-118.

Kim, M. J., Futai, K., Jo, J., Hayashi, Y., Cho, K. & Sheng, M. (2007). Synaptic Accumulation of PSD-95 and Synaptic Function Regulated by Phosphorylation of Serine-295 of PSD-95. *Neuron,* Vol.56, pp. 488–502

Klyubin, I., Betts, V., Welzel, A. T., Blennow, K., Zetterberg, H., Wallin, A., Lemere, C. A. , Cullen, W. K., Peng, Y., Wisniewski, T., Selkoe, D. J., Anwyl, R., Walsh, D. M. & Rowan, M. J. (2008). Amyloid beta protein dimer-containing human CSF disrupts synaptic plasticity: prevention by systemic passive immunization. *J. Neurosci.,* Vol. 28, No.16, pp. 4231-7, ISSN 0270-6474/08/284231-07.

Konradi, C. & Heckers, S. (2003). Molecular aspects of glutamate dysregulation: implications for schizophrenia and its treatment. *Pharmacol. Ther.,* Vol.97, pp. 153–79, ISSN 0163-7258.

Kullmann, D. M. & Lamsa, K. (2008). Roles of distinct glutamate receptors in induction of anti-hebbian long-term potentiation. *J. Physiol,* Vol.586, No.6, pp. 1481-6.

Kumar, A. (2011). Long-term potentiation at CA3–CA1 hippocampal synapses with special emphasis on aging, disease, and stress. *Front. Ag. Neurosci.,* Vol3, Article 7, doi: 10.3389/fnagi.2011.00007

Lamprecht, R. & LeDoux, J. (2004). Structural plasticity and memory. *Nature Reviews Neuroscience,* Vol.5, pp. 45-54.

Lamsa, K. P., Heeroma, J. H., Somogyi, P., Rusakov, D. A. & Kullmann, D. M. (2007). Anti-hebbian long-term potentiation in the hippocampal feedback inhibitory circuit. *Science,* Vol.315, No.5816, pp. 1262-6.

Lee, H. K., Barbaroise, M., Kameyama, K., Bear, M. F. & Huganhir, R. L. (2000). Regulation of distinct AMPA receptor phosphorylation sites during bidirectional synaptic plasticity. *Nature,* Vol.405, pp. 955-959.

Lev- Ram, V., Wong, S. T., Storm, D. R. & Tsein, R. Y. (2002). A new form of cerebellar long term potentiation is postsynaptic and depends on nitric oxide but not cAMP. *Proc. Natl. Acad. Sci. USA.,* Vol 99, pp. 8389-8393.

Levy, W. B. & Steward, O. (1979). Synapses as associative memory elements in the hippocampal formation. *Brain Res.,* Vol.175, No.2, pp. 233-45.

Li, S., Hong, S., Shepardson, N. E., Walsh, D.M., Shankar, G. M. & Selkoe, D. (2009). Soluble oligomers of amyloid β protein facilitate hippocampal long-term depression by disrupting neuronal glutamate uptake. *Neuron,* Vol.62, No6, pp. 788–801.

Lisman, J., Grace, A. A. & Duzel, E. (2011). A neohebbian framework for episodic memory; role of dopamine-dependent late LTP. *Trends in Neurosciences.*

Lisman, J., Schulman, H. & Cline, H. (2002). The molecular basis of CaMKII function in synaptic and behavioural memory. *Nat. Rev. Neurosci.,* Vol.3, pp.1 75-190.

Lu, J. T., Li, C. Y., Zhao, J. P., Poo, M. M. & Zhang, X. H. (2007). Spike-timing-dependent plasticity of neocortical excitatory synapses on inhibitory interneurons depends on target cell type. *J. Neurosci.,* Vol.27, No.36, pp. 9711-20.

Lu,Y., Ji,Y., Ganeshan, S., Schloesser, R., Martinowich, K., Sun, M., Mei, F., Chao, M, V. & Lu, B. (2011) TrkB as a Potential Synaptic and Behavioral Tag. *The journal of Neuroscience,* Vol.31(33), pp. 11762-11771.

Mahan, A. L. & Ressler, K. J. (2011). Fear conditioning, synaptic plasticity and the amygdala: implications for post traumatic stress disorder, *Trends in Neurosciences*,(Article in press), ISSN 0166-2236

Malenka, R. C. & Bear, M. F. (2004). LTP and LTD: An embarrassment of riches. *Neuron,* Vol.44, No(1), pp. 5-21.

Malenka, R. C. (2002). Synaptic plasticity. *Neuropsychopharmacology: The Fifth Generation of Progress,* pp. 147-157.

Malenka, R. C. (2003). The long-term potential of LTP. *Nat. Rev. Neurosci.,* Vol.4, No.11, pp. 923-6.

Markram, H. (1997). Regulation of Synaptic Efficacy by Coincidence of Postsynaptic APs and EPSPs. *Science,* Vol.275, pp. 213.

Marr, D. (1969). Theory of cerebellar cortex. *J. Physiol.,* Vol.202, pp. 437-455.

Martin, S. J., Grimwood, P. D. & Morris, R. G. (2000). Synaptic plasticity and memory: An evaluation of the hypothesis. *Annu. Rev. Neurosci.,* Vol.23, pp. 649-711.

Molnar, E. (2011). Long-term potentiation in cultured hippocampal neurons. *Seminars in Cell and Developmental Biology,*article in press, ISSN 1084-9521

Montoya, D. A. C. (2011). Synaptic plasticity in Alzheimer's disease: Toward early detection using non-invasive protocols. *Rev. Neurocience.* (Article in press).

Moosmang, S., Haider, N., Klugbauer, N., Adelsberger, H., Langwieser, N., Muller, J., Stiess, M., Marais, E., Schulla, V., Lacinova, L., Goebbels, S., Nave, K. A., Storm, D. R., Hofmann, F. & Kleppisch, T. (2005). Role of hippocampal Cav1.2 Ca^{2+} channels in NMDA receptor-independent synaptic plasticity and spatial memory. *J. Neurosci.,* Vol.25, No 43, pp. 9883-92.

Morshita, W., Connor, J. H., Xia, H., Quinlan E, M., Shenolikar, S. & Malenka R. C. (2001). Regulation of Synaptic Strength by Protein Phosphatase 1. *Neuron,* Vol.32, pp.1 133–1148.

Mucke, L., Masliah, E., Yu, G. Q., Mallory, M., Rockenstein, E. M., Tatsuno, G., Hu, K., Kholodenko, D., Johnson-Wood, K. & McConlogue, L. (2000). High-level neuronal expression of A beta 1-42 in wild-type human amyloid protein precursor transgenic mice: synaptotoxicity without plaque formation, *J. Neurosci.,* Vol.20, No.11, pp. 4050–4058, ISSN 0270-6474.

Mulkey, R. M., Herron, C. E. & Malenka, R. C. (1993). An essential role for protein phosphatases in hippocampal long-term depression. *Science,* Vol.261, pp. 1051–1055.

Nguyen, P. V. & Woo, N. H. (2003). Regulation of hippocampal synaptic plasticity by cyclic amp-dependent protein kinases. *Prog. Neurobiol.,* Vol.71, No.6, pp. 401-37.

Nguyen, P. V., Abel, T. & Kandel, E. R. (1994). Requirement of a critical period of transcription for induction of a late phase of ltp. *Science,* Vol.265, No.5175, pp. 1104-7.

Nicoll, R. A. & Schmitz, D. (2005). Synaptic plasticity at hippocampal mossy fibre synapses. *Nat. Rev. Neurosci.,* Vol.6, No.11, pp. 863-76.

Nosyreva, E. D. & Huber, K. M. (2005). Developmental switch in synaptic mechanisms of hippocampal metabotropic glutamate receptor-dependent long-term depression. *J. Neurosci.,* Vol.25, pp. 2992–3001.

Olds, J., Disterhoft, J. F., Segal, M., Kornblith, C. L. & Hirsh, R. (1972). Learning centers of rat brain mapped by measuring latencies of conditioned unit responses. *J. Neurophysiol.,* Vol.35, No.2, pp. 202.

O'Leary, H., Liu, W. H., Rorabaugh, J. M., Coultrap, S. J. & Bayer, K. U. (2011). Nucleotides and phosphorylation bi-directionally modulate Ca^{2+}/calmodulin-dependent protein kinase II (CaMKII) binding to the N-methyl-D-aspartate (NMDA) receptor subunit GluN2B. *J. Biol. Chem.* Vol.286, pp. 31272-31281

Omkumar, R. V., Kiely, M., Rosentein, A. J., Min, K. T. & Kennedy, M. B. (1996). Identification of a phosphorylation site for calcium/calmodulin dependent protein kinase II in the NR2B subunit of the N-methyl-D-aspartate receptor. *J. Biol. Chem.*, Vol.271, pp. 31670-31678

Otmakhov, N., Khibnik, L., Otmakhova, N., Carpenter, S., Riahi, S., Asrican, B. & Lisman, J. (2004). Forskolin-induced LTP in the ca1 hippocampal region is NMDA receptor dependent. *J. Neurophysiol.*, Vol.91, No.5, pp. 1955-62.

Palop, J. J., Chin, J., Roberson, E. D., Wang, J., Thwin, M. T, Bien-Ly, N., Yoo, J., Ho, K. O., Yu, G. Q, Kreitzer, A., Finkbeiner, S., Noebels, J. L. & Mucke, L. (2007). Aberrant excitatory neuronal activity and compensatory remodeling of inhibitory hippocampal circuits in mouse models of Alzheimer's disease. *Neuron,* Vol.55, pp. 697–711.

Palop, J. J. & Mucke, L. (2010). Amyloid-β-induced neuronal dysfunction in Alzheimer's disease: from synapses toward neural networks. *Nat. Neurosci.*, Vol.13, No.7, pp. 812- 818.

Park, S., Park, M. J., Kim, S., Kim, J., Shepherd, J. D., Smith- Hicks, C .L., Chowdhury, S., Kaufmann, W., Kuhl, D., Ryazanov, A. G., Huganir, R. L, Linden, D. J. & Worley, P.F. (2008). Elongation Factor 2 and Fragile X Mental Retardation Protein Control the Dynamic Translation of Arc/Arg3.1 Essential for mGluR-LTD. *Neuron,* Vol.59, pp. 70–83.

Paz, R. D., Tardito, S., Atzori, M. & Tseng, K. Y. 2008. Glutamatergic dysfunction in schizophrenia: from basic neuroscience to clinical psychopharmacology. *Eur. Neuropsychopharmacol,* Vol.18, pp. 773–86.

Pradeep, K. K., Cheriyan, J., Suma Priya, S. D., Rajeevkumar, R., Mayadevi, M., Praseeda, M. & Omkumar R, V. (2009). Regulation of Ca^{2+}/calmodulin-dependent protein kinase II catalysis by N-methyl-D-aspartate receptor subunit 2B. *Biochem. J.*, Vol.419, pp. 123-32.

Proctor, D.T., Coulson, E. J. & Dodd, P. R. (2011). Post-synaptic scaffolding protein interactions with glutamate receptors in synaptic dysfunction and Alzheimer's disease, *Progress in Neurobiology,* Vol.93, pp. 509–521, ISSN 0301-0082.

Rajeevkumar, R., Suma Priya, S., Mayadevi, M., Mathew Steephan, Santoshkumar ,T. R., John Cheriyan, Sanalkumar, R., Pradeep, K. K., Jackson James & Omkumar, R. V. (2009). Phosphorylation status of NR2B subunit of NMDA receptor regulates its interaction with Calcium/calmodulin dependent protein kinase II. *J. Neurochem.*, Vol.110, pp. 92-105.

Ramnani, N. (2006). The primate cortico-cerebellar system: anatomy and function. *Nat. Rev. Neurosci.*, Vol.7, pp. 511-522.

Raymond, C. R. (2008). Different requirements for action potentials in the induction of different forms of long-term potentiation. *J. Physiol,* Vol.586, No.7, pp. 1859-65.

Reymann, K. G. & Frey, J. U. (2007). The late maintenance of hippocampal LTP: Requirements, phases, 'synaptic tagging', 'late-associativity' and implications. *Neuropharmacology,* Vol.52, No.1, pp. 24-40.

Roberson, E. D., Halabisky, B., Jong, W., Yoo., Yao, J., Chin, J., Yan, F., Wu, T., Hamto, P., Devidze, N., Yu, G., Palop, J. J., Noebels, J. L. & Mucke, L. (2011). Amyloid-β/Fyn-induced synaptic, network, and cognitive impairments depend on tau levels in multiple mouse, models of Alzheimer's disease, *The Journal of Neuroscience,* Vol.31, No.2, pp. 700 -711, ISSN 0270-6474.

Rygh, L, J., Svendsen, F., Fiska, A., Haugan, F., Hole, K. & Tjølsen, A. (2005). Long-term potentiation in spinal nociceptive systems—how acute pain may become chronic. *Psychoneuroendocrinology,* Vol.30, pp. 959-964.

Schonewille, M., Gao, Z., Henk-Jan Boele., Vinueza Veloz M, F., Amerika W, E., Simek A. A. M., De Jeu, M. T., Steinberg, J. P., Takamiya, K., Hoebeek, F. E., Linden, D. J,. Huganir, R. L. & De Zeeuw, C. I. (2011). Reevaluating the Role of LTD in Cerebellar Motor Learning, *Neuron,* Vol.70, pp. 43–50.

Scoville, W. B. & Milner, B. (1957). Loss of recent memory after bilateral hippocampal lesions. *Journal of Neurology, Neurosurgery & Psychiatry,* Vol.20, No.1, pp. 11.

Selkoe, D. J. (2008). Soluble oligomers of the amyloid beta-protein impair synaptic plasticity and behavior. *Behav. Brain Res.,* Vol.192, pp. 106–113, ISSN 0166-4328.

Sgobio, C., Ghiglieri, V., Cinzia Costa, C., Bagetta, V., Siliquini, S., Barone, I.,Filippo, M., Gardoni, F., Gundelfinger, E. D., Di Luca, M., Picconi, B. & Calabresi, P. (2010). Hippocampal synaptic plasticity, memory, and epilepsy: Effects of long-term valproic acid treatment, *Biol. Psychiatry.,* Vol.67, pp. 567–574, ISSN 0006-3223.

Shankar, G. M., Bloodgood, B. L., Townsend, M., Walsh, D. M., Selkoe, D. J. & Sabatini, B. L (2007). Natural oligomers of the Alzheimer amyloid-beta protein induce reversible synapse loss by modulating an NMDA-type glutamate receptor-dependent signaling pathway. *J. Neurosci.,* Vol.27, pp. 2866–2875, ISSN 0270-6474.

Shankar, G. M., Li, S., Mehta, T. H., Garcia-Munoz, A., Shepardson, N. E., Smith, I., Brett, F. M., Farrell, M. A., Rowan M. J. & Lemere C. A. (2008). Amyloid- protein dimers isolated directly from Alzheimer's brains impair synaptic plasticity and memory. *Nature medicine,* Vol.14, pp. 837-842.

Shepherd, J. D. & Bear, M. F. (2011). New views of Arc, a master regulator of synaptic plasticity, *Nature Neuroscience,* Vol.14, No.3, pp. 279-284.

Shipton, O. A., Leitz, J. R., Dworzak, J., Christine, E. J. Acton,C. E., Tunbridge, E. M., Denk, F., Hana, N., Dawson, H. N, Vitek, M. P, Wade-Martins, R., Paulsen, O. & Vargas-Caballero, M. (2011). Tau protein is required for amyloid β-induced impairment of hippocampal long-term potentiation, *J. Neurosci,* Vol.31, No.5, pp. 1688 -1692, ISSN 0270-6474.

Smith, C. C. & Mcmahon, L. L. (2005). Estrogen-induced increase in the magnitude of long-term potentiation occurs only when the ratio of NMDA transmission to AMPA transmission is increased. *J. Neurosci,* Vol.25, No.34, pp. 7780-91.

Snyder, E. M., Philpot, B. D., Huber, K. M.,Dong, X., Fallon, J. R., & Bear, M. F. (2001). Internalization of ionotropic glutamate receptors in response to mGluR activation. *Nat. Neurosci.,* Vol.4. pp. 1079–1085.

Stephan, A., Laroche, S. & Davis, S. (2001). Generation of aggregated b-Amyloid in the rat hippocampus impairs synaptic transmission and plasticity and causes memory deficits, *J. Neurosci*, Vol.21, No.15, pp. 5703–5714.

Strack, S., McNeill R. B & Colbran, R. J. (2000). Mechanism and regulation of calcium/calmodulin dependent protein kinase II targeting to the NR2B subunit of the N-methyl-D-aspartate receptor. *J. Biol. chem.*, Vol.273, pp. 23789-23806.

Sweatt, J. D. (2010). *Mechanisms of memory*. Academic press, U.K., 2 nd Edition, ISBN 978-012-374951-2.

Tackenberg, C. & Brandt, R. (2009). Divergent pathways mediate spine alterations and cell death induced by amyloid-β, wild-type tau, and R406W tau, *J. Neurosci.*, Vol.29, No.46, pp. 14439 -14450, ISSN 0270-6474/09/291443.

Tergau, F., Naumann, U., Paulus, W. & Steinhoff, B. J. (1999). Low-frequency repetitive transcranial magnetic stimulation improves intractable epilepsy. *Lancet*, Vol.353, pp. 2209.

Teyler, T. J. & Discenna, P. (1987). Long-term potentiation. *Annu Rev Neurosci*, Vol.10, pp. 131-61.

Tiron ,A. & Wibrand, K. (2010). The Arc of synaptic memory. *Exp. Brain Res.*, Vol.200, pp. 125-140.

Ueda, K., Shinohara, S., Yagami, T., Asakura, K. & Kawasaki, K. (1997). Amyloid beta protein potentiates Ca $^{2+}$ influx through L-type voltage-sensitive Ca^{2+} channels: A possible involvement of free radicals. *J. Neurochem.*, Vol.68, pp. 265–271.

Vogt, K. E. & Canepari, M. (2010). On the Induction of Postsynaptic Granule Cell - Purkinje Neuron LTP and LTD. *The Cerebellum*,Vol.9, No.3, pp. 284-90.

Walsh, D. M., Klyubin, I., Fadeeva, J. V., Cullen, W. K., Anwyl, R., Wolfe, M. S, Rowan, M. J. & Selkoe, D. J. (2002). Naturally secreted oligomers of amyloid β protein potently inhibit hippocampal long-term potentiation in vivo, *Nature*, Vol.416, pp. 535-539.

Wang, H. W., Pasternak, J. F., Kuo, H., Ristic, H., Lambert, M. P., Chromy, B., Viola, K. L., Klein, W. L., Stine, W. B., Krafft, G. A. & Trommer, B. L. (2002). Soluble oligomers of beta amyloid (1-42) inhibit long-term potentiation but not long-term depression in rat dentate gyrus, *Brain Res.*, Vol.924, No.2, pp. 133–140, ISSN 0006-8993.

Wang, Q., Rowan, M. J. & Anwy, l. R. (2004). Beta-amyloid-mediated inhibition of NMDA receptor-dependent long-term potentiation induction involves activation of microglia and stimulation of inducible nitric oxide synthase and superoxide. J. *Neurosci.*, Vol.24, No.27, pp. 6049–6056, ISSN 0270-6474/04/246049-08.

West, A. E., Chen, W. G., Dalva, M. B., Dolmetsch, R. E., Kornhauser, J. M., Shaywitz, A. J., Takasu, M. A., Tao, X. & Greenberg, M. E. (2001). Calcium regulation of neuronal gene expression. *Proc. Natl. Acad. Sci. USA.*, Vol.98, No.20, pp. 11024-31.

Williams, J. H., Errington, M. L., Lynch, M. A. & Bliss, T. V. (1989). Arachidonic acid induces a long-term activity-dependent enhancement of synaptic transmission in the hippocampus. *Nature*, Vol.341, No.6244, pp. 739-42.

Woo, N. H., Teng, H. K., Siao, C. J., Chiaruttini, C., Pang, P. T ., Milner, T. A., Hempstead, B. L. & Bai Lu. (2005). Activation of p75NTR by proBDNF facilitates hippocampal long-term depression. *Nature Neuroscience*, Vol.8, pp. 1069 - 1077.

Wyneken, U., Marengo, J. J., Villanueva, S., Soto, D. Sandoval, R. Gundelfinger, E. D. & Orrego, F. (2003). Epilepsy-induced changes in signaling systems of human and rat postsynaptic densities, *Epilepsia,* Vol.44, No.2, pp. 243–246.

Xia, W. (2010). Brain amyloid β protein and memory disruption in Alzheimer's disease, *Neuropsychiatric Disease and Treatment,* Vol.6, pp. 605–612.

Xia, J., Chung, H. J., Wihler, C., Huganir, R. L. & Linden, D. J. (2000). Cerebellar long term depression requires PKC-regulated interactions between GluR2/3 and PDZ domain containing proteins. *Neuron,* Vol.28, pp. 499-510.

Yasuda, H., Barth, A. L., Stellwagen, D. & Malenka, R. C. (2003). A developmental switch in the signaling cascades for LTP induction. *Nat Neurosci,* Vol.6, No.1, pp. 15-6.

Zeng, Y., Zhao, D. & Xie, C. W. (2010). Neurotrophins enhance CaMKII activity and rescue amyloid-beta induced deficits in hippocampal synaptic plasticity. *J. Alzheimers Dis.,* Vol.21, No.3, pp. 823-831.

Zukin R. S., Richter J. D. & Bagni, C. (2009) Signals, synapses and synthesis: how new proteins control plasticity. *Frontiers in neural circuits,* Vol.3, No.14, pp. 1-8.

14

Brain Energy Metabolism in Health and Disease

Felipe A. Beltrán, Aníbal I. Acuña,
María Paz Miró and Maite A. Castro*
*Instituto de Bioquímica y Microbiología, Facultad de Ciencias,
Universidad Austral de Chile, Valdivia,
Chile*

1. Introduction

Living cells require energy to perform work, to maintain their organized structures, to synthesize cellular components, to generate electric currents and many other processes. Energy metabolism is a highly coordinated cellular activity in which enzymes are organized into discrete metabolic pathways that cooperate in degrading energy-rich nutrients from the environment. Glucose is the principal metabolic substrate for living cells including brain cells. It is rich in potential energy and is also a versatile precursor, giving rise to metabolic intermediaries for biosynthetic reactions. Glycogen is a polymer of glucose and is the form in which glucose is stored. The mammalian brain contains glycogen, which is located predominantly in astrocytes (Brown & Ransom, 2007). In particular situations, substrates other than glucose can be utilized by the brain. β-hydroxybutyrate, acetoacetate and acetone are ketone bodies produced in the liver from Acetyl-CoA. Ketone bodies are an important source of brain energy in breast-fed neonates and during starvation when carbohydrates are scarce. However, it has been proposed that part of brain energy comes from the conversion of glucose to lactate at one location (within one cell) and part comes from the oxidation of lactate to pyruvate at another location (within the same cell or in a different cell).

The brain makes up 2% of a person's weight. Despite this, even at rest, the brain consumes 25% of the body's energy. Most of the energy consumed in the brain is attributable to restoration of the membrane gradient following neuronal depolarization. Neurotransmitter recycling, intracellular signaling and dendritic and axonal transport also require energy (Attwell & Laughlin, 2001). Even though neurons are responsible for massive energy consumption, the brain is made up of many cells, including neurons, glial and ependymal cells. Every brain cell has a specific function and thus every brain cell has different metabolic needs. Many of these specific functions are concerned with maintainance of neuronal transmission. For example, astrocytes play a central role in supporting neurons metabolically by producing lactate, through glycolysis and activation of glycogen catabolism (Brown & Ransom, 2007). Another critical factor for maintenance of neuronal

*Corresponding Author

transmission is an adequate supply of nutrients and oxygen from blood. Neurotransmitters stimulate neurovascular messenger production in astrocytes and neurons. These molecules induce the local constriction and dilation of smooth muscle around the neighboring arterioles (Attwell et al., 2010).

There have been several reports of metabolic impairment in a variety of neurodegenerative disorders such as Alzheimer's disease, Huntington's disease, amyotrophic lateral sclerosis and Parkinson's disease, among others (Mosconi et al., 2005, Leenders et al., 1986, Kuwert et al., 1993, Hattingen et al., 2009). Because brain is an expensive organ in energetic terms, disruptions in energy production may affect neuronal transmission and thus, neuronal survival. Moreover, deregulation of energy metabolism could be implicated in an increased production of oxidative species. Indeed, oxidative damage has been proposed in such disorders (Mazziotta et al., 1987, Navarro et al., 2009).

2. Metabolic sources and principal metabolic pathways for brain energy metabolism

There are two barriers protecting the brain from toxic metabolites: the blood-brain barrier and the blood-CSF barrier formed by epithelial cells of the choroid plexus. These barriers protect the brain from possible changes in the concentration of blood metabolites. In the same way, they work as selective filters to allow for controlled delivery of metabolic substrates into the brain. These metabolic substrates are mainly glucose, ketone bodies and some metabolic intermediaries such as lactate and pyruvate.

2.1 Use of glucose in brain

Glucose is an essential energy source for the adult human brain. According to *in vivo* studies using labeled 2-deoxyglucose or 2-fluorodeoxyglucose there is a correlation between brain function and brain metabolism (Sokoloff et al., 1977). Glucose is rich in potential energy and thus, it is a good metabolic fuel. In any tissue glucose can follow several metabolic pathways. In brain, glucose is almost entirely oxidized through sequential glycolysis and the tricarboxylic cycle (TCA) associated with oxidative phosphorylation. Glucose can also be stored as the polysaccharide, glycogen. Glucose is not only an excellent energetic fuel, it is also a remarkably versatile precursor supplying metabolic intermediaries for biosynthetic reactions. In brain most of these intermediaries serve to synthesize neurotransmitters and gliotransmitters, as well as other molecules of biological significance. Glucose oxidation via glycolysis provides metabolic intermediaries besides producing ATP. Glucose can be oxidized through an alternative pathway: the pentose phosphate pathway (PPP). Glucose oxidation through PPP provides 5-carbon monosaccharides for nucleic acid synthesis and NADPH for reductive biosynthetic processes and for mantainance of the redox balance in the cell.

2.1.1 Glycolysis

In glycolysis, a molecule of glucose is oxidized to two molecules of pyruvate. This oxidation occurs through ten enzyme-catalyzed reactions (Figure 1). The first step in glycolysis is phosphorylation of glucose at C-6, by hexokinase, to yield glucose-6-phosphate. Most of the glucose-6-phosphate is degraded to pyruvate. But glucose-6-phosphate can be used to generate glucose-1-phosphate, which in turn is used to synthesize glycogen (see below) or to generate NADPH and ribose-5-phosphate through PPP (see below). Myo-inositol is also synthesized from glucose-6-phosphate and serves as a precursor for phosphatidylinositide signaling molecules. The first step in glycolysis and the next nine enzymatic reactions occur in all brain cells (Lowry & Passonneau, 1964).

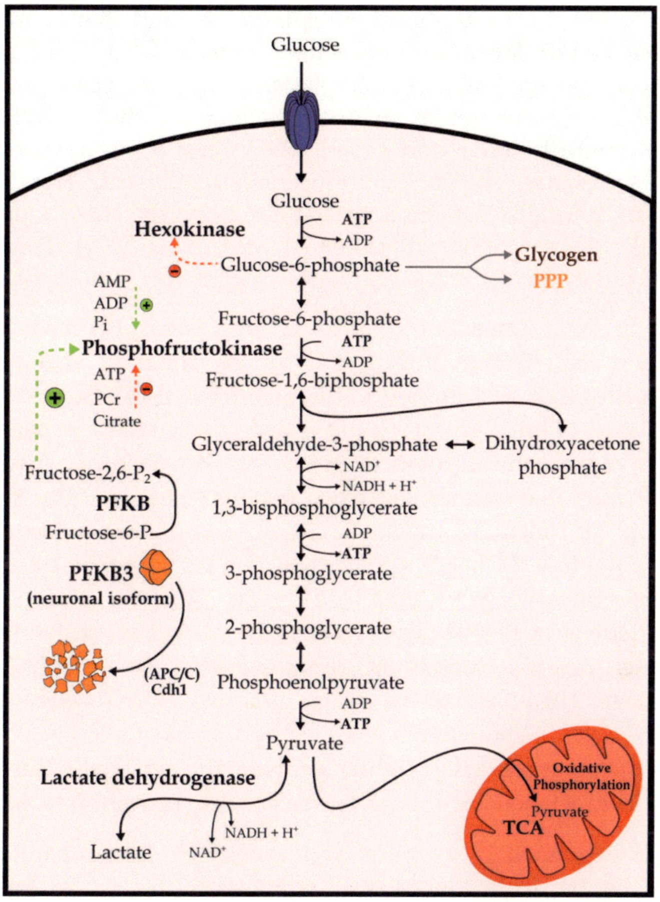

Fig. 1. Glycolysis. The first step in glycolysis is phosphorylation of glucose to glucose-6-phosphate by hexokinase, an enzyme inhibited by the same glucose-6-phosphate. Glucose must be phosphorylated to glucose-6-phosphate for it to enter glycolysis. The most important step in the control of glycolytic flux is a reaction catalyzed by phosphofructokinase (PFK). PFK is inhibited by compounds that accumulate when energy status is high (ATP, citrate) and it is activated by products of functional metabolic activity (AMP, ADP). PFK1 in neurons is not activated by fructose 2,6-bisphosphate (Fructose-2,6-P_2) because the enzyme that catalyzes F2,6BP production is constantly degraded.

Major sites for the control of glycolytic flux are hexokinase (EC 2.7.1.1), phosphofructokinase 1 (PFK1, EC 2.7.1.11) and pyruvate kinase (EC 2.7.1.40; Lowry & Passoneau, 1964). Hexokinase catalyzes the transfer of a phosphate group from one molecule of ATP to glucose (Figure 1). Type-I hexokinase is the predominant isoenzyme in brain (Wilson, 1995). This reaction is irreversible under intracellular conditions., Type-I hexokinase is normally saturated with substrate and strongly inhibited by its product, glucose-6-phosphate (Wilson, 2003). Type-I hexokinase binds to the outer mitochondrial membrane via a hydrophobic N-terminal sequence (Wilson, 1997). Type-I hexokinase interacts with porin (also named voltage-dependent anion channel) which is a membrane protein located at the outer mitochondrial membrane. When type-I hexokinase binds to mitochondria, the K_i for glucose-6-phosphate is increased and the K_m for ATP is reduced, suggesting that the bound form is more active (Wilson, 2003). This association occurs alongside changes in the cellular metabolic state. It has also been proposed that type-I hexokinase can bind to microtubules in order to increase their activity. Indeed, under mitogenic stimulus, mitochondria and type-I hexokinase colocalization decreases, while tubulin and type-I hexokinase colocalization increases in glial cells (Sanchez-Alvarez et al., 2004). These changes in localization are accompanied by an increase in glucose transporters (GLUTs) and hexokinase expression (Sanchez-Alvarez et al., 2004). Therefore, hexokinase and GLUTs should be key factors in the regulation of glycolytic flux capacity.

All three isotypes of PFK1 (muscle [M], liver [L] and brain [B]) have been observed by immunohistochemical analysis in neurons and astrocytes. The three isoenzymes differ in their allosteric properties and their distribution in different brain cells. These differences might be important for regulation of brain glycolysis in the different cellular compartments. Regulation of PFK activity is a major control point for glycolysis (Passoneau & Lowry, 1964). PFK1 is inhibited by compounds that accumulate when energy status is high (ATP, citrate) and is activated by products of functional metabolic activity (AMP, ADP). The powerful allosteric activator of PFK1 is fructose 2,6-bisphosphate, which is produced by the enzymatic reaction catalyzed by phosphofructokinase 2 (PFK2 or PFKB, EC 2.7.1.105). PFKB3 is the main isoform expressed in brain. However, PFKB3 has been described as being constantly degraded via the E3 ubiquitin ligase anaphase-promoting complex/cyclosome (APC/C)-Cdh1 (Herrero-Mendez et al., 2009). Therefore, glycolysis in neurons is not activated. Indeed, when mitochondrial respiration is inhibited, astrocytes upregulate their glycolytic rates through fructose 2,6-bisphosphate production, while neurons die quickly. Thus glucose must be oxidized through other metabolic pathways, such as PPP, in neurons (see below).

Pyruvate kinase is expressed in neurons and astrocytes. But apparently, in brain, the reaction catalyzed by pyruvate kinase does not appear to be a major control point in glycolysis (Lowry & Passoneau, 1964).

2.1.2 Glycogen metabolism

Glucose can be stored in the form of glycogen in brain. Glycogen is synthesized from glucose-6-phosphate via glucose-1-phosphate and UDPglucose. Glycogen stores may only sustain brain metabolic turnover for a few minutes at most. Glycogen metabolism is regulated by two enzyme reactions, catalyzed by glycogen synthase and glycogen phosphorylase (Figure 2). Most, if not all, glycogen is localized in astrocytes (Vilchez et al., 2007). However, neuronal cells express enzymatic machinery for glycogen synthesis. Glycogen synthase is expressed in cultured neurons in a highly phosphorylated (inactive) state (Vilchez et al., 2007). Glycogen synthase phosphorylation is achieved by glycogen synthase kinase 3 (EC 2.7.11.26). The abnormal activation of glycogen synthase is responsible for abnormal glycogen deposits in neurons, a feature observed in Lafora disease. Lafora disease is an autosomal recessive form of epilepsy which has been associated with mutations in malin and laforin genes. The malin-laforin complex induces the degradation of both PTG (regulatory subunit of protein phosphatase 1 that activates glycogen synthase) by dephosphorylation, and glycogen synthase. Interaction of malin and laforin is a regulated process that is modulated by the AMP-activated protein kinase (Solaz-Fuster et al., 2008).

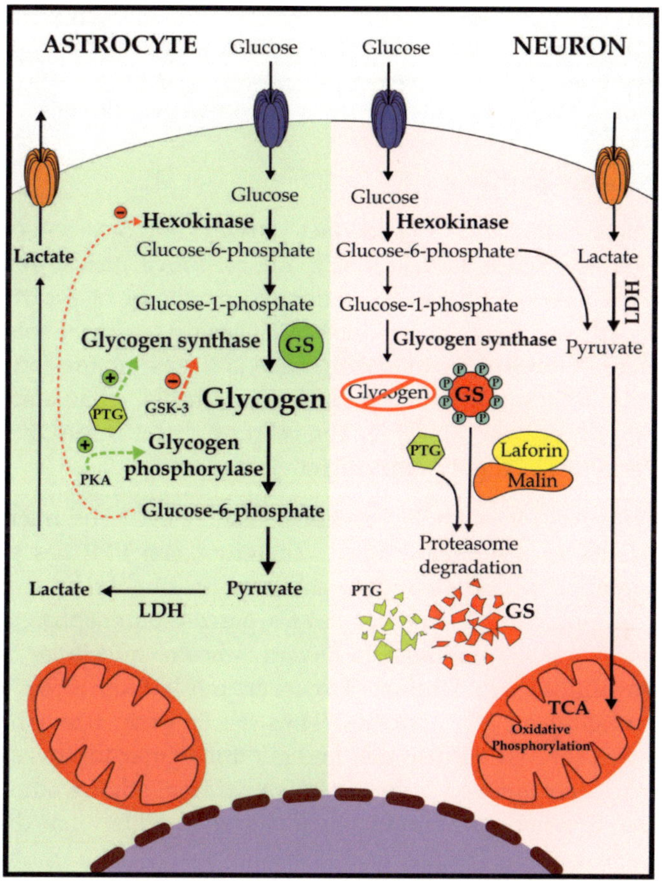

Fig. 2. Glycogen metabolism. Glycogen is synthesized in astrocytes by glycogen synthase (GS). Glycogenolysis is mediated by glycogen phosphorylase (GP). Both GS and GP are regulated in opposite directions by phosphorylation. GS is activated by protein phosphatase-1 and inhibited by GS kinase-3 (GSK-3). Both GS and protein phosphatase-1 interact with glycogen via protein targeting to glycogen (PTG). In neurons, GS is present in a highly phosphorylated, inactive state and, together with PTG, is targeted for proteasome-dependent degradation by the laforin-malin complex. Glycogenolysis in astrocytes depends on GP, which is activated by phosphorylation by several kinases, including the cyclic adenosine monophosphate (cAMP)-activated protein kinase A (PKA) in response to several neurochemical signals. Glycogenolysis in astrocytes leads to the production of lactate, which serves as an energy substrate for oxidative metabolism in the active neurons.

On the other hand, astrocytic glycogen is good for the brain. During synaptic activity, breakdown of astrocytic glycogen is stimulated by neurotransmitters such as glutamate and norepinephrine (Walls et al., 2008). Adrenergic agents cause protein kinase A (PKA) activation in astrocytes through metabotropic receptor binding. Glycogenolysis in astrocytes depends on glycogen phosphorylase, which is activated by phosphorylation of several kinases, including PKA (Benarroch, 2010). Glycogenolysis produces glucose-6-phosphate. It has been proposed that glucose-6-phosphate is used to produce metabolic substrates such as lactate, which can be exported from astrocytes to neuronal cells (Benarroch, 2010; Walls et al., 2008). It has also been proposed that glucose-6-phosphate from glycogen in astrocytes inhibits glycolysis (by hexokinase inhibition) and thus, glucose consumption is favored by neurons (DiNuzzo et al., 2011). In any case, glycogen is important for brain. Indeed glycogen metabolism in astrocytes only occurs in mature astrocytic cells.

2.1.3 Pentose phosphate pathway

The pentose phosphate pathway (PPP) generates NADPH and 5-carbon carbohydrates. PPP has two distinct phases (Figure 3). The first is the oxidative phase, in which NADPH is generated, and in the second phase, non-oxidative synthesis of 5-carbon carbohydrates occurs. Even if this pathway involves oxidation of glucose, its primary role is anabolic rather than catabolic. Glucose-6-phosphate dehydrogenase is the regulatory enzyme in PPP. It is regulated by the NADPH:$NADP^+$ ratio and is allosterically stimulated by nicotinamide adenine dinucleotide phosphate ($NADP^+$). The ratio of NADPH:$NADP^+$ is normally high. Thus, this makes the cytosol a highly-reducing environment.

$NADP^+$ is a coenzyme used in anabolic reactions, such as lipid and nucleic acid synthesis, which require NADPH as a reducing agent. Therefore, the PPP has a more prominent function in developing brain compared to adult brain due to lipogenesis and myelin formation during development. Astrocytes have a glucose-6-phosphate dehydrogenase K_i 10-times lower than glioma cells because PPP is an indicator of cellular biosynthesis, while glycolysis indicates cellular proliferation. However, adult brain slices from several age groups have shown similar PPP capacities. Thus, adult brain has a high PPP capacity. NADPH could be used for neurotransmitter and gliotransmitter turnover and to metabolize aldehydes and peroxides produced by monoamine oxidase, among other enzymes. In this way, NADPH is used to regenerate glutathione (GSH) from glutathione disulfide, which is a product of peroxide scavenging (Baquer et al., 1988).

As was mentioned previously, neurons are unable to increase glycolysis due to the lack of PFKB3. PFKB3 is constantly degraded in neuronal cells and thus glucose should be directed mainly to the PPP to generate NADPH and regenerate GSH (Bolaños et al., 2010). Recently, it has been demonstrated that glucose metabolism and glycogen utilization is impaired in astrocytes with a chronic GSH deficit (Lavoie et al., 2011). So, PPP activity is important in other brain cells besides neurons.

2.1.4 Tricarboxylic acid cycle and oxidative phosphorylation

The tricarboxylic acid (TCA) cycle, also called the citric acid cycle or Krebs cycle, includes eight enzyme-catalysed chemical reactions, which are of central importance in all living cells. The purpose of the TCA is the complete oxidation of acetyl carbons from acetyl coenzyme A (Acetyl-CoA) with the subsequent formation of NADH and $FADH_2$ (Figure 4). The TCA cycle is closely linked to oxidative phosphorylation. In oxidative phosphorylation NADH and $FADH_2$ are reoxidized. NADH and $FADH_2$ electrons are transferred from electron

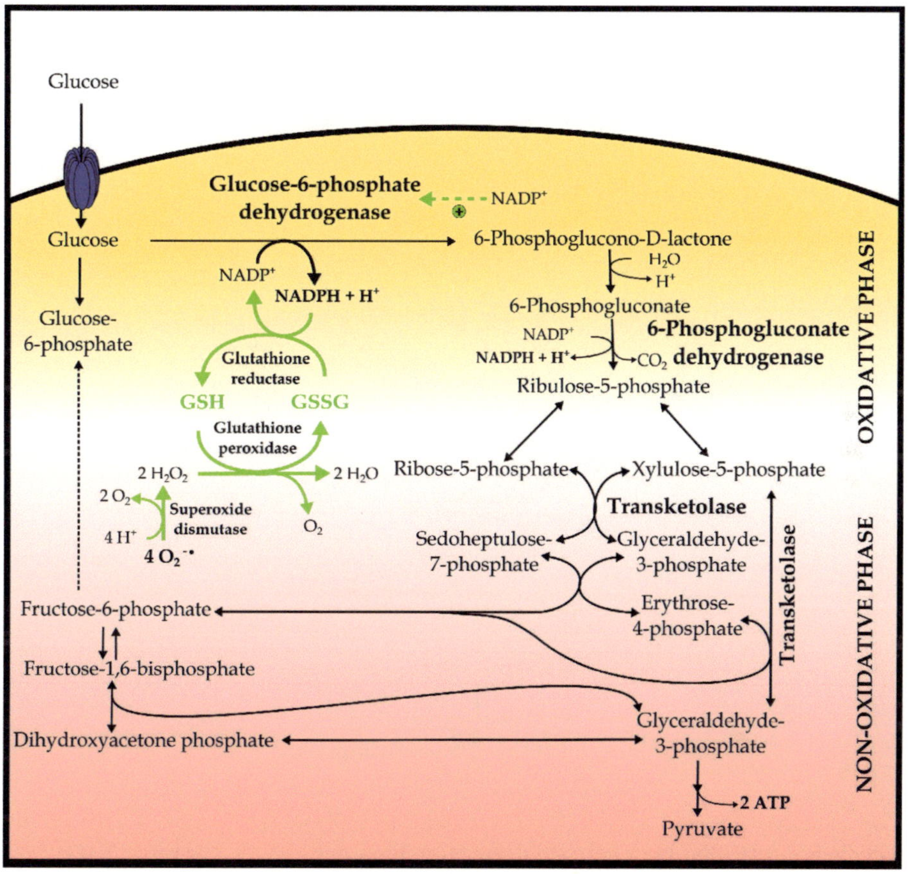

Fig. 3. The pentose phosphate pathway and glutathione. In the oxidative branch of the pentose phosphate pathway, two NADPH are generated per glucose-6-phosphate. The only limiting reaction of the pathway is catalyzed by glucose-6-phosphate dehydrogenase (G6PDH), which is allosterically activated by $NADP^+$. G6PDH catalyzes glucose-6-phosphate oxidation and the production of the first NADPH. This NADPH is oxidized and thus glutathione is reduced. The second NADPH is generated through the oxidative decarboxylation of 6-phosphogluconate, a reaction catalyzed by glucose-6-phosphogluconate dehydrogenase. The nonoxidative branch of the pentose phosphate pathway provides a reversible link with glycolysis by regenerating the two glycolytic intermediates glyceraldehyde-3-phosphate and fructose-6-phosphate.

donors to consecutive electron acceptors, in which the last electron acceptor is oxygen (oxygen is reduced to H_2O, Figure 4). The energy released by electrons flowing through this electron transport chain is used to transport protons across the inner mitochondrial membrane, generating a potential energy (as an electrochemical gradient). This energy is used to synthesize ATP in a enzyme reaction catalyzed by a large enzyme called ATP synthase.

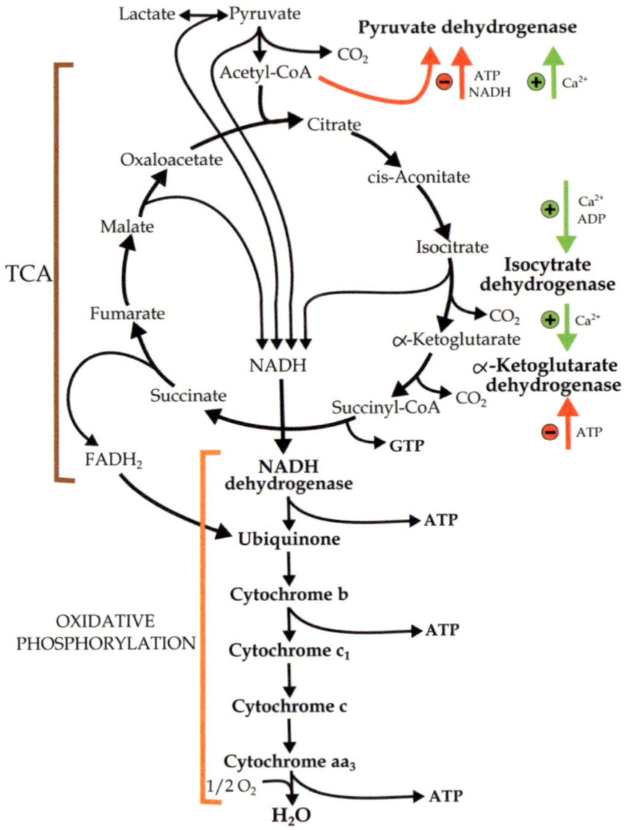

Fig. 4. The tricarboxylic acid cycle (TCA) and oxidative phosphorylation. Pyruvate entry into the cycle is controlled by pyruvate dehydrogenase activity that is inhibited by ATP and NADH. Two other regulatory steps in the cycle are controlled by isocitrate and α-ketoglutarate dehydrogenase, whose activity is controlled by the levels of high-energy phosphates. All dehydrogenases are stimulated by Ca^{2+}. NADH and $FADH_2$ produced in TCA are reoxidized by the donation of their electron to the electron transport chain, the final goal of which is reduction of oxygen to water. Electron flux is responsible for the necessary energy to drive ATP synthesis.

2.1.4.1 Formation of Acetyl-CoA

Acetyl-CoA is produced mainly from pyruvate, the product of glycolysis. Pyruvate enters the mitochondrion and it is oxidized via an enzyme reaction catalyzed by the pyruvate dehydrogenase complex. This is composed of three different enzymes that catalyse seven reactions in order to oxidize pyruvate to Acetyl-CoA. Pyruvate dehydrogenase complex K_m for Acetyl-CoA is approximately 0.05 mM. which is similar to pyruvate concentrations in brain. The enzyme complex also requires a variety of substrates and cofactors: pyruvate, NAD^+, thiamine pyrophosphate, FAD, lipoic acid and coenzyme A. Activity of pyruvate dehydrogenase complex is regulated by phosphorylation state and Ca^{2+} concentration among other factors (Huang et al., 1998). Pyruvate dehydrogenase complex immunoreactivity has been observed in neuronal cells (Calingasan et al., 1994). A low pyruvate dehydrogenase complex enzyme activity and immunoreactivity has been described in neurons following ischemia and reperfusion. This could explain the reduced cerebral glucose and oxygen consumption that occurs after cerebral ischemia (Martin et al., 2005).

Although brain Acetyl-CoA is mainly derived from pyruvate, it can also be synthesized form fatty acids, ketone bodies (see below), monocarboxylate acids, such as lactate (see below) and acetate. Fatty acids are mainly oxidized inside the mitochondria through β-oxidation to produce Acetyl-CoA, NADH and $FADH_2$.

2.2 Use of lactate and ketone bodies

The transport of lactate and ketone bodies is accomplished by the monocarboxylate transporters (MCTs). Although BBB cells express MCT1, monocarboxylates cross the BBB with poor efficiency under physiological conditions. Only under extreme conditions, like starvation or prolonged exercise, could these compounds be important exogenous sources of metabolic fuel for the brain (Quistorff et al. 2008).

2.2.1 Lactate formation and lactate oxidation

Normally, when the glycolysis rate exceeds the rate of triose entry into the TCA cycle, pyruvate can be reduced to lactate by lactate dehydrogenase (LDH, EC 1.1.1.27) which catalyzes a reversible reaction (Figure 1). Lactate must be released because local lactate accumulation would be an opposing driving force that would influence many reversible NAD^+/NADH-coupled redox reactions.

Extracellular lactate is transported into the cell and is oxidized to pyruvate because LDH catalyzes the reversible interconversion between pyruvate and lactate. Two distinct subunits combine to form the five tetrameric isoenzymes of LDH. The LDH-5 subunit (muscle type, also termed the A or M subunit) has a higher maximal velocity (V_{max}) and is present in glycolytic tissues, favoring the formation of lactate from pyruvate, while the LDH-1 subunit (heart type, also referred to as the B or H subunit) favors the reaction towards the production of pyruvate. The different catalytic properties of the five isoenzymes of LDH (H4 or LDH-1, H3M or LDH-2, H2M2 or LDH-3, HM3 or LDH-4, and M4 or LDH-5) are in proportion to the ratio of LDH-5 to LDH-1 subunits. It has been demonstrated that neurons contain predominantly LDH-1, while astrocytes express LDH-5 (Bittar et al. 1996). In this way, lactate synthesized within astrocytes and released into the interstitial space in brain may serve as energy fuel for neurons. Astrocytes release lactate at a greater rate than neurons and lactate is preferentially metabolized in neural cells to produce energy and in oligodendrocytes to synthesize lipids (to make myelin, Sanchez-Abarca et al., 2001).

2.2.2 Ketone bodies formation and oxidation

Glucose is the main energetic fuel for brain. However, under certain conditions the brain can meet its energetic needs using ketone bodies. During ketosis, glucose brain consumption decreases by about 10% per each mM of plasma ketone bodies (LaManna et al., 2009). Ketone bodies are produced from Acetyl-CoA. Lipids are not a major energy source for the brain. Astrocytes are able to oxidize fatty acids and ketone bodies, while neurons and oligodendrocytes can only use ketone bodies.

Ketone bodies are synthesized mainly in the liver. Ketone body synthesis is activated after exhaustion of cellular carbohydrate stores (glycogen). Fatty acids are broken down via β-oxidation to Acetyl-CoA, NADH and $FADH_2$. Normally, Acetyl-CoA is completely oxidized via the TCA cycle. However, if the amount of Acetyl-CoA generated in fatty-acid β-oxidation increases disproportionately, the processing capacity of the TCA cycle will start to drop due to low levels of intermediates. Acetyl-CoA will then be used instead for biosynthesis of acetoacetate, β-hydroxybutyrate and acetone (ketone bodies) through four enzymatic reactions (Figure 4). The utilization of ketones bodies is controlled by leptin through AMPK inhibition in the hypothalamic region (Narishima et al., 2011).

During starvation, during chronic feeding with high fat/low carbohydrate or in pathophysiological conditions as diabetes, glucose stores are depleted and ketone body synthesis is stimulated. Under these conditions, the concentration of ketone bodies in blood increases and MCT expression increases at the blood brain barrier. Within the brain, ketone bodies may be used because all brain cells express MCTs and because the enzymatic reactions of ketone body synthesis are reversible (except for spontaneous decarboxylation of acetoacetate to acetone). Thus brain cells obtain Acetyl-CoA from ketone bodies and Acetyl-CoA may be oxidized for those cells through the TCA cycle. The starving brain also extracts fatty acids from blood. Astrocytes can degrade fatty acids by β-oxidation to provide neurons with ketone bodies (Edmond, 1992). Moreover, ketone body oxidation must be important during the first postnatal period. Knockout animals for the ketolytic enzyme succinyl-CoA: 3-oxoacid CoA-transferase exhibit normal prenatal development, but develop ketoacidosis, hypoglycemia, and reduced plasma lactate concentrations within the first 48 h of birth (Cotter et al., 2011).

A ketogenic diet has been proposed for treatment of epilepsy. This diet is a strict high fat, low protein, low carbohydrate diet, and is anticonvulsant in many drug-resistant epileptic children. The diet is also effective in mice. The mechanism by which this diet controls intractable seizures is unknown. The diet does not affect behavorial performance or synaptic plasticity. Ketone bodies not only function as an energy substrate, but also as intermediates for the synthesis of lipids and neurotransmitters. Because of this, a link has been proposed between ketone bodies, brain function and polyunsaturated fatty acids (Pifferi et al., 2008). Another proposed mechanism to explain the neuroprotective effect of the ketogenic diet is via mitochondrial improvement by scavenging of reactive species and regulation of gene expression to increase neuronal survival (Beskow et al., 2008). Ketone bodies are also proposed as protectors from neurotoxicity in other pathologies, such as Parkinson's disease and Alzheimer's disease (Kashiwaya et al., 2000).

3. Metabolic pathways during brain activation

The resting brain is not really at rest. It demonstrates continuous cognitive and sensory activity. For example, when we listen music, auditive areas of the brain are selectively activated. Over 120 years ago, brain activation was shown to produce an increase en blood flow in specific brain areas. The increased blood flow has been shown to be accompanied by an increase in glucose utilization (Sokoloff et al., 1977). A mechanism that couples neuronal metabolism with blood flow should thus exist. An increase in extracellular K^+, adenosine, and lactate and related changes in pH are all a consequence of increased neuronal activity. All of them have been considered mediators of neurovascular coupling because they have vasoactive effects (Villringer & Dirnagl, 1995). Astroglial cells seem to be protagonists in the coupling of neuron metabolism and blood flow. Astrocytes, like neurons, are organized into networks, although glial cells are organized as a syncytium, linked to each other by gap junctions (Giaume et al., 2010). Neuronal cells exchange information through chemical and electrical synapses. Astrocyte gap junctions are regulated by extra- and intracelullar signals. Astrocytes release molecules that induce local constriction or dilation of smooth muscle cells surrounding endothelial cells forming arterioles (Attwell et al., 2010). Astrocytes also release molecules in response to neuronal activation. These molecules can modulate synaptic transmission and neuronal excitability (a concept referred to as the tripartite synapse, Perea & Araque, 2010). So, during brain activation, blood flow is increased due to several interactions between brain cells. We will discuss below the metabolic pathways that function during brain activation in neuronal and astroglial cells. We will then discuss the neuroglial interation and molecular mechanisms that modulate the interaction.

3.1 Neuron metabolism during activity periods

In a chemical synapse, neurotransmitters released from the presynaptic neuron bind to ionotropic receptors in the postsynaptic membrane increasing the open probability of these ion channels. The ion flow can produce membrane depolarization (excitatory action potentials) or hyperpolarization (inhibitory action potentials). Excitatory action potentials are produced by the sequential opening of voltage-sensitive Na^+ channels, followed by the delayed opening of K^+ channels. This permits movement of positive charges from and into the neuronal cytosol. According to the biophysical properties of neuronal membranes, a theoretical minimum positive charge transfer (carried by Na^+) was predicted per propagating action potential of 121 nC/cm^2. This was corroborated by Alle and colleagues (2009) who calculated that charging of membrane capacitance requires 153 nC/cm^2 only 1.3 times more than the theoretical minimum. Action potentials are thus energy-efficient, minimizing their contribution to activity-dependent metabolism. But human brain has billions of neurons and each neuron maintains a large number of synaptic connections to other neurons. Even though action potentials are energy-efficient, this is consistent with the fact that neuronal activity accounts for 80% of brain energy consumption (Sibson et al., 1998). Most of the energy consumed in the brain is attributable to restoration of the membrane resting potential following depolarization. This is accomplished by the Na^+/K^+-ATPase (EC 3.6.1.3, Attwell & Laughlin, 2001). Other energy-consuming processes are neurotransmitter recycling and axonal and dendritic transport (Ames, 2000). Because glutamate synapses represent at least 80% of cortical synapses, glutamate-mediated neurotransmission consumes most of the energy expended in the brain.

Electrical stimulation opens Na^+ channels in neuronal populations. An increase in intracellular Na^+ concentration activates the Na^+/K^+-ATPase at its Na^+-sensitive intracellular site. The activation of Na^+/K^+-ATPase is accompanied by a decrease in the ATP/ADP ratio and glycolysis activation (Figure 6, probably via allosteric activation of PFK1 by ADP). Glycolysis activation is accompanied by a Ca^{2+} increase and an increase in pyruvate and $NADH/NAD^+$ concentrations. TCA and oxidative phosphorylation are also stimulated (Figure 6). Indeed, mitochondrial dehydrogenases are activated by an increase in intracellular Ca^{2+} (Figure 4). During glutamatergic activity, glutamate binds to ionotropic receptors and metabotropic channels in these cells. Both produce an increase in intracellular Ca^{2+}. Glucose oxidation (determined by CO_2 production) has been shown to be produced by an increased intracellular Na^+ concentration in neuronal-enriched cultures. However, neuronal cells are unable to stimulate glycolysis via fructose 2,6-bisphosphate (see above, Herrero-Mendez et al., 2009). It has thus been proposed that, when energy needs are overcome by glycolytic activity stimulated by ADP, neuronal cells preferentially consume lactate. Astrocytes release lactate in response to synaptic activation (see below, Magistretti et al., 2000) and neuronal cells oxidize this lactate through the TCA and oxidative phosphorylation via a mechanism named the neuron lactate shuttle hypothesis (ANLSH, see below, Magistretti et al., 1999; Allaman et al., 2010). To facilitate lactate use, glycolysis must be inhibited. We will discuss below the details of neuron-glia coupling and the inhibition of glucose use.

The pentose phosphate pathway (PPP) supplies red blood cells with NADPH, which in turn maintains the reduced state of glutathione (GSH). GSH has antioxidant properties since the thiol group in its cysteine moiety is a reducing agent and can be reversibly oxidized and reduced. In cells, GSH is maintained in the reduced form by the enzyme glutathione reductase. Regeneration of reduced *GSH* requires *NADPH*. Therefore, PPP is important for maintenance of adequate levels of GSH (Figure 6). Neurons are thought to be particularly vulnerable to damage by reactive oxygen and nitrogen species. Nitrogen species stimulate the PPP rate (Bolaños et al., 2010). The brain is a specific source of oxidative species such as those coming from metabolism of excitatory amino acids and neurotransmitters. During glutamatergic activity, glutamate binds ionotropic receptors and metabotropic channels in these cells. Both produce an increase on intracellular Ca^{2+}. The high and constant use of oxygen results in oxidative stress through the production of superoxide. Finally, other sources of free radicals are produced by Cytochrome P450 and monoamine oxidase activity. It is thus not surprising that neuronal cells oxidize glucose through the PPP (Figure 5 and Figure 6), especially, considering that neurons are unable to increase glycolysis activity via allosteric activation of PFK1 by fructose 2,6-bisphosphate (Figure 1, Herrero-Mendez et al., 2009).

3.2 Metabolic activation in astrocytes

Extracellular K^+ activates the Na^+/K^+-ATPase via its extracellular K^+-sensitive site in cultured astrocytes but not in neurons (Grisar et al. 1979; Hajek et al. 1996). Na^+/K^+-ATPase activation produces a decrease in the ATP/ADP ratio, and thus glycolysis activation (see above, Figure 7, Sokoloff et al., 1996). Extracellular K^+ concentrations of between 5 and 12 mM increase glucose phosphorylation in cultured astrocytes (Hof et al., 1988). The Na^+/K^+-ATPase can also be activated by increased intracellular Na^+ concentration (Denton et al., 1988). An increase in intracellular Na^+ concentration in astrocytes can be stimulated by the presence of glutamate. Glutamate uptake is carried out by excitatory amino acid transporters. This transport by excitatory amino acid transporters is dependent on the electrochemical gradient of sodium ions. Glutamate uptake can induce metabolic activation in astrocytes and can also be used as energetic fuel. Glutamate can be transformed into α-ketoglutarate through a reaction catalyzed by the enzyme aspartate amino transferase (EC 2.6.1.1, Fonnum, 1967) and thus, glutamate carbons can be oxidized through the TCA.

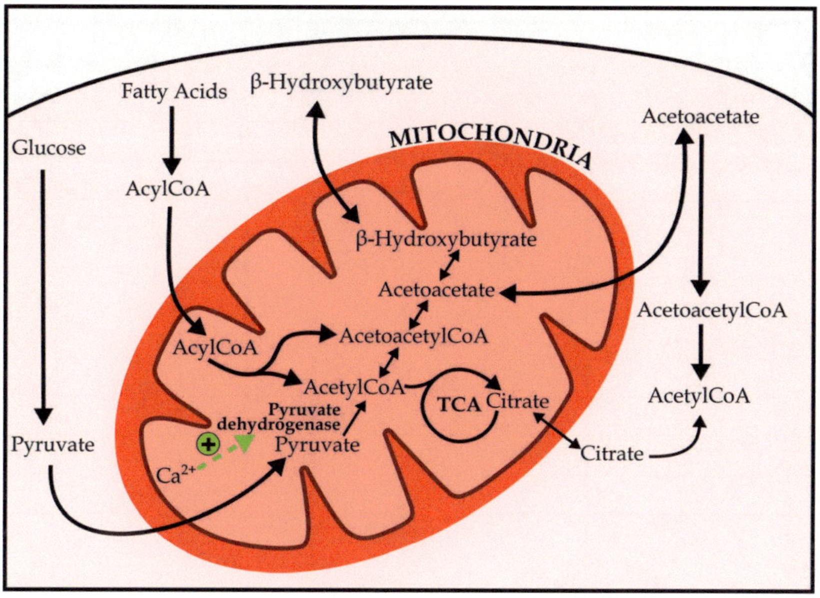

Fig. 5. Relationship between lipid metabolism and the TCA cycle. Under particular dietary conditions, such as lactation in newborns or fasting in adults, the ketone bodies acetoacetate and β-hydroxybutyrate and circulating fatty acids can provide substrates to the TCA cycle after their conversion to Acetyl-CoA. Carbon atoms for lipid synthesis can be provided by glucose through citrate produced in the TCA cycle, a particularly relevant process for the developing brain.

Glycogen stores may also be mobilized during astrocytic activation (Figure 7). During brain activation, neurotransmitters such as noradrenaline can stimulate PTG expression and thus, glycogen synthesis (Allaman et al., 2010). However, at the same time, Na^+/K^+-ATPase activation induces a decrease in the ATP/ADP ratio and glycogen catabolism activation. Serotonin and other neurotransmitters induce an increase in intracellular concentrations of Ca^{2+} (via IP_3 production) and thus, activate glycogenolysis (Chen & Hertz, 1999). Activation of glycogen synthesis and degradation is termed the glycogen shunt (Walls et al., 2008). Glucose-6-phosphate from glycogen can be oxidized through glycolysis to produce lactate which is exported to neurons (Figure 7). It has, in fact, been demonstrated that glycogen is required for sustaining glutamatergic neurotransmission and for long-term memory formation (Suzuki et al., 2011).

Besides glutathione, the brain also uses ascorbic acid to protect itself from oxidant species. Ascorbic acid is highly concentrated in brain (Kratzing et al. 1982). In aqueous solutions, ascorbic acid is a powerful reductant and is oxidized to dehydroascorbic acid. The regeneration of ascorbic acid from dehydroascorbic acid is not spontaneous. Reduction is mainly an enzymatically catalyzed reaction, which may be glutathione-dependent (Ishikawa et al. 1998). Astrocytes are thought to be involved in ascorbic acid recycling (Figure 10, Astuya et al. 2005). During synaptic activity, ascorbic acid is released from intracellular reservoirs (O'Neill et al. ,1984; Ghasemzadeh et al., 1991; Yusa, 2001). The molecular basis of ascorbic acid efflux is not yet well known. Neurons can take up ascorbic acid efficiently because they express SVCT2 (Castro et al., 2001). Ascorbic acid is oxidized within neurons

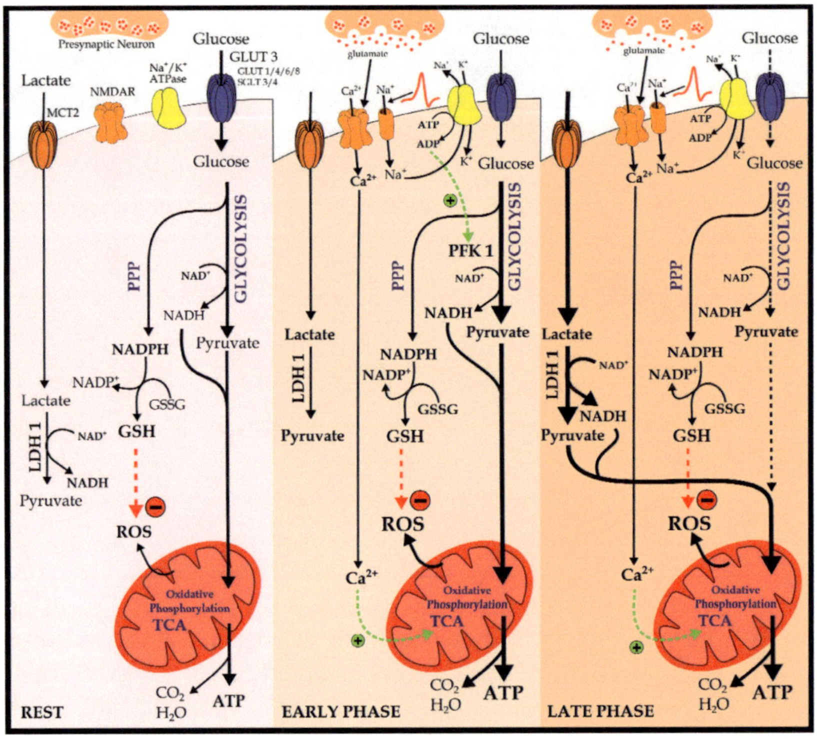

Fig. 6. Neuron metabolism during synaptic activity. Electrical stimulation opens Na^+ channels in neuronal cells. An increase in intracellular Na^+ concentration is able to activate Na^+K^+-ATPase at its Na^+-sensitive intracellular site (early phase). This activation produces a decrease in ATP/ADP ratio and thus, glycolysis activation by allosteric activation of PFK1 by ADP. Glycolysis activation is accompanied by Ca^{2+} increase and therefore, mitochondrial oxidative metabolism activation. In the late phase of synaptic activation, glycolysis activity is inhibited and lactate uptake is stimulated (see Figure 10 for details of inhibition of glucose utilization and stimulation of lactate transport in synaptically-active neurons). PPP is always present in neuronal cells because NADPH is required to maintain the redox balance in these cells. During synaptic activity, PPP becomes more important because synaptic activity produces oxidant species. NADPH is used to regenerate GSH and thus, to reduce oxidant species.

because during synaptic activity many oxidant species are generated. Neuronal oxidized ascorbic acid (dehydroascorbic acid) can be released through glucose transporters, GLUT1 or GLUT3 (because dehydroascorbic acid is a substrate for GLUTs; Vera et al., 1993). Astrocytes uptake dehydroascorbic acid through GLUT1 and thus, they reduce dehydroascorbic acid to ascorbic acid through mechanisms that require GSH. GSH regeneration and PPP activation under synaptic transmission conditions should thus be important for astrocytes (Figure 7, Figure 10).

Astrocytic cells also express metabotropic glutamate receptors (mGluRs). Thus, during excitatory brain activation, glutamate is not only taken up by excitatory amino acid transporters, but glutamate activates mGluRs, which produce and increase intracellular Ca^{2+}

and the production of arachidonic acid and prostaglandins. These substances stimulate dilation or constriction of adjacent arterioles and permit that the correct nutrients and oxygen supply are present in order to sustain neurotransmission (Peppiat & Attwell, 2004).

3.3 Neuron-glia metabolic coupling

As we discuss above, the key to neuron-glia metabolic coupling is the excitatory neurotransmitter glutamate and a rise in extracellular K^+. Glutamatergic synaptic activity is necessary to maintain a low glutamate concentration in the extracellular space for efficient and successful synaptic transmission to occur and to prevent excitotoxicity. Glutamate uptake in astrocytes occurs via excitatory amino acid transporters. Within the cell, glutamate is then converted to glutamine by glutamine synthetase (EC 6.3.1.2). Glutamine is released into the extracellular space and is taken up by adjacent neurons that synthesize glutamate from glutamine in a reaction catalyzed by glutaminase (EC 3.5.1.2). This recycling of glutamate is named the glutamate–glutamine cycle (Figure 10, Sibson et al., 1997).

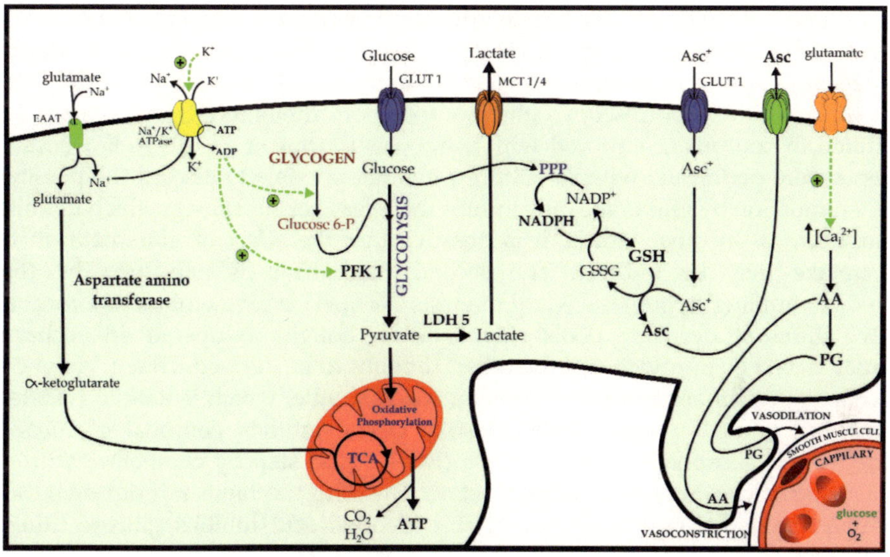

Fig. 7. Metabolic activation of astrocytes. Synaptic activity produces an increase in extracellular K^+, which stimulates Na^+K^+-ATPase by binding of its extracellular K^+-sensitive site. The excitatory neurotransmitter glutamate is taken up by astrocytes through excitatory amino acid transporters. This kind of transport produces an increase in intracellular Na^+, which stimulates Na^+K^+-ATPase by binding of its intracellular Na^+-sensitive site. Na^+K^+-ATPase activation produces a decrease in ATP/ADP ratio and, thus glycolysis and glycogenolysis activation. In addition, glucose is oxidized by PPP to produce NADPH and to maintain the redox balance, reducing glutathione and ascorbic acid (Asc). Ascorbic acid released by astrocytes is taken up by neurons to protect themselves from oxidant species (ascorbic acid is oxidized in neurons). Oxidized ascorbic acid (dehydroascorbic acid, Asc^+) is released from neurons and taken up by astrocytes through GLUT1. Finally, in astrocytes, glutamate is able to bind ionotropic receptors, which are predominantly calcium channels. This Ca^{2+} increase cooperates with TCA activation and produces arachidonic acid (AA) and prostaglandin (PG) which stimulate the constriction and dilation of capillaries, respectively.

According to ANLSH, glutamate uptake also stimulates glucose uptake (Pellerin & Magistretti, 1994), glycolysis and lactate release in astrocytes (Pellerin & Magistretti, 1994; Demestre et al., 1997). In a similar way, glycolysis and glucose uptake is activated by an increase in the extracellular concentration of K^+ (Pellerin & Magistretti, 1994; Gegelashvili et al., 2007). An increased extracellular K^+ concentration stimulates 2-deoxyglucose phosphorylation (Hof et al., 1988) and lactate formation and release of lactate (Walz & Mukerji, 1988) in cultured astrocytes. Neurons take up the lactate released from astrocytes (Figure 10, Magistretti et al., 2000; Allaman et al., 2010). Lactate flow happens would be possible because there are a differential MCTs and LDH isoenzymes expression between neuronal and astroglial cells. However, use of neuronal lactate has been strongly debated in studies that support the idea that glucose is the main metabolic substrate for these cells (Chih & Roberts, 2003; Dienel, 2009; Gjedde, 2002; Hertz, 2004; Hertz et al., 2007; Mangia et al., 2003; Mangia et al., 2009).

Activation of glycolysis produces an increase in pyruvate and proton concentrations that are accompanied by a decrease in the $NAD^+/NADH$ ratio. Neuronal LDH1 should catalyze reduction of pyruvate to lactate. So, lactate utilization by neurons would only be possible if the consumption of glucose, either at the transport or the glycolysis stage, were inhibited. To explain this, at least four different (though coexistent) ideas have been proposed (Figure 10). Firstly, using real-time microscopy, glucose transport inhibition by glutamate has been demonstrated in neurons co-cultured with astrocytes (Porras et al., 2008). But because these experiments were performed with co-cultures, it is not possible to discard the possibility that astrocytic stimulation by glutamate may induce the release of substances which inhibit glucose uptake in neurons. In other words, it is possible that the effect of glutamate on neuronal glucose uptake may be indirect. The second mechanism is explained by the redox switch/redox coupling hypothesis (Cerdan et al., 2006). This idea embraces a mechanism in which two different pyruvate pools exist: one is thought to operate in exchange with extracellular lactate or pyruvate and the other, thought to be derived from glycolytic activity. This mechanism considers a lactate/pyruvate redox shuttle, which is able to transfer lactate from astrocytes to neurons. So, high cytosolic lactate inhibits neuronal glycolysis at the glyceraldehyde- 3-phosphate dehydrogenase (EC 1.2.1.12) step by competing with cytosolic NAD^+, favoring oxidation of extracellular lactate. The third mechanism is our own theory. We have demonstrated that neuronal intracellular ascorbic acid inhibits glucose utilization in neurons (Castro et al., 2009) through GLUT3 inhibition (Figure 8, Beltrán et al., 2011). This mechanism is supported by the idea of ascorbic acid recycling in brain (see above, Figure 10, Astuya et al., 2005). Using primary cultures of cortical neurons treated with a specific shRNA (to block GLUT3 expression) and a fluorescent glucose analogue, we have shown that this transporter is important, using real-time experiments (Figure 7). At the same time, intracellular ascorbic acid is able to stimulate lactate transport in neurons and in cells that express GLUT3 (Figure 9, Castro et al., 2008). Because ascorbic acid is able to change metabolic substrate preferences, we have termed this mechanism the ascorbic acid metabolic switch (Castro et al., 2009). The fourth proposed mechanism relates to the inability of neuronal cells to overactivate glycolysis (Herrero-Mendez et al., 2009; Bolaños et al., 2010). This idea is supported by elegant experimental data that demonstrate that in neurons, it is not possible to produce the allosteric activator of PFK1 (and therefore glycolysis activator) fructose 2,6-bisphosphate. The enzyme that catalyzes fructose-2,6-bisphosphate in neurons, PFK3B, has a very short half-life as it is being constantly degraded (Herrero-Mendez et al., 2009). This mechanism does not exclude basal glycolytic activity however.

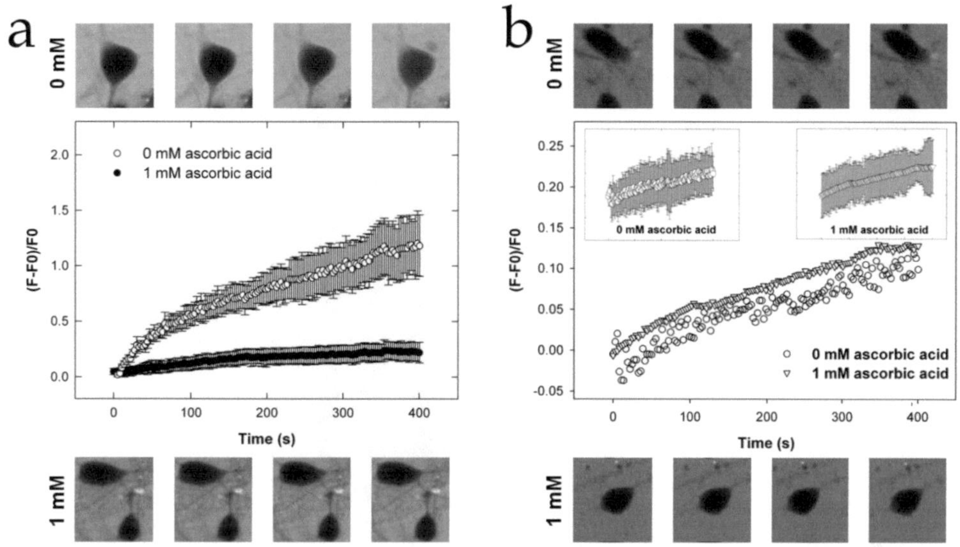

Fig. 8. Intracellular ascorbic acid only inhibits transport of 2-NBDG in cells expressing GLUT3. A: Time course of uptake of 2-NBDG (2-[N-(7-nitrobenz-2-oxa-1,3-diazol-4-yl)amino]-2-deoxyglucose). 2-NBDG transport in cortical neurons in the presence (closed circles) or absence (open circles) of intracellular ascorbic acid. B: Time course of uptake of 2-NBDG transport in neuronal cells treated with shRNA to knock down GLUT3 expression in the presence (triangles) or absence (circles) of intracellular ascorbic acid. The data represent the mean ± SD of four experiments (14 control cells and 10 shRNA-treated cells). The images represent one control experiment and one experiment with shRNA-treated cells, in the presence or absence of ascorbic acid. Adapted from Beltran et al. (2011) with permission of the publisher.

4. Metabolic failure in neurodegenerative diseases

Neurodegenerative disease is a broad term for a range of conditions which primarily affect neurons in the brain. Progression of neurodegenerative diseases is accompanied by loss of neuronal cell structure and function and even cell death. These diseases have many similarities at a sub-cellular level including atypical protein assemblies, failure of normal protein degradation pathways, induced cell death, impaired axonal transport and metabolic failures (Rubinsztein et al., 2006; De Vos et al., 2008; Bredesen et al., 2006; Lin & Beal, 2006). A better knowledge of how these failures arise may offer fresh hope for development of therapies that improve treatment of these diseases.

Directly or indirectly, energy is necessary for many, if not all, cellular processes. It is thus possible to speculate that metabolic failure is an early event in neurodegenerative disease. Indeed, there are neurodegenerative diseases caused by a deficiency of metabolic enzymes. One of these is pyruvate dehydrogenase complex deficiency (Brown et al., 1994). This condition has similar characteristics to those of other neurodegenerative diseases. Several neurodegenerative disorders, such as Alzheimer's disease, Huntington's disease and Parkinson's disease, show metabolic failure represented by altered patterns of expression of nutrient transporters, metabolic enzymes and molecular components of cellular respiration.

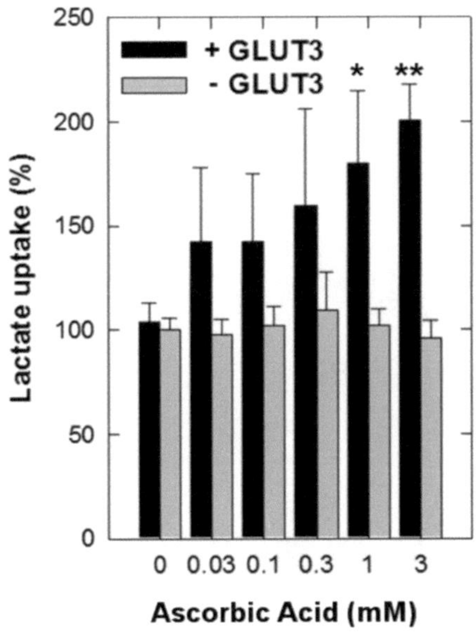

Fig. 9. Intracellular ascorbic acid stimulates lactate uptake in cells expressing GLUT3. Substrate dependence for the inhibition of 0.1 mM lactate transport (10 s, 20 °C) by intracellular ascorbic acid (cells were preloaded with ascorbic acid at the concentrations indicated) in cultured cortical astrocytes (gray bars) and cultured cortical astrocytes expressing GLUT3-EGFP (black bars). Cortical astrocytes were transfected through electroporation. The data represent the mean ± SD of three experiments.

Metabolic failure is also represented by altered activities of the enzymes involved in energy metabolism. Mitochondria are the main platform for oxidative metabolism. They participate in cell metabolism, they produce ATP and they are important regulators of cytosolic calcium, which in turn, is related to whether or not programmed cell death occurs. Neurodegenerative diseases trigger programmed cell death and thus the role of mitochondria is key, from beginning to end of the disease, from the initial failure in energy metabolism to the later onset of cell death.

4.1 Alzheimer's disease

Alzheimer's disease is the most common cause of dementia. It is characterized by progressive cognitive dysfunction. The Alzheimer's disease brain appears atrophied. The temporal lobe, parietal lobe, frontal cortex and cingulate gyrus show degeneration and loss of cellular mass (Wenk, 2003). Parkinson's disease is characterized by loss of neurons and synapses in the cerebral cortex and in some subcortical regions. Genetically, Alzheimer's disease is heterogeneous and complex, showing no simple mode of inheritance. The causes of most Alzheimer's disease cases are still unknown, though in 1-5% of cases, genetic differences have been described. There are two neuropathological changes that can be correlated with an Alzheimer's disease diagnosis. First of all, neurofibrillary tangles (NFTs) accumulate in neuronal cytosol. And secondly, extracellular amyloid deposits appear in the form of senile plaques containing amyloid peptide (Duyckaerts et al., 2008).

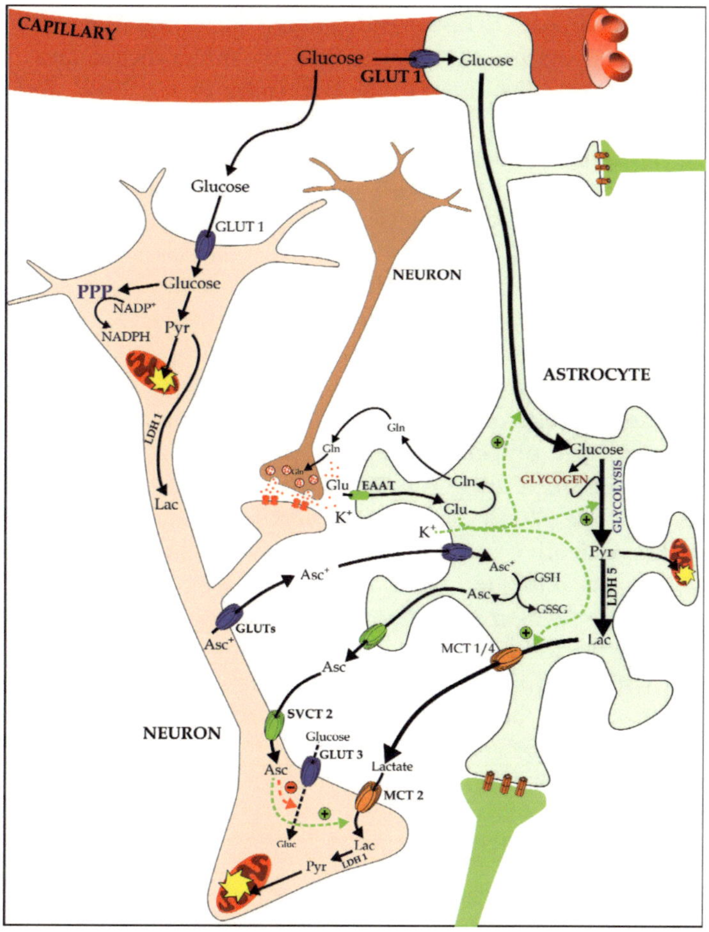

Fig. 10. Neuron-glia metabolic coupling. During glutamatergic synaptic activity, increases in extracellular glutamate and K+ concentration are produced. This metabolically activates these cells (see Figure 7 for details of astrocytic metabolic activation). Astrocytes uptake glutamate and convert it into glutamine. Glutamine is released and taken up by neuronal cells to glutamate resynthesis (glutamate-glutamine shuttle). Metabolic activation of astrocytes produces an increase in glycolysis, glycogenolysis activities and lactate production. Lactate is taken up by neurons to support their energetic needs (astrocyte-neuron lactate shuttle). Lactate uptake and lactate oxidation in neurons is possible because these cells are not able to activate glycolysis through fructose 2,6-bisphosphate production (see Figure 6 for details of metabolism in synaptically-active neuronal cells). Glutamate also stimulates ascorbic acid release form astrocytes. Neuronal cells take up ascorbic acid through SVCT2. Intracellular ascorbic acid inhibits glucose transport through GLUT3 inhibition and stimulates lactate transport (ascorbic acid metabolic switch). Synaptic activity is accompanied by production of oxidant species. Thus ascorbic acid is oxidized to reduce that species. Dehydroascorbic acid (oxidized ascorbic acid, Asc+) is released by neurons and taken up by astrocytes through GLUT1. Astrocytes reduce dehydroascorbic acid to ascorbic acid via gluthathione-dependent reductases (ascorbic acid recycling). Glu: glutathione, Gluc: glucose, Gln: glutamine, Lac: lactate, Pyr: pyruvate.

Type 2 diabetes mellitus appears to be a significant risk factor for Alzheimer's disease (Bosco et al., 2011). Alzheimer's disease is characterized by a significant and pre-symptomatic reduction of brain glucose utilization (Table 1, Ferreira et al., 2010). Indeed, it has been proposed that early diagnosis of Alzheimer's disease will be rendered possible through a combination of imaging modalities (such as *magnetic resonance imaging,* MRI and *positron emission tomography,* PET; Mosconi et al., 2005). There is a correlation between impairment of glucose cerebral metabolism, decreased GLUT expression and cerebral spinal fluid tau protein levels. (Liu et al., 2008; Cevarolo et al., 2008). Indeed, patients show decreased GLUT3 levels (Liu et al., 2008, Harr et al., 1995). A decrease in glycolytic enzyme levels and activity, PFK1 and glyceraldehyde-3-phosphate dehydrogenase (EC 1.2.1.12) has also been described. Decreased glycolysis could be related to an increase in glycogen synthesis. Pharmacological glycogen synthase kinase 3 inhibition improves behavioral dysfunction and decreases tau phosphorylation (Onishi et al., 2011). A spatial correlation between brain glycolysis without oxidative mitochondrial metabolism and amyloid deposition has been described (Vlassenko et al., 2010). Aggregate forms of amyloid can modify glucose metabolism and oxidative stress in astrocytes, affecting neuronal cells and probably contributing to neuronal death (Allaman et al., 2010). Indeed, reduction of GLUT1 and MCT expression, as well as the retraction of of astrocyte endfeet occurs in Alzheimer's disease producing uncoupling of the neurovascular unit (Merlini et al., 2011). The activity of PPP is increased in Alzheimer's disease. Increased oxidative stress markers in Alzheimer's disease samples correlated with enhanced PPP activity suggesting that PPP activity could play a role in the response against brain pro-oxidant activity in Alzheimer's disease. Finally, mitochondrial dysfunction (Schapira et al., 2006), decreased expression of oxidative phosphorylation and reduced activity of cytochrome oxidase were all observed in Alzheimer's disease.

4.2 Huntington's disease

Huntington's disease is a progressive, autosomal dominant, neurodegenerative disorder. It can affect individuals of all ages, from infancy to old age and develops over a period of 15-20 years. Motor dysfunction and cognitive abnormalities are common symptoms. The disease is caused by an expanded polyglutamine (polyQ) stretch in the corresponding causal gene. Huntington's disease represents one of a growing number of polyQ repeat diseases that cause region-specific neuronal degeneration, including spinobulbar muscular atrophy and spinocerebellar ataxias (Pennuto et al., 2009). In Huntington's disease, polyQ expansion affects the *Huntingtin* gene, resulting in major cell loss in the striatum, a region of the basal ganglia that integrates cortical information for behavioral output. Huntington's disease is characterized by widespread neurodegeneration with preferential deterioration of medium-sized spiny neurons (MSSNs) in the striatum (Penney & Young, 1998). The major excitatory input to MSSNs comes from the cortex (corticostriatal pathway) and the thalamus. Huntington's disease also causes dysfunction and subsequent death of neurons in other brain regions, including the cortex.

The *Huntingtin* gene codes for a protein called the huntingtin protein (Htt). It is a soluble 384 kDa protein, essential for embriogenesis, and ubiquitously expressed in moderate amounts in the nervous system as well as in other systems (Cattaneo et al., 2001). Htt is associated with various intracellular organelles, including the nucleus, endoplasmic reticulum, Golgi complex, microtubules and endosomal compartments. Wild-type (normal) huntingtin has an important role in the intracellular transport of vesicles, organelles and traffic of proteins to the cell surface (Caviston et al., 2009). Expansion of a glutamine stretch within the Htt protein to more than 40 repeats appears to confer a dominant toxic property that is deleterious to neurons and detrimental to normal Htt biological activities. The precise actions of the mutant huntingtin are still not clearly understood.

Huntington's disease is characterized by a failure in brain energy metabolism (Table 1). Defects in energy metabolism may even extend to presymptomatic subjects. Positron emission tomography studies have demonstrated marked reductions in glucose metabolism in the basal ganglia (Mazziotta et al., 1987), and in the cerebral cortex of symptomatic Huntington's disease patients (Leenders et al., 1986; Kuwert et al., 1993). However, Oláh and colleagues (2008) described an increase in several glycolytic enzymes and ATP production in brain from Huntington's disease animals. By contrast, the same authors described a marked decrease in glyceraldehyde-3-phosphate dehydrogenase activity. An impairment in enzyme activity of the TCA cycle (Lim et al., 2008) and oxidative phosphorylation has also been described. A key role for proliferator-activated receptor gamma coactivator-1 α has been proposed in the control of energy metabolism in the early stages of Huntington's disease pathogenesis. Proliferator-activated receptor gamma coactivator-1 α is a transcriptional coactivator that regulates several metabolic processes, including mitochondrial biogenesis and oxidative phosphorylation (Finck & Kelly, 2006). Although the origin of metabolic impairment is unknown, it is proposed that a systematic downregulation of persoxisome proliferator-activated receptor-γ plays a critical role in the deregulation of energy homeostasis observed in Huntington's disease (Chiang et al., 2010). Metabolic failure in Huntington's disease not only occurs in brain. Htt is a ubiquitous protein and thus energetic failure may also be observed in peripheral tissues. Huntington's disease patients do show progressive weight loss and development of diabetes (Aziz et al., 2010). These symptoms may be related to an impairment of insulin secretion (Smith et al., 2009).

Finally, oxidative damage has been shown (Mazziotta et al., 1987), as well as impaired SOD activity (Mazziotta et al., 1987) and impaired ascorbic acid homeostasis (Rebec et al., 1994) in Huntington's disease animal models. Our group has been making steady progress with respect to the function of ascorbic acid in neuronal metabolism (Castro et al., 2008; Castro et al., 2009; Beltrán et al., 2011, see above). Ascorbic acid, the reduced form of vitamin C, modulates neuronal metabolism between resting state and brain activation periods.

4.3 Parkinson's disease

Parkinson's disease is the most common neurodegenerative movement disorder of central nervous system. Clinical symptoms are due to the progressive degeneration of dopaminergic neurons in the substantia nigra and other monoaminergic neurons in the brainstem (Braak et al., 2003). The pathology of this disease is characterized by the accumulation of α-synuclein into inclusions called Lewy bodies in neurons. Although Parkinson's disease is a sporadic condition of uncertain ethiology, there is some evidence that mitochondrial dysfunction considerably contributes to the pathogenesis of this disorder (Schapira, 2008). Mutations in several genes are found in Parkinson's disease. Point mutations, duplications and triplications in the α-synuclein gene and mutations in the leucine-rich repeat kinase 2 (LRRK2). Mutations have also been described in genes coding

CNS DISEASE	METABOLIC FAILURE	REFERENCES
Alzheimer's Disease (AD)	Reduced glucose metabolism in AD patients and animal models via measurement of CMRgl by FDG-PET. Early hypometabolism in posterior associative cortical areas and prefrontal areas. Increased activity of G6PDH in temporal cortex of AD patients. Increased G6PDH levels in pyramidal neurons from hippocampus. Mitochondrial dysfunction including: mtDNA mutation, decreased mRNA levels for complex I-IV subunits of the electron transport chain. Decreased activities of glycolytic enzymes, lower pyruvate synthesis, lower pyruvate dehydrogenase activity, lower Acetyl-CoA production and impaired cycloxygenase activity. Decreased expression of GLUT1 and MCT1 in blood brain barrier of AD animal models, decreased GLUT1 and GLUT3 in AD brains. Decreased amount of GLUT-1 transporter in the hippocampus and cerebral cortex of AD patients.	Browen et al., 1979 Ferreira et al., 2010; Harr et al., 1995; Hooijimans et al., 2007; Horwood & Davies, 1994; Kalaria & Harik,1989;; Langbaum et al., 2009; Liu et al., 2008; Merlini et al., 2011; Mooradian et al., 1997;; Nicholson et al., 2010; Ojaimi et al., 1999; Parker et al., 1994; Schapira et al., 2006; Shima et al., 2011; Simpson et al., 1994; Sims et al., 1983; Sorbi et al., 1983; Villain, 2010.
Huntington's disease (HD)	Reduced glucose metabolism in the basal ganglia and cerebral cortex of symptomatic HD patients. Deficiency in activities of respiratory chain complexes II, III and IV in caudate nucleus. Decreased cAMP levels in HD postmortem brain and Hdh^{Q111} striatum. Decreased ATP and ATP/ADP ratio. Defective mitochondrial oxidative phosphorylation. Cytochrome oxidase subunit I (COI) mRNA levels are reduced within neurons of the putamen and globus pallidus. Expression of mHTT in hypothalamus causes metabolic imbalance in mice. Decreased GLUT1 and GLUT3 transporter expression in caudate of postmortem HD brains.	Gamberino & Brennan, 1994; Gourfinkel-An et al., 2002; Gu et al., 1996; Hult et al., 2011; Kuwert et al., 1990; Kuwert et al., 1993; Leenders et al., 1986; Lim et al., 2007; Mann et al., 1990; Martin et al., 1992; Mazziotta et al., 1987;
Parkinson's disease (PD)	Hypometabolism in striatal, thalamic, and motor regions in PD animal models with significant alterations in striatal and cortical function (FDG-PET). PD patients showed patterns of decreased metabolism in bilateral inferior, medial frontal and right parietal lobes, caudate nucleus and visual cortex. Deficiency in the activity of complex I in mitochondria of substantia nigra. Glucose metabolism is decreased in the caudate, putamen and thalamus in a primate PD model.	Bohnen et al., 2011; Borghammer et al., 2011 Brownell et al., 2003; Feng et al., 2008; Hattingen et al., 2009; Hou et al., 2010; Hyu Lee et al., 2009; Lee et al., 2010; Lyoo et al., 2008; Perneczky et al., 2008; Schapira et al., 1989.

Table 1. Metabolic failures in neurodegenerative diseases.

for Parkin, DJ-1, PINK1 and ATP13A2 (Biskup et al., 2008). The exact role of α-synuclein remains unknown, but it is thought to participate in maintenance of vesicle pools. Parkin directs ubiquitination of α-synuclein (Haywood & Staveley, 2004). Ubiquitin tagged α-synuclein is directed to proteosome and degraded. The parkin protein thus promotes Parkinson's disease by enhancing the failure in normal protein degradation. Mutations in PINK1 and DJ1 genes are related to mitochondrial dysfunction in Parkinson's disease. Oxidative stress also occurs in Parkinson's disease. Dopamine metabolism produces oxidant species. In this way, the α-synuclein mutation contributes to oxidative stress because in the presence of mutated α-synuclein, dopamine remains in the cytosol instead of being loaded into synaptic vesicles (Henchcliffe, 2008).

A hypometabolism of glucose has been described in Parkinson's disease patients (Huang et al., 2007; Yong et al., 2007; Perneczy et al., 2008; Hosokai et al., 2009; Lee et al., 2008; Lee et al., 2010; Bohnen et al., 2011; Borghammer et al., 2011). However, there is only limited molecular evidence to support this feature. Defects in oxidative phophorylation with a decreased activity of complex I have been reported (Navarro et al., 2009; Hattingen et al., 2009). This evidence leads us to speculate that in Parkinson's disease, mitochondrial dysfunction by redox imbalance precedes metabolic failure. However, a role for glycogen synthase kinase 3-3, an enzyme participating in glycogen metabolism (see below) has been proposed in Parkinson's disease pathogenesis (as for Alzheimer's disease pathogenesis, Nagao et al., 2008; Garcia-Gorotiaga et al., 2009).

5. Conclusions

The metabolic cost of brain activity is high. Neuronal activity accounts for 80% of brain energy consumption. Glucose is an essential energy source for the adult human brain. It can be used to obtain energy and to produce metabolic intermediaries for biosynthesis of compound of biological interest. Glucose can also be stored in brain, in the form of glycogen. Glucose oxidation via glycolysis occurs in all brain cells. However, the ability of neuronal cells to activate this metabolic pathway is poor. Astrocytic glycolysis and glycogenolysis is activated in response to synaptic activation with the subsequent formation of lactate. Thus, during glutamatergic synaptic activity neurons preferably consume lactate released from glia. The energetic coupling between neuronal and astroglial cells is essential to meet energy brain needs in an efficient way. Astrocytes interact with each other and with endothelial cells from the blood brain barrier and smooth muscle cells surrounding arterioles. Under fasting conditions, during intense exercise and in suckling infants, ketone bodies are a significant source of energetic fuel for brain. Metabolic failure has been described in several neurodegenerative diseases. These diseases present atypical protein assemblies, failures in normal protein degradation pathways, induced cell death, impaired axonal transport and metabolic failures. Almost all cellular processes need energy. It is thus possible that metabolic failure is an early event in these pathologies. This hypothesis is supported by evidence that shows metabolic failure in pre-symptomatic patients suffering from diseases such as Alzheimer's disease and Huntington's disease.

6. Acknowledgements

We gratefully acknowledge the helpful suggestions of T. Valencia and S. Brauchi. This work was supported by Chilean grant FONDECYT 1110571.

7. References

Allaman, I., Gavillet, M., Bélanger, M., Laroche, T., Viertl, D., Lashuel, H.A, & Magistretti, Pierre J. (2010). Amyloid-beta aggregates cause alterations of astrocytic metabolic phenotype: impact on neuronal viability. *J Neurosci*, 30(9), 3326-38.

Alle H., Roth A., Geiger J.R. (2009) Energy-efficient action potentials in hippocampal mossy fibers. *Science*. 11;325(5946):1405-8.

Ames A. III (2000) CNS energy metabolism as related to function. *Brain Res.* Rev. 34, 42–68.

Araque, A., Parpura, V., Sanzgiri, R. P., & Haydon, P. G. (1999). Tripartite synapses: glia, the unacknowledged partner. *Trends Neurosci*, 22(5), 208-215.

Astuya, A., Caprile, T., Castro, M., Salazar, K., García, M. D. L. A., Reinicke, K., Rodríguez, F. (2005). Vitamin C uptake and recycling among normal and tumor cells from the central nervous system. *J Neurosci Res*, 79(1-2), 146-56.

Attwell D. and Laughlin S. B. (2001) An energy budget for signaling in the grey matter of the brain. *J. Cereb. Blood Flow Metab*. 21,1133–1145.

Attwell, D., Buchan, A. M., Charpak, S., Lauritzen, M., Macvicar, B., & Newman, E., (2010). Glial and neuronal control of brain blood flow. *Nature*,468(7321),232-43.

Aziz, N. A., Pijl, H., Frölich, M., Snel, M., Streefland, T. C. M., Roelfsema, F., & Roos, R. a C. (2010). Systemic energy homeostasis in Huntington's disease patients. *J Neurol, Neuros Psychiatry*, 81(11),1233-7.

Baquer NZ, Hothersall JS, McLean P. (1988) Function and regulation of the pentose phosphate pathway in brain. Curr Top Cell Regul, 29:265-89.

Beltrán, F. A., Acuña, A. I., Miró, M. P., Angulo, C., Concha, I. I., & Castro, M. A. (2011). Ascorbic acid-dependent GLUT3 inhibition is a critical step for switching neuronal metabolism. *J Cel Phys*, 226(12):3286-94.

Benarroch, E. E.(2010).Glycogen metabolism:metabolic coupling between astrocytes and neurons. *Neurology*,74(11),919-23.

Beskow, A. P., Fernandes, C. G., Leipnitz, G., da Silva, L. D. B., Seminotti, B., Amaral, A. U., Wyse, A. T. S., et al. (2008).Influence of ketone bodies on oxidative stress parameters in brain of developing rats in vitro. *Metab Brain Dis*, 23(4), 411-25.

Biskup, S., Gerlach, M., Kupsch, A., Reichmann, H., Riederer, P., Vieregge, P. Gasser, T. (2008). Genes associated with Parkinson syndrome. *J Neurol*, 255 Suppl 5, 8-17.

Bittar P. G., Charnay Y., Pellerin L., Bouras C., Magistretti P. J. (1996) Selective distribution of lactate dehydrogenase isoenzymes in neurons and astrocytes of human brain. *J Cereb Blood Flow Metab*, 16(6):1079-89.

Bohnen, N. I., Koeppe, R. a, Minoshima, S., Giordani, B., Albin, R. L., Frey, K. a, & Kuhl, D. E. (2011). Cerebral glucose metabolic features of Parkinson disease and incident dementia:longitudinal study. *Soc Nucl Med*, 52(6),848-55.

Bolaños, J. P., & Almeida, A. (2010). The pentose-phosphate pathway in neuronal survival against nitrosative stress. *IUBMB life*, 62(1), 14-8.

Bolaños, J. P., Almeida, A., & Moncada, S. (2010). Glycolysis: a bioenergetic or a survival pathway? *Bioch Scien*, 35(3), 145-9.

Borghammer, P., Hansen, S. B., Eggers, C., Chakravarty, M., Vang, K., Aanerud, J., Hilker, R., et al. (2011). Glucose metabolism in small subcortical structures in Parkinson's disease. *Acta Neurol Scandinavica*, 1-8

Bosco, D., Fava, A., Plastino, M., Montalcini, T., & Pujia, A. (2011). Possible implications of insulin resistance and glucose metabolism in Alzheimer's disease pathogenesis. *J Cell Mol Med,* 15(9), 1807-1821.

Braak, H., Del Tredici, K., Rub, U., de Vos, R. A., Jansen Steur, E. N., & Braak, E. (2003). Staging of brain pathology related to sporadic Parkinson's disease. *Neurobiol Aging,* 24(2), 197-211.

Bredesen, D. E., Rao, R. V., & Mehlen, P. (2006). Cell death in the nervous system. *Nature,* 443(7113), 796-802.

Brown, G. K., Otero, L. J., Legris, M., & Brown, R. M. (1994). Syndrome of the month Pyruvate dehydrogenase deficiency. *Amino Acids,* 875-879.

Brown AM & Ransom BR. (2007). Astrocyte glycogen and brain energy metabolism. *Glia* 55(12):1263-71.

Bröer, S., Rahman, B., Pellegri, G., Pellerin, L, Martin, J. L., Verleysdonk, S., Hamprecht, B. (1997).Comparison of lactate transport in astroglial cells and monocarboxylate transporter 1 (MCT1) expressing Xenopus laevis oocytes. Expression of two different monocarboxylate transporters in astroglial cells and neurons. *J Biol Chem,* 272(48), 30096- 102.

Calingasan NY, Baker H, Sheu KF, Gibson GE (1994). Distribution of the alpha-ketoglutarate dehydrogenase complex in rat brain. J *Comp Neuron* 346(3):461-79.

Castro M., Caprile T., Astuya A. et al. (2001) High-affinity sodium–vitamin C co-transporters (SVCT) expression in embryonic mouse neurons. *J. Neurochem.* 78, 815–823

Castro, M. A, Angulo, C., Brauchi, S., Nualart, F., & Concha, I. I. (2008). Ascorbic acid participates in a general mechanism for concerted glucose transport inhibition and lactate transport stimulation. *Pflügers Archiv : Eur J Phys,* 457(2), 519-28.

Castro, M. A, Beltrán, F. A, Brauchi, S., & Concha, I. I. (2009). A metabolic switch in brain: glucose and lactate metabolism modulation by ascorbic acid. *J Neuroch,*110(2), 423-40.

Cattaneo, E., Rigamonti, D., Goffredo, D., Zuccato, C., Squitieri, F., & Sipione, S. (2001). Loss of normal huntingtin function: new developments in Huntington's disease research. *Trends Neurosci,* 24(3), 182-188.

Caviston, J. P., & Holzbaur, E. L. (2009). Huntingtin as an essential integrator of intracellular vesicular trafficking. *Trends Cell Biol,* 19(4), 147-155.

Cerdán, S., Rodrigues, T. B., Sierra, A., Benito, M., Fonseca, L. L., Fonseca, C. P., & García-Martín, M. L. (2006). The redox switch/redox coupling hypothesis. *Neurochem Internat,* 48(6-7),523-30.

Ceravolo, R., Borghetti, D., Kiferle, L., Tognoni, G., Giorgetti, a, Neglia, D., Sassi, N., et al. (2008). CSF phosporylated TAU protein levels correlate with cerebral glucose metabolism assessed with PET in Alzheimer's disease. *Brain Res Bul,* 76(1-2), 80-4.

Chen, Y., & Hertz, L. (1999). Noradrenaline effects on pyruvate decarboxylation: correlation with calcium signaling. *J Neurosci Res,* 58(4), 599-606.

Chen, C. M. (2011). Mitochondrial dysfunction, metabolic deficits, and increased oxidative stress in Huntington's disease. *Chang Gung Med J, 34*(2), 135-152.

Chiang, M.-C., Chen, C.-M., Lee, M.-R., Chen, H.-W., Chen, H.-M., Wu, Y.-S., Hung, C.-H., et al. (2010). Modulation of energy deficiency in Huntington's disease via activation of the peroxisome proliferator-activated receptor gamma. *Hum Mol Gen,* 19(20), 4043-58.

Chih, C. P., & Roberts Jr, E. L. (2003). Energy substrates for neurons during neural activity: a critical review of the astrocyte-neuron lactate shuttle hypothesis.*J Cereb Blood Flow Metab,* 23(11), 1263-1281.

Choi D. W. (1988) Glutamate neurotoxicity and diseases of the nervous system. *Neuron* 1, 623–634.

Cotter, D. G., d' Avignon, D. A., Wentz, A. E., Weber, M. L., & Crawford, P. a. (2011). Obligate role for ketone body oxidation in neonatal metabolic homeostasis. J *Biol Chem,* 286(9), 6902-10.

Demestre, M., Boutelle, M., & Fillenz, M. (1997). Stimulated release of lactate in freely moving rats is dependent on the uptake of glutamate. *J Physiol,* 499 (Pt 3), 825-832.

Denton, R. M., Rutter, G. a, Midgley, P. J., & McCormack, J. G. (1988). Effects of Ca2+ on the activities of the calcium-sensitive dehydrogenases within the mitochondria of mammalian tissues. *J Cardiov Pharm,* 12 Suppl 5, S69- 72.

Devraj, K., Klinger, M. E., Myers, R. L., Mokashi, A., Hawkins, R. a, & Simpson, Ian a. (2011). GLUT-1 glucose transporters in the blood-brain barrier: Differential phosphorylation. *J Neuros Res,* 000, 1-13.

Dienel, G. A., & Cruz, N. F. (2009). Exchange-mediated dilution of brain lactate specific activity: implications for the origin of glutamate dilution and the contributions of glutamine dilution and other pathways. *J Neurochem,* 109 Suppl 1, 30-37.

DiNuzzo, M., Maraviglia, Bruno, & Giove, Federico. (2011). Why does the brain (not) have glycogen? *BioEssays* : 33(5), 319-26.

Duchen, M. R. (2000). Mitochondria and Ca(2+)in cell physiology and pathophysiology. *Cell Calcium,* 28(5-6), 339-348.

Duyckaerts, C., Potier, M. C., & Delatour, B. (2008). Alzheimer disease models and human neuropathology: similarities and differences. *Acta Neuropathol,* 115(1), 5-38.

Ferreira, I L, Resende, R., Ferreiro, E., Rego, A C, & Pereira, C. F. (2010). Multiple Defects in Energy Metabolism in Alzheimer's Disease. *Current,* 1193-1206.

Finck, B. N., & Kelly, D. P. (2006). PGC-1 coactivators: inducible regulators of energy metabolism in health and disease. *J Clin Invest,* 116(3), 615-622.

Fonnum, F. (1968). The distribution of glutamate decarboxylase and aspartate transaminase in subcellular fractions of rat and guinea-pig brain. *Biochem J,* 106(2), 401-12.

Gegelashvili, M., Rodriguez-kern, A., Sung, L., Shimamoto, K., & Gegelashvili, G. (2007). Glutamate transporter GLAST/EAAT1 directs cell surface expression of FXYD2/g subunit of Na, K-ATPase in human fetal astrocytes, 50,916-920.

Ghasemzadeh, B., Cammack, J., & Adams, R. N. (1991). Dynamic changes in extracellular fluid ascorbic acid monitored by in vivo electrochemistry. *Brain Res,* 547(1), 162-166.

Giaume, C., & Theis, M. (2010). Pharmacological and genetic approaches to study connexin-mediated channels in glial cells of the central nervous system. *Brain Res Rev,* 63(1-2), 160-76.

Gjedde, A., Marrett, S., & Vafaee, M. (2002). Oxidative and nonoxidative metabolism of excited neurons and astrocytes. *J Cereb Blood Flow Metab,* 22(1), 1-14.

Goldberg N. D., Passonneau J. V. and Lowry O. H. (1966) Effects of changes in brain metabolism on the levels of citric acid cycle intermediates. *J. Biol. Chem.* 241, 3997–4003.

Grisar T., Frere J. M. and Franck G. (1979) Effect of K+ ions on kinetic properties of the (Na+, K+)-ATPase (EC 3.6.1.3) of bulk isolated glial cells, perikarya and synaptosomes from rabbit brain cortex. *Brain Res.* 165, 87–103.

Gunter, T. E., Yule, D. I., Gunter, K. K., Eliseev, R. a, & Salter, J. D. (2004). Calcium and mitochondria. *FEBS letters,* 567(1), 96-102.

Hajek I., Subbarao K. V. and Hertz L. (1996) Acute and chronic effects of potassium and noradrenaline on Na+, K+-ATPase activity in cultured mouse neurons and astrocytes. *Neurochem. Int.* 28, 335–342.

Harr, S. D., Simonian, N. A., & Hyman, B. T. (1995). Functional alterations in Alzheimer's disease: decreased glucose transporter 3 immunoreactivity in the perforant pathway terminal zone. *J Neuropathol Exp Neurol,* 54(1), 38-41.

Hattingen, E., Magerkurth, J., Pilatus, U., Mozer, A., Seifried, C., Steinmetz, H., Zanella, F., (2009). Phosphorus and proton magnetic resonance spectroscopy demonstrates mitochondrial dysfunction in early and advanced Parkinson's disease. Brain : *J Neur,* 132(Pt 12), 3285-97.

Haywood, S., Muller, T., Muller, W., Heinz-Erian, P., Tanner, M. S., & Ross, G. (2001). Copper-associated liver disease in North Ronaldsay sheep: a possible animal model for non-Wilsonian hepatic copper toxicosis of infancy and childhood. *J Pathol,* 195(2), 264-269.

Haywood, A. F., & Staveley, B. E. (2004). Parkin counteracts symptoms in a Drosophila model of Parkinson's disease. *BMC Neurosci,* 5, 14.

Henchcliffe, C., & Beal, M. F. (2008). Mitochondrial biology and oxidative stress in Parkinson disease pathogenesis. *Nat Clin Pract Neurol,* 4(11), 600-609.

Herrero-Mendez, A., Almeida, A., Fernández, E., Maestre, C., Moncada, S., & Bolaños, J. P. (2009). The bioenergetic and antioxidant status of neurons is controlled by continuous degradation of a key glycolytic enzyme by APC/C-Cdh1. *Nat Cell Biol,* 11(6), 747-52.

Hertz, L. (2004). The astrocyte-neuron lactate shuttle: a challenge of a challenge. *J Cereb Blood Flow Metab,* 24(11),1241-1248.

Hertz, L., & Kala, G. (2007). Energy metabolism in brain cells: effects of elevated ammonia concentrations. *Metab Brain Dis,* 22(3-4), 199-218

Hof, P. R., Pascale, E., & Magistretti, P. J. (1988). K+ at concentrations reached in the extracellular space during neuronal activity promotes a Ca2+-dependent glycogen hydrolysis in mouse cerebral cortex. *J Neurosci,* 8(6), 1922-1928.

Huang B, Gudi R, Wu P, Harris RA, Hamilton J, Popov KM. (1998). Isoenzymes of pyruvate dehydrogenase phosphatase. DNA-derived amino acid sequences, expression, and regulation. *J Biol Chem* 273(28):17680-8.

Huang, C., Mattis, P., Tang, C., Perrine, K., Carbon, M., & Eidelberg, D. (2007).Metabolic brain networks associated with cognitive function in Parkinson's disease. *NeuroImage,* 34(2), 714-23.

Ishikawa, T., Kuo, M. T., Furuta, K., & Suzuki, M. (1998). A new aspect on glutathione-associated biological function of MRP/GS-X pump and its gene expression. *Cytotechnology,*27(1-3), 81-93.

Kashiwaya, Y., Takeshima, T., Mori, N., Nakashima, K., Clarke, K., & Veech, R. L. (2000). - NL - Hydroxybutyrate protects neurons in models of Alzheimer's and Parkinson's disease. *PNAS* 97: 5440-5444.

Kratzing, C. C., Kelly, J. D., & Oelrichs, B. A. (1982). Ascorbic acid in neural tissues. *J Neurochem,* 39(3), 625-627.

Ksiezak-Reding H., Blass J. P., Gibson G. E. (1982) Studies on the pyruvate dehydrogenase complex in brain with the arylamine acetyltransferase-coupled assay. *J Neurochem,* 38(6):1627-36.

Kuwert, T., Boecker, H., Titz, H., Herzog, H., Wang, B.-C., Nayak, U., Feinendegen, L.E.(1993). Striatal glucose consumption in chorea-free subjects at risk of Huntington's disease. *J Neurol* 241(1), 31-36.

LaManna J. C., Salem N., Puchowicz M., Erokwu B., Koppaka S., Flask C., Lee Z. (2009) Ketones suppress brain glucose consumption. *Adv Exp Med Biol,* 645:301-6.

Lavoie, S., Allaman, I., Petit, J.-marie, Do, K. Q., & Magistretti, Pierre J. (2011). Altered Glycogen Metabolism in Cultured Astrocytes from Mice with Chronic Glutathione Deficit; Relevance for Neuroenergetics in Schizophrenia. *Metab Clin Exp,* 6(7).

Lee, M. S., Lyoo, C. H., Ryu, Y. H., Lim, H. S., Nam, C. M., Kim, H. S., & Rinne, J. O. (2011). The effect of age on motor deficits and cerebral glucose metabolism of Parkinson's disease. *Acta Neurol Scand,* 124(3), 196-201.

Leenders KL, Frackowiak RS, Quinn N, Marsden CD (1986).Brain energy metabolism and dopaminergic function in Huntington's disease measured in vivo using positron emission tomography. *Mov Disord.*;1(1):69-77.

Lim, D., Fedrizzi, L., Tartari, M., Zuccato, C., Cattaneo, E., Brini, M., & Carafoli, E. (2008). Calcium homeostasis and mitochondrial dysfunction in striatal neurons of Huntington disease. *J Biol Chem, 283*(9), 5780-9.

Lin, M. T., & Beal, M Flint. (2006). Mitochondrial dysfunction and oxidative stress in neurodegenerative diseases. *Nature,* 443(7113), 787-95.

Liu, Y., Liu, F., Iqbal, K., Grundke-Iqbal, I., & Gong, C.-X. (2008). Decreased glucose transporters correlate to abnormal hyperphosphorylation of tau in Alzheimer disease. *FEBS letters,* 582(2), 359-64.

Loreck, D. J., Galarraga, J., Van der Feen, J., Phang, J. M., Smith, B. H., & Cummins, C. J. (1987). Regulation of the pentose phosphate pathway in human astrocytes and gliomas. *Metab Brain Dis,* 2(1), 31- 46.

Lowry O. H. and Passonneau J. V. (1964) The relationships between substrates and enzymes of glycolysis in brain. *J. Biol. Chem.* 239, 31–42.

Magistretti, P J. (2000). Cellular bases of functional brain imaging: insights from neuron-glia metabolic coupling. *Brain research,* 886(1-2), 108-112.

Mangia, S., Giove, F, Bianciardi, M., Di Salle, F., Garreffa, G., & Maraviglia, B. (2003). Issues concerning the construction of a metabolic model for neuronal activation. *J Neurosci Res*, 71(4), 463-7.

Mangia, S., Simpson, I. A., Vannucci, S. J., & Carruthers, A (2009). The in vivo neuron-to-astrocyte lactate shuttle in human brain: evidence from modeling of measured lactate levels during visual stimulation. *J Neurochem*, 109 Suppl 1, 55-62.

Martin E, Rosenthal RE, Fiskum G.(2005) Pyruvate dehydrogenase complex: metabolic link to ischemic brain injury and target of oxidative stress. *J Neurosci Res*. 79(1-2):240-7.

Mazziotta JC, Phelps ME, Pahl JJ, Huang SC, Baxter LR, Riege WH, Hoffman JM, Kuhl DE, Lanto AB, Wapenski JA. (1987).Reduced cerebral glucose metabolism in asymptomatic subjects at risk for Huntington's disease.*N Engl J Med*. 12;316(7):357-62.

Merlini, M., Meyer, E. P., Ulmann-Schuler, A., & Nitsch, R. M. (2011). Vascular β-amyloid and early astrocyte alterations impair cerebrovascular function and cerebral metabolism in transgenic arcAβ ice. *Acta Neuropath*, 122(3), 293-311.

Mochel, F., & Haller, R. G. (2011). Energy deficit in Huntington disease: why it matters. Energy, 121(2), 493-499.

Mosconi, L., Tsui, W.-H., De Santi, S., Li, J., Rusinek, H., Convit, a, Li, Y., et al. (2005). Reduced hippocampal metabolism in MCI and AD: automated FDG-PET image analysis. *Neurology*, 64(11), 1860-7.

Myers, R. H., Vonsattel, J. P., Stevens, T. J., Cupples, L. A., Richardson, E. P., Martin, J. B., & Bird, E. D. (1988). Clinical and neuropathologic assess ment of severity in Huntington's disease. *Neurology*, 38(3), 341-347.

Nagao, M., & Hayashi, H. (2009). Glycogen synthase kinase-3beta is as so ciated with Parkinson's disease. *Neurosci lett*, 449(2), 103-7.

Navarro, A., & Boveris, A. (2009). Brain mitochondrial dysfunction and oxidative damage in Parkinson's disease. *J Bioenerg Biomemb*, 41(6), 517-21.

Narishima, R., Yamasaki, M., Hasegawa, S., Yoshida, S., Tanaka, S., & Fukui, T. (2011). Leptin controls ketone body utilization in hypothalamic neuron. *Neurosci lett*, 490(3), 185-90.

Olah, J., Klivenyi, P., Gardian, G., Vecsei, L., Orosz, F., Kovacs, G. G., Ovadi, J. (2008). Increased glucose metabolism and ATP level in brain tissue of Huntington's disease transgenic mice. *FEBS J, 275*(19), 4740-4755

O'Neill, R. D., Fillenz, M., Sundstrom, L., & Rawlins, J. N. (1984). Voltammetrically monitored brain ascorbate as an index of excitatory amino acid release in the unrestrained rat. *Neurosci Lett*, 52(3), 227-233.

Onishi, T., Iwashita, H., Uno, Y., Kunitomo, J., Saitoh, M., Kimura, E., Fujita,H., et al. (2011). A Novel Glycogen Synthase Kinase 3Inhibitor2- methyl-5-(3-{4[(S)methylsulfinyl] phenyl}-1- benzofuran- 5-yl)- 1,3,4-oxadiazole (MMBO) Decreases Tau Phosphorylation and Ameliorates Cognitive Deficits in a Transgenic Model of Alzheimer's Disease. *J Neurochem*, 2-17.

Pellerin, L, & Magistretti, P J. (1994). Glutamate uptake into astrocytes stimulates aerobic glycolysis: a mechanism coupling neuronal activity to glucose utilization.

Proceedings of the National Academy of Sciences of the United States of America, 91(22), 10625-9.

Pellerin, Luc. (2008). Brain energetics (thought needs food). *Curr Op Clin Nutr Metab Care,* 11(6), 701-5.

Pennuto, M., Palazzolo, I., & Poletti, A. (2009). Post-translational modifications of expanded polyglutamine proteins: impact on neurotoxicity. *Hum Mol Genet,* 18(R1), R40-47.

Peppiatt, C., & Attwell, D. (2004). Neurobiology: feeding the brain. *Nature,* 431(7005), 137-138.

Perneczky, R., Drzezga, A., Boecker, Henning, Ceballos- Baumann, A. O., Granert, O., Förstl, H., Kurz, A., et al. (2008). Activities of daily living, cerebral glucose metabolism, and cognitive reserve in Lewy body and Parkinson's disease. *Dem Geriatr Cognit* Dis,26(5), 475-81.

Pifferi, F., Tremblay, S., Plourde, M., Tremblay-Mercier, J., Bentourkia, M., & Cunnane, S. C. (2008). Ketones and brain function: possible link to polyunsaturated fatty acids and availability of a new brain PET tracer, 11C-acetoacetate. *Epilepsia,* 49 Suppl 8, 76-9.

Polakis PG& Wilson JE. An intact hydrophobic N-terminal sequence is critical for binding of rat brain hexokinase to mitochondria (1985). *Arch Biochem Biophys.* 236(1):328-37.

Porras, O. H., Ruminot, I., Loaiza, A., & Barros, L. F. (2008). Na(+)-Ca(2+) cosignaling in the stimulation of the glucose transporter GLUT1 in cultured astrocytes. *Glia,* 56(1), 59-68.

Quistorff, B., Secher, N. H., & Van Lieshout, J. J. (2008). Lactate fuels the human brain during exercise. *FASEB J* , 22(10), 3443-9.

Rebec G. V. and Pierce R. C. (1994) A vitamin as neuromodulator:ascorbate release into the extracellular luid of the brain regulates opaminergic and glutamatergic transmission. *Prog. Neurobiol.* 43,537–565.

Roy, C. S., and Sherrington, C. S. (1890). On the regulation of the blood supply of the brain. *J. Physiol.* (Lond.) 11, 85–108.

Rubinsztein, D. C. (2006). The roles of intracellular protein- degradation pathways in neurodegeneration. *Nature,* 443(7113), 780-6.

Sánchez-Abarca L. I., Tabernero A., Medina J. M. (2001). Oligodendrocytes use lactate as a source of energy and as a precursor of lipids. *Glia,* 36(3):321-9.

Sánchez-Alvarez R., Tabernero A., Medina J. M. (2004). Endothelin-1 stimulates the translocation and upregulation of both glucose transporter and hexokinase in astrocytes: relationship with gap junctional communication. *J Neurochem,* 89(3):703-14.

Schapira, A. H. V. (2006). Review Mitochondrial disease. *Lancet,* 70-82.

Schapira, A. H. (2008). Mitochondrial dysfunction in neurodegenerative diseases. *Neurochem Res,* 33(12), 2502-2509.

Sherrington, A. (1979). Fluoridation. *Can J Public Health,* 70(4), 219.

Sibson, N. R., Dhankhar, a, Mason, G. F., Rothman, D. L., Behar, K. L., & Shulman, R. G. (1998). Stoichiometric coupling of brain glucose metabolism and glutamatergic neuronal activity. *Nat Acad Scien United St Am,* 95(1), 316-21.

Sokoloff L., Reivich M., Kennedy C. (1977) The [14C]deoxyglucose method for the measurement of local cerebral glucose utilization: theory, procedure, and normal values in the conscious and anesthetized albino rat. *J. Neurochem.* 28, 897–916.

Sokoloff, L., Takahashi, S., Gotoh, J., Driscoll, B. F., & Law, M. J. (1996). Contribution of astroglia to functionally activated energy metabolism. *Dev Neurosci,* 18(5-6), 344-352.

Solaz-Fuster, M. C., Gimeno-Alcañiz, J. V., Ros, S., Fernandez-Sanchez, M. E., Garcia-Fojeda, B., Criado Garcia, O., Vilchez, D., et al. (2008). Regulation of glycogen synthesis by the laforin-malin complex is modulated by the AMP-activated protein kinase pathway. *Hum Mol Gen,* 17(5), 667-78.

Smith, R., Bacos, K., Fedele, V., Soulet, D., Walz, H. A, Obermüller, S., Lindqvist, A., et al. (2009). Mutant huntingtin interacts with {beta}- tubulin and disrupts vesicular transport and insulin secretion. *Hum Mol Gen,* 18(20), 3942-54.

Twelvetrees, A. E., Yuen, E. Y., Arancibia-Carcamo, I. L., MacAskill, A. F., Rostaing, P., Lumb, M. J., Humbert, S., et al. (2010). Delivery of GABAARs to synapses is mediated by HAP1-KIF5 and disrupted by mutant huntingtin. *Neuron,* 65(1), 53-65.

Vera J. C., Rivas C. I., Fischbarg J. and Golde D. W. (1993) Mammalian facilitative hexose transporters mediate the transport of dehydroascorbic acid. *Nature* 364, 79–82.

Villringer, a, & Dirnagl, U. (1995). Coupling of brain activity and cerebral blood flow: basis of functional neuroimaging. Cereb Brain Metab Rev, 7(3), 240-76.

Vlassenko, A. G., Vaishnavi, S. N., Couture, L., Sacco, D., Shannon, B. J., Mach, R. H., Morris, J. C., (2010). Spatial correlation between brain aerobic glycolysis and amyloid-β (Aβ) deposition. *October* 107(41), 17763-17767.

De Vos, K. J., Grierson, A. J., Ackerley, S., & Miller, C. C. J. (2008). Role of axonal transport in neurodegenerative diseases. *Annual Rev Neurosci,* 31, 151-73.

Walls A. B., Sickmann H. M., Brown A., Bouman S. D., Ransom B., Schousboe A., Waagepetersen H. S. (2008). Characterization of 1,4-dideoxy-1,4-imino-d-arabinitol (DAB) as an inhibitor of brain glycogen shunt activity. *J Neurochem,* 105(4):1462-70.

Walz, W., & Mukerji, S. (1988). Lactate production and release in cultured astrocytes. *Neurosci Lett,* 86(3), 296-300.

Wenk, G. L. (2003). Neuropathologic changes in Alzheimer's disease. *J Clin Psychiatry,* 64 Suppl 9, 7-10.

Wilkin G. P. and Wilson J. E. (1977) Localization of hexokinases in neuronal tissue: light microscopic studies with immunofluorescence and histochemical procedures. *J. Neurochem.* 29, 1039-1051.

Wilson J. E. (1995) Hexokinases. *Rev. Physiol. Biochem. Pharmacol.* 126, 65–198

Wilson JE. Homologous and heterologous interactions between hexokinase and mitochondrial porin: evolutionary implications. (1997). *J Bioenerg Biomembr.* 29(1):97-102.

Wilson M. C., Jackson V. N., Heddle C., Price N. T., Pilegaard H., Juel C., Bonen A., Montgomery I., Hutter O. F. and Halestrap A. P. (1998) Lactic acid efflux from white skeletal muscle is catalyzed by the monocarboxylate transporter isoform MCT3. *J. Biol. Chem.* 273, 15920–15926.

Wright E. M., Loo D. D., Panayotova-Heiermann M. et al. (1994) 'Active' sugar transport in eukaryotes. *J. Exp. Biol.* 196, 197–212.

Yusa, T. (2001). Increased extracellular ascorbate release reflects glutamate re-uptake during the early stage of reperfusion after forebrain ischemia in rats. *Brain Res,* 897(1-2), 104-113.

15

Tau and Amyloid-β Conformational Change to β-Sheet Structures as Effectors in the Development of Alzheimer's Disease

Martha A. De Anda-Hernández[1*], Karla I. Lira-De León[1*], Raúl Mena[2], Victoria Campos-Peña[3] and Marco A. Meraz-Ríos[1]
Center of Research and Advanced Studies, CINVESTAV-IPN,
[1]Molecular Biomedicine Department, CINVESTAV-IPN,
[2]Physiology, Biophysics and Neurosciences Department, CINVESTAV-IPN,
[3]Experimental Laboratory of Neurodegenerative Diseases, Neurology and Neurosurgery National Institute (INNN),
Mexico

1. Introduction

The pathology of Alzheimer Disease (AD) has been intensely studied in the last 20 years (Duyckaerts et al., 2009) because it is a progressive neurodegenerative disorder that causes dementia in approximately 10% of individuals older than 65 years (Hampel et al., 2010). AD occurs gradually; starting with the so called mild cognitive impairment (MCI) recognized by mild memory disturbances and noticed difficulties in performing more demanding cognitive tasks. With disease progression the decline in memory and cognition become more expressed and are accompanied by changes in personality and behaviour. In later stages of the disease loss of speech and movement is followed by total disability and finally death. A person with AD lives on average eight years after the onset of symptoms (Zerovnik, 2010). Actual studies are focused in many strategies for markers of susceptibility, early diagnostic, understanding of molecular mechanism, effective treatment and preventing strategies. According to Duyckaerts and coworkers (2009) AD could be divided in three broad chapters: lesions related to abnormal accumulation of proteins, those that are due to neural losses and finally those that are due to the reactive processes. According to abnormal accumulations proteins, AD is characterized by the presence of two types of neuropathological hallmarks: neurofibrillary tangles (NFTs) and neuritic plaques (NP). NFTs are intraneuronal aggregates of abnormally modified Tau (phosphorylated at non physiological sites, truncation, etc). NP are extracellular and mainly composed of amyloid β-peptide (AB) deposits (Martin et al., 2011). The most of the cases of AD are reported as "sporadic" pathway, because we still do not know what could be the factors that lead to this disease. Many hypotheses has been proposed, including immune system participation (Solomon &Frenkel, 2010), pathogens (Miklossy, 2011), oxidative stress responses, and more. At the end, in patients we can always find NFTs and NP in several regions of the brain

* Both authors contributed in the same manner

(Braak &Braak, 1991). About these lesions, Braak and Braak (1991) established a relationship between the appearance of NP and NFTs with cognitive decline in post-mortem studies (Braak &Braak, 1991).

At the moment, AD can be diagnosed conclusively only post-mortem. However, advances in neuroimaging by magnetic resonance imaging (MRI) and by positron electron tomography (PET) allow researchers to see accumulation of amyloid plaques and NFTs in the living brain. In such a way, the course of the disease at various time points can be followed and an early diagnosis obtained. One, in principle, could even monitor the development/progression of the disease (Zerovnik, 2010). Several evidences demonstrate that under the formation of these lesions, are implicated in an important manner, conformational changes for Tau and amyloid β-peptide. Understanding the process at the molecular level is important for toxic aggregates could be stopped from forming or, alternatively, their removal could be accelerated. Antibodies directed against a common structural epitope shared by the prefibrillar oligomers could serve such a role. Common structural characteristics of amyloid fibrils are: predominantly β-sheet secondary structure, detected by specific dyes, and binding and a characteristic pattern seen by X-ray diffraction. By electron microscopy amyloigenic fibrils also are visualized allowing morphological studies (Zerovnik, 2010). In this chapter we focus on the importance of changes in conformation of both proteins during abnormal aggregation associated to AD.

2. Amyloid β

A growing body of evidence suggests that altered processing of amyloid precursor protein (APP) is one of the early events in the pathogenesis of AD. APP is a transmembrane glycoprotein of type 1 from 120 to 200 kD wich are ubiquitously expressed, but are most abundant in the brain (Selkoe, 1994). The APP gene is located on the long arm of chromosome 21 in humans (Kang 1987) and contains 18 exons (figure 1A) through alternative splicing of exons 7, 8 and 15 are generated 8 isoforms that have pattern cell specific expression and are designated by the number of amino acids they contain. The size of the isoforms can vary from 563 to 770 amino acids (Coulson et al., 2000). In central nervous system express only 4 isoforms: PPA695, PPA714, PPA751 and PPA770, PPA695 of which is the most abundant isoform in neurons, while that PPA751 and PPA770 isoforms are expressed mainly in glial cells (Yoshikai et al., 1990; Zheng &Koo, 2006). Only isoforms PPA695, PPA751 and PPA770 contains the sequence encoding the amyloid-β (AB) peptide (Golde et al., 1990; Kang et al., 1987). The full-length APP (APP 770) consists of 18 exons, where exon 17 resembles the membrane spanning domain. APP 695 lacking both, exon 7 and exon 8 is primarily expressed by neurons and is the most abundant APP transcript in the brain (Neve 1988). APP 751 (lacking exon 8), APP 714 (lacking exon 7) and APP 770 were first identified in peripheral organs but are also expressed in brain glial cells. Other alternatively generated splice variants of APP involving exon 15 were recently discovered in peripheral leucocytes and in microglial cells and therefore denoted as leukocyte- derived APP (L-APP) (Konig et al., 1992). The AB fragment is part of exon 16 and 17 (figure 1B) and begins 99 amino acid residues from the carboxy terminus and extends 12-15 residues into the hydrophobic membrane domain (Estus et al., 1992). The APP protein is composed of three regions: a large extracellular domain in the N-terminal region that forms a globular structure, a transmembrane region, which contains part of the AB sequence, and a small cytoplasmic domain laregion C-terminal (figure 1B). The overall structure includes the position of a heparin binding domain, metal binding domains, sites of phosphorylation and glycosylation. Two of the isoforms (APP 751 and APP 770) have a domain Kunitz-type protease inhibior (KPI) and a signal peptide (De Strooper, 2010).

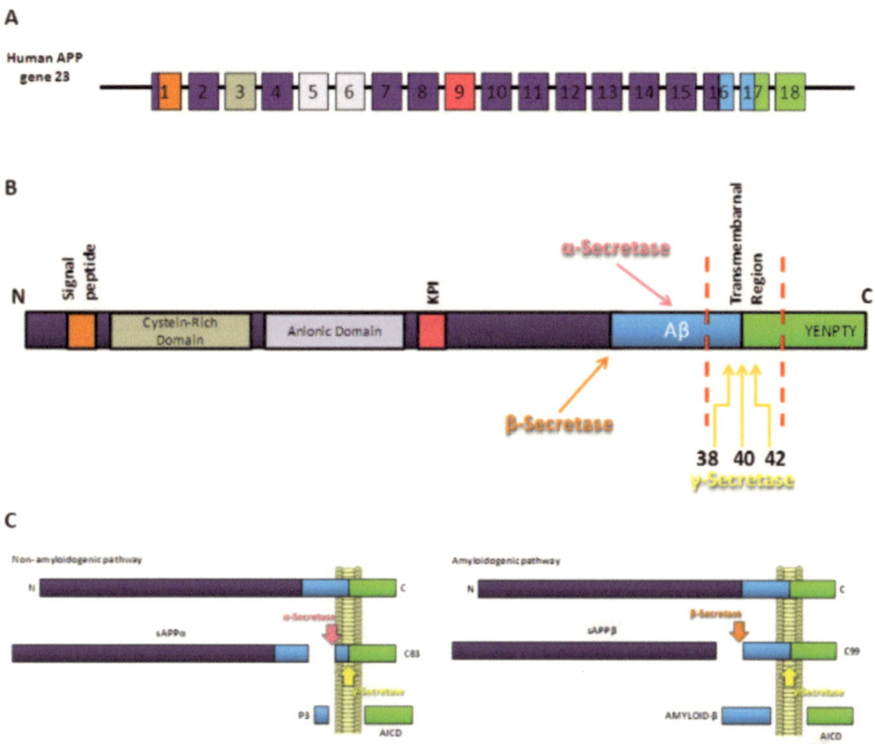

Fig. 1. Characteristics of APP and processing (A) Exon structure of human APP gene 23. Exons are indicated by rectangles. Alternatively spliced exons are 7, 8 and 15. Functional protein domains are indicated by different colors. Distances between exons are not representative. (B) Schematic representation of human APP protein including the relative position of the α-, β- and γ-secretase cleavage sites. KPI: Kunitz-type protease inhibitor domain, AICD: APP intracellular domain, YENPTY: motif that binds he phosphotyrosine binding (PTB) domain of X11. (C) Schematic diagram of APP processing pathways. APP proteolytic catabolism includes two different pathways: an amyloidogenic pathway and a non-amyloidogenic pathway (constitutive secretary pathway). The different APP fragments are generated after secretase cleavage.

In brain tissue, APP can be processed in two ways: non-amyloidogenic and amyloidogenic pathway. In the non-amyloidogenic pathway, APP is first cleaved by α-secretase within the AB sequence, which releases the sAPPα ectodomain. Further processing of the resulting carboxyl terminal by γ-secretase results in the release of the p3 fragment and AICD (figure 1C) (Greenwald &Riek, 2010). The most prevalent area of research in AD studies the proteolytic generation of AB from APP. The β-secretase and γ-secretase cleave APP in the so-called amyloidogenic pathway β-secretase release the ectodomain sAPPβ, and the remaining APP carboxy-terminal fragment (C99) is subsequently cleaved by the γ-secretase liberating the secreted AB peptide(s) and the APP intracellular domain (AICD) (figure 1C). The biological functions of sAPPβ, AB, and the AICD remain rather elusive, although AB release is associated with synaptic activity, depression excitatory synaptic transmission onto neurons. The production of AB occurs naturally inside the human brain, these fragment possesses and amphiphilic structure with hydrophilic N- and hydrophobic C- terminus, however the C-terminal end is variable ranging at least from 37 to 42 residues; the most studied forms are AB 1-40 and AB 1-42 that consist of 40 and 42 residues respectively (Fandrich et al., 2011). Under physiological conditions, the ratio of AB42 to AB40 is about 1:10. AB42 plays a critical role in the pathogenesis of AD since its aggregative ability and neurotoxicity are much greater than those of AB40 (De Strooper, 2010).

About APP function, the analysis sequence and structure indicate that the protein is organized into different domains, because it is believed that APP is important for functions as neuronal survival, synaptogenesis, cell adhesion, inhibition of clotting factors, inhibiting platelet activation and in the modulation of copper homeostasis (Chow et al., 2010; De Strooper, 2010). The precise function of various APP isoforms in the brain is still unknown. It has been suggested that APP plays a role in establishing or maintaining cell-cell contacts which is also consistent with preferential localization of APP at nerve terminals, because have been shown their interaction with extracellular matrix proteins and heparin sulfate proteoglycans through E1 and E2 regions of APP (Schubert et al., 1995; Small et al., 1999). The function of APP as a cell surface receptor has been proposed for the evidence of AB could bind to APP and also the similarities of their secondary structure with Notch receptor (Zheng &Koo, 2011). About the neuronal survival and synaptogenesis functions of APP the reports showed that APP expression is upregulated during neuronal maturation and differentiation, also induced after traumatic brain injury, these results are reinforced because the reduction of APP is associated with neuronal impairment (Hung et al., 1992; Leyssen et al., 2005). The APP can be phosphorylated at multiple sites resulted in several consequence such as localization to the growth cones and neuritis (Muresan &Muresan, 2005). Other contrasting activity of soluble APP is the cytotoxic properties of C99 fragment as result of β-secretase cleaveage (Neve et al., 1996). Meanwhile, the functional properties of AB peptides have not been fully clarified to date, although numerous studies suggest that peptides have a number of neurotrophic and neurotoxic properties (Tycko, 2011). It is suggested that AB soluble plays an important role in neuronal growth, survival, and synaptic modulation, while the oligomers and fibrils have toxic properties (Kamenetz et al., 2003; Plant et al., 2003; Puzzo et al., 2008). Studies have shown that AB oligomers are able to induce increased cell death and apoptosis soluble or fibrillar forms, suggesting that the structural conformation peptide is important in determining its physiological action (Small et al., 2001).

2.1 Amyloid β structure and aggregation

Recent biophysical investigations using electron microscopy, Fourier Transform Infrared Resonance (FTIR) studies and Circular Dicroism (CD) spectroscopy showed that AB fibrils adopt a β-sheet structure (Serpell et al., 2000). However, a high-resolution structural analysis of AB fibrils has yet to be conducted since single crystal X-ray crystallography and solution nuclear magnetic resonance (NMR) cannot be applied to insoluble AB fibrils (Greenwald &Riek, 2010). AB peptides generated can exist as monomers, dimers and oligomers with aggregation and eventually produce protofibrils fibrils, they acquire a conformation which β-pleated sheet. The AB peptide has a spontaneous tendency to oligomerization, forming toxic species which can even add intracellularly and therefore believed to play a role this fundamental neurotoxicity in AD (Klein et al., 2001; Murray et al., 2009). Recent experiments have established that the main structure adopted by these peptides depends on the environment. The monomers contain a amphipathic sequence that favors the α-helix structure in solution but preferred aqueous β-pleated structure (Greenwald &Riek, 2010).

The structures of β-sheets are parallel or anti-parallel alignments of two or more β-stranded peptides that are held together by inter-strand hydrogen bonds. The β-sheet is not an unusual structure with more than 30% of the secondary structure of all proteins. The structure consisting of strands aligned in parallel feature twelve-membered hydrogen bonded rings, while those with strands in anti-parallel arrays are characterized by alternating 10- and 14-membered H-bonded rings. Dihedral angles commonly found in parallel ($\varphi = -119°$, $\psi = 113°$) and anti-parallel ($\varphi = -139°$, $\psi = 135°$) β-sheets are closer to those of the fully extended single-strand conformation ($\varphi = \psi = \pm 180°$) than β-turns or α-helices. The β-sheet usually acts as a scaffold to stabilize protein architecture, but it is also an important recognition motif in some protein–protein and protein–DNA interactions that mediate biological processes and some notable diseases (Harrison et al., 2007; Jenkins &Pickersgill, 2001). The peptide self-assembly to AB fibrils is a widespread phenomenon in nature; these structures are associated with protein aggregation pathologies such as AD. Therefore the structural analysis of AB fibrils is one of the most promising ways of revealing the mechanism involved in this event. Investigations showed a conserved evolutionarily protein motifs. The description of a common cross-β structure consists of β-strand peptides aligned in either parallel or antiparallel orientations to provide β-sheet structures that ultimately laminate to form fibrillar architectures. This process is mediated by noncovalent forces such as hydrophobic and hydrogen bonding interactions. However, the contribution of these forces is poorly understood (Bemporad et al., 2006; Tycko, 2011). Other critical interactions in cross-β peptide self-assembly are aromatic π-π, frequent in aromatic amino acids in the core of amyloid sequences, because mutations o deletions cause the loss of the structure (Bowerman et al., 2011; Marshall et al., 2011). Fibrils of AB42 and AB10-35 show a strong dependence of pH on morphology observed; at pH 7.4 protofilaments of AB42 exist singly and in pairs, but protofilaments of AB10-35 exist in pairs only. Studies on NMR indicate a parallel β-sheet organization on AB42 fibrils, consistent with supramolecular structures of other fibrils of AB10-35 and AB40. Although, there is a disagreement in the results obtained for fibrils formed by AB10-35 and AB40 with parallel organization, while the observations in AB42 fibril showed an antiparallel β-sheet structure. The explanation is that amyloid fibrils do not have a universal supramolecular organization. Also the results obtained of electronic microscopy and diffraction support a tubular structure for AB fibrils (Antzutkin et al., 2002). Analysis of the amyloidogenic regions in fibril-forming proteins showed a high occurrence of the aromatic residues phenylalanine and tyrosine, which have a high propensity to stack the delocalized π-electron rings in a parallel manner. Studies with short peptides have confirmed that even two consecutive phenylalanine residues are sufficient to facilitate assembly into nanotube-like structures, and stacks of aromatic residues were observed in crystal structures (Nerelius et al., 2010).

Also it has been suggested that the amphiphilicity of the peptide plays a significant role in determining whether peptide strands within the fibril are parallel or anti-parallel. Parallel β-sheets in proteins usually adjoin α-helices, suggesting that they are intrinsically less stable on their own than are anti-parallel β-sheets. The AB40 and AB10–35 peptides both have hydrophobic C-termini, and their reported assembly into parallel β-sheets allows the juxtaposition of the hydrophobic portions of the peptides, shielding them from aqueous solution. An anti-parallel disposition would be costly energetically because of the forced association of hydrophobic and hydrophilic regions. AB16–22 and AB34–42 both have a centrally located hydrophobic segment and thus no advantage of sequestration of hydrophobic regions provided by either a parallel or antiparallel arrangement. The anti-parallel β-sheet arrangements found for these two peptides may then be the result of favorable charge interactions between side chains or termini, or improved H-bonding (Harrison et al., 2007). A model proposed for this structure is a parallel β-helix consisting of an extended polypeptide chain wrapping around a cylindrical template, where adjacent strands of the helix are connected through H-bonds and is based on two key features of the polyglutamine diffraction data; the absence of a 10-Å reflection and the presence of a weak, low-angle reflection of 31 Å (Perutz et al., 2002).

The crucial region for the formation of crossed-β fibrils is found in 15-23 residues (QKLVFFAED) (figure 2A), substitution of Thr for Phe19 can abolish plaque-forming competence of the mutant peptide and that the mutant peptide was significantly less folded in aqueous buffer than the wild-type peptide. Further, the Phe19 in the AB antiparallel β-sheet is key in determining the properties of the fibril, because the observation that the Thr for Phe19 substitution lacks fibril-forming competence. Also the Lys16 in AB is positioned for electrostatic interaction with the charged sulfate groups of inductors of aggregation such as Congo Red (Carter &Chou, 1998). The KLVFFAED motif, a known amyloidogenic sequence of the AB, which contains positively and negatively charged residues (figure 2B) and has a high β-strand propensity (figure 2C). As mentioned above, minor alterations in sequence, such as replacement of Val or Phe with Leu or Ala, can abolish fibril formation and that the amyloidogenic properties of short peptides can be abolished by introduction of adjacent sequence motifs such as β-turns. These data indicate that both the amino acid sequence as such and its structural context affect the ability to form amyloid fibrils (Nerelius et al., 2010). In macromolecular level, aggregates are typically fibrillar in electron microscopy images generally with linear (figure 2D), unbranched fibrils of variable length. Each fibril is thought to consist of several protofilaments, the number being specific to the particular amyloid protein. Improved imaging of protofilaments has revealed that certain fibrils are clearly helical, with the protofilaments slowly twisting around each other. For Aβ34–42 fibrils, the twisted fibril "unwinds" under denaturing conditions and for Aβ40 at high pH, suggesting that these protofilaments are associated through both electrostatic and hydrophobic interactions (Fraser et al., 1992; Halverson et al., 1990). Amyloids are typically large (Megadalton) elongated structures with varying lengths and often varying ultrastructural appearances (Toyama &Weissman, 2011). Here we describe some of the most commonly used techniques employed in amyloid structure characterization. Electron microscopy and atomic force microscopy (AFM) are the two most widely used microscopy techniques employed in the study of amyloids. Both provide a nanometer-resolution perspective of the ultrastructural characteristics of amyloids. This includes amyloid fiber length and width, morphology such as curvature and persistence length, surface characteristics such as periodic twists, and higher-order assembly. Electron microscopy and AFM helped establish many of the common ultrastructural characteristics of amyloid fibers, such as the long, relatively straight and unbranched nature of the fibers; the typical fiber width of 5–15 nm; the periodic twist often observed; and the conclusion that many amyloid fibers are made up of the bundling of thinner protofibrils. To better understand the higher-order assembly of amyloid fibers, scanning transmission electron microscopy (STEM) and tilted-beam transmission electron microscopy, both forms of electron microscopy, have provided data that describe the amount of mass-per-unit length (MPL) of amyloids. These data are particularly valuable in determining how many monomers make up a single layer of the fiber structure. AFM has also been used to determine the relative fiber rigidity by monitoring its propensity to bend. Electron microscopy and AFM both have the advantage of being single-fiber approaches, which are useful in visualizing structural heterogeneity within a single-fiber preparation (Chen et al., 2009; Shirahama &Cohen, 1965).

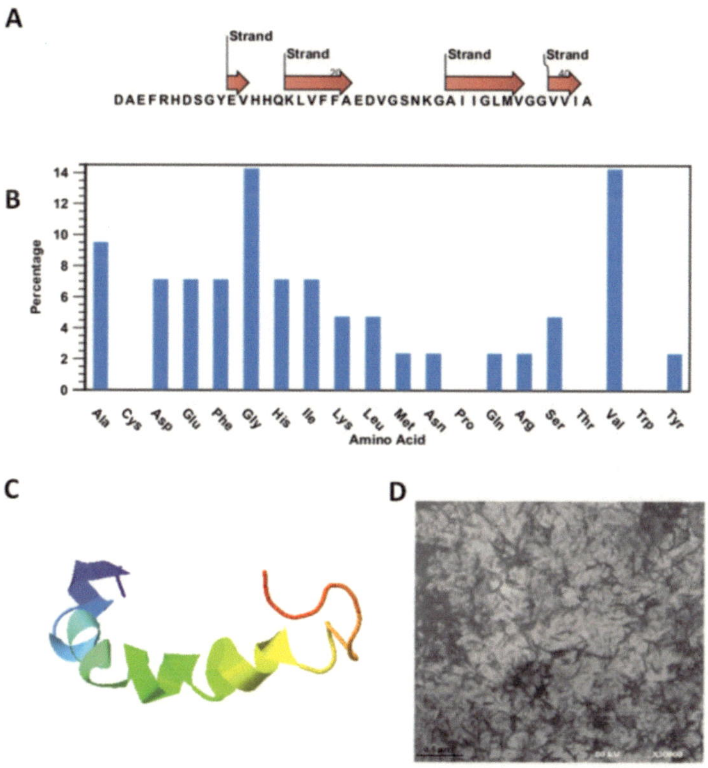

Fig. 2. Characteristics of Amyloid β. (A) Structure diagram and amino acid sequence of AB42. (B) Amino acid distribution histogram of AB42. (C) Proposed AB42 structure based on predicted β-strand propensities (Displayed in Jmol). (D) Electron Microscopy photograph of *in vitro* AB42 aggregates.

Fiber X-ray diffraction was one of the first structural techniques that provided a substantial clue to the overall fold of amyloid fibers. In this method, fibrous samples are bombarded with X-ray radiation, and diffraction patterns result from interference patterns from any regularly spaced structural features present in the fibers. As alluded to above, this technique established the cross-β diffraction pattern interpreted as β-sheets parallel to the fiber axis, with β-strands perpendicular. It has also aided in testing the validity of particular model structures. Here, a theoretical Xray fiber diffraction pattern is calculated on the basis of a particular model and then is compared to an actual diffraction pattern (Makin et al., 2005). FTIR and CD are absorptive spectroscopic techniques that measure nonsymmetrical or chiral molecular systems in bulk, FTIR spectroscopy measuring molecular bond vibrational frequencies and CD the differential absorption of left versus right circular polarized light. Both of these properties are highly sensitive to secondary structure, and therefore, deconvoluted FTIR and CD spectrum provide accurate estimations of the contribution of β-sheets, α-helices, and loops to the overall structure (Berthomieu &Hienerwadel, 2009; Ranjbar &Gill, 2009). Cryoelectron Microscopy: is a technique that positions itself as a capable alternative to conventional X-ray crystallography and solution NMR in amyloid structure determination. Unlike X-ray crystallography, proteins of interest need not be in a crystalline form for cryoelectron microscopy; rather, structural data can be acquired on single particles. Furthermore, amyloid preparations do not need to be labeled with stable isotopes, is the case with NMR, nor do they even need to be highly pure preparations. This is particularly advantageous owing to the inherent heterogeneous nature of the amyloid conformation (Mizuno et al., 2011). X-Ray Crystallography: although the large and heterogeneous nature of amyloid fibers would seem to be incompatible with X-ray crystallography, Eisenberg and colleagues have been able to acquire adequate diffraction data from microcrystals of short peptides (6–7 residues) that formed amyloid-like structures. Based on X-ray crystallography showed that structures bore strong resemblance to many existing models of amyloid fibers, suggesting they may in fact represent the structure of the amyloid fold. Since this initial study, multiple amyloidogenic peptides have been successfully crystallized and their structures solved (Nelson et al., 2005; Wiltzius et al., 2009).

AB early aggregates also can showed a globular appearance that further organize into beaded chains, globular annular "doughnut" shaped assemblies eventually giving mature protofilaments and fibrils. Pre-fibrilar aggregates may interact with reconstituted phospholipid membranes and with cell membranes where they form aspecific channels (pores) disrupting cellular homeostasis (figure 5). The latter possible mechanism of toxicity is similar to that displayed by antimicrobial peptides, pore-forming eukaryotic proteins and bacterial toxins and newly synthesised cyclic peptide antibiotics (Stefani &Dobson, 2003).

The cell membrane could be a nucleating center for amyloid aggregation. The evidence showed that AB species are tight binding to GM1 ganglioside (GM1), in the brain showing early pathological changes of AD. The ganglioside-bound AB (GAB) possessed unique characteristics, including its altered immunoreactivity, which suggests its distinct conformation from native AB, and its strong potency to accelerate Aβ assembly into fibrils. The hypothesis is that AB adopts an altered conformation following interaction with GM1, leading to the generation of GAB, and then GAβ acts as an endogenous seed for Alzheimer amyloid in the brain. GAB is favorably generated in the unique ganglioside-enriched (clustered), raft-like microdomains; moreover, amyloid fibrils formed in the presence of gangliosides are neurotoxic. Probably the ganglioside binding is the initial and common step in the development of a part of human misfolding-type amyloidoses, including AD (Matsuzaki et al., 2010). Recent reports supports that soluble oligomers of AB may be the key neurotoxic species associated with the progression of AD and that the process of AB aggregation may drive this event. Recent data obtained in our laboratory suggest that the presence of soluble oligomers in rat hippocampus promotes localized mechanism of inflammatory responses (unpublished data). Is alspo reported that soluble oligomers of AB and Tau accumulate in the lipid rafts of brains from AD patients through an as yet unknown mechanism. In cell culture models the exogenously applied AB in the form of oligomers can be trafficked on the neuronal membrane and accumulate in lipid rafts. The oligomers induced dynamic alterations in lipid raft protein composition were found to facilitate this movement. There is a clear association between AB accumulation and redistribution on the neuronal membrane and alterations in the protein composition of lipid rafts. Also the reports showed that fyn is a key protein on AB redistribution and accumulation in lipid rafts as and mediating the cell death induced by the AB oligomers and defines a mechanism by which oligomers of AB and Tau accumulate in lipid rafts (Williamson et al., 2008).

3. Tau protein

Tau is a microtubule-associated protein (MAP) that is believed to stabilise microtubules and to promote microtubule assembly. Of the neuronal MAPs, it is one of the most abundant (Goedert &Spillantini, 2011). Tau protein is found in many animal species such as *Caenorhabditis elegans, Drosophila,* goldfish, bullfrog, rodents, bovines, goat, monkeys and humans (Buee et al., 2000). In humans, Tau is encoded by a single-copy gene located on chromosome 17q21.1 in humans (figure 3A). It produces three transcripts of 2, 6 and 9 kb which are differentially expressed in the nervous system, depending upon stage of neuronal maturation and neuron type. The 2 and 6 kb Tau mRNAs arise from utilization of two alternative polyadenylation sites separated by ~4 Kbp. So far, one promoter has been mapped for the Tau gene in both human and rat, located directly upstream of Tau exon -1. However, the 6 kb Tau transcript is responsive to NGF, whereas the 9 kb one is not. Also, the 6 and 9 kb transcripts are restricted to neuronal tissues, whereas the 2 kb Tau transcript is ubiquitous (Andreadis, 2005; Andreadis et al., 1996). Tau primary transcript contains 16 exons, but two of them (exons 4A and 8) are not present in mRNA in human brain. Exon 4A is present in peripheral nervous system not only in humans, also in bovine and rodent peripherial tissues. On the other hand, exon 8 has not been described in humans. Exon -1 is part of the promoter, transcribed but not translated, just like exon 14 (Buee et al., 2000). Exon 3 is never found without exon 2, and as exon 10, are present in an adult-specific manner (figure 1B), but their ratios differ in various central nervous system compartments (Andreadis, 2011; Takuma et al., 2003). All six possible product combinations of the 2/3/10 splicing events have been observed (figure 3B), indicating that separate factors govern their splicing (Andreadis, 2011). Alternative splicing of hinge-region exon 6 gives rise to Tau variants that lack the domain responsible of microtubule binding, and is mentioned that alters Tau function (Andreadis, 2011; Luo et al., 2004). Saitohin (STH), an intronless gene encoding an open reading frame of 128 amino acids, is located in the intron between exons 9 and 10 of the human Tau gene (Wang et al., 2011). Recently has been associated the existence of a polymorphic form with AD, but is still under research. In the 6 principal human Tau protein isoforms are present two domains (Figure 2C): the projection domain located in the amino-terminal and is composed of an acidic region and a proline rich region (PRR). The other domain is named microtubule binding domain (MTBD), which contain the C-termini *per se*, and a microtubule binding region (MTBR), conformed indeed by the presence from three (3R) to four repeats (4R) (Buee et al., 2000). They differ from each other by the presence or absence of 29- or 58-amino acid inserts located in the amino-terminal half and an additional 31-amino acid repeat in the carboxy-terminal half (Goedert &Spillantini, 2011). Tau is enriched in axons of growing and mature neurons and is critical for neuronal function. Among its many roles, Tau promotes neurite outgrowth, organizes axonal microtubules (MTs) and is involved in kinesin-dependent axonal transport (Andreadis, 2011; Hirokawa et al., 1988; LaPointe et al., 2009). Additionally, the interaction of Tau with diverse structural and functional proteins suggests that Tau may play crucial roles not only in normal architecture but also in signal transduction of the neurons (Wang &Liu, 2008). The acidic sequences may be involved in cation binding and in iron binding site motif, also is

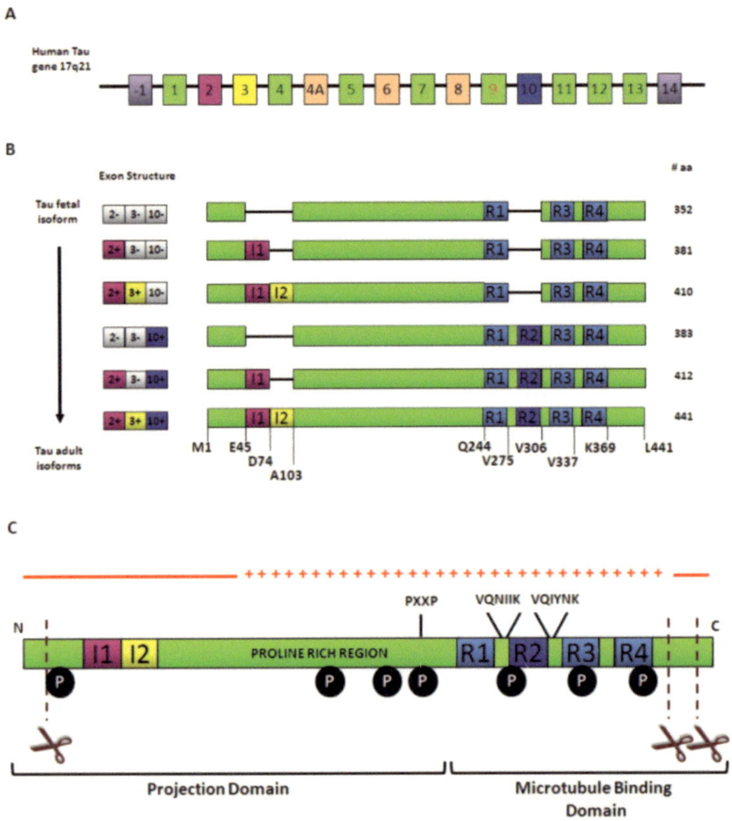

Fig. 3. Characteristics of human Tau protein. (A) Human Tau gene presents 14 exons and -1 is part of the Tau gen promotor: -1 and 14 can be transcribed but not translated; in human CNS are not normally expressed exons 4A, 6 and 8. In all isoforms are expressed exons 1, 4, 5, 7, 9, 11, 12 and 13. Exons 2, 3 and 10 can be excluded depending of Tau isoform. In exon 9 is codified the protein Saitohin. Exons are indicated by rectangles. Distances between exons are representative. (B) Tau isoforms expressed in human CNS, showing number of aminoacids and inserts that differ each of them. Functional protein domains are indicated by different colors (C) Domains contained in most of the isoforms of human Tau protein: the N-terminal is named projection domain and is subdivided in acidic domain and proline rich regions; also here is a PXXP motif for SH3 domain interactions. The C-terminal, also named microtubule binding domain (MTBD) contains the MTBR and the C-terminus *per se*; in 4R isoforms is present 2 sequences with β sheet structure tendency adjacent to the second and third repeats. P= phosphorylation sites; ✂= truncations sites.

proposed that the motif KKXK is involved in heparing binding (Ávila et al., 2002) and actin interaction (Zmuda &Rivas, 2000). In this regions is present various PPXXP or PXXP motifs which allow Tau protein to interacts with SH3 domains of diverse proteins such as Src family members like Fyn, Lck, Src (Lee, 2005; Lee et al., 1998; Scales et al., 2011) and others like PCL-γ (Hwang et al., 1996; Jenkins &Johnson, 1998). Is also mentioned that STH interacts with Tau and Abl and influences in Abl phosphorylation (Wang et al., 2011), but this phenomena needs further research.

The efficacy of Tau to binding MTs is influenced by the degree of phosphorylation and the exclusion/inclusion of exon 10. The affinity of Tau against MTs is weaker in 3R isoforms than 4R isoforms, perhaps leading to differential regulation of microtubule behaviour (Eckermann et al., 2007; Goode et al., 2000; Lu &Kosik, 2001). Another important factor influences Tau-MTs interaction: site-specific phosphorylation. This is due to the high frequency of phosphorylatable residues (45 S, 35 T and 5 Y in the largest isoform), combined with the open structure of Tau which renders it accessible to many kinases (Mandelkow et al., 2007). The majority of the phosphorylation sites are Serine or Threonine residues followed by Prolines (SP/TP motifs) that lie in the domains flanking the repeats and can be phosphorylated by several Proline-directed kinases and by neuronal kinases MARK (affecting the KXGS motifs within Tau's repeat domain) (Eckermann et al., 2007; Trinczek et al., 1995). Among the kinases responsible for Tau phosphorylation are Glycogen Synthase Kinase 3β (Lin et al., 2007), cyclin-dependent kinase 5 (Cdk5), MT-affinity regulatory kinase, cAMP-dependent protein kinase (Johnson &Stoothoff, 2004), dual-specificity tyrosine-phosphorylated and regulated kinase 1A, Tau–tubulin kinase 1, and calmodulin-dependent protein kinase 2 (Meraz-Ríos et al., 2010)

3.1 Tau conformational changes in physiological and pathological conditions

Tau is a highly flexible and extended protein, natively unfolded and with hydrophilic and basic character, highly soluble shown by sequence analysis and CD experiments (Eckermann et al., 2007; Shkumatov et al., 2011). Firstly was suggested that Tau in solution may be as much as 77% random coil and behave like "Gaussian coils" or "worm like-chains", in which the direction of the polypeptide backbone chain varies in a more-or-less random fashion (Goode et al., 2000). However, a potential β-pleated region has been proposed for the microtubule binding region (Ávila et al., 2002). When Tau is attached to MTs, is suggested to assume an "L" conformation, meaning that MTBR interacts with the MTs and the N-termini is projected to cytosol, where can interacts with other proteins (Hirokawa et al., 1988; Mandelkow et al., 2007; Sillen et al., 2007).

On the other hand, is suggested by fluorescence resonance energy transfer (FRET), electron paramagnetic resonance (EPR) and small-angle X-ray scattering that Tau can adopt a global hairpin (paperclip) structure in solution (when is not attached to MTs) (Jeganathan et al., 2008a; Mandelkow et al., 2007; Mylonas et al., 2008). From a structural perspective, the folding of the N- and C-domains over the repeat domain would be expected to protect against aggregation, and indeed Tau forms aggregates more readily when the non-repeat domains are cleaved off (Mylonas et al., 2008). The conversion of certain soluble peptides and proteins into insoluble filaments or misfolded amyloid proteins is believed to be the central event in the etiology of a majority of neurodegenerative diseases (Nonaka et al.,

2010). Tau protein is not the exception. Despite its random coil appearance in solution, Tau assembles into well-defined fibbers, the Paired Helical Filaments (PHFs) (von Bergen et al., 2000). The appearance of conformational changes in Tau as early alterations in AD neuropathology has been eloquently confirmed in several studies (Ávila et al., 2002). Even when is reported that α-helix structures are present in PHFs (Sadqi et al., 2002), the β-sheet structure seems to be the major structure involved in Tau aggregation. Two hexapeptides, ^{275}VQJINK^{280} and ^{306}VQJVYK^{311} which are respectively located at the beginning of the second and third MTBR are prominent in generating β-sheet structures during Tau aggregation process (Martin et al., 2011). These hexapeptides structure are well characterized by several methodologies, like FTIR, AFM and CD (Chaudhary et al., 2009). Another reports mention that proline is frequently involved in a β-turn by reason of its restricted ø angle and that the Pro-Gly motif is favored to make a Type II β-turn and the SPXX motif is known to stabilize β-turns, independent of X. Also is predicted that Tau contains 54 β-turns involving about 35% the protein sequence (Goux, 2002). For the conformational studies, Goux (2002) mentions that is important to consider factors as temperature or solvent-induced changes in Tau to the *cis-trans* proline distribution of isomers, resulting in a change in protein conformation, also mentioned by other authors for the two hexapeptides mentioned before (Chaudhary et al., 2009; Goux, 2002).

As a general view for aggregation studies, conformational changes have been studied by the use of aggregations inducers or punctual mutations in the MTBR. The other manner is by promoting post-translational modifications in Tau molecule, such as phosphorylations or truncations or by the analysis of PHFs. In the presence of pro-aggregatory factors as polyanions, stimuli the assembly of full lenght Tau, 3R or 4R, and when mutations forms associated to other Tauopathies seem to be a faster process of filament formation. In both are reported the presence of β-sheet enriched structures (Friedhoff et al., 2000). The β-strands usually run perpendicular to the helix axis forming a cross-β motif. By *in vitro* assays, is suggested that β-sheet structures might be stabilized by the presence of salt bridges or by hydrogen bonds, which promote forming a continuous β-sheet extending along the axis (Berriman et al., 2003; Jeganathan et al., 2008b). Such structures can be stained with certain dyes such as Congo red (CR), Thioflavine S (TS) or Thiazine Red (TR) which are thought to interact with the repeating β strands (Glenner et al., 1972; Luna-Muñoz et al., 2008; Zilka et al., 2006). Planar aromatic dyes as CR, TR, and TS also are capable of inducing Tau fibrillization *in vitro*. In our group we developed a cellular model to study the particularities of these dyes at *in vivo* Tau aggregation. The SH-SY5Y cells were incubated with each dye and our results showed that three dyes gave rise to aggregates of Tau with different morphological characteristics. This method can be used to test related drugs with inhibitory potential for Tau abnormal polymerization (Lira-De León et al, unpublished data).

Alternatively, Tau can indeed adopt distinct conformations has been observed in sequential phosphorylation reactions. This theory is supported by biophysical evidence showing that Tau paracrystals become longer and stiffer following phosphorylation, suggesting a conformational change of the protein upon phosphorylation; specifically NMR and CD evidence shows that a Tau peptide undergoes a conformational change following phosphorylation at Thr231 and Ser235 (Goux, 2002). Moreover, where the AD-specific phosphoepitope of antibody AT-100 in the proline-rich region can only be generated by a sequential phosphorylation of Tau first by GSK-3β (at Thr212) and then by PKA (at Ser214), indicating that pre-phosphorylation at certain sites can alter the conformation such that other phosphorylation reactions are no longer possible (Friedhoff et al., 2000). Tau abnormal phosphorylation at specific sites are strongly associated to other post-translational modifications such endogenous proteolysis or truncation. This abnormal process is defined as a protein cutting that could also promote aberrant aggregation (Ávila et al., 2004) In the case of Tau molecule, the lost of any of its C- and N-extremes leads to a change of properties of the molecule. The lost of the N-terminal has been proposed as an early event in Tau aggregation process because of the capability of this extreme of inhibit Tau oligomerization *in vitro* (Ghoshal et al., 2002; Horowitz et al., 2006) On the other hand, C-terminal proteolysis is strongly correlated with neuropathological lesions and cognitive impairment (García-Sierra et al., 2001; Meraz-Ríos et al., 2010). Latest years many reports have demonstrated the relationship between site-specific phosphorylation at sites Ser199, Ser202, Thr205, Thr212, Ser214, located in proline-rich region, and Ser396 and Ser 404, located near C-termini. These impact in conformation of Tau, and perhaps expose sites for further specific proteolysis in Asp421 and Glu391 (Fischer et al., 2009; Jeganathan et al., 2008a; Luna-Muñoz et al., 2007; Mondragon-Rodriguez et al., 2008). Specific Tau-phosphorylation also alters microtubule-binding capacity and increase rate of filament nucleation (Chang et al., 2011; Fischer et al., 2009). With this issue, is proposed the sequential relationship between phosphorylation→ conformational change→ truncation, which can be repeated until Tau protein lost their N- and C-termini, exposing a minimal resistance protease region named PHF-core (figure 3) (Binder et al., 2005; García-Sierra et al., 2008; Wischik et al., 1985; Wischik et al., 1996). The dense core of PHFs is compound of the repeat region of the Tau protein, forming a fuzzy coat beside the filament with N- and C-termini of the protein(Skrabana et al., 2004). According to *in vitro* assays, this PHF-core is able to promote Tau aggregation (Campos-Peña et al., 2009; Wischik et al., 1996).

Considering these data, is important to use diverse strategies for the study of this phenomena. For elucidated this issue is used conformational-specific antibodies. The Alz-50 and MC-1, two conformational sensitive antibodies, have been demonstrated to recognize a pathological conformation of Tau molecule in NFTs (Jicha et al., 1997; Lin et al., 2007). Either antibody recognizes the N-termini nearby C-termini, determinate by fluorescence lifetime imaging and other techniques (Hyman et al., 2005). Even these antibodies recognize a region in the N-termini (7-9) and C-termini (312-342), both conserved in all Tau human isoforms, in tissue they have a distinct pattern of signal (Jicha et al., 1997). In AD brain, MC1 stains "pretangle neurons", and its immunopositivity is indicative of very early neuronal pathological changes. Alz50 stains both pretangle neurons, as well as early-formed paired-helical filaments (Nogalska et al., 2011). Moreover, a number of studies have proposed that the phosphorylation modification at S-P or T-P motifs in Tau might cause Tau conformational change and the *cis-trans* isomerisation, made by the prolyl-peptide isomerise Pin-1, might regulate Tau function. This association is dependent on a folding of the Tau molecule, this bend occurring locally in the vicinity of Thr231-P motif, and actually recognized by TG3 antibody (Friedhoff et al., 2000; Lin et al., 2007; Luna-Muñoz et al., 2005; Weaver et al., 2000). The antibody Tau-66 is another conformational-associated antibody, recognizing residues between 155-244 and 305-314. This antibody recognizes NFT, and also cytoplasmic points on some non-fibrillary neurons, mostly associated to truncated N- and C-termini (García-Sierra et al., 2003). During this study, they suggest there is a progression from Alz-50 to Tau-66 conformation during NFTs evolution. Related to this, Goux based on PHFs extraction and CD assays, mention that Tau has a structure containing 31-37% helix,

15-20% β-sheet, 20-23% turn, and 26-29% unordered structure (Goux, 2002), perhaps influencing in this "specific-antibody" conformation. It was also mentioned by Barghorn and co-workers that for aggregation issues, Tau must adopt a specific conformation that allows a subsequent fibril formation (Barghorn &Mandelkow, 2002). Recent studies use mAb423 antibody, which recognize truncated Tau in Glu391, as a tool for structural studies directed to the PHF core (from 297-391 of 441 isoform), allowing to estimate the enrichment of β-sheet structures (Sevcik et al., 2007; Skrabana et al., 2010; Wischik et al., 1985). In this aim, antibodies have probe been an important tool for recognize conformational changes in Tau during aggregation events.

3.2 Impact of Tau conformational change during aggregation process

Partially folded or misfolded states often tend to aggregate because these forms typically expose hydrophobic amino acid residues and regions of unstructured polypeptide backbone, features that are largely buried in the native state. Like intramolecular folding, aggregation, i.e., the association of two or more non-native protein molecules, is driven by hydrophobic forces and predominantly results in the formation of amorphous structures that lack long range order. Although the toxic principle operating in the age-of-onset diseases is far from being understood, a consensus is emerging that oligomeric, soluble states of the respective disease protein are the primary cytotoxic species (Vabulas et al., 2010). Tau proteins fibrillize efficiently *in vitro* into β-pleated sheet structures with biochemical and biophysical properties of amyloid fibrils (figure 4A-B), but they do so only in the presence of negatively charged cofactors such as heparin, RNA, or DNA. The kinetic profile of Tau fibrillization *in vitro* generally resembles that of other amyloid proteins, when is important an increase of β-sheet structures (figure 4C), with a lag phase during which time nucleating units are believed to be formed followed by rapid fibril growth (Congdon et al., 2008; Matthes et al., 2011; von Bergen et al., 2000; Xu et al., 2010). Covalently linked dimers can be formed by disulfide cross-linking and by electronic microscopy it seems as rod-like particles (Friedhoff et al., 2000). The dimers of Tau molecules become subunits of filaments, forming protomers, adopting the parallel, in register cross-β-sheet structure typical of amyloid aggregates. On the basis of morphology and mass-per-unit length measurements, mature Tau filaments (PHFs) consist of two protofilaments wound around each other (Congdon et al., 2008). This has led to several proposed "nucleation-elongation" models of Tau fibril assembly (figure 5). In the classic equilibrium nucleation-elongation model elaborated for linear polymer formation, assembly-competent monomer is in rapid equilibrium with a thermodynamically unstable species termed the nucleus, in Tau case, probably the PHF-core (figure 4D). Once assembly-competent conformations are adopted (Weaver et al., 2000), the rate-limiting step in the reaction becomes dimerization, with subsequent aggregate growth occurring through monomer addition. When the critical nucleus cluster size is reached, subsequent additions to the nascent filament end are energetically favorable, and elongation proceeds efficiently (figure 5). This pathway leads to peaked distributions of filament lengths early in the reaction time series followed by slow relaxation toward exponential distributions at equilibrium. Finally, aggregation rates can be limited by secondary nucleation events, which occur on existing aggregates (Congdon et al., 2008). In addition, an alternative linear colloidal aggregation model has been proposed for Tau in which the protein forms colloidal spheres that serve as nucleation units that, through charge-dipole and dipole-dipole interactions, go on to form linear fibers (Xu et al., 2010). Either pathway seems that adoption of assembly competent conformations, perhaps associated with enriched β-sheet content, can be driven by small diffusible ligands in a process that approximates homogeneous nucleation (Congdon et al., 2008).

Pathologic Tau fibrils show diverse morphologies in diseased brains, where transmission electron microscopy (TEM) images typically reveal PHFs in AD NFTs or neuropil threads, although straight filaments (SFs) and twisted ribbons (TRs) are also seen (Xu et al., 2010). Those protofibrils seem to be wound around one another exposing a crossover repeat of~80 nm, a maximal width of ~22 nm, and a narrow waist of ~12 nm. The twisted appearance is variable as follows: ~10% of Tau fibrils are straight filaments (Wegmann et al., 2010). Additional morphologic variants of Tau fibrils have been observed in other Tauopathies

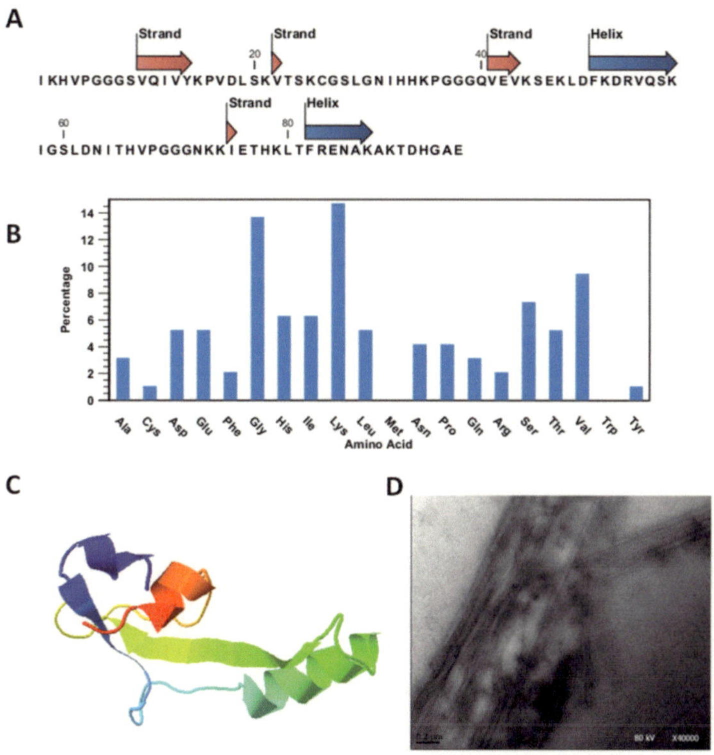

Fig. 4. Characteristics of PHF-core. (A) Structure diagram and amino acid sequence of PHF core (Tau441). Although Tau presents a secondary random coil structure, the R2 and R3 of MTBD showed a motif with regional trend to β-sheet structure. (B) Amino acid distribution histogram of PHF core; they are partially hydrophobic; (C) Proposed core structure based on predicted β-strand propensities (Displayed in Jmol). (D) Electron Microscopy photograph of Tau aggregates induced by the presence of the PHF core.

such as progressive supranuclear palsy (PSP), corticobasal degeneration (CBD), Pick's disease, and FTDP-17 syndromes. It seems that in these pathologies the crossover repeat is ~160 nm. Likewise, Tau fibrils reassembled *in vitro* can display a variable twist between filaments assembled from different variants of Tau proteins (e.g. different splicing variants) or even within a given filament (Wegmann et al., 2010). In the cellular environment protein expression, protein folding, and protein degradation are highly regulated processes. Protein over-expression can lead to protein aggregation, which also is a regulated process. The molecular machines, from the microtubular transport system which assists protein folding and prevents aggregation, to the ubiquitin proteasome system and autophagic vacuoles, which degrade normal and aggregated proteins all work in concert. In a healthy cell they can maintain the equilibrium between synthesis, folding, function and degradation (Zerovnik, 2010). Recent evidence suggests that proteins that are able to constrain the structural freedom of Tau are essential for Tau processing and participate in its accumulation. Interactions of Tau with a specific family of proteins termed *cis-trans* peptidyl-prolyl isomerases (PPIases) has already revealed the importance of this protein family to regulate Tau phosphorylation cycles and its overall stability (Koren et al., 2011). Pin-1 is demostrated to interact with Tau through Thr231-P, promoting a conformational change that allows the action of phospatase PP2A over Tau (Bulbarelli et al., 2009). Recent findings suggest that FKBP51 has a similar activity to Pin1; however, unlike Pin1, FKBP51 coordinates with Hsp90 to isomerize Tau. It also cooperates with distinct protein phosphatases that may also be novel participants in Tau biology. Recently is also suggested the participation of another isomerases like cyclophilin family, but is under research (Koren et al., 2011). In this matter chaperones, specially Hsp90, also can be necessary to maintain Tau in a non-aggregated state, a consequence that may ultimately be deleterious for the brain under pathological conditions (Koren et al., 2009).

The phenomena are not stopped there. The accumulation and propagation of amyloidogenic proteins like Tau are believed to occur through nucleation-dependent polymerization and propagate in an extracellular manner. Tau may be released to the extracellular space upon neuron degeneration, where it could be toxic to other neurons (Ávila, 2010; Gómez-Ramos et al., 2006). This suggests that high molecular weight protein aggregates or amyloid seeds shed from one cell may easily be propagated to others (e.g. neurons or glial cells) under pathological conditions (e.g. alteration in membrane permeability due to aging or virus infection, impairment of membrane function as a result of physical interaction or abnormal membrane depolarization) that favor intracellular deposition of protein fibrils (Nonaka et al., 2010). Further investigation about this must be done. Until now, there is still an incomplete understanding of the sequence of events leading to Tau fibrillization, and it is unclear how the different structural variants of Tau fibrils arise or if these variants (PHFs, SFs, TRs) are interconvertible (Xu et al., 2010). And as a recent issue, the importance of extracellular misfolded Tau during aggregation issues and cellular components such as plasma membrane or mislocalization (Campos-Peña et al., 2009; Lira-De León, 2009), need more investigations. With this last purpose, in cell-models we noticed the enrichment of β-sheet structures in cells expressing PHF-core with a signal promoting the localization of it into Plasma membrane associated to presence of 441-Tau (Campos-Peña et al., 2009). Further investigation in this aim needs complementary studies.

4. Conclusion

Structural studies of amyloidogenic fibrils are crucial. The insolubility and stability of fibrils makes difficult to work with by conventional methods. The research has concentrated on the use of peptides for structural studies, but the information obtained is complex for the different conditions used in the assembly of amyloidogenic fibrils in Tau or AB proteins. There is a minimum sequence with amino acids partially hidrofobic that trend to form a β-sheet structure, this region nucleating amyloidogenic fibril formation and is extremely insoluble.

Analysis of the amyloidogenic regions showed a high occurrence of the aromatic residues phenylalanine and tyrosine, which have a high propensity to stack the delocalized π-electron rings. Studies with short peptides have confirmed that even two consecutive phenylalanine residues are sufficient to facilitate assembly into nanotube-like structures. Protofibrils have been identified which appear to be fibrillar precursors to amyloidogenic fibril formation, and these are preceded by the appearance of small oligomers of Tau and AB. Whether these small intermediates interact directly to form protofibrils and then these elongate to form the fully formed fibril (figure 5). This process can be favored by interaction with membranes rich in negative charged surface, whereas the hydrophobic interior strengthens electrostatic secondary interactions and favors monomer recruitment with increase of local concentration, resulting in aggregate nucleation and membrane disassembly. Developing techniques for directly visualizing amyloidogenic fibrils at high resolution is promising solution to answer many key questions remain to be addressed. Elucidating these questions will undoubtedly reveal novel insights into diseases pathogenesis.

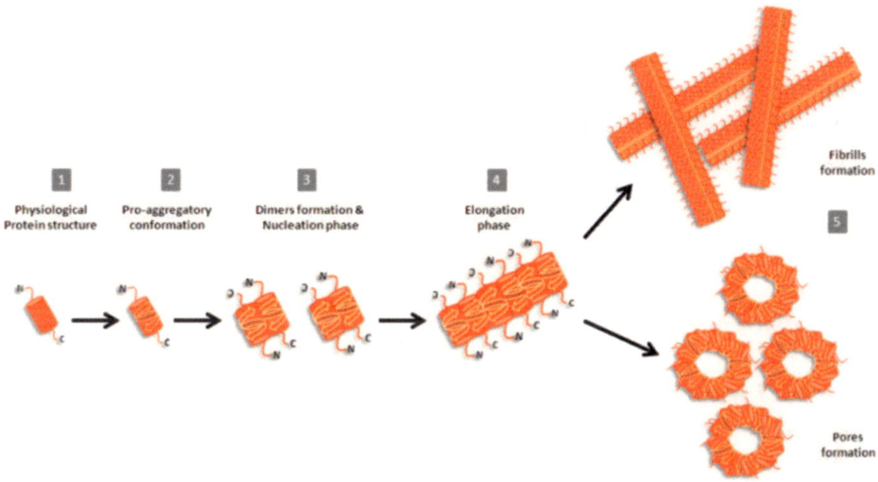

Fig. 5. Common fibrillization pathway of amyloid-β and Tau protein. Under physiological conditions, both proteins adopt a basal conformation (1), but when this is altered, they can adopt a pro-aggregatory conformation (enriched in β-sheet structures). This abnormal conformation (2) allows the formation of dimers and the beginning of a nucleation phase (3). Continuous recruitment of pro-aggregatory forms lead to an elongation phase (4); which finally ends in the formations of fibrills or pores (5).

5. Acknowledgment

To Carmen Silva-Lucero, MSc. for the assistant of this writing. Financials support by CONACyT- México to MD-H and KL-D grants.

6. References

Andreadis, A. (2005). Tau gene alternative splicing: expression patterns, regulation and modulation of function in normal brain and neurodegenerative diseases. Biochim Biophys Acta 1739(2-3): 91-103.

Andreadis, A. (2011). Tau splicing and the intricacies of dementia. J Cell Physiol. May 20. doi: 10.1002/jcp.22842. [Epub ahead of print]

Andreadis, A., Wagner, B. K., Broderick, J. A. & Kosik, K. S. (1996). A tau promoter region without neuronal specificity. J Neurochem 66(6): 2257-2263.

Antzutkin, O. N., Leapman, R. D., Balbach, J. J. & Tycko, R. (2002). Supramolecular structural constraints on Alzheimer's beta-amyloid fibrils from electron microscopy and solid-state nuclear magnetic resonance. Biochemistry 41(51): 15436-15450.

Ávila, J. (2010). Intracellular and extracellular tau. Front Neurosci 4: 49.

Ávila, J., Lim, F., Moreno, F., Belmonte, C. & Cuello, A. C. (2002). Tau function and dysfunction in neurons: its role in neurodegenerative disorders. Mol Neurobiol 25(3): 213-231.

Ávila, J., Lucas, J. J., Pérez, M. & Hernández, F. (2004). Role of tau protein in both physiological and pathological conditions. Physiol Rev 84(2): 361-384.

Barghorn, S. & Mandelkow, E. (2002). Toward a unified scheme for the aggregation of tau into Alzheimer paired helical filaments. Biochemistry 41(50): 14885-14896.

Bemporad, F., Calloni, G., Campioni, S., Plakoutsi, G., Taddei, N. & Chiti, F. (2006). Sequence and structural determinants of amyloid fibril formation. Accounts of chemical research 39(9): 620-627.

Berriman, J., Serpell, L. C., Oberg, K. A., Fink, A. L., Goedert, M. & Crowther, R. A. (2003). Tau filaments from human brain and from in vitro assembly of recombinant protein show cross-beta structure. Proc Natl Acad Sci U S A 100(15): 9034-9038.

Berthomieu, C. & Hienerwadel, R. (2009). Fourier transform infrared (FTIR) spectroscopy. Photosynthesis research 101(2-3): 157-170.

Binder, L. I., Guillozet-Bongaarts, A. L., García-Sierra, F. & Berry, R. W. (2005). Tau, tangles, and Alzheimer's disease. Biochim Biophys Acta 1739(2-3): 216-223.

Bowerman, C. J., Liyanage, W., Federation, A. J. & Nilsson, B. L. (2011). Tuning beta-sheet peptide self-assembly and hydrogelation behavior by modification of sequence hydrophobicity and aromaticity. Biomacromolecules 12(7): 2735-2745.

Braak, H. & Braak, E. (1991). Neuropathological stageing of Alzheimer-related changes. Acta Neuropathol 82(4): 239-259.

Buee, L., Bussiere, T., Buee-Scherrer, V., Delacourte, A. & Hof, P. R. (2000). Tau protein isoforms, phosphorylation and role in neurodegenerative disorders. Brain Res Brain Res Rev 33(1): 95-130.

Bulbarelli, A., Lonati, E., Cazzaniga, E., Gregori, M. & Masserini, M. (2009). Pin1 affects Tau phosphorylation in response to Abeta oligomers. Mol Cell Neurosci 42(1): 75-80.

Campos-Peña, V., Tapia-Ramírez, J., Sanchez-Torres, C. & Meraz-Ríos, M. A. (2009). Pathological-like assembly of tau induced by a paired helical filament core expressed at the plasma membrane. J Alzheimers Dis 18(4): 919-933.

Carter, D. B. & Chou, K. C. (1998). A model for structure-dependent binding of Congo red to Alzheimer beta-amyloid fibrils. Neurobiol Aging 19(1): 37-40.

Congdon, E. E., Kim, S., Bonchak, J., Songrug, T., Matzavinos, A. & Kuret, J. (2008). Nucleation-dependent tau filament formation: the importance of dimerization and an estimation of elementary rate constants. J Biol Chem 283(20): 13806-13816.

Coulson, E. J., Paliga, K., Beyreuther, K. & Masters, C. L. (2000). What the evolution of the amyloid protein precursor supergene family tells us about its function. Neurochem Int 36(3): 175-184.

Chang, E., Kim, S., Schafer, K. N. & Kuret, J. (2011). Pseudophosphorylation of tau protein directly modulates its aggregation kinetics. Biochim Biophys Acta 1814(2): 388-395.

Chaudhary, N., Singh, S. & Nagaraj, R. (2009). Morphology of self-assembled structures formed by short peptides from the amyloidogenic protein tau depends on the solvent in which the peptides are dissolved. J Pept Sci 15(10): 675-684.

Chen, B., Thurber, K. R., Shewmaker, F., Wickner, R. B. & Tycko, R. (2009). Measurement of amyloid fibril mass-per-length by tilted-beam transmission electron microscopy. Proc Natl Acad Sci U S A 106(34): 14339-14344.

Chow, V. W., Mattson, M. P., Wong, P. C. & Gleichmann, M. (2010). An overview of APP processing enzymes and products. Neuromolecular medicine 12(1): 1-12.

De Strooper, B. (2010). Proteases and proteolysis in Alzheimer disease: a multifactorial view on the disease process. Physiol Rev 90(2): 465-494.

Duyckaerts, C., Delatour, B. & Potier, M. C. (2009). Classification and basic pathology of Alzheimer disease. Acta Neuropathol 118(1): 5-36.

Eckermann, K., Mocanu, M. M., Khlistunova, I., Biernat, J., Nissen, A., Hofmann, A., Schonig, K., Bujard, H., Haemisch, A., Mandelkow, E., Zhou, L., Rune, G. & Mandelkow, E. M. (2007). The beta-propensity of Tau determines aggregation and synaptic loss in inducible mouse models of tauopathy. J Biol Chem 282(43): 31755-31765.

Estus, S., Golde, T. E., Kunishita, T., Blades, D., Lowery, D., Eisen, M., Usiak, M., Qu, X. M., Tabira, T., Greenberg, B. D. & et al. (1992). Potentially amyloidogenic, carboxyl-terminal derivatives of the amyloid protein precursor. Science 255(5045): 726-728.

Fandrich, M., Schmidt, M. & Grigorieff, N. (2011). Recent progress in understanding Alzheimer's beta-amyloid structures. Trends in biochemical sciences 36(6): 338-345.

Fischer, D., Mukrasch, M. D., Biernat, J., Bibow, S., Blackledge, M., Griesinger, C., Mandelkow, E. & Zweckstetter, M. (2009). Conformational changes specific for pseudophosphorylation at serine 262 selectively impair binding of tau to microtubules. Biochemistry 48(42): 10047-10055.

Fraser, P. E., Nguyen, J. T., Inouye, H., Surewicz, W. K., Selkoe, D. J., Podlisny, M. B. & Kirschner, D. A. (1992). Fibril formation by primate, rodent, and Dutch-hemorrhagic analogues of Alzheimer amyloid beta-protein. Biochemistry 31(44): 10716-10723.

Friedhoff, P., von Bergen, M., Mandelkow, E. M. & Mandelkow, E. (2000). Structure of tau protein and assembly into paired helical filaments. Biochim Biophys Acta 1502(1): 122-132.

García-Sierra, F., Ghoshal, N., Quinn, B., Berry, R. W. & Binder, L. I. (2003). Conformational changes and truncation of tau protein during tangle evolution in Alzheimer's disease. J Alzheimers Dis 5(2): 65-77.

García-Sierra, F., Mondragon-Rodriguez, S. & Basurto-Islas, G. (2008). Truncation of tau protein and its pathological significance in Alzheimer's disease. J Alzheimers Dis 14(4): 401-409.

García-Sierra, F., Wischik, C. M., Harrington, C. R., Luna-Muñoz, J. & Mena, R. (2001). Accumulation of C-terminally truncated tau protein associated with vulnerability of the perforant pathway in early stages of neurofibrillary pathology in Alzheimer's disease. J Chem Neuroanat 22(1-2): 65-77.

Ghoshal, N., García-Sierra, F., Wuu, J., Leurgans, S., Bennett, D. A., Berry, R. W. & Binder, L. I. (2002). Tau conformational changes correspond to impairments of episodic memory in mild cognitive impairment and Alzheimer's disease. Exp Neurol 177(2): 475-493.

Glenner, G. G., Eanes, E. D. & Page, D. L. (1972). The relation of the properties of Congo red-stained amyloid fibrils to the -conformation. J Histochem Cytochem 20(10): 821-826.

Goedert, M. & Spillantini, M. G. (2011). Pathogenesis of the Tauopathies. J Mol Neurosci. Jul 23. [Epub ahead of print]

Golde, T. E., Estus, S., Usiak, M., Younkin, L. H. & Younkin, S. G. (1990). Expression of beta amyloid protein precursor mRNAs: recognition of a novel alternatively spliced form and quantitation in Alzheimer's disease using PCR. Neuron 4(2): 253-267.

Gómez-Ramos, A., Diaz-Hernández, M., Cuadros, R., Hernández, F. & Ávila, J. (2006). Extracellular tau is toxic to neuronal cells. FEBS Lett 580(20): 4842-4850.

Goode, B. L., Chau, M., Denis, P. E. & Feinstein, S. C. (2000). Structural and functional differences between 3-repeat and 4-repeat tau isoforms. Implications for normal tau function and the onset of neurodegenetative disease. J Biol Chem 275(49): 38182-38189.

Goux, W. J. (2002). The conformations of filamentous and soluble tau associated with Alzheimer paired helical filaments. Biochemistry 41(46): 13798-13806.

Greenwald, J. & Riek, R. (2010). Biology of amyloid: structure, function, and regulation. Structure 18(10): 1244-1260.

Halverson, K., Fraser, P. E., Kirschner, D. A. & Lansbury, P. T., Jr. (1990). Molecular determinants of amyloid deposition in Alzheimer's disease: conformational studies of synthetic beta-protein fragments. Biochemistry 29(11): 2639-2644.

Hampel, H., Blennow, K., Shaw, L. M., Hoessler, Y. C., Zetterberg, H. & Trojanowski, J. Q. (2010). Total and phosphorylated tau protein as biological markers of Alzheimer's disease. Exp Gerontol 45(1): 30-40.

Harrison, R. S., Sharpe, P. C., Singh, Y. & Fairlie, D. P. (2007). Amyloid peptides and proteins in review. Reviews of physiology, biochemistry and pharmacology 159: 1-77.

Hirokawa, N., Shiomura, Y. & Okabe, S. (1988). Tau proteins: the molecular structure and mode of binding on microtubules. J Cell Biol 107(4): 1449-1459.

Horowitz, P. M., LaPointe, N., Guillozet-Bongaarts, A. L., Berry, R. W. & Binder, L. I. (2006). N-terminal fragments of tau inhibit full-length tau polymerization in vitro. Biochemistry 45(42): 12859-12866.

Hung, A. Y., Koo, E. H., Haass, C. & Selkoe, D. J. (1992). Increased expression of beta-amyloid precursor protein during neuronal differentiation is not accompanied by secretory cleavage. Proc Natl Acad Sci U S A 89(20): 9439-9443.

Hwang, S. C., Jhon, D. Y., Bae, Y. S., Kim, J. H. & Rhee, S. G. (1996). Activation of phospholipase C-gamma by the concerted action of tau proteins and arachidonic acid. J Biol Chem 271(31): 18342-18349.

Hyman, B. T., Augustinack, J. C. & Ingelsson, M. (2005). Transcriptional and conformational changes of the tau molecule in Alzheimer's disease. Biochim Biophys Acta 1739(2-3): 150-157.

Jeganathan, S., Hascher, A., Chinnathambi, S., Biernat, J., Mandelkow, E. M. & Mandelkow, E. (2008a). Proline-directed pseudo-phosphorylation at AT8 and PHF1 epitopes induces a compaction of the paperclip folding of Tau and generates a pathological (MC-1) conformation. J Biol Chem 283(46): 32066-32076.

Jeganathan, S., von Bergen, M., Mandelkow, E. M. & Mandelkow, E. (2008b). The natively unfolded character of tau and its aggregation to Alzheimer-like paired helical filaments. Biochemistry 47(40): 10526-10539.

Jenkins, J. & Pickersgill, R. (2001). The architecture of parallel beta-helices and related folds. Progress in biophysics and molecular biology 77(2): 111-175.

Jenkins, S. M. & Johnson, G. V. (1998). Tau complexes with phospholipase C-gamma in situ. Neuroreport 9(1): 67-71.

Jicha, G. A., Bowser, R., Kazam, I. G. & Davies, P. (1997). Alz-50 and MC-1, a new monoclonal antibody raised to paired helical filaments, recognize conformational epitopes on recombinant tau. J Neurosci Res 48(2): 128-132.

Johnson, G. V. & Stoothoff, W. H. (2004). Tau phosphorylation in neuronal cell function and dysfunction. J Cell Sci 117(Pt 24): 5721-5729.

Kamenetz, F., Tomita, T., Hsieh, H., Seabrook, G., Borchelt, D., Iwatsubo, T., Sisodia, S. & Malinow, R. (2003). APP processing and synaptic function. Neuron 37(6): 925-937.

Kang, J., Lemaire, H. G., Unterbeck, A., Salbaum, J. M., Masters, C. L., Grzeschik, K. H., Multhaup, G., Beyreuther, K. & Muller-Hill, B. (1987). The precursor of Alzheimer's disease amyloid A4 protein resembles a cell-surface receptor. Nature 325(6106): 733-736.

Klein, W. L., Krafft, G. A. & Finch, C. E. (2001). Targeting small Abeta oligomers: the solution to an Alzheimer's disease conundrum? Trends in neurosciences 24(4): 219-224.

Konig, G., Monning, U., Czech, C., Prior, R., Banati, R., Schreiter-Gasser, U., Bauer, J., Masters, C. L. & Beyreuther, K. (1992). Identification and differential expression of a novel alternative splice isoform of the beta A4 amyloid precursor protein (APP) mRNA in leukocytes and brain microglial cells. J Biol Chem 267(15): 10804-10809.

Koren, J., 3rd, Jinwal, U. K., Davey, Z., Kiray, J., Arulselvam, K. & Dickey, C. A. (2011). Bending tau into shape: the emerging role of peptidyl-prolyl isomerases in tauopathies. Mol Neurobiol 44(1): 65-70.

Koren, J., 3rd, Jinwal, U. K., Lee, D. C., Jones, J. R., Shults, C. L., Johnson, A. G., Anderson, L. J. & Dickey, C. A. (2009). Chaperone signalling complexes in Alzheimer's disease. J Cell Mol Med 13(4): 619-630.

LaPointe, N. E., Morfini, G., Pigino, G., Gaisina, I. N., Kozikowski, A. P., Binder, L. I. & Brady, S. T. (2009). The amino terminus of tau inhibits kinesin-dependent axonal transport: implications for filament toxicity. J Neurosci Res 87(2): 440-451.

Lee, G. (2005). Tau and src family tyrosine kinases. Biochim Biophys Acta 1739(2-3): 323-330.

Lee, G., Newman, S. T., Gard, D. L., Band, H. & Panchamoorthy, G. (1998). Tau interacts with src-family non-receptor tyrosine kinases. J Cell Sci 111 (Pt 21): 3167-3177.

Leyssen, M., Ayaz, D., Hebert, S. S., Reeve, S., De Strooper, B. & Hassan, B. A. (2005). Amyloid precursor protein promotes post-developmental neurite arborization in the Drosophila brain. EMBO J 24(16): 2944-2955.

Lin, Y. T., Cheng, J. T., Liang, L. C., Ko, C. Y., Lo, Y. K. & Lu, P. J. (2007). The binding and phosphorylation of Thr231 is critical for Tau's hyperphosphorylation and functional regulation by glycogen synthase kinase 3beta. J Neurochem 103(2): 802-813.

Lira-De León, K. I., De Anda-Hernández, M.A., Campos-Peña, V. and Meraz-Ríos, MA. (2009). Plasma membrane-associated PHF-core could be the trigger for Tau aggregation in Alzheimer's Disease.in *Current Hypotheses and Research Milestones in Alzheimer's Disease*. Maccioni, R. & Perry, G. Springer New York. ISBN: 978-0-387-87994-9, 93-100

Lu, M. & Kosik, K. S. (2001). Competition for microtubule-binding with dual expression of tau missense and splice isoforms. Mol Biol Cell 12(1): 171-184.

Luna-Muñoz, J., Chávez-Macias, L., García-Sierra, F. & Mena, R. (2007). Earliest stages of tau conformational changes are related to the appearance of a sequence of specific phospho-dependent tau epitopes in Alzheimer's disease. J Alzheimers Dis 12(4): 365-375.

Luna-Muñoz, J., García-Sierra, F., Falcon, V., Menendez, I., Chávez-Macias, L. & Mena, R. (2005). Regional conformational change involving phosphorylation of tau protein at the Thr231, precedes the structural change detected by Alz-50 antibody in Alzheimer's disease. J Alzheimers Dis 8(1): 29-41.

Luna-Muñoz, J., Peralta-Ramírez, J., Chávez-Macias, L., Harrington, C. R., Wischik, C. M. & Mena, R. (2008). Thiazin red as a neuropathological tool for the rapid diagnosis of Alzheimer's disease in tissue imprints. Acta Neuropathol 116(5): 507-515.

Luo, M. H., Tse, S. W., Memmott, J. & Andreadis, A. (2004). Novel isoforms of tau that lack the microtubule-binding domain. J Neurochem 90(2): 340-351.

Makin, O. S., Atkins, E., Sikorski, P., Johansson, J. & Serpell, L. C. (2005). Molecular basis for amyloid fibril formation and stability. Proc Natl Acad Sci U S A 102(2): 315-320.

Mandelkow, E., von Bergen, M., Biernat, J. & Mandelkow, E. M. (2007). Structural principles of tau and the paired helical filaments of Alzheimer's disease. Brain Pathol 17(1): 83-90.

Marshall, K. E., Morris, K. L., Charlton, D., O'Reilly, N., Lewis, L., Walden, H. & Serpell, L. C. (2011). Hydrophobic, aromatic, and electrostatic interactions play a central role in amyloid fibril formation and stability. Biochemistry 50(12): 2061-2071.

Martin, L., Latypova, X. & Terro, F. (2011). Post-translational modifications of tau protein: implications for Alzheimer's disease. Neurochem Int 58(4): 458-471.

Matsuzaki, K., Kato, K. & Yanagisawa, K. (2010). Abeta polymerization through interaction with membrane gangliosides. Biochim Biophys Acta 1801(8): 868-877.

Matthes, D., Gapsys, V., Daebel, V. & de Groot, B. L. (2011). Mapping the conformational dynamics and pathways of spontaneous steric zipper Peptide oligomerization. PLoS One 6(5): e19129.

Meraz-Ríos, M. A., Lira-De León, K. I., Campos-Peña, V., De Anda-Hernández, M. A. & Mena-López, R. (2010). Tau oligomers and aggregation in Alzheimer's disease. J Neurochem 112(6): 1353-1367.

Miklossy, J. (2011). Emerging roles of pathogens in Alzheimer disease. Expert Rev Mol Med 13: e30.

Mizuno, N., Baxa, U. & Steven, A. C. (2011). Structural dependence of HET-s amyloid fibril infectivity assessed by cryoelectron microscopy. Proc Natl Acad Sci U S A 108(8): 3252-3257.

Mondragon-Rodriguez, S., Mena, R., Binder, L. I., Smith, M. A., Perry, G. & García-Sierra, F. (2008). Conformational changes and cleavage of tau in Pick bodies parallel the early processing of tau found in Alzheimer pathology. Neuropathol Appl Neurobiol 34(1): 62-75.

Muresan, Z. & Muresan, V. (2005). Coordinated transport of phosphorylated amyloid-beta precursor protein and c-Jun NH2-terminal kinase-interacting protein-1. J Cell Biol 171(4): 615-625.

Murray, M. M., Bernstein, S. L., Nyugen, V., Condron, M. M., Teplow, D. B. & Bowers, M. T. (2009). Amyloid beta protein: Abeta40 inhibits Abeta42 oligomerization. Journal of the American Chemical Society 131(18): 6316-6317.

Mylonas, E., Hascher, A., Bernado, P., Blackledge, M., Mandelkow, E. & Svergun, D. I. (2008). Domain conformation of tau protein studied by solution small-angle X-ray scattering. Biochemistry 47(39): 10345-10353.

Nelson, R., Sawaya, M. R., Balbirnie, M., Madsen, A. O., Riekel, C., Grothe, R. & Eisenberg, D. (2005). Structure of the cross-beta spine of amyloid-like fibrils. Nature 435(7043): 773-778.

Nerelius, C., Fitzen, M. & Johansson, J. (2010). Amino acid sequence determinants and molecular chaperones in amyloid fibril formation. Biochemical and biophysical research communications 396(1): 2-6.

Neve, R. L., Boyce, F. M., McPhie, D. L., Greenan, J. & Oster-Granite, M. L. (1996). Transgenic mice expressing APP-C100 in the brain. Neurobiol Aging 17(2): 191-203.

Nogalska, A., D'Agostino, C., Engel, W. K. & Askanas, V. (2011). Novel demonstration of conformationally modified tau in sporadic inclusion-body myositis muscle fibers. Neurosci Lett.

Nonaka, T., Watanabe, S. T., Iwatsubo, T. & Hasegawa, M. (2010). Seeded aggregation and toxicity of {alpha}-synuclein and tau: cellular models of neurodegenerative diseases. J Biol Chem 285(45): 34885-34898.

Perutz, M. F., Finch, J. T., Berriman, J. & Lesk, A. (2002). Amyloid fibers are water-filled nanotubes. Proc Natl Acad Sci U S A 99(8): 5591-5595.

Plant, L. D., Boyle, J. P., Smith, I. F., Peers, C. & Pearson, H. A. (2003). The production of amyloid beta peptide is a critical requirement for the viability of central neurons. J Neurosci 23(13): 5531-5535.

Puzzo, D., Privitera, L., Leznik, E., Fa, M., Staniszewski, A., Palmeri, A. & Arancio, O. (2008). Picomolar amyloid-beta positively modulates synaptic plasticity and memory in hippocampus. J Neurosci 28(53): 14537-14545.

Ranjbar, B. & Gill, P. (2009). Circular dichroism techniques: biomolecular and nanostructural analyses- a review. Chemical biology & drug design 74(2): 101-120.

Sadqi, M., Hernández, F., Pan, U., Pérez, M., Schaeberle, M. D., Ávila, J. & Muñoz, V. (2002). Alpha-helix structure in Alzheimer's disease aggregates of tau-protein. Biochemistry 41(22): 7150-7155.

Scales, T. M., Derkinderen, P., Leung, K. Y., Byers, H. L., Ward, M. A., Price, C., Bird, I. N., Perera, T., Kellie, S., Williamson, R., Anderton, B. H. & Reynolds, C. H. (2011). Tyrosine phosphorylation of tau by the SRC family kinases lck and fyn. Mol Neurodegener 6: 12.

Schubert, D., Behl, C., Lesley, R., Brack, A., Dargusch, R., Sagara, Y. & Kimura, H. (1995). Amyloid peptides are toxic via a common oxidative mechanism. Proc Natl Acad Sci U S A 92(6): 1989-1993.

Selkoe, D. J. (1994). Alzheimer's disease: a central role for amyloid. J Neuropathol Exp Neurol 53(5): 438-447.

Serpell, L. C., Blake, C. C. & Fraser, P. E. (2000). Molecular structure of a fibrillar Alzheimer's A beta fragment. Biochemistry 39(43): 13269-13275.

Sevcik, J., Skrabana, R., Dvorsky, R., Csokova, N., Iqbal, K. & Novak, M. (2007). X-ray structure of the PHF core C-terminus: insight into the folding of the intrinsically disordered protein tau in Alzheimer's disease. FEBS Lett 581(30): 5872-5878.

Shirahama, T. & Cohen, A. S. (1965). Structure of amyloid fibrils after negative staining and high-resolution electron microscopy. Nature 206(985): 737-738.

Shkumatov, A. V., Chinnathambi, S., Mandelkow, E. & Svergun, D. I. (2011). Structural memory of natively unfolded tau protein detected by small-angle X-ray scattering. Proteins 79(7): 2122-2131.

Sillen, A., Barbier, P., Landrieu, I., Lefebvre, S., Wieruszeski, J. M., Leroy, A., Peyrot, V. & Lippens, G. (2007). NMR investigation of the interaction between the neuronal protein tau and the microtubules. Biochemistry 46(11): 3055-3064.

Skrabana, R., Dvorsky, R., Sevcik, J. & Novak, M. (2010). Monoclonal antibody MN423 as a stable mold facilitates structure determination of disordered tau protein. J Struct Biol.

Skrabana, R., Kontsek, P., Mederlyova, A., Iqbal, K. & Novak, M. (2004). Folding of Alzheimer's core PHF subunit revealed by monoclonal antibody 423. FEBS Lett 568(1-3): 178-182.

Small, D. H., Clarris, H. L., Williamson, T. G., Reed, G., Key, B., Mok, S. S., Beyreuther, K., Masters, C. L. & Nurcombe, V. (1999). Neurite-outgrowth regulating functions of the amyloid protein precursor of Alzheimer's disease. J Alzheimers Dis 1(4-5): 275-285.

Small, D. H., Mok, S. S. & Bornstein, J. C. (2001). Alzheimer's disease and Abeta toxicity: from top to bottom. Nat Rev Neurosci 2(8): 595-598.

Solomon, B. & Frenkel, D. (2010). Immunotherapy for Alzheimer's disease. Neuropharmacology 59(4-5): 303-309.

Stefani, M. & Dobson, C. M. (2003). Protein aggregation and aggregate toxicity: new insights into protein folding, misfolding diseases and biological evolution. Journal of molecular medicine 81(11): 678-699.

Takuma, H., Arawaka, S. & Mori, H. (2003). Isoforms changes of tau protein during development in various species. Brain Res Dev Brain Res 142(2): 121-127.

Toyama, B. H. & Weissman, J. S. (2011). Amyloid structure: conformational diversity and consequences. Annual review of biochemistry 80: 557-585.

Trinczek, B., Biernat, J., Baumann, K., Mandelkow, E. M. & Mandelkow, E. (1995). Domains of tau protein, differential phosphorylation, and dynamic instability of microtubules. Mol Biol Cell 6(12): 1887-1902.

Tycko, R. (2011). Solid-state NMR studies of amyloid fibril structure. Annual review of physical chemistry 62: 279-299.

Vabulas, R. M., Raychaudhuri, S., Hayer-Hartl, M. & Hartl, F. U. (2010). Protein folding in the cytoplasm and the heat shock response. Cold Spring Harb Perspect Biol 2(12): a004390.

von Bergen, M., Friedhoff, P., Biernat, J., Heberle, J., Mandelkow, E. M. & Mandelkow, E. (2000). Assembly of tau protein into Alzheimer paired helical filaments depends on a local sequence motif ((306)VQIVYK(311)) forming beta structure. Proc Natl Acad Sci U S A 97(10): 5129-5134.

Wang, J. Z. & Liu, F. (2008). Microtubule-associated protein tau in development, degeneration and protection of neurons. Prog Neurobiol 85(2): 148-175.

Wang, Y., Gao, L., Conrad, C. G. & Andreadis, A. (2011). Saitohin, which is nested within the tau gene, interacts with tau and Abl and its human-specific allele influences Abl phosphorylation. J Cell Biochem.

Weaver, C. L., Espinoza, M., Kress, Y. & Davies, P. (2000). Conformational change as one of the earliest alterations of tau in Alzheimer's disease. Neurobiol Aging 21(5): 719-727.

Wegmann, S., Jung, Y. J., Chinnathambi, S., Mandelkow, E. M., Mandelkow, E. & Muller, D. J. (2010). Human Tau isoforms assemble into ribbon-like fibrils that display polymorphic structure and stability. J Biol Chem 285(35): 27302-27313.

Wiltzius, J. J., Landau, M., Nelson, R., Sawaya, M. R., Apostol, M. I., Goldschmidt, L., Soriaga, A. B., Cascio, D., Rajashankar, K. & Eisenberg, D. (2009). Molecular mechanisms for protein-encoded inheritance. Nature structural & molecular biology 16(9): 973-978.

Williamson, R., Usardi, A., Hanger, D. P. & Anderton, B. H. (2008). Membrane-bound beta-amyloid oligomers are recruited into lipid rafts by a fyn-dependent mechanism. The FASEB journal : official publication of the Federation of American Societies for Experimental Biology 22(5): 1552-1559.

Wischik, C. M., Crowther, R. A., Stewart, M. & Roth, M. (1985). Subunit structure of paired helical filaments in Alzheimer's disease. J Cell Biol 100(6): 1905-1912.

Wischik, C. M., Edwards, P. C., Lai, R. Y., Roth, M. & Harrington, C. R. (1996). Selective inhibition of Alzheimer disease-like tau aggregation by phenothiazines. Proc Natl Acad Sci U S A 93(20): 11213-11218.

Xu, S., Brunden, K. R., Trojanowski, J. Q. & Lee, V. M. (2010). Characterization of tau fibrillization in vitro. Alzheimers Dement 6(2): 110-117.

Yoshikai, S., Sasaki, H., Doh-ura, K., Furuya, H. & Sakaki, Y. (1990). Genomic organization of the human amyloid beta-protein precursor gene. Gene 87(2): 257-263.

Zerovnik, E. (2010). Protein conformational pathology in Alzheimer's and other neurodegenerative diseases; new targets for therapy. Curr Alzheimer Res 7(1): 74-83.

Zheng, H. & Koo, E. H. (2006). The amyloid precursor protein: beyond amyloid. Mol Neurodegener 1: 5.

Zheng, H. & Koo, E. H. (2011). Biology and pathophysiology of the amyloid precursor protein. Mol Neurodegener 6(1): 27.

Zilka, N., Filipcik, P., Koson, P., Fialova, L., Skrabana, R., Zilkova, M., Rolkova, G., Kontsekova, E. & Novak, M. (2006). Truncated tau from sporadic Alzheimer's disease suffices to drive neurofibrillary degeneration in vivo. FEBS Lett 580(15): 3582-3588.

Zmuda, J. F. & Rivas, R. J. (2000). Actin disruption alters the localization of tau in the growth cones of cerebellar granule neurons. J Cell Sci 113 (Pt 15): 2797-2809.

16

Alzheimer's Disease: Approaches to Pathogenesis in the Genomic Age

Greg T. Sutherland and Jillian J. Kril
Disciplines of Pathology and Medicine,
Sydney Medical School,
University of Sydney,
Australia

1. Introduction

The prevalence of Alzheimer's disease (AD), the most common form of dementia, is rising rapidly worldwide. A seemingly imminent epidemic is predicted to have wide reaching societal and economic consequences, becoming the leading health issue for many countries by the middle of this century. This epidemic is driven by an ageing world population in combination with a lack of disease modifying treatments or preventive strategies. The popular amyloid cascade hypothesis suggests that AD is precipitated by the dysregulated metabolism of the amyloid precursor protein resulting in the accumulation of the beta-amyloid peptide (Aβ) in the brain. This hypothesis is the basis for most experimental treatments currently in clinical trials. However, not all evidence supports a precipitating role of abnormal Aβ accumulation in the common forms of AD.

The completion of the human genome project in 2001 has ushered in a dramatic increase in the technologies available to biologists and these have been applied to understanding the pathogenesis of complex disorders, like AD. Genome-wide association and expression (transcriptomic) studies are now commonplace creating a more immediate and dynamic, but invariably more complex, research environment.

Transcriptomic studies in particular have the potential to greatly influence our understanding of complex diseases like AD, but to date they have provided quite discordant results. There are a number of potential reasons for this including our incomplete understanding of the complex nature of the human brain at the molecular level. It is now known that the evolutionary advances in our cognitive capacity have largely originated at the level of transcription with substantial increases in both coding and non-coding RNA variants. Until recently transcriptomic platforms only assayed a proportion of the coding RNA species, but with the introduction of next generation sequencing the whole transcriptome, both coding and non-coding, can now be investigated.

In this chapter we undertake a review of the clinical and pathological characteristics of AD before considering the impact of new technologies on AD research and their future role in finding a cure for this important disease.

2. Alzheimer's disease

2.1 Overview

The term dementia encapsulates a number of separate diseases that clinically manifest as a progressive decline in cognitive function. Alzheimer's disease (AD) is the most common form of dementia accounting for approximately 60% of all cases. It is estimated that the current 36 million sufferers worldwide will increase to 115 million by 2050 (Alzheimer's Disease International, 2009). In countries like Australia, dementia will become the number one health cost by the middle of this century exceeding both heart disease and cancer (Access Economics, 2009). These surprising predictions result from the additive effects of an ageing world population, the duration of the disease and the extended period where the patient is totally dependent on caregivers. The societal trend in Western countries towards professional aged care services accounts for the majority of the current and predicted costs.

More importantly, AD is a cruel disease that robs patients of their sense of self and places considerable physical and psychological strain on caregivers, who are often isolated from society themselves. As the currently available treatments only provide transient improvement, an AD epidemic will only be halted with the development of new therapies. It has been predicted that a novel therapeutic agent that delays disease onset and progression by just one year would result in nine million fewer cases by 2050 (Brookmeyer *et al.*, 2007).

The other approach to reducing the worldwide burden of AD is prevention. This would be based on either avoiding identified risk factors or augmenting the impact of protective factors. Unfortunately finding such factors through epidemiological studies has proved extremely difficult to date.

The completion of the human genome project in 2001 ushered in a dramatic increase in the technologies that have subsequently been applied to understanding the pathogenesis of complex disorders, like AD. Genome-wide association and expression studies are now commonplace in AD research creating a more immediate and dynamic research environment. The application of these technologies to clinical, pathological and epidemiological studies of AD is starting to bear fruit although effective treatments are not necessarily close at hand.

2.2 The history of AD

Emil Kraepelin first used the name Alzheimer's disease in 1910 in recognition of Alois Alzheimer (1864-1915), the German psychiatrist and neuropathologist, who had originally described the clinical and pathological features of the disease. Kraepelin was keen to make the distinction between the presenile form of dementia (described by Alzheimer) and the more common senile variant.

Alzheimer's findings were originally published in 1907, in the form of a conference abstract where he described a delusional woman (Auguste D) who had slowly lost her cognitive function and died at 55 years of age (Alzheimer, 1907). According to a later translation of the original manuscript Auguste D suffered from reduced comprehension and memory as well as psychotic symptoms including paranoia that resulted in her psychosocial impairment (Maurer *et al.*, 1997). The first formal description of Auguste D was by Perusini in 1909 in a textbook edited by Nissl and Alzheimer (Perusini, 1909). Alzheimer himself only published a detailed clinical and pathological report in 1911 along with his findings from a second case (Johan F) (Alzheimer, 1911). Interestingly Alzheimer described Auguste D as having both the pathologies that we now know as plaques and tangles in her cerebral cortex but Johan F as having only plaques. Graeber and colleagues re-examined Alzheimer's original sections 90 years later and confirmed the original histopathological findings for Johann F (Graeber *et al.*, 1997) and Auguste D (Graeber *et al.*, 1998). In accordance with Kraepelin's original classification the term Alzheimer's disease or Alzheimer's presenile dementia continued to be exclusively used for a rare disease of mid-life until the 1970's when neuropathologists realised that the more common senile dementia and the type described by Alzheimer were indistinguishable (Terry and Katzman, 1983).

2.3 Prevalence and cost

The mean age at onset of AD is around 75 years of age and the overall prevalence is about 1% in most developed nations. If AD prevalence is divided into different age bands then we see a rapid increase from 1% in the 60-64 year age group to greater than 25% in individuals over 85 years of age (Jorm and Jolley, 1998).

A comprehensive estimate of worldwide prevalence was recently reported with age- and gender-specific prevalence and projections out to 2050 (Alzheimer's Disease International, 2009). This suggested that the current worldwide burden of 35.6 million dementia sufferers would nearly double every 20 years, to 65.7 million in 2030, and 115.4 million in 2050. The authors attributed this increase to population growth and demographic ageing.

Alzheimer's Disease International (ADI) has addressed the current cost of dementia worldwide and predicted its future economic impact (Alzheimer's Disease International, 2010). They suggested that the currents cost of US$604 billion would increase by 85% to US$1000 billion by 2030. They noted considerable disparity between high-income and low-income countries largely due to formal care facilities in the former, rather than direct health costs. Direct health costs amounted to only 16% of the average $32,000 per annum costs in the USA. ADI considered that stigmatisation played a role here where cognitive decline was often the precipitant for institutionalisation as opposed to individuals with severe physical disabilities who are often supported at home by community services.

In terms of care-giving an important indirect effect of AD and dementia that may often be missed in such reports is the physical and psychological toll on the caregivers themselves. It is estimated that a person with dementia requires more than 7 hours of close supervision per day (Wimo *et al.*, 2007). Caregivers are commonly spouses or first-degree relatives, and for long periods of time will be as socially isolated as the patients themselves. They are estimated to experience between a three- and 40-fold increase in their risk of major depression (Cuijpers, 2005). Caregivers who choose to support a dementia patient at home also are likely to suffer a huge financial burden, through lost of income, disability-friendly renovations and the hiring of respite care. These costs are only partially off set by government allowances or pensions in most cases.

2.4 Clinical findings

The term dementia refers to the main clinical manifestation of AD but also occurs with other diseases including frontotemporal dementia (FTD), vascular dementia (VaD) and dementia with Lewy bodies (DLB). Dementia is a progressive decline in cognition that impairs social and/or occupational function. The deficits in a particular individual will reflect the regions in which neuronal loss occurs.

AD sufferers will usually present to a general physician because of their own concern about deteriorating cognition or the concerns of an informant (often their spouse or work colleague). A general physician may refer the patient to a specialist geriatrician or neurologist but many patients remain under the primary care of their general practitioners. The loss of short-term memory is often the earliest cognitive phenotype for AD (Dubois and Albert, 2004).

2.5 Diagnosis

The criteria for a clinical diagnosis of AD were established in 1984 and have remained unchanged for the past 27 years (McKhann *et al.,* 1984). The diagnosis of AD is currently based on clinical examination and neuropsychological testing although a definitive diagnosis can only made by postmortem examination. However, the latter is uncommon outside a research setting. A diagnosis of 'Probable AD' is made when there is worsening memory function, particularly episodic memory, accompanied by deficits in two or more other cognitive domains such as executive function, attention, language or visuospatial skills.

A diagnosis of AD would be supported by a positive family history, a normal electroencephalogram, normal cerebrospinal fluid (CSF) analysis and atrophy on computer-assisted tomography (CAT) imaging (the only neuroimaging modality available in 1984). An alternative diagnosis of 'possible AD' was suggested when there was a general dementia syndrome but with variations in onset and clinical course (McKhann *et al.,* 1984). Exclusion criteria for AD included the rapid onset of dementia, an early prominence of gait abnormalities or a focal neurological deficit.

In 2011, these criteria were updated, prompted by some inconsistent clinical-pathological correlations and a need to incorporate the likely prodromal periods of AD and biomarkers (biological markers) (Jack et al., 2011). The new criteria propose a continuum of impairment but also delineate three stages along this spectrum: preclinical AD, mild cognitive impairment (MCI) and clinical AD. The basis for these stages is that the pathophysiological process of AD can be reliably represented by biomarkers. The existing 'probable' and 'possible' categories are now expanded to (1) Probable AD dementia, (2) Possible AD dementia, and (3) Dementia with evidence of the AD pathophysiological process. An example of the latter would be an individual with a less typical clinical presentation but with AD-like biomarkers on their neuroimaging or CSF analysis (McKhann *et al.,* 2011). However, biomarkers continue to only support a clinical diagnosis of AD while definitive diagnosis still requires a postmortem examination.

The differentiation of AD from MCI rests on the determination of whether or not there is significant interference in the ability to function at work or in usual daily activities (Albert *et al.,* 2011). MCI is not a definite stage on the progression to AD because some individuals will never develop dementia or will develop other forms such as VaD. However, pathological studies suggest that the majority of individuals with MCI have typical AD pathology, but just in a lesser amount to those who become clinically demented (Haroutunian *et al.,* 2009).

The definition of preclinical AD remains a research-only paradigm based on the promise that biomarkers faithfully reflect the underlying pathophysiological processes (Sperling *et al.*, 2011). As will be discussed below this preclinical diagnostic paradigm is firmly based on one, albeit prominent, working hypothesis for AD pathogenesis.

2.6 Clinical heterogeneity

The review of the clinical diagnostic criteria was prompted in part by increasing reports of variations in the classic presentation of AD. It has even been suggested that the term Alzheimer's syndrome is more appropriate than AD (Zellner *et al.*, 2009). In addition to the classic amnestic presentation of AD described above, a "visual variant" of AD, often called posterior cortical atrophy, a "language variant" called logopenic/phonological aphasia (Gorno-Tempini *et al.*, 2011) and a frontal/behavioural variant are occasionally observed (Johnson *et al.*, 1999). The latter two are also considered sub-categories of frontotemporal dementia hinting that there might be considerable overlap in clinicopathological correlates between the current clinical dementia categories. This is supported by a recent study that found AD to be the primary pathological diagnosis in a range of focal cortical syndromes including 50% of corticobasal disease and 44% progressive non-fluent aphasia, another language variant of frontotemoporal dementia (Alladi *et al.*, 2007). This clinical or phenotypic heterogeneity in AD suggests variation in both aetiology and pathogenesis and the potential ramifications of this will be discussed in greater detail below.

2.7 Current treatment options

There are two classes of drugs that are currently used to treat moderate to severe cases of AD. They are the acetylcholinesterases inhibitors (ChEIs) and glutaminergic receptor antagonists. The cholinergic (acetylcholine producing) neurons of the basal forebrain nuclei such as the nucleus basalis of Meynert are among the earliest lost in AD (Cullen and Halliday, 1998). These neurons synapse in the prefrontal cortex and the hippocampus where they release acetylcholine to modulate circuits involved in learning and memory (Gold, 2003).

Acetylcholinesterases are enzymes responsible for the rapid breakdown of acetylcholine in the synaptic cleft. ChEIs are postulated to maximise the residual acetylcholine modulating these memory circuits in the AD brain and there are three types in current use donepezil, rivastigmine and galantamine. Meta-analyses of randomised control trials for the three ChEIs suggest that all show moderate improvements in cognitive function over placebo but the incidence of adverse events is lowest for donepezil (Birks, 2006; Hansen *et al.*, 2008)

The other drug in common use is called memantine, a low affinity glutamate NMDA receptor antagonist. The postulated mechanism of action for memantine is the prevention of glutamate-mediated excitatory neurotoxicity (McShane *et al.*, 2006). As with the ChEIs, meta-analyses report a significant but marginal improvement (Raina *et al.*, 2008) with particular attenuation of behavioural symptoms (Gauthier *et al.*, 2008). Memantine is less efficacious in mild to moderate compared to severe AD (MMSE >15) (McShane *et al.*, 2006; Schneider *et al.*, 2011).

Unfortunately there is no evidence that either of these treatments significantly alters disease progression (Golde *et al.*, 2011). Hence there is enormous research effort aimed at finding alternative treatment strategies, some of which have already reached Phase II and III human clinical trials. These potential treatments are discussed below.

2.8 Neuropathology

As discussed in the section above, a definitive diagnosis of AD can only be made at postmortem examination. Unfortunately the number of autopsies has declined markedly in the last three decades depriving clinicians and researchers alike of an important source of medical knowledge. Neuropathological examinations are now largely restricted to a research environment with the potential issue that clinically confirmed cases are not be representative of the AD spectrum in the greater population.

As with the clinical diagnosis, there are established criteria for the pathological diagnosis of AD (Hyman and Trojanowski, 1997) although these too are currently being revised. Interestingly, although postmortem examination is required for a definitive diagnosis of AD the pathological criteria again, only suggests that AD is 'probable' or 'possible'. In order to understand how these criteria have been derived it is useful to give a brief overview of the characteristic or pathognomonic aspects of AD.

2.8.1 Gross pathology

The gross pathology of the end-stage AD brain is characterised by widespread atrophy due to the extensive neuronal loss. There is narrowing of gyri and widening of sulci with atrophy of the temporal cortices and a disproportionate atrophy of the entorhinal cortex, amygdala and hippocampus in particular. The remaining cortical regions are generally atrophic, but to a lesser extent than the temporal lobe, although there are also regions seemingly spared from neuronal loss such as the inferior frontal cortex (Halliday *et al.*, 2003) (Fig. 1(a-b)).

2.8.2 Plaques and tangles

The neuropathology of AD is characterised by two pathognomonic entities; the intraneuronal neurofibrillary tangle (NFT) and the extracellular plaque. NFTs are chiefly composed of hyperphosphorylated fibrillar forms of a protein called microtubule associated protein tau (MAPT or tau), while plaques are predominantly composed of fibrils of peptides collectively termed beta-amyloid (Aβ) (Fig. 1 (c-d)).

For most individuals, there is a good correlation between spread of NFT pathology from the medial temporal lobe to the association and finally primary cortices, and the probability of dementia (Newell *et al.*, 1999). In comparison the regional distribution of plaques tends to be highly variable between patients (Braak and Braak, 1991). Similarly plaques vary more in their cortical laminar pattern whereas NFTs are found mainly in layers III and V coinciding with the corticocortical projection (pyramidal) neurons (Lewis *et al.*, 1987). Plaques also vary in their structure and are referred to as 'diffuse' (lacking associated inflammatory cells and dystrophic neurites) and 'cored' or 'neuritic' plaques. It is generally considered that diffuse plaques eventually become cored but an alternative explanation suggests that the amyloid of diffuse and cored plaques are derived from blood vesssels and neurons respectively (D'Andrea and Nagele, 2010).

Extracellular Aβ deposition is considered to be the most likely precipitating event in the disease (Hardy and Selkoe, 2002). In comparison, NFT formation is a subsequent but necessary step in neurodegeneration of AD with intracellular tangles becoming 'ghost tangles' when the neuron eventually succumbs and the insoluble tau protein is left behind in the parenchyma. Presumably the brain macrophages find these extracellular tangles too difficult to phagocytose or they are relatively inert.

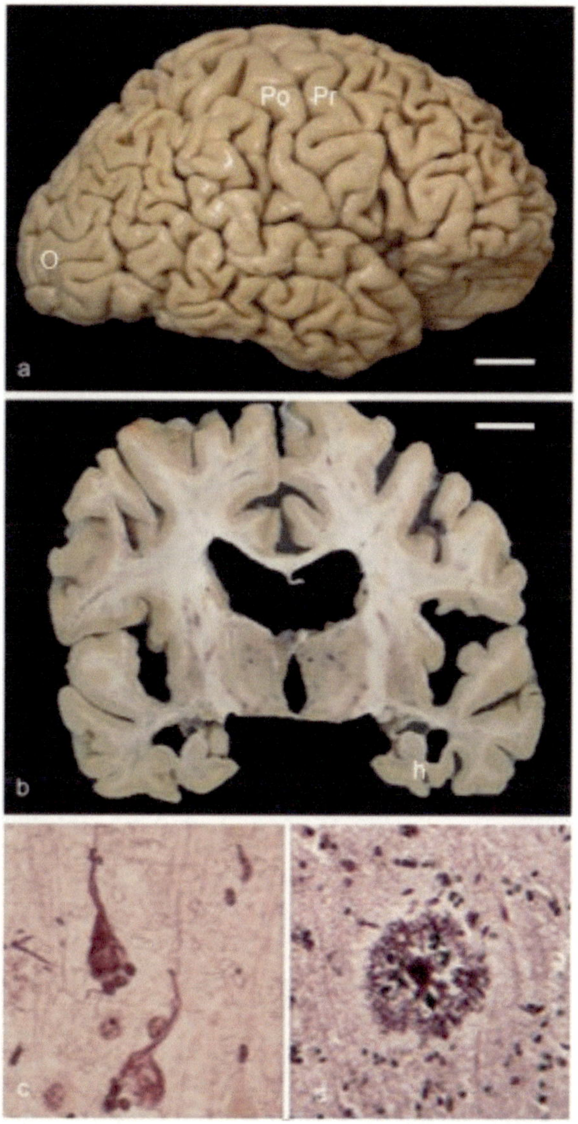

Fig. 1. The neuropathological features of Alzheimer's disease. A series of macro-and microscopic images show the pathological features of Alzheimer's disease (a) A lateral view of the right cerebral hemisphere shows extensive atrophy of the temporal and frontal lobes. There are also regions spared in this case including the precentral (Pr) and and postcentral (Po) gyri and the occipital pole (O), size bar = 2cm (b) A coronal view at the level of the lateral geniculate body demonstrates the severe atrophy in the temporal lobe including the hippocampus (h), along with enlargement of the Sylvian fissure, and third and lateral ventricles, size bar = 2cm (c) A modified Bielschowsky's silver stain shows neurofibrillary tangles in two cortical pyramidal neurons, magnification = 400x and (d) a cored plaque, with its dense amyloid core surrounded by diffuse amyloid, dystrophic neurites and cellular debris, magnification = 200x.

2.8.3 Neuronal loss

The hippocampal CA1 (1st cornus ammonis or Ammon's horn) region experiences the greatest loss of neurons in AD of approximately 70%. The CA1 is anatomically and functional connected to the entorhinal cortex where the earliest development of NFTs and neuronal loss in AD is thought to occur. The locus coeruleus (noradrenalin production), nucleus basalis of Meynert and the Raphe nuclei can also experience losses of greater than 50% as does the majority of the temporal lobe (Kril and Halliday, 2001). The loss of neurons in the nucleus basalis of Meynert is similar to the number of ghost tangles but in the hippocampus (Kril *et al.*, 2002) and entorhinal cortex (Gomez-Isla *et al.*, 1996) neuron loss actually exceeds the number of ghost tangle suggesting other neurodegenerative mechanisms are at work. The spread of pathology and associated neuronal loss in AD dictates the symptomology. The reader will note the early involvement of the hippocampus, a key region in both memory generation and consolidation. Interestingly the eventual spread of AD pathology mirrors the anatomical boundaries of the default network - the "brain system active when individuals are not focused on their external environment" (Buckner *et al.*, 2008). The default network is involves with the process of internal mentation or self-relevant mental simulation. This peculiarly human activity could explain the regional selectivity of neuronal loss in AD while deficits in the network are certainly consistent with the loss of self-awareness in moderate to severe stages of the disease (Buckner *et al.*, 2008).

2.8.4 Chronic inflammation

AD is also characterised by a chronic inflammatory process that is commonly called reactive gliosis. Markers of inflammation such as MHC II expression are higher in demented patients than those in nondemented individuals with AD pathology and may be better correlated with synaptic dysfunction than either plaques or NFTs (Lue *et al.*, 1996). Essentially when we refer to reactive gliosis we mean reactive microgliosis, a hyperplastic and hypertrophic response of the resident macrophages in the brain. There is also astrocyte pathology but this remains less well defined in AD (Beach and McGeer, 1988). The increased expression of the cytosketal protein glial fibrillary acidic protein (GFAP) that characterised 'reactive' astrocytes has been described in AD brains although this was not correlated with either plaques or NFTs (Simpson *et al.*). Microglia are originally derived from the haemopoietic system and migrate to the brain during the early embryological period. Reactive microglia in AD are closely associated with plaques and studies with immunomodulatory therapies suggest that they are relatively effective, at least early in the disease process, at phagocytosing Aβ plaques (Perlmutter *et al.*, 1990; Edison *et al.*, 2008). However neuroinflammation appears to exacerbate AD pathogenesis (Krause and Muller, 2010) and anti-inflammatory medication use is associated with a reduced risk of AD (Vlad *et al.*, 2008). This apparent paradox might be explained by microglia initially serving a protective role but eventually becoming overstimulated and producing excessive reactive oxygen species that lead to neurotoxicity (Innamorato *et al.*, 2009). Nevertheless anti-inflammatory medications do not reduce the progression of AD pathology (Halliday *et al.*, 2000). As microglia are now known to have physiological functions in the brain such the maintenance of synaptic plasticity and it has been suggested that they may be more 'victim' than 'villain' in AD (Graeber and Streit, 2010).

2.8.5 Diagnostic criteria

The current pathological criteria are based on the quantity of both plaques and NFTs (Hyman and Trojanowski, 1997) and incorporate a staging scheme for the neuropathological progression of NFTs ('Braak staging scheme') (Braak and Braak, 1991). The likelihood of AD is high if there are frequent neocortical plaques and NFTs consistent with Braak stage V/VI; is intermediate if plaques are moderate with Braak stage III/VI and low if neocortical plaques are sparse with Braak stage is I/II.

2.9 The ageing brain

One of the reasons that the AD neuropathological diagnostic criteria are a probability scale is the occurrence of both plaques and NFTs, either independently or together, in a proportion of aged subjects without dementia. Diffuse plaques are seen in as many as 30% of all brains examined (Braak and Braak, 1997; Davis *et al.*, 1999). A similar percentage of cognitively normal individuals have tau-positive neuritic pathology (Knopman *et al.*, 2003) although tau pathology confined to the hippocampal formation appears to be seen in most, if not all, aged brains (Troncoso *et al.*, 1996). As discussed above the quantity of AD pathology tends to correlate relatively closely to the level of dementia and many researchers consider that the presence of mild pathology is representative of preclinical AD (Price *et al.*, 2009). Dementia then occurs when the quantity of AD pathology crosses a particular threshold. Two issues with this idea are that some individuals with Aβ will not develop dementia prior to death (incidental AD pathology) and these Aβ clinicopathological correlations tend to breakdown in the oldest old (>90 years of age) (Kril, 2009).

As will be discussed further below, the common occurrence of incidental AD and AD-type pathology in nondemented controls could also be a factor in the small effect sizes and lack of reproducibility seen in AD association studies to date (Sutherland *et al.*, 2011b).

3. The genomic era and its new technologies

The last decade has seen an incredible advance in the biologist's armamentarium for investigating complex diseases. This biological revolution has its roots in the development of molecular biology techniques such as gene cloning using restriction enzymes (Nathans and Smith, 1975), DNA hybridisation (Southern, 1975), Sanger sequencing (Sanger *et al.*, 1977) and the polymerase chain reaction (PCR) (Saiki *et al.*, 1985; Mullis and Faloona, 1987). However, it was human genome project that provided the real impetus.

3.1 The human genome project

The human genome project began in 1989 and was initially headed by the co-founder of DNA's structure and Nobel laureate, James D Watson. He was succeeded by Francis Collins who headed the public sequencing effort while a private consortium (Celera) also undertook the challenge of sequencing the entire (haploid) human genome, an estimated three billion base pairs. The twin consortia announced the completion of the draft human genome in late 2000 (public (Lander *et al.*, 2001) and Celera (Venter *et al.*, 2001)) although a so-called completed version was only announced in 2003. The templates for these human genomes were pooled DNA samples while the entire genome of a single individual was only published in 2007 (Levy *et al.*, 2007). However it is currently estimated that actually only 93% of the human genome has been sequenced with repeat regions within telomeres and centromeres remaining outstanding. The public contribution to the first human genome is estimated to have cost US$3 billion.

It was predicted prior to and during the project that the human genome would contain between 40,000 and 100,000 protein coding genes and this number would greatly exceed other mammals, explaining, in particular, our cognitive uniqueness. However, it now appears that we have only about 20,000 to 25,000 protein-coding genes (1-2% of the entire genome), a figure that is, not only similar to other mammals, but dwarfed by some plant species (International Human Genome Sequencing Consortium, 2004).

In disease research we are particularly interested in the genetic variation between affected and unaffected individuals. As the sequencing of whole genomes for all the individuals in a research cohort remains prohibitively expensive, researchers have had use to methods that can approximate the total genetic variation.

3.2 Genetic variation

In monogenic forms of diseases such as AD, single, rare genetic polymorphisms that we commonly call mutations cause the disease. These mutations generally segregate in families or very rarely originate *de novo* in the germ line of our patient of interest (proband). The former have been, and will continue to be for the next few years at least, discovered by gene linkage studies in multi-generational families.

In contrast most AD cases are regarded as sporadic with no familial or geographic clustering. They are also called idiopathic (literally unknown pathogenesis). However despite lacking a Mendelian pattern of inheritance we do know that genetics contributes to the susceptibility of sporadic AD. What we do not know for any particular sufferer is the magnitude of that genetic contribution or the number of genes involved. The 'common variant' hypothesis for complex diseases states that a variable number of commonly occurring gene variants combine to make up the genetic component of disease causation. A common variant or polymorphism is defined as one where the minor allele frequency is greater than 1% in the population.

The most numerous genetic variants are single nucleotide polymorphisms (SNPs) and there are thought to be around 30 million SNPs in total meaning that two unrelated persons, chosen at random, will differ at about 1 in every 1,200 to 1,500 bases. In 2002 the National Institutes of Health started a $138 million project called the HapMap Project to catalogue the common SNPs in European, East Asian (Han Chinese and Japanese and African (Yoruba)) populations. By 2010 HapMap had released details of SNPs and inferred copy number polymorphisms in 1300 individuals from these four ethnic groups (Altshuler *et al.*, 2010). As will be discussed below, this detailed data on human genetic variation combined with gene chip technology allows the simultaneous testing of more than 2 million SNPs in what are called genome wide-association studies (GWAs).

The remaining 'uncatalogued' common variants will consist of rarer SNPs and smaller copy number variations (<500 base pairs) (Conrad *et al.*, 2010). The '1000 human genome project' aims to use next generation sequencing (NGS) to bridge this gap (The 1000 Genomes Project

Consortium, 2010). NGS has many current and potential applications in studying complex diseases and will be a recurring theme for the remainder of this chapter.

3.3 Microarrays

Microarrays (a generic term for a gene chip) are utilised for GWAs but they are more commonly known as a platform in genome-wide expression or transcriptomic studies. Microrrays were initially manufactured by printing the cDNAs of interest onto a glass microscope slide but now short oligonucleotides (probes) complementary to known exonic regions are directly synthesised onto a glass microscope slide or microscopic beads. Probes are typically designed to complement (bind to) the 3′ untranslated regions of transcripts although newer generation arrays have multiple probes across whole genes. The detection of signal with the microarray platform relies on probe-hybridisation and non-specific binding can potentially affect the relative detection of lowly expressed transcripts. Modern microarrays have around 50,000 probes representing the approximately 20,000 known protein coding genes, meaning there is redundancy for some genes. The accompanying software will usually report only the maximally expressed or maximally differentiated probe for each gene. The ability to make 20,000 comparisons in a single experiment is an extremely powerful and seductive tool that importantly makes no *a priori* hypotheses to the importance of any one gene. However, this number of comparisons always exceeds the number of individuals being sampled creating statistical dilemmas for the confident detection of real differences. This 'curse of multidimensionality' similarly affects the analysis of GWAs or any -omic platform (Somorjai *et al.*, 2003).

3.4 Next generation sequencing

The sequencing of the human genome project was carried out using a technique called dye terminator chemistry developed by Fred Sanger 30 years before (Sanger *et al.*, 1977). This technique relies on the amplification of the DNA sequence with incorporation of terminating dideoxynucleotides and the subsequent arrangement of all the fragments (now by software) to derive the final sequence. Although capable of long accurate reads (up to 1500 bases) and eventually automated with capillary technology the technique was, by today's standards, very slow.

The term next generation sequencing (NGS) generically refers to platforms that allow the sequencing of several hundred thousand templates simultaneously (Margulies et al., 2005). For most NGS platforms the multiple templates are sequentially exposed to a known nucleotide whose attachment to its complementary base generates ATP, which is subsequently used to produce a luminescent signal. The signals across the array are captured as an image, before the excess nucleotides are washed away and the process repeated. The actual cycle number or read length is platform-dependent, but will vary from 75 to about 400 bases. This in-parallel sequencing is obviously much quicker than the single-sample Sanger method and now allows relatively small laboratories with a single instrument to perform whole genome sequencing that was, until very recently, the domain of dedicated sequencing centres. There are now also third generation sequencing systems based on single-molecule analysis. These promise to be quicker and cheaper than NGS platforms and more accurate due to longer read lengths although they may still not quite achieve the lengths seen with Sanger sequencing.

One of the major applications of NGS is full-length mRNA sequencing called RNA-Seq. Unlike microarrays RNA-Seq provides a digital readout of all transcripts including those that are lowly expressed and it does not rely on prior knowledge of the genome for probe design. Most current preparatory methods for RNA-Seq continue to use a PolyA fraction (mRNA) but total RNA methods, which require the deletion of the abundant architectural RNA species (ribosomal and transfer RNA), are improving. The latter allows the full repertoire of both coding and non-coding RNA to be quantified.

3.5 Proteomics

The term proteome describes the full complement of proteins, including post-translational variants, produced in a particular cell or tissue (Wilkins *et al.,* 1996). For many biologists, proteins remain the key functional entities that can only be approximated by transcriptomic analyses. Certainly there is not necessarily a linear relationship between mRNA and proteins levels. In a generic proteomic analysis, the lysate would be separated by two-dimensional gel electrophoresis and the 'spots' of interest excised, digested, and the resultant peptide fragments subjected to mass spectroscopy (MS). Individual spectra are compared to databases to derive peptide identity and by computation, the likely parent protein. This process is also referred to peptide mass fingerprinting. It is now more common to use tandem MS where a specific peptide is further fragmented and fragments subjected to MS (peptide fragmentation fingerprinting). Proteomics can be made semi-quantitative by spiking in stable isotopes as reporter ions allowing the relative abundance of the peptides in the overall spectra to be calculated.

4. Pathogenesis

Pathogenesis is defined as the series of events and mechanisms that result in the clinical manifestation of a disease. It encompasses the aetiological agent, its entry into the host and the subsequent host responses to that agent over time. In general the greater the 'dose' of an aetiological agent, the more rapid will be the disease onset and severity. Host resistance or compensatory mechanisms will act to maintain homeostasis and so delay the disease onset and its impact, but an over exuberant or aberrant host response could also be a major factor in the clinical manifestation of the disease itself. Neurodegenerative diseases tend to be late-onset, around 75 years in the case of AD, with preclinical or prodromal periods of extended, but unknown, lengths. This type of disease history presents a number of pathogenic possibilities. In one scenario the aetiological agent(s) are extremely subtle and require a long time period to overcome host resistance. Alternatively host resistance may be entirely capable of dealing with the neurodegenerative agent until it fails due to old age. In the latter case a much shorter prodromal period would be expected. A variation on the latter theme is that rather than a foreign agent inducing the pathogenic process, it is a physiological process that goes awry because suitable checks and balances fail with advancing age. If the latter proved to be the case with AD then treatment strategies might be plagued by unwanted side effects.

In the introduction we discussed that there are two major forms of AD, monogenic and sporadic. These types of AD are sometimes referred to early-onset (EOAD) and late onset

(LOAD), with 60 years of age often given as the arbitrary cut off. With reference to monogenic forms of AD we might think of mutations as an increased 'dose' (severity) of an aetiological agent and monogenic AD can present as young as 20 years of age. In fact, very rarely, AD-causing mutations are actually gene multiplications with direct gene dosage effects.

Sporadic forms of a disease are defined by having no familial or geographic clustering but this term is slightly misleading because there is certainly a genetic component in these common forms of AD. Epidemiological studies suggest that AD sufferers have a 2.5 fold greater likelihood of family history of the disease (Sutherland *et al.*, 2011b). In our 'dose' analogy above the late-onset nature of these common forms of AD would be consistent with common genetic variants, conferring only slight alterations to protein function or expression, being the causative agent. We also generally assume that the genetic component will be multifaceted with both additive and interactive relationships with environmental exposures. The latter refers to a scenario where a potential genetic risk factor only modifies disease risk if that individual has been exposed to a certain environmental stress. We will return to the discussion of AD genetics shortly but it is useful at this stage to introduce the amyloid precursor protein (APP) and its metabolite Aβ.

4.1 APP metabolism

The Aβ peptide was initially purified from amyloid-containing AD brain tissue (Glenner and Wong, 1984) and the cored plaques of AD and Down syndrome patients (Masters *et al.*, 1985). The parent protein, APP, was then isolated from a human brain cDNA library (Kang *et al.*, 1987). The predicted 695 amino acid long protein with a single transmembrane domain was described as being similar to the prion protein, a hypothesised neuronal surface receptor. There are three major APP isoforms, 695, 751 and 770 amino acids in length with APP_{695} being the most common in neural tissue (Yoshikai *et al.*, 1990).

Following translation the APP protein is retained in the secretory pathway, and is transported to the cell membrane. The protein is subsequently degraded via proteolytic cleavage by either α-, and γ-secretases or alternatively β- and γ-secretases at the cell membrane or following the endocytosis of APP as part of normal membrane turnover (LaFerla *et al.*, 2007). In addition a variable fraction of APP undergoes post-translational proteolytic cleavage within the secretory pathway. The γ-secretase is a multi-unit enzyme, that includes either the presenilin 1 (PS1) or presenilin 2 (PS2) proteins and it cleaves APP (and other proteins such as Notch) within its transmembrane domain. α-secretase activity is carried out by a family of proteins (including ADAM 9) and this cleavage results in the secretion of an extracellular fragment of APP (sAPP-α) and the retention of a C-terminal fragment (CTF) of 83 amino acids (Fig. 2). sAPPα appears to act as a neuroprotectant, and has neurotrophic effects on synaptic plasticity (Postina, 2008). Alternatively, and mutually exclusive to α-secretase cleavage, the β-secretase enzyme (BACE1, also called Asp2, memapsin 2, is the major form in the brain) cleaves APP at variable sites about 16 amino acids proximal to the α-secretase site (Vassar *et al.*, 2009). The combination of β-secretase and γ-secretase cleavages releases a variety of peptides that are collectively called Aβ (1,2,3 to 39-43) (Fig. 2).

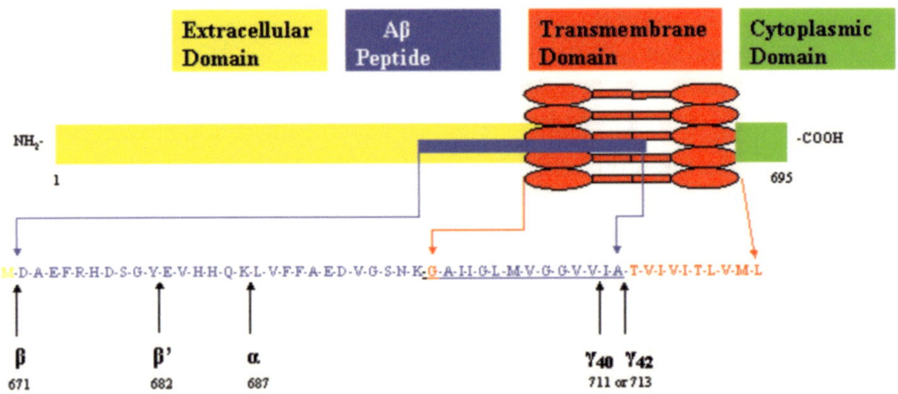

Fig. 2. The structure of the amyloid precursor protein (APP_{770}). This is a schematic diagram of the longest APP isoform (APP_{770}). The α-, β-and γ-secretase sites are shown. APP undergoes physiological cleavage through two alternative pathways; α-secretase or β-secretase. The latter pathway involves the cleavage of APP at β and γ sites and results in the production of various Aβ peptides. Cleavage at the α site prohibits the formation of the Aβ peptides. The hydrophobic 29-40(2) segment of the Aβ peptide is part of the transmembrane domain of APP and is likely to confer both aggregative and membrane-binding behaviour to these peptides (Sutherland, 2003, PhD thesis).

The β-secretase pathway is also called the amyloidogenic pathway because the major products $A\beta_{1-40}$ and $A\beta_{1-42}$ will rapidly aggregate with themselves *in vitro* and *in vivo* with $A\beta_{1-42}$ in particular capable of rapid self-assembly. $A\beta_{1-42}$ is known to be neurotoxic *in vitro* (Lorenzo and Yankner, 1994) and *in vivo* (see animal models below) and thought to be central to AD pathogenesis.

Amyloid structures are composed of pairs of anti-parallel β -strands or β-pleated sheets of Aβ. It was these fibrillar forms of Aβ that were originally presumed to be pathogenic although oligomers are now generally regarded as the pathogenic form of Aβ (Walsh *et al.*, 2002). Interestingly Aβ is produced in proportion to synaptic activity and has the opposite effect to sAPPα on synaptic connections (Selkoe, 2002). This could suggest an useful antagonistic action although Aβ is still generally regarded purely as a degradative product. Aβ is normally removed from the brain by the perivascular drainage of interstitial fluid to the cervical lymphatics (Weller *et al.*, 2008) but is also actively secreted into the CSF.

4.2 Monogenic forms

The first AD family presenting with an apparent Mendelian pattern of inheritance was described in 1932 (Schottky, 1932). In more modern times a family was reported with 51 affected persons in 8 generations (Nee *et al.*, 1983). Down syndrome individuals who are trisomic for chromosome 21 (C21) and have 3 copies of the APP gene also develop Aβ pathology (Heston, 1977). A gene dosage model was proposed for Down syndrome patients as an explanation for early presentation with AD-like pathological changes (Tanzi, 1989).

Early linkage studies of multiple large kindreds mapped a common genetic defect to the *APP* region of C21 (St George-Hyslop, 1987 #8988) although *APP* did not initially appear to be involved (Tanzi *et al.*, 1987a; Tanzi *et al.*, 1987b). Missense mutations in *APP* was eventually described in 1991(Goate *et al.*, 1991) while the predicted duplications in the APP gene, given the gene dosage hypothesis for Down syndrome, were only discovered later (Rovelet-Lecrux *et al.*, 2006). These cases also showed cerebral amyloid angiopathy, a disease entity that can occur independently of AD but is present in 80% of sporadic AD cases (Ellis *et al.*, 1996). APP mutations themselves are very rare and it is the PSEN1 gene (encoding presenilin 1) where the majority of AD mutations have been detected (Sherrington, 1995 #674). Mutations in the PSEN2 gene were also found in 1995 (Levy-Lahad *et al.*, 1995) but these are also relatively uncommon (Bekris *et al.*, 2010). In comparison to *PSEN1* mutation carriers the PSEN 2 cases had a more variable phenotype, a later onset of disease and a reduced penetrance, but the ratio of $A\beta_{1\text{-}42}$:$A\beta_{1\text{-}40}$ is increased in all monogenic AD brains.

One of the PSEN1 families (N141I mutation) was descended from Volga Germans who had immigrated to the USA. It was later suggested that these individuals were likely to originate from the same region of Germany as Auguste D (Yu, 2010 #8999) and perhaps she had the same mutation.

4.3 Amyloid cascade hypothesis

There is almost irrefutable proof that monogenic forms of AD result from the aberrant production or metabolism of the Aβ peptides and these rare forms are, apart from the earlier age at onset, phenotypically very similar to the sporadic forms (Shepherd *et al.*, 2009). This similarity was the major driver for Hardy and Higgins to propose the amyloid cascade hypothesis for the pathogenesis of sporadic AD in 1992. This hypothesis suggested that the neurotoxic Aβ sets up a cascade of events in adjacent neurons resulting in NFT formation and neuronal death. How Aβ actually precipitates these events was not articulated but most interpreted the hypothesis as suggesting that it was Aβ fibrils in the form of plaques that were the neurotoxic entity. Later amendments to the hypothesis suggested that it was more likely to be $A\beta_{1\text{-}42}$ oligomers rather than fibrils but whether these interact directly with the neuronal cell membrane or via receptors was still unknown (Hardy and Selkoe, 2002). The cascade hypothesis remains the most popular working hypothesis for AD pathogenesis and is the underlying basis for proposed preclinical diagnostic criteria and the vast majority of treatments under development (Sperling *et al.*, 2011). Nevertheless, it is not quite unanimously accepted. Distracters, in particular, point to the fact that NFTs rather than amyloid are initially deposited in the memory-associated hippocampus and that the regional progression of NFTs is a better correlate of disease symptoms and severity (Braak and Braak, 1991). Furthermore the latest GWAs also hint at Aβ-independent mechanisms for sporadic forms of the disease (discussed below).

The monogenic forms of AD have also allowed the production of animal models, the main research workhorse towards understanding pathogenesis. A brief synopsis of the mice models is given below but the area has been extensively reviewed by Gotz and Ittner (Gotz and Ittner, 2008) including a thorough consideration of how invertebrate models such the fruitfly (*Drosophila melogaster*) and the worm, *Caenorhabditis elegans*, have also impacted on AD research.

The transgenic expression of human mutant APP in mice (Games *et al.*, 1995) caused plaques and inflammatory responses but not tangles or any substantial neuronal loss. These mice were subsequently crossed with a variety of gene knockout strains including an apolipoprotein E (APOE) null mouse where a dramatic reduction in Aβ load was seen (Bales *et al.*, 1997). As we will discuss shortly, the possession of the ε4 variant of the APOE gene is a leading risk factor for sporadic AD. Holtzman and colleagues were then able to show in these mice that the additional expression of human APOE ε4 produced a 10-fold greater increase in Aβ deposits than APOE ε3 (Holtzman *et al.*, 2000). A double transgenic mouse was subsequently developed with both APP and PSEN1 mutant forms and this showed both an acceleration of Aβ deposition and an increased quantity of Aβ load over either parent mutant mouse (Holcomb *et al.*, 1998).

Aβ-orientated studies have dominated the AD field but there has always been a sub-community of researchers that have investigated the role of tau. The first tau transgenic mouse was produced in 1995 and showed that exogenous tau was redistributed away from the axon and hyperphosphorylated in a 'pre-tangle' state (Gotz *et al.*, 1995). Although no mutations in the tau gene (MAPT) have been found in AD patients, tau mutations have been described in a familial form of frontotemporal dementia proving that mutant tau is sufficient for neurodegeneration (Hutton *et al.*, 1998). The first mutant tau mouse strain was produced in 2000 (Lewis *et al.*, 2000) and then a double mutant APP/tau cross was produced in 2001 with the expectation that this would be an accurate phenocopy of AD (Lewis *et al.*, 2001). This double mutant showed the same Aβ pathology as the APP mutant mouse but greater NFT pathology than the parent mutant tau mouse strain and greater neuronal loss. This suggested a potential interaction between Aβ and tau, a possibility strengthened by the demonstration that the intracerebral injection of $A\beta_{1\text{-}42}$, had the same precipitating effect on tau pathology in a second mutant tau strain (Gotz *et al.*, 2001)

It was with the generation of a triple transgenic mouse (APP /tau/PSEN1) that a model that closely recapitulated human AD pathology became available (Oddo *et al.*, 2003). Furthermore Aβ deposition preceded tangle formation in this model supporting the amyloid cascade hypothesis.

The cascade hypothesis does not suggest a direct interaction between tau and Aβ but rather that an extracellular Aβ build up eventually results in altered neuronal tau kinase and phosphatase activity precipitating tau hyperphosphorylation (Hardy and Selkoe, 2002). However support for such a direct interaction came from *in vitro* studies where Aβ in the presence of tau forms fibrillar aggregates containing both molecules (Giaccone *et al.*, 1996). Of course such an interaction would require the intraneuronal build up of Aβ, a hypothesis that remains largely left field despite reasonable evidence supporting it (D'Andrea *et al.*, 2001; LaFerla *et al.*, 2007; Gouras *et al.*, 2010).

A particularly interesting finding was that 'neurotoxic' Aβ failed to cause degeneration of neuronal cultures from tau null mice (Rapoport *et al.*, 2002). In 2007 a similar effect was demonstrated in a mouse over-expressing human APP where behavioral deficits were attenuated on a tau null background (Roberson *et al.*, 2007). As tau did not reduce the levels of APP or Aβ the authors surmised that it must 'uncouple Aβ from downstream pathogenic mechanisms'. They were able to rule out Aβ-mediated modifications of tau such as hyperphosphorylation or truncation as the mechanism. It seemed that tau was sensitising the mice to Aβ-mediated over excitation and potential excitotoxicity.

Excitotoxicity in the brain can result from overactivation of N-methyl-D-aspartate (NMDA) receptors (NRs) and it has been postulated that Aβ causes excitotoxicity through a NR-mediated mechanism (Snyder *et al.,* 2005). Under normal conditions the phosphorylation of these NRs by kinases such as Fyn facilitate interactions with post-synaptic density protein 95, the necessary conduit in the perpetuation of the excitatory signal. Interestingly increased Fyn expression was known to exacerbate toxicity in APP transgenic mice (Chin *et al.,* 2005). These factors all appeared unrelated until Ittner and colleagues showed in a dysfunctional tau mouse model, that when the tau-mediated dendritic transport of Fyn was prevented, Aβ-mediated excitotoxicity and premature lethality was attenuated (Ittner *et al.,* 2010).

It remains unclear how Aβ actually decreases the threshold for glutamate excitotoxicity but it is not thought to be through direct binding to the NRs (Snyder *et al.,* 2005). Nevertheless the NR antagonist, memantine is considered to act by blocking Aβ-neurotoxicity (Miguel-Hidalgo *et al.,* 2002).

4.4 Sporadic forms and the APOE ε4 genotype

There are very few factors, genetic or environmental, that have reproducibly been shown to modify the risk for sporadic forms of AD. Age, family history, female gender, low education, head injury and type II diabetes seem to increase risk. While long-term anti-inflammatory use and performing mental and physical activity seems to be protective. This area has been recently reviewed (Sutherland *et al.,* 2011b). The finding of AD prevalence being inversely associated with education led to the idea of non-demented aged individuals having a 'cognitive reserve' (Stern *et al.,* 1994). This hypothesis suggests that the more our brains are utilised the better they are able to withstand or perhaps more accurately compensate for, increasing AD pathology. Nevertheless, apart from ageing itself, all these factors have been shown to have very minor effects on AD risk.

One notable exception here is the possession of the *APOE* ε4 allele which could account for as much as 50% of the attributed risk in AD (Ashford, 2004). This effect was first described in 1993 (Corder *et al.,* 1993) but it is still not known how this common variant actually modifies disease risk. ApoE is the major apolipoprotein of the brain and its primary role is the delivery of lipids and particularly cholesterol to neurons from astrocytes. There are three major protein isoforms (ε2/3/4) based on their respective positions when separated by isoelectric focussing (IEF) (Zellner *et al.,* 2009). The variants are generated by two non-synonymous single nucleotide polymorphisms (SNPs) in exon 3 of the gene, rs429358 and rs7412. Alternative cytosine or thymine bases at these sites leads to either arginine or cysteine at positions 112 and 158 in apoE protein, respectively. The apoE ε4 isoform has arginine at both positions and varies from the common ε3 isoform in both its binding affinities (Weisgraber *et al.,* 1982) and degradation properties (Fukumoto *et al.,* 2003; Riddell *et al.,* 2008). The risk of sporadic AD increases with the dose of the APOE ε4 allele; heterozygotes are at a two-fold higher risk but ε4 homozygotes are at a greater than 12-fold risk (Corder *et al.,* 1993). There is a similar effect on the age at disease onset with an estimated decrease of 7-9 years per allele (Chapman *et al.,* 2001). However, possession of this allele is neither essential nor sufficient for AD. ApoE ε4 has an increased binding efficiency for Aβ (Strittmatter *et al.*, 1993) and can accelerate Aβ fibril formation *in vitro* (Castano *et al.*, 1995). It is therefore generally interpreted that the apoE ε4 isoform modifies AD risk by accelerating the development of plaques although it is probably a more complex association between neuronal lipid content and amyloid precursor protein metabolism (Grosgen *et al.*, 2010).

Before the arrival of GWAs, a meta-analysis of single candidate gene studies showed that, apart from APOE, very few other gene loci modified AD risk and their effects were all very modest (odds ratios ~1.25) (Bertram *et al.*, 2008). The first GWAs in 2007 essentially confirmed these findings (Grupe *et al.*, 2007; Reiman *et al.*, 2007)

Subsequent GWAs would concentrate on defining the non-*APOE* genetic component of AD and in 2009 two independent studies reported an association with a second apolipoprotein-encoding gene, CLU, which encodes clusterin or apoJ and a gene called PiCALM (which encodes phosphatidylinositol binding clathrin assembly protein) (Harold *et al.*, 2009; Lambert *et al.*, 2009). Clusterin is best known as a chaperone protein but as its alternative name suggests it is also found in lipoprotein particles and regulates cholesterol and lipid metabolism in the brain (Nuutinen *et al.*, 2009). A feature of these later GWAs were their two-tiered approach where only SNPs deemed significant in a first cohort were tested in an additional independent cohort and only those replicated in both reported as significant. This strategy reduced the multidimensionality of the study and theoretically the risk of generating false positives. Lambert and colleagues also found an additional association with the CR1 gene, encoding a complement receptor (Lambert *et al.*, 2009).

In 2011 two further GWAs were reported that combined these multi-tier approaches with meta-analyses of additional data sets to further increase their detection sensitivity (Hollingworth *et al.*, 2011; Naj *et al.*, 2011). In combination these 2011 studies confirmed 10 significant loci associated with sporadic AD included the genes previously described (APOE, CLU, PICALM and CR1). One of the co-authors from these studies suggested that these 10 genes implicate three pathways in AD pathogenesis, immune system function, cholesterol metabolism and synaptic cell membrane processes (Morgan, 2011). He further suggested that these pathways appear to be largely Aβ-independent. However Aβ is known to inhibit synaptic activity and Aβ can bind to membranes where it may actually modulate the lipid make-up including cholesterol content (Grimm *et al.*, 2005).

Morgan considers that GWAs have now accounted for up to 50% of genetic risk in sporadic AD (Morgan, 2011). The question remains what has happened to the missing heritability? SNP arrays detect common variants (SNP directly and copy number variants by inference) but there is an alternative hypothesis that a large proportion of AD cases will result from rare variants in many different genes (Pritchard, 2001). Alternatively, Cooper and Shendure argue that it is not the GWAs technology that is limiting detection of common variants but rather our interpretation of the data (Cooper and Shendure, 2011). They maintain that an improvement in 'probability' is required before such studies will reach their maximum detection potential. This means that the analysis needs to be limited to functional entities only to reduce the number of tests carried out. They admit that defining which SNPs are functional (or in close linkage disequilibrium with such SNPs) remains a 'work in progress' but report steady advances in both computational approaches that predict changes in protein structure in non-synonymous SNPs and multiplex experimental approaches that combine mutagenesised libraries, *in vitro* transcription and RNA-Seq.

Two other factors potentially lowering the power of GWAs are not platform-related at all. As discussed above AD pathology is present in 30% or more of our age-matched controls and there are variations in the clinical presentation of AD. In particular it seems highly probable that individuals who develop clinical variations such as posterior cortical atrophy or logopenic aphasia will have different underlying genetic susceptibilities. It is hoped that biomarkers will be able to facilitate more focused comparisons of AD sub-groups or allow the dichotomous case-control paradigm to be replaced by an investigations of a continuous variable such as amyloid load using positive electron tomography (PET) (Sutherland *et al.*, 2011b).

4.5 Transcriptomics and brain tissue

Most readers will associate the term 'microarray' with whole genome expression studies. Microarray (expression) studies have been extensively used over the last decade for the analysis of human tissue and animal models. As discussed above, researchers were expecting a relatively high 40 to 100,000 protein-encoding genes in the human genome. This expectation was largely based on the evolutionarily complex human brain. However comparative genomic analyses have now shown that the increase in complexity and specialisation of the human brain is largely derived at the level of transcription (Enard *et al.*, 2002). This includes the utilisation of variable length 3' untranslated regions (Ramskold *et al.*, 2009) and alternatively spliced isoforms (Pan *et al.*, 2008; Wang *et al.*, 2008). This transcriptomic diversity will underlie both brain function and presumably dysfunction, making the transcriptomic analysis of postmortem human brain tissue a seemingly ideal experimental paradigm to find pathogenic clues in AD.

A meta-analysis of microarray studies in AD utilising brain tissue has not been undertaken but a review of reported finding suggests that these studies have been largely discordant and disappointingly have not provided novel clues about AD pathogenesis (Courtney *et al.*, 2010). These divergent findings may be due to a number of different factors. High RNA quality is the major factor in the subsequent quality of microarray data. Brain tissue pH is the major determinant of RNA quality but unfortunately it is the agonal period that is critical in determining pH, and this is both long in neurodegenerative disease and out of the control of the researcher. In comparison to animal or cell culture models RNA quality is invariably poorer from postmortem brain tissue (Preece and Cairns, 2003). The study of postmortem tissue is also inherently a retrospective analysis. The time component of neurodegenerative diseases means many rounds of tissue insult and compensatory host responses will have occurred, particularly in regions such as the entorhinal cortex in AD. The pathology in the postmortem brain may have little informative value on what precipitated the disease at the transcriptomic level. In other words it becomes impossible to delineate disease 'cause' from 'effect'.

Variability in microarray studies may also reflect limitations in the technology itself (Sutherland *et al.*, 2011a). A new NGS-based platform promises to address most of these issues and is discussed immediately below, but prior to this let us briefly look at a combination of the two main methodologies discussed above, GWA and expression studies. These can be combined to derive expression quantitative trait loci (eQTL). In a direct experiment approach genomic DNA of a case-control cohort will be assayed by SNP array while expression analysis will be carried out on say, RNA from peripheral leucocytes of the same individuals. The expression of each individual transcript can be regarded as an independent variable and tested against all the SNPs on the GWAs array. This experiment can detect 'cis' effects of SNPs influencing the expression of their own gene but also 'trans' effects of SNPs that are spatially disparate from the gene of interest.

Alternatively an indirect approach can be used where the expression analysis is carried out in the brain tissue of neuropathologically confirmed cases and controls while the GWAs is in an independent AD cohort from (ideally) the same population. Such an indirect study has been carried out in AD and their major findings were three SNPs that associated significantly with IDE (insulin degrading enzyme) expression levels. This is a very interesting finding as IDE actually degrades Aβ (Kurochkin and Goto, 1994) and a meta-analysis, although not the latest GWAs, suggests that it is associated with sporadic AD (Bertram *et al.*, 2007). Presumably such studies will soon be reported with the partial or complete use of NGS.

4.6 RNA-Seq

As will be seen in the next section of this chapter NGS will influence nearly all aspects of research on disease pathogenesis. However it may have the greatest impact in trancriptomic analysis (Sutherland *et al.*, 2011a). In comparison to microarrays, RNA-Seq with its linear dynamic range and sensitivity for expression changes in low-abundant transcripts, provides a much more accurate (digital) signal. All transcripts can be confidently assumed to be present regardless of their level of expression. Second, microarrays rely on known genomic sequences for their probe design whereas RNA-Seq, with no such limitation, can detect novel transcripts (Cloonan and Grimmond, 2008). Third, microarrays generally quantify only the total transcripts for each gene but RNA-Seq, with its single base resolution, can detect the exact location of transcription boundaries allowing all transcriptional outputs to be quantified. This includes variants due to alternative promoter usage, splicing patterns and 3' UTR lengths that are unique to the human brain. A recent 'proof of concept' RNA-Seq study compared commercial RNA samples from AD patients with pooled control samples (Twine *et al.*, 2011). One of their major findings was the dysregulation of *APOE* transcription in the temporal lobe of an AD patient. SNPs in and around the APOE gene seemingly associate with AD independently of the ε4 effect, although there is a 7 kb linkage disequilibrium block that covers the entire APOE gene locus (Belbin *et al.*, 2007). It is anticipated that more RNA-Seq studies of postmortem brain tissue will appear in the literature in the near future.

4.7 Proteomics

The application of proteomics to AD has involved analyses of CSF, plasma and postmortem brain tissue. The driver for this research is to find biomarkers or a proteomic signature to improve AD diagnosis and potentially allow preclinical diagnosis (Zellner *et al.*, 2009).

It has been known for sometime that there are protein-based alterations in the CSF profile of AD patients. Given the role of excess $A\beta_{1\text{-}42}$ in the disease it is perhaps surprisingly to see that this specific peptide is reduced in patient (clinical) analytes (Blennow and Hampel, 2003). This has been explained by the pathogenic retention of $A\beta_{1\text{-}42}$ in the parenchyma facilitating plaque development. However there are increases seen in both phosphorylated tau species and total tau in AD patients' CSF.

A proteomic study that utilised two-dimensional gel electrophoresis (2-DE) found 23 differentially expressed proteins in the CSF of AD patients (Finehout *et al.*, 2007). These included a down-regulation of apoE (but they did not identify Aβ or tau). The sampling of CSF is relatively straightforward but it is not without risk of infection or spinal cord damage. There are also important ethical considerations in consenting dementia patients for such procedures although this issue also extends across the breadth of potential clinical research.

Researchers and clinicians are therefore keen to find brain-specific (and disease-specific) patterns of expression in serum or plasma samples that are more easily sampled and can be sampled repeatedly during the course of the disease. A disease-specific pattern in peripheral samples could reflect a number of scenarios; pathogenic species have drained or potentially leaked from the brain, there are systemic manifestations of the disease process or the functional consequences of underlying genetic susceptibility can be detected peripherally. As the brain is behind the relatively impermeable blood-brain barrier, leaked metabolites are unlikely to contribute greatly to plasma. Nevertheless the proteins, complement factor H and α-2 macroglobulin have been detected in plasma using by 2-DE and immunochemical assays although their sensitivity (62%) and specificity (60%) is far below those required for a biomarker (Hye *et al.*, 2006). In a recent study the reduced levels of apoE seen in the CSF, have also been seen in plasma of early stage AD sufferers, and particularly in *APOE* ε4 carriers. The decrease in apoE levels was inversely correlated with Aβ load seen on PET (Gupta *et al.*, 2011).

5. Future

As we contemplate the future of research in AD, it is worthwhile reiterating that there are currently no treatments that slow the progression of the disease. At their first clinical presentation AD sufferers will already have significant neuronal loss. Ideally, neuroprotective agents are required but these would still be relatively ineffective if only implemented at the onset of clinical signs. A successful treatment regime is dependent on the co-discovery of a therapeutic target(s) and a preclinical biomarker(s). These, in turn, are both predicated on gaining a greater understanding of early pathogenic events.

5.1 Advances in understanding pathogenesis

Without doubt the major technological advance in biology is NGS. It seems only a matter of time before the much-anticipated '$1000 genome' is standard practice in both research and clinical practice (Pareek *et al.*, 2011). Furthermore NGS is about to become third generation sequencing where nucleic acids are sequenced without the need for preparatory PCR amplification of templates, a procedure that potentially introduces biases. These 'third-gen' technologies run at nanoscale proportions and rely on either detecting the exonuclease cleavage of a specific nucleotide from the template or their incorporation into a newly synthesised DNA strand. It is predicted that these new platforms will achieve read lengths of around 1000 base pairs making the subsequent alignment to a reference genome a more rapid and accurate process.

In terms of AD research, NGS will spell the end of the current design of GWAs. All study subjects will soon be sequenced directly allowing both the 'rare' and 'common variant' hypotheses to be simultaneously tested. We are already seeing an intermediate combination of SNP global analyses with more focused sequencing efforts (Lupton *et al.,* 2011). For example, an investigation of hypertriglyceridemic patients by GWAs followed by the resequencing of candidate genes uncovered a significant burden of rare variants (Johansen *et al.,* 2010).

It is interesting to postulate whether the knowledge of all genetic variation between affected and unaffected individuals (in a cohort) will deliver us the complete understanding of AD pathogenesis. There is no doubt that we will uncover hitherto unknown genetic clues that could increase our focus towards one defective pathway. However the single mutation in the autosomal-dominant inherited Huntington's disease was discovered in 1993 (The Huntington's Disease Collaborative Research Group, 1993) and much remains to be known about the functional ramifications of that defect.

In terms of transcriptomics, RNA-Seq templates usually involve polyA pre-selection so that only the mRNA fraction is sequenced however total RNA approaches are available where ribosomal RNA, which accounts for as much as 90% of the transcriptome, is selectively depleted. The move to total RNA approaches seems prudent given the increasing importance of non-coding and non-polyadenylated RNA species in biology (Mattick *et al.,* 2010) and the human brain in particular (Mattick, 2011). Non-coding RNA is transcribed from what was previously called 'junk' DNA and there is an amazingly diverse and continually expanding list of different RNA species being discovered. Perhaps more daunting is that single RNA molecules can also exist as structural variants with different functional roles (Wan *et al.,* 2011). Notwithstanding the latter, the RNA-Seq platform finally gives us the opportunity to comprehensively investigate the transcriptome of the human brain (Sutherland *et al.,* 2011a).

5.2 Diagnosis

When the first comprehensive criteria for clinical diagnosis were formulated in 1984, the only imaging modality in routine use in neurology was computer-assisted tomography. Neuroimaging has come a long way since then with volumetric magnetic resonance imaging (MRI), functional MRI including diffusion tensor imaging, single-photon emission computed tomography (SPECT) and PET with the amyloid-binding ligand, ^{11}C-Pittsburgh Compound B (PiB-PET) and brain glucose metabolism (FDG-PET)) all been applied to AD patients. Neuroimaging in AD has recently been the subject of a large international public/private partnership, based in the USA (Weiner *et al.,* 2010). Established in 2004, the Alzheimer's disease neuroimaging initiative (ADNI) seeks to validate MRI and PET images, in combination with CSF/blood biomarkers, as predictors and outcomes for use in clinical trials of AD treatments. They had a particular interest in establishing the criteria for preclinical AD and so recruited elderly controls and MCI patients, as well as AD sufferers, and followed them prospectively. ADNI consider, as per the amyloid cascade hypothesis, that the earliest detectable changes in at risk individuals are related to Aβ. Moreover there is a detectable initial increase in CSF $A\beta_{1-42}$ (preclinical) and amyloid deposition using PiB-PET. As discussed above these changes have been included in preclinical criteria but only for use in a research context at this stage (Sperling *et al.*, 2011). When this detectable change in Aβ metabolism actually begins is unknown but decreases in CSF $A\beta_{1\text{-}42}$ are seen as early as the 6th decade in apoE ε4 carriers and their age-related decrease is more severe (Peskind *et al.*, 2006). Similarly PiB imaging of nondemented aged persons in Australia suggested that 33% of healthy controls had high PiB binding (Rowe *et al.*, 2010). Interesting a correlation between PiB binding and cognition was only seen in *APOE* ε4 carriers.

The increases in CSF phosphorylated and total tau are generally considered a later disease marker of the disease representative of neuronal degeneration, and likely to coincide with brain atrophy, hypometabolism or hypoperfusion on imaging (Weiner *et al.*, 2010). However at least one study of MCI suggests that by this stage there are already decreases in CSF $A\beta_{1\text{-}42}$ and increases in tau (Herukka *et al.*, 2005). Rowe and colleagues suggested that Aβ deposition (and increased CSF tau) are probably inevitable with ageing and other factors are involved in conversion to dementia (Rowe *et al.*, 2010).

5.3 Treatments in development

Although not the subject of this chapter it would seem remiss not to touch on the excitement currently generated by stem cell technology in medical research. The possibility of regenerative medicine in neurodegenerative disease has been stimulated by the demonstration of neurogenesis in the human adult brain (Eriksson *et al.*, 1998), the induction of stem cells from differentiated adult cells (Takahashi *et al.*, 2007) and the conversion of these cells to mature phenotypes such as dopaminergic (Soldner *et al.*, 2009) and motor neurons (Dimos *et al.*, 2008). Regenerative medicine or cell transplantation therapies may prove efficacious in many diseases although the chances in AD, with its extensive neuronal loss, do appear more remote. A therapy promoting endogenous neurogenesis looks more promising and its stimulation through physical activity or environmental enrichment seen in animal models may yet underlie the 'cognitive reserve' hypothesis. Furthermore the potential for modelling AD using patient-derived cell lines is an exciting field with applications in understanding basic pathogenesis through to preclinical drug screening and clinical toxicity studies (Sutherland and Sidhu, 2011).

The mechanism of action for the majority of drugs in current Phase II or III clinical trials is limiting the production or increasing the clearance of Aβ (Gravitz, 2011). These include antibodies to Aβ, inhibitors of Aβ aggregation and inhibitors of γ-secretase. In comparison inhibitors of β-secretase have proved more difficult to develop because of difficulties crossing the blood-brain-barrier and their poor affinity for the catalytic site, but two reports suggest that these roadblocks may have been solved (Atwal *et al.*, 2011; Yu *et al.*, 2011).

Two of the four drugs in Phase III trials, bapineuzumab and solanezumab are humanised monoclonal antibodies (derived from murine antibodies). These passive immunisation strategies were developed when initial studies testing an aggregated Aβ vaccine were abandoned due to 6% of the participants developing sterile meningoencephalitis (Orgogozo *et al.*, 2003). An Aβ vaccine had previously removed and prevented plaques in mutant APP transgenic mice, (Schenk *et al.*, 1999) and reversed their learning deficits (Janus *et al.*, 2000; Dodart *et al.*, 2002). Passive immunisation seemed to have a similar effect in mice but the earliest reports from human trials suggest that, despite reducing amyloid load, these strategies have no effect on cognitive function (Rinne *et al.,* 2010). Furthermore trials determining the efficacy and safety of the γ-secretase inhibitor, semagacestat, had to be terminated due to actual cognitive decline (Cummings, 2010).

These results have been seen by some as serious threats to the validity of the amyloid cascade hypothesis in sporadic AD, although proponents have countered these criticisms by arguing that Aβ therapy is failing because it is instituted too late in the disease process (Gandy, 2011; Golde *et al.*, 2011). They maintain that Aβ therapy needs to be instituted as a prophylaxis and this, of course, means the preclinical identification of future AD patients and the treatment, or at least testing, of individuals without symptoms (Golde *et al.*, 2011).

According to Golde, Schneider and Koo, and based on the findings from imaging and CSF biomarker studies described above, individuals destined to have AD show detectable Aβ deposition at least 10 years earlier. Furthermore amyloid plaques visualized by radioligand imaging and low CSF $A\beta_{1-42}$ can be monitored throughout potential trials of Aβ therapies. It is not clear how an original cohort might be selected but aged *APOE* ε4 carriers were suggested for screening (Golde *et al.,* 2011). This hypothesized approach raises some very interesting ethical questions, not to mention changes required to regulatory criteria that are currently based on clinical symptoms.

5.4 Preventive health

Epidemiological studies were instrumental in establishing the connection between serum lipid levels, particularly high cholesterol, and coronary heart disease. Proponents of prophylactic Aβ immunotherapy might argue that their proposal is similar to the current use of statins in reducing blood cholesterol. However epidemiological studies have been relatively unsuccessful in finding factors that modify the risk for AD, meaning that any proposed preventative strategies remain speculative at best.

The statins story is an interesting one because individuals in the initial trials for heart disease appeared to have a reduced incidence of AD (Jick *et al.*, 2000; Wolozin *et al.*, 2000). This led to considerable research into cardiovascular risk factors in AD including hypertension, elevated serum cholesterol, smoking middle age obesity and type II diabetes. Interesting only type II diabetes survives meta-analyses (Sutherland *et al.*, 2011b).

Remaining physically and mentally active does seem to be relatively effective but it is likely that a cognitive reserve allows individuals to starve off the effects of AD pathology rather than decreasing the pathology itself. Of course this would still be an effective method to reduce the societal burden of AD.

Despite all the research, the current situation in AD could still be summarised by the following paragraph from a recent commentary in the Journal supplement, Nature Outlook:

"A big part of the problem is that researchers don't know enough about the biology of Alzheimer's disease to identify the right targets. The disease is the result of a long chain of events, but some of the links in that chain are still a mystery – nobody is certain which link to cut to stop disease progression" (Gravitz, 2011).

6. Conclusion

Given the passage above the reader may become overly pessimistic about the possibilities for a cure of Alzheimer's in the immediate future. In its general use the term 'cure' implies that there is a readily identifiable agent that causes AD and that this agent can be attenuated or even removed without any serious deleterious effects to the sufferer.

All AD research to date suggests that there is no clear single aetiology for the majority of sufferers. The major pathogenic hypothesis is that in susceptible individuals, on a background of ageing, there is an increased production or decreased clearance (Mawuenyega *et al.*, 2010) of a normal 'degradative' product called Aβ whose build up in the brain becomes neurotoxic.

An alternative or adjunctive interpretation is that Aβ has a physiological role in the brain, perhaps synaptic pruning or inhibiting excitatory activity and that Aβ metabolism itself becomes dysregulated in response to an unknown aetiological factor. The individuals who develop AD may have a greater propensity to deposit Aβ or are less resistance to its downstream effects. In the latter scenario, monogenic forms of AD could still explained by a greater propensity to oligomerisation and deposition. The caveat is that prophylactic Aβ immunotherapy may prove to have more serious side effects than if Aβ is just a degradative product.

The amyloid cascade hypothesis is a very good one that no doubt encapsulates important aspects of the pathogenesis of sporadic AD. However technological advances such as GWAs suggests that Aβ-independent mechanisms are (also) important in AD while RNA-Seq is only now offering a methodology where the transcriptome of the human brain can actually be comprehensively examined. It therefore seems too premature to place all our therapeutic eggs in the Aβ cascade basket.

7. References

Access Economics (2009). Keeping Dementia Front of Mind: Incidence and Prevalence 2009 - 2050. Report for Alzheimer's Australia. Canberra.

Albert MS, DeKosky ST, Dickson D, Dubois B, Feldman HH, Fox NC, Gamst A, Holtzman DM, Jagust WJ, Petersen RC, Snyder PJ, Carrillo MC, Thies B and Phelps CH (2011). The diagnosis of mild cognitive impairment due to Alzheimer's disease: recommendations from the National Institute on Aging-Alzheimer's Association workgroups on diagnostic guidelines for Alzheimer's disease. *Alzheimers Dement* 7(3): 270-279.

Alladi S, Xuereb J, Bak T, Nestor P, Knibb J, Patterson K and Hodges JR (2007). Focal cortical presentations of Alzheimer's disease. *Brain* 130(Pt 10): 2636-2645.

Altshuler DM, Gibbs RA, Peltonen L, Dermitzakis E, Schaffner SF, Yu F, Bonnen PE, de Bakker PI, Deloukas P, Gabriel SB, Gwilliam R, Hunt S, Inouye M, Jia X, Palotie A, Parkin M, Whittaker P, Chang K, Hawes A, Lewis LR, Ren Y, Wheeler D, Muzny DM, Barnes C, Darvishi K, Hurles M, Korn JM, Kristiansson K, Lee C, McCarrol SA, Nemesh J, Keinan A, Montgomery SB, Pollack S, Price AL, Soranzo N, Gonzaga-Jauregui C, Anttila V, Brodeur W, Daly MJ, Leslie S, McVean G, Moutsianas L, Nguyen H, Zhang Q, Ghori MJ, McGinnis R, McLaren W, Takeuchi F, Grossman SR, Shlyakhter I, Hostetter EB, Sabeti PC, Adebamowo CA, Foster MW, Gordon

DR, Licinio J, Manca MC, Marshall PA, Matsuda I, Ngare D, Wang VO, Reddy D, Rotimi CN, Royal CD, Sharp RR, Zeng C, Brooks LD and McEwen JE (2010). Integrating common and rare genetic variation in diverse human populations. *Nature* 467(7311): 52-58.

Alzheimer A (1907). Ueber eine eigenartige Erkrankung der Himrinde. *Allg. Z. Psychiat. Med.* 64: 146-148.

Alzheimer A (1911). Ueber eigenartige Krankheitsfalle des spateren *Alters. Z. Ges. Neurol. Psychiat.* 4: 356-385.

Alzheimer's Disease International (2009). World Alzheimer Report 2010. Prince M. London.

Alzheimer's Disease International (2010). 2010 Alzheimer's disease facts and figures. *Alzheimers Dement* 6(2): 158-194.

Ashford JW (2004). APOE genotype effects on Alzheimer's disease onset and epidemiology. *J Mol Neurosci* 23(3): 157-165.

Atwal JK, Chen Y, Chiu C, Mortensen DL, Meilandt WJ, Liu Y, Heise CE, Hoyte K, Luk W, Lu Y, Peng K, Wu P, Rouge L, Zhang Y, Lazarus RA, Scearce-Levie K, Wang W, Wu Y, Tessier-Lavigne M and Watts RJ (2011). A therapeutic antibody targeting BACE1 inhibits amyloid-beta production in vivo. *Sci Transl Med* 3(84): 84ra43.

Bales KR, Verina T, Dodel RC, Du Y, Altstiel L, Bender M, Hyslop P, Johnstone EM, Little SP, Cummins DJ, Piccardo P, Ghetti B and Paul SM (1997). Lack of apolipoprotein E dramatically reduces amyloid beta-peptide deposition. *Nat Genet* 17(3): 263-264.

Beach TG and McGeer EG (1988). Lamina-specific arrangement of astrocytic gliosis and senile plaques in Alzheimer's disease visual cortex. *Brain Res* 463(2): 357-361.

Bekris LM, Yu CE, Bird TD and Tsuang DW (2010). Genetics of Alzheimer disease. *J Geriatr Psychiatry Neurol* 23(4): 213-227.

Belbin O, Dunn JL, Ling Y, Morgan L, Chappell S, Beaumont H, Warden D, Smith DA, Kalsheker N and Morgan K (2007). Regulatory region single nucleotide polymorphisms of the apolipoprotein E gene and the rate of cognitive decline in Alzheimer's disease. *Hum Mol Genet* 16(18): 2199-2208.

Bertram L, Lange C, Mullin K, Parkinson M, Hsiao M, Hogan MF, Schjeide BM, Hooli B, Divito J, Ionita I, Jiang H, Laird N, Moscarillo T, Ohlsen KL, Elliott K, Wang X, Hu-Lince D, Ryder M, Murphy A, Wagner SL, Blacker D, Becker KD and Tanzi RE (2008). Genome-wide association analysis reveals putative Alzheimer's disease susceptibility loci in addition to APOE. *Am J Hum Genet* 83(5): 623-632.

Bertram L, McQueen MB, Mullin K, Blacker D and Tanzi RE (2007). Systematic meta-analyses of Alzheimer disease genetic association studies: the AlzGene database. *Nat Genet* 39(1): 17-23.

Birks J (2006). Cholinesterase inhibitors for Alzheimer's disease. *Cochrane Database Syst Rev*(1): CD005593.

Blennow K and Hampel H (2003). CSF markers for incipient Alzheimer's disease. *Lancet Neurol* 2(10): 605-613.

Braak H and Braak E (1991). Neuropathological stageing of Alzheimer-related changes. *Acta Neuropathol* (Berl) 82(4): 239-259.

Braak H and Braak E (1997). Frequency of stages of Alzheimer-related lesions in different age categories. *Neurobiol Aging* 18(4): 351-357.

Brookmeyer R, Johnson E, Ziegler-Graham K and Arrighi HM (2007). Forecasting the global burden of Alzheimer's disease. *Alzheimers Demen*t 3(3): 186-191.

Buckner RL, Andrews-Hanna JR and Schacter DL (2008). The brain's default network: anatomy, function, and relevance to disease. *Ann N Y Acad Sci* 1124: 1-38.

Castano EM, Prelli F, Wisniewski T, Golabek A, Kumar RA, Soto C and Frangione B (1995). Fibrillogenesis in Alzheimer's disease of amyloid beta peptides and apolipoprotein E. *Biochem J* 306 (Pt 2): 599-604.

Chapman J, Korczyn AD, Karussis DM and Michaelson DM (2001). The effects of APOE genotype on age at onset and progression of neurodegenerative diseases. *Neurology* 57(8): 1482-1485.

Chin J, Palop JJ, Puolivali J, Massaro C, Bien-Ly N, Gerstein H, Scearce-Levie K, Masliah E and Mucke L (2005). Fyn kinase induces synaptic and cognitive impairments in a transgenic mouse model of Alzheimer's disease. *J Neurosci* 25(42): 9694-9703.

Cloonan N and Grimmond SM (2008). Transcriptome content and dynamics at single-nucleotide resolution. *Genome Biol* 9(9): 234.

Conrad DF, Pinto D, Redon R, Feuk L, Gokcumen O, Zhang Y, Aerts J, Andrews TD, Barnes C, Campbell P, Fitzgerald T, Hu M, Ihm CH, Kristiansson K, Macarthur DG, Macdonald JR, Onyiah I, Pang AW, Robson S, Stirrups K, Valsesia A, Walter K, Wei J, Tyler-Smith C, Carter NP, Lee C, Scherer SW and Hurles ME (2010). Origins and functional impact of copy number variation in the human genome. *Nature* 464(7289): 704-712.

Cooper GM and Shendure J (2011). Needles in stacks of needles: finding disease-causal variants in a wealth of genomic data. *Nat Rev Genet* 12(9): 628-640.

Corder EH, Saunders AM, Strittmatter WJ, Schmechel DE, Gaskell PC, Small GW, Roses AD, Haines JL and Pericak-Vance MA (1993). Gene dose of apolipoprotein E type 4 allele and the risk of Alzheimer's disease in late onset families. *Science* 261(5123): 921-923.

Courtney E, Kornfeld S, Janitz K and Janitz M (2010). Transcriptome profiling in neurodegenerative disease. *J Neurosci Methods* 193(2): 189-202.

Cuijpers P (2005). Depressive disorders in caregivers of dementia patients: a systematic review. *Aging Ment Health* 9(4): 325-330.

Cullen KM and Halliday GM (1998). Neurofibrillary degeneration and cell loss in the nucleus basalis in comparison to cortical Alzheimer pathology. *Neurobiol Aging* 19(4): 297-306.

Cummings J (2010). What can be inferred from the interruption of the semagacestat trial for treatment of Alzheimer's disease? *Biol Psychiatry* 68(10): 876-878.

D'Andrea MR and Nagele RG (2010). Morphologically distinct types of amyloid plaques point the way to a better understanding of Alzheimer's disease pathogenesis. *Biotech Histochem* 85(2): 133-147.

D'Andrea MR, Nagele RG, Wang HY, Peterson PA and Lee DH (2001). Evidence that neurones accumulating amyloid can undergo lysis to form amyloid plaques in Alzheimer's disease. *Histopathology* 38(2): 120-134.

Davis DG, Schmitt FA, Wekstein DR and Markesbery WR (1999). Alzheimer neuropathologic alterations in aged cognitively normal subjects. *J Neuropathol Exp Neurol* 58(4): 376-388.

Dimos JT, Rodolfa KT, Niakan KK, Weisenthal LM, Mitsumoto H, Chung W, Croft GF, Saphier G, Leibel R, Goland R, Wichterle H, Henderson CE and Eggan K (2008). Induced pluripotent stem cells generated from patients with ALS can be differentiated into motor neurons. *Science* 321(5893): 1218-1221.

Dodart JC, Bales KR, Gannon KS, Greene SJ, DeMattos RB, Mathis C, DeLong CA, Wu S, Wu X, Holtzman DM and Paul SM (2002). Immunization reverses memory deficits without reducing brain Abeta burden in Alzheimer's disease model. *Nat Neurosci* 5(5): 452-457.

Dubois B and Albert ML (2004). Amnestic MCI or prodromal Alzheimer's disease? *Lancet Neurol* 3(4): 246-248.

Edison P, Archer HA, Gerhard A, Hinz R, Pavese N, Turkheimer FE, Hammers A, Tai YF, Fox N, Kennedy A, Rossor M and Brooks DJ (2008). Microglia, amyloid, and cognition in Alzheimer's disease: An [11C](R)PK11195-PET and [11C]PIB-PET study. *Neurobiol Dis* 32(3): 412-419.

Ellis RJ, Olichney JM, Thal LJ, Mirra SS, Morris JC, Beekly D and Heyman A (1996). Cerebral amyloid angiopathy in the brains of patients with Alzheimer's disease: the CERAD experience, Part XV. *Neurology* 46(6): 1592-1596.

Enard W, Khaitovich P, Klose J, Zollner S, Heissig F, Giavalisco P, Nieselt-Struwe K, Muchmore E, Varki A, Ravid R, Doxiadis GM, Bontrop RE and Paabo S (2002). Intra- and interspecific variation in primate gene expression patterns. *Science* 296(5566): 340-343.

Eriksson PS, Perfilieva E, Bjork-Eriksson T, Alborn AM, Nordborg C, Peterson DA and Gage FH (1998). Neurogenesis in the adult human hippocampus. *Nat Med* 4(11): 1313-1317.

Finehout EJ, Franck Z, Choe LH, Relkin N and Lee KH (2007). Cerebrospinal fluid proteomic biomarkers for Alzheimer's disease. *Ann Neurol* 61(2): 120-129.

Fukumoto H, Ingelsson M, Garevik N, Wahlund LO, Nukina N, Yaguchi Y, Shibata M, Hyman BT, Rebeck GW and Irizarry MC (2003). APOE epsilon 3/ epsilon 4 heterozygotes have an elevated proportion of apolipoprotein E4 in cerebrospinal fluid relative to plasma, independent of Alzheimer's disease diagnosis. *Exp Neurol* 183(1): 249-253.

Games D, Adams D, Alessandrini R, Barbour R, Berthelette P, Blackwell C, Carr T, Clemens J, Donaldson T, Gillespie F and et al. (1995). Alzheimer-type neuropathology in transgenic mice overexpressing V717F beta-amyloid precursor protein. *Nature* 373(6514): 523-527.

Gandy S (2011). Perspective: prevention is better than cure. *Nature* 475(7355): S15.

Gauthier S, Loft H and Cummings J (2008). Improvement in behavioural symptoms in patients with moderate to severe Alzheimer's disease by memantine: a pooled data analysis. *Int J Geriatr Psychiatry* 23(5): 537-545.

Giaccone G, Pedrotti B, Migheli A, Verga L, Perez J, Racagni G, Smith MA, Perry G, De Gioia L, Selvaggini C, Salmona M, Ghiso J, Frangione B, Islam K, Bugiani O and Tagliavini F (1996). beta PP and Tau interaction. A possible link between amyloid and neurofibrillary tangles in Alzheimer's disease. *Am J Pathol* 148(1): 79-87.

Glenner GG and Wong CW (1984). Alzheimer's disease and Down's syndrome: sharing of a unique cerebrovascular amyloid fibril protein. *Biochem Biophys Res Commun* 122(3): 1131-1135.

Goate A, Chartier-Harlin MC, Mullan M, Brown J, Crawford F, Fidani L, Giuffra L, Haynes A, Irving N, James L and et al. (1991). Segregation of a missense mutation in the amyloid precursor protein gene with familial Alzheimer's disease. *Nature* 349(6311): 704-706.

Gold PE (2003). Acetylcholine modulation of neural systems involved in learning and memory. *Neurobiol Learn Mem* 80(3): 194-210.

Golde TE, Schneider LS and Koo EH (2011). Anti-abeta therapeutics in Alzheimer's disease: the need for a paradigm shift. *Neuron* 69(2): 203-213.

Gomez-Isla T, Price JL, McKeel DW, Jr., Morris JC, Growdon JH and Hyman BT (1996). Profound loss of layer II entorhinal cortex neurons occurs in very mild Alzheimer's disease. *J Neurosci* 16(14): 4491-4500.

Gorno-Tempini ML, Hillis AE, Weintraub S, Kertesz A, Mendez M, Cappa SF, Ogar JM, Rohrer JD, Black S, Boeve BF, Manes F, Dronkers NF, Vandenberghe R, Rascovsky K, Patterson K, Miller BL, Knopman DS, Hodges JR, Mesulam MM and Grossman M (2011). Classification of primary progressive aphasia and its variants. *Neurology* 76(11): 1006-1014.

Gotz J, Chen F, van Dorpe J and Nitsch RM (2001). Formation of neurofibrillary tangles in P301l tau transgenic mice induced by Abeta 42 fibrils. Science 293(5534): 1491-1495.

Gotz J and Ittner LM (2008). Animal models of Alzheimer's disease and frontotemporal dementia. *Nat Rev Neurosci* 9(7): 532-544.

Gotz J, Probst A, Spillantini MG, Schafer T, Jakes R, Burki K and Goedert M (1995). Somatodendritic localization and hyperphosphorylation of tau protein in transgenic mice expressing the longest human brain tau isoform. *EMBO J* 14(7): 1304-1313.

Gouras GK, Tampellini D, Takahashi RH and Capetillo-Zarate E (2010). Intraneuronal beta-amyloid accumulation and synapse pathology in Alzheimer's disease. *Acta Neuropathol* 119(5): 523-541.

Graeber MB, Kosel S, Egensperger R, Banati RB, Muller U, Bise K, Hoff P, Moller HJ, Fujisawa K and Mehraein P (1997). Rediscovery of the case described by Alois Alzheimer in 1911: historical, histological and molecular genetic analysis. *Neurogenetics* 1(1): 73-80.

Graeber MB, Kosel S, Grasbon-Frodl E, Moller HJ and Mehraein P (1998). Histopathology and APOE genotype of the first Alzheimer disease patient, Auguste D. Neurogenetics 1(3): 223-228.

Graeber MB and Streit WJ (2010). Microglia: biology and pathology. *Acta Neuropathol* 119(1): 89-105.

Gravitz L (2011). Drugs: a tangled web of targets. *Nature* 475(7355): S9-11.

Grimm MO, Grimm HS, Patzold AJ, Zinser EG, Halonen R, Duering M, Tschape JA, De Strooper B, Muller U, Shen J and Hartmann T (2005). Regulation of cholesterol and sphingomyelin metabolism by amyloid-beta and presenilin. *Nat Cell Biol* 7(11): 1118-1123.

Grosgen S, Grimm MO, Friess P and Hartmann T (2010). Role of amyloid beta in lipid homeostasis. *Biochim Biophys Acta* 1801(8): 966-974.

Grupe A, Abraham R, Li Y, Rowland C, Hollingworth P, Morgan A, Jehu L, Segurado R, Stone D, Schadt E, Karnoub M, Nowotny P, Tacey K, Catanese J, Sninsky J, Brayne C, Rubinsztein D, Gill M, Lawlor B, Lovestone S, Holmans P, O'Donovan M, Morris JC, Thal L, Goate A, Owen MJ and Williams J (2007). Evidence for novel susceptibility genes for late-onset Alzheimer's disease from a genome-wide association study of putative functional variants. *Hum Mol Genet* 16(8): 865-873.

Gupta VB, Laws SM, Villemagne VL, Ames D, Bush AI, Ellis KA, Lui JK, Masters C, Rowe CC, Szoeke C, Taddei K and Martins RN (2011). Plasma apolipoprotein E and Alzheimer disease risk: the AIBL study of aging. *Neurology* 76(12): 1091-1098.

Halliday GM, Double KL, Macdonald V and Kril JJ (2003). Identifying severely atrophic cortical subregions in Alzheimer's disease. *Neurobiol Aging* 24(6): 797-806.

Halliday GM, Shepherd CE, McCann H, Reid WG, Grayson DA, Broe GA and Kril JJ (2000). Effect of anti-inflammatory medications on neuropathological findings in Alzheimer disease. *Arch Neurol* 57(6): 831-836.

Hansen RA, Gartlehner G, Webb AP, Morgan LC, Moore CG and Jonas DE (2008). Efficacy and safety of donepezil, galantamine, and rivastigmine for the treatment of

Alzheimer's disease: a systematic review and meta-analysis. *Clin Interv Aging* 3(2): 211-225.

Hardy J and Selkoe DJ (2002). The amyloid hypothesis of Alzheimer's disease: progress and problems on the road to therapeutics. *Science* 297(5580): 353-356.

Harold D, Abraham R, Hollingworth P, Sims R, Gerrish A, Hamshere ML, Pahwa JS, Moskvina V, Dowzell K, Williams A, Jones N, Thomas C, Stretton A, Morgan AR, Lovestone S, Powell J, Proitsi P, Lupton MK, Brayne C, Rubinsztein DC, Gill M, Lawlor B, Lynch A, Morgan K, Brown KS, Passmore PA, Craig D, McGuinness B, Todd S, Holmes C, Mann D, Smith AD, Love S, Kehoe PG, Hardy J, Mead S, Fox N, Rossor M, Collinge J, Maier W, Jessen F, Schurmann B, van den Bussche H, Heuser I, Kornhuber J, Wiltfang J, Dichgans M, Frolich L, Hampel H, Hull M, Rujescu D, Goate AM, Kauwe JS, Cruchaga C, Nowotny P, Morris JC, Mayo K, Sleegers K, Bettens K, Engelborghs S, De Deyn PP, Van Broeckhoven C, Livingston G, Bass NJ, Gurling H, McQuillin A, Gwilliam R, Deloukas P, Al-Chalabi A, Shaw CE, Tsolaki M, Singleton AB, Guerreiro R, Muhleisen TW, Nothen MM, Moebus S, Jockel KH, Klopp N, Wichmann HE, Carrasquillo MM, Pankratz VS, Younkin SG, Holmans PA, O'Donovan M, Owen MJ and Williams J (2009). Genome-wide association study identifies variants at CLU and PICALM associated with Alzheimer's disease. *Nat Genet* 41(10): 1088-1093.

Haroutunian V, Hoffman LB and Beeri MS (2009). Is there a neuropathology difference between mild cognitive impairment and dementia? *Dialogues Clin Neurosci* 11(2): 171-179.

Herukka SK, Hallikainen M, Soininen H and Pirttila T (2005). CSF Abeta42 and tau or phosphorylated tau and prediction of progressive mild cognitive impairment. *Neurology* 64(7): 1294-1297.

Heston LL (1977). Alzheimer's disease, trisomy 21, and myeloproliferative disorders: associations suggesting a genetic diathesis. *Science* 196(4287): 322-323.

Holcomb L, Gordon MN, McGowan E, Yu X, Benkovic S, Jantzen P, Wright K, Saad I, Mueller R, Morgan D, Sanders S, Zehr C, O'Campo K, Hardy J, Prada CM, Eckman C, Younkin S, Hsiao K and Duff K (1998). Accelerated Alzheimer-type phenotype in transgenic mice carrying both mutant amyloid precursor protein and presenilin 1 transgenes. *Nat Med* 4(1): 97-100.

Hollingworth P, Harold D, Sims R, Gerrish A, Lambert JC, Carrasquillo MM, Abraham R, Hamshere ML, Pahwa JS, Moskvina V, Dowzell K, Jones N, Stretton A, Thomas C, Richards A, Ivanov D, Widdowson C, Chapman J, Lovestone S, Powell J, Proitsi P, Lupton MK, Brayne C, Rubinsztein DC, Gill M, Lawlor B, Lynch A, Brown KS, Passmore PA, Craig D, McGuinness B, Todd S, Holmes C, Mann D, Smith AD, Beaumont H, Warden D, Wilcock G, Love S, Kehoe PG, Hooper NM, Vardy ER, Hardy J, Mead S, Fox NC, Rossor M, Collinge J, Maier W, Jessen F, Ruther E, Schurmann B, Heun R, Kolsch H, van den Bussche H, Heuser I, Kornhuber J, Wiltfang J, Dichgans M, Frolich L, Hampel H, Gallacher J, Hull M, Rujescu D, Giegling I, Goate AM, Kauwe JS, Cruchaga C, Nowotny P, Morris JC, Mayo K, Sleegers K, Bettens K, Engelborghs S, De Deyn PP, Van Broeckhoven C, Livingston G, Bass NJ, Gurling H, McQuillin A, Gwilliam R, Deloukas P, Al-Chalabi A, Shaw CE, Tsolaki M, Singleton AB, Guerreiro R, Muhleisen TW, Nothen MM, Moebus S, Jockel KH, Klopp N, Wichmann HE, Pankratz VS, Sando SB, Aasly JO, Barcikowska M, Wszolek ZK, Dickson DW, Graff-Radford NR, Petersen RC, van Duijn CM, Breteler MM, Ikram MA, Destefano AL, Fitzpatrick AL, Lopez O, Launer LJ, Seshadri S, Berr C, Campion D, Epelbaum J, Dartigues JF, Tzourio C,

Alperovitch A, Lathrop M, Feulner TM, Friedrich P, Riehle C, Krawczak M, Schreiber S, Mayhaus M, Nicolhaus S, Wagenpfeil S, Steinberg S, Stefansson H, Stefansson K, Snaedal J, Bjornsson S, Jonsson PV, Chouraki V, Genier-Boley B, Hiltunen M, Soininen H, Combarros O, Zelenika D, Delepine M, Bullido MJ, Pasquier F, Mateo I, Frank-Garcia A, Porcellini E, Hanon O, Coto E, Alvarez V, Bosco P, Siciliano G, Mancuso M, Panza F, Solfrizzi V, Nacmias B, Sorbi S, Bossu P, Piccardi P, Arosio B, Annoni G, Seripa D, Pilotto A, Scarpini E, Galimberti D, Brice A, Hannequin D, Licastro F, Jones L, Holmans PA, Jonsson T, Riemenschneider M, Morgan K, Younkin SG, Owen MJ, O'Donovan M, Amouyel P and Williams J (2011). Common variants at ABCA7, MS4A6A/MS4A4E, EPHA1, CD33 and CD2AP are associated with Alzheimer's disease. *Nat Genet* 43(5): 429-435.

Holtzman DM, Bales KR, Tenkova T, Fagan AM, Parsadanian M, Sartorius LJ, Mackey B, Olney J, McKeel D, Wozniak D and Paul SM (2000). Apolipoprotein E isoform-dependent amyloid deposition and neuritic degeneration in a mouse model of Alzheimer's disease. *Proc Natl Acad Sci U S A* 97(6): 2892-2897.

Hutton M, Lendon CL, Rizzu P, Baker M, Froelich S, Houlden H, Pickering-Brown S, Chakraverty S, Isaacs A, Grover A, Hackett J, Adamson J, Lincoln S, Dickson D, Davies P, Petersen RC, Stevens M, de Graaff E, Wauters E, van Baren J, Hillebrand M, Joosse M, Kwon JM, Nowotny P, Che LK, Norton J, Morris JC, Reed LA, Trojanowski J, Basun H, Lannfelt L, Neystat M, Fahn S, Dark F, Tannenberg T, Dodd PR, Hayward N, Kwok JB, Schofield PR, Andreadis A, Snowden J, Craufurd D, Neary D, Owen F, Oostra BA, Hardy J, Goate A, van Swieten J, Mann D, Lynch T and Heutink P (1998). Association of missense and 5'-splice-site mutations in tau with the inherited dementia FTDP-17. *Nature* 393(6686): 702-705.

Hye A, Lynham S, Thambisetty M, Causevic M, Campbell J, Byers HL, Hooper C, Rijsdijk F, Tabrizi SJ, Banner S, Shaw CE, Foy C, Poppe M, Archer N, Hamilton G, Powell J, Brown RG, Sham P, Ward M and Lovestone S (2006). Proteome-based plasma biomarkers for Alzheimer's disease. *Brain* 129(Pt 11): 3042-3050.

Hyman BT and Trojanowski JQ (1997). Consensus recommendations for the postmortem diagnosis of Alzheimer disease from the National Institute on Aging and the Reagan Institute Working Group on diagnostic criteria for the neuropathological assessment of Alzheimer disease. *J Neuropathol Exp Neurol* 56(10): 1095-1097.

Innamorato NG, Lastres-Becker I and Cuadrado A (2009). Role of microglial redox balance in modulation of neuroinflammation. *Curr Opin Neurol* 22(3): 308-314.

International Human Genome Sequencing Consortium (2004). Finishing the euchromatic sequence of the human genome. *Nature* 431(7011): 931-945.

Ittner LM, Ke YD, Delerue F, Bi M, Gladbach A, van Eersel J, Wolfing H, Chieng BC, Christie MJ, Napier IA, Eckert A, Staufenbiel M, Hardeman E and Gotz J (2010). Dendritic Function of Tau Mediates Amyloid-beta Toxicity in Alzheimer's Disease Mouse Models. *Cell* 142(3): 387-397.

Jack CR, Jr., Albert MS, Knopman DS, McKhann GM, Sperling RA, Carrillo MC, Thies B and Phelps CH (2011). Introduction to the recommendations from the National Institute on Aging-Alzheimer's Association workgroups on diagnostic guidelines for Alzheimer's disease. *Alzheimers Dement* 7(3): 257-262.

Janus C, Pearson J, McLaurin J, Mathews PM, Jiang Y, Schmidt SD, Chishti MA, Horne P, Heslin D, French J, Mount HT, Nixon RA, Mercken M, Bergeron C, Fraser PE, St George-Hyslop P and Westaway D (2000). A beta peptide immunization reduces behavioural impairment and plaques in a model of Alzheimer's disease. *Nature* 408(6815): 979-982.

Jick H, Zornberg GL, Jick SS, Seshadri S and Drachman DA (2000). Statins and the risk of dementia. *Lancet* 356(9242): 1627-1631.

Johansen CT, Wang J, Lanktree MB, Cao H, McIntyre AD, Ban MR, Martins RA, Kennedy BA, Hassell RG, Visser ME, Schwartz SM, Voight BF, Elosua R, Salomaa V, O'Donnell CJ, Dallinga-Thie GM, Anand SS, Yusuf S, Huff MW, Kathiresan S and Hegele RA (2010). Excess of rare variants in genes identified by genome-wide association study of hypertriglyceridemia. *Nat Genet* 42(8): 684-687.

Johnson JK, Head E, Kim R, Starr A and Cotman CW (1999). Clinical and pathological evidence for a frontal variant of Alzheimer disease. Arch Neurol 56(10): 1233-1239.

Jorm AF and Jolley D (1998). The incidence of dementia: a meta-analysis. *Neurology* 51(3): 728-733.

Kang J, Lemaire HG, Unterbeck A, Salbaum JM, Masters CL, Grzeschik KH, Multhaup G, Beyreuther K and Muller-Hill B (1987). The precursor of Alzheimer's disease amyloid A4 protein resembles a cell-surface receptor. Nature 325(6106): 733-736.

Knopman DS, Parisi JE, Salviati A, Floriach-Robert M, Boeve BF, Ivnik RJ, Smith GE, Dickson DW, Johnson KA, Petersen LE, McDonald WC, Braak H and Petersen RC (2003). Neuropathology of cognitively normal elderly. *J Neuropathol Exp Neurol* 62(11): 1087-1095.

Krause DL and Muller N (2010). Neuroinflammation, microglia and implications for anti-inflammatory treatment in Alzheimer's disease. *Int J Alzheimer Dis.* 2010; 2010: 732806.

Kril JJ (2009). Alzheimer disease: Alzheimer disease neuropathology in the oldest old. *Nat Rev Neurol* 5(8): 411-412.

Kril JJ and Halliday GM (2001). Alzheimer's disease: its diagnosis and pathogenesis. *Int Rev Neurobiol* 48: 167-217.

Kril JJ, Patel S, Harding AJ and Halliday GM (2002). Neuron loss from the hippocampus of Alzheimer's disease exceeds extracellular neurofibrillary tangle formation. *Acta Neuropathol* 103(4): 370-376.

Kurochkin IV and Goto S (1994). Alzheimer's beta-amyloid peptide specifically interacts with and is degraded by insulin degrading enzyme. *FEBS Lett* 345(1): 33-37.

LaFerla FM, Green KN and Oddo S (2007). Intracellular amyloid-beta in Alzheimer's disease. *Nat Rev Neurosci* 8(7): 499-509.

Lambert JC, Heath S, Even G, Campion D, Sleegers K, Hiltunen M, Combarros O, Zelenika D, Bullido MJ, Tavernier B, Letenneur L, Bettens K, Berr C, Pasquier F, Fievet N, Barberger-Gateau P, Engelborghs S, De Deyn P, Mateo I, Franck A, Helisalmi S, Porcellini E, Hanon O, de Pancorbo MM, Lendon C, Dufouil C, Jaillard C, Leveillard T, Alvarez V, Bosco P, Mancuso M, Panza F, Nacmias B, Bossu P, Piccardi P, Annoni G, Seripa D, Galimberti D, Hannequin D, Licastro F, Soininen H, Ritchie K, Blanche H, Dartigues JF, Tzourio C, Gut I, Van Broeckhoven C, Alperovitch A, Lathrop M and Amouyel P (2009). Genome-wide association study identifies variants at CLU and CR1 associated with Alzheimer's disease. *Nat Genet* 41(10): 1094-1099.

Lander ES, Linton LM, Birren B, Nusbaum C, Zody MC, Baldwin J, Devon K, Dewar K, Doyle M, FitzHugh W, Funke R, Gage D, Harris K, Heaford A, Howland J, Kann L, Lehoczky J, LeVine R, McEwan P, McKernan K, Meldrim J, Mesirov JP, Miranda C, Morris W, Naylor J, Raymond C, Rosetti M, Santos R, Sheridan A, Sougnez C, Stange-Thomann N, Stojanovic N, Subramanian A, Wyman D, Rogers J, Sulston J, Ainscough R, Beck S, Bentley D, Burton J, Clee C, Carter N, Coulson A, Deadman R, Deloukas P, Dunham A, Dunham I, Durbin R, French L, Grafham D, Gregory S,

Hubbard T, Humphray S, Hunt A, Jones M, Lloyd C, McMurray A, Matthews L, Mercer S, Milne S, Mullikin JC, Mungall A, Plumb R, Ross M, Shownkeen R, Sims S, Waterston RH, Wilson RK, Hillier LW, McPherson JD, Marra MA, Mardis ER, Fulton LA, Chinwalla AT, Pepin KH, Gish WR, Chissoe SL, Wendl MC, Delehaunty KD, Miner TL, Delehaunty A, Kramer JB, Cook LL, Fulton RS, Johnson DL, Minx PJ, Clifton SW, Hawkins T, Branscomb E, Predki P, Richardson P, Wenning S, Slezak T, Doggett N, Cheng JF, Olsen A, Lucas S, Elkin C, Uberbacher E, Frazier M, Gibbs RA, Muzny DM, Scherer SE, Bouck JB, Sodergren EJ, Worley KC, Rives CM, Gorrell JH, Metzker ML, Naylor SL, Kucherlapati RS, Nelson DL, Weinstock GM, Sakaki Y, Fujiyama A, Hattori M, Yada T, Toyoda A, Itoh T, Kawagoe C, Watanabe H, Totoki Y, Taylor T, Weissenbach J, Heilig R, Saurin W, Artiguenave F, Brottier P, Bruls T, Pelletier E, Robert C, Wincker P, Smith DR, Doucette-Stamm L, Rubenfield M, Weinstock K, Lee HM, Dubois J, Rosenthal A, Platzer M, Nyakatura G, Taudien S, Rump A, Yang H, Yu J, Wang J, Huang G, Gu J, Hood L, Rowen L, Madan A, Qin S, Davis RW, Federspiel NA, Abola AP, Proctor MJ, Myers RM, Schmutz J, Dickson M, Grimwood J, Cox DR, Olson MV, Kaul R, Shimizu N, Kawasaki K, Minoshima S, Evans GA, Athanasiou M, Schultz R, Roe BA, Chen F, Pan H, Ramser J, Lehrach H, Reinhardt R, McCombie WR, de la Bastide M, Dedhia N, Blocker H, Hornischer K, Nordsiek G, Agarwala R, Aravind L, Bailey JA, Bateman A, Batzoglou S, Birney E, Bork P, Brown DG, Burge CB, Cerutti L, Chen HC, Church D, Clamp M, Copley RR, Doerks T, Eddy SR, Eichler EE, Furey TS, Galagan J, Gilbert JG, Harmon C, Hayashizaki Y, Haussler D, Hermjakob H, Hokamp K, Jang W, Johnson LS, Jones TA, Kasif S, Kaspryzk A, Kennedy S, Kent WJ, Kitts P, Koonin EV, Korf I, Kulp D, Lancet D, Lowe TM, McLysaght A, Mikkelsen T, Moran JV, Mulder N, Pollara VJ, Ponting CP, Schuler G, Schultz J, Slater G, Smit AF, Stupka E, Szustakowski J, Thierry-Mieg D, Thierry-Mieg J, Wagner L, Wallis J, Wheeler R, Williams A, Wolf YI, Wolfe KH, Yang SP, Yeh RF, Collins F, Guyer MS, Peterson J, Felsenfeld A, Wetterstrand KA, Patrinos A, Morgan MJ, de Jong P, Catanese JJ, Osoegawa K, Shizuya H, Choi S and Chen YJ (2001). Initial sequencing and analysis of the human genome. *Nature* 409(6822): 860-921.

Levy S, Sutton G, Ng PC, Feuk L, Halpern AL, Walenz BP, Axelrod N, Huang J, Kirkness EF, Denisov G, Lin Y, Macdonald JR, Pang AW, Shago M, Stockwell TB, Tsiamouri A, Bafna V, Bansal V, Kravitz SA, Busam DA, Beeson KY, McIntosh TC, Remington KA, Abril JF, Gill J, Borman J, Rogers YH, Frazier ME, Scherer SW, Strausberg RL and Venter JC (2007). The Diploid Genome Sequence of an Individual Human. *PLoS Biol* 5(10): e254.

Levy-Lahad E, Wasco W, Poorkaj P, Romano DM, Oshima J, Pettingell WH, Yu CE, Jondro PD, Schmidt SD, Wang K and et al. (1995). Candidate gene for the chromosome 1 familial Alzheimer's disease locus. *Science* 269(5226): 973-977.

Lewis DA, Campbell MJ, Terry RD and Morrison JH (1987). Laminar and regional distributions of neurofibrillary tangles and neuritic plaques in Alzheimer's disease: a quantitative study of visual and auditory cortices. J Neurosci 7(6): 1799-1808.

Lewis J, Dickson DW, Lin WL, Chisholm L, Corral A, Jones G, Yen SH, Sahara N, Skipper L, Yager D, Eckman C, Hardy J, Hutton M and McGowan E (2001). Enhanced neurofibrillary degeneration in transgenic mice expressing mutant tau and APP. *Science* 293(5534): 1487-1491.

Lewis J, McGowan E, Rockwood J, Melrose H, Nacharaju P, Van Slegtenhorst M, Gwinn-Hardy K, Paul Murphy M, Baker M, Yu X, Duff K, Hardy J, Corral A, Lin WL, Yen SH, Dickson DW, Davies P and Hutton M (2000). Neurofibrillary tangles, amyotrophy and progressive motor disturbance in mice expressing mutant (P301L) tau protein. *Nat Genet* 25(4): 402-405.

Lorenzo A and Yankner BA (1994). Beta-amyloid neurotoxicity requires fibril formation and is inhibited by congo red. *Proc Natl Acad Sci U S A* 91(25): 12243-12247.

Lue LF, Brachova L, Civin WH and Rogers J (1996). Inflammation, A beta deposition, and neurofibrillary tangle formation as correlates of Alzheimer's disease neurodegeneration. *J Neuropathol Exp Neurol* 55(10): 1083-1088.

Lupton MK, Proitsi P, Danillidou M, Tsolaki M, Hamilton G, Wroe R, Pritchard M, Lord K, Martin BM, Kloszewska I, Soininen H, Mecocci P, Vellas B, Harold D, Hollingworth P, Lovestone S and Powell JF (2011). Deep sequencing of the Nicastrin gene in pooled DNA, the identification of genetic variants that affect risk of Alzheimer's disease. *PLoS One* 6(2): e17298.

Margulies M, Egholm M, Altman WE, Attiya S, Bader JS, Bemben LA, Berka J, Braverman MS, Chen YJ, Chen Z, Dewell SB, Du L, Fierro JM, Gomes XV, Godwin BC, He W, Helgesen S, Ho CH, Irzyk GP, Jando SC, Alenquer ML, Jarvie TP, Jirage KB, Kim JB, Knight JR, Lanza JR, Leamon JH, Lefkowitz SM, Lei M, Li J, Lohman KL, Lu H, Makhijani VB, McDade KE, McKenna MP, Myers EW, Nickerson E, Nobile JR, Plant R, Puc BP, Ronan MT, Roth GT, Sarkis GJ, Simons JF, Simpson JW, Srinivasan M, Tartaro KR, Tomasz A, Vogt KA, Volkmer GA, Wang SH, Wang Y, Weiner MP, Yu P, Begley RF and Rothberg JM (2005). Genome sequencing in microfabricated high-density picolitre reactors. *Nature* 437(7057): 376-380.

Masters CL, Simms G, Weinman NA, Multhaup G, McDonald BL and Beyreuther K (1985). Amyloid plaque core protein in Alzheimer disease and Down syndrome. *Proc Natl Acad Sci U S A* 82(12): 4245-4249.

Mattick JS (2011). The central role of RNA in human development and cognition. *FEBS Lett* 585(11): 1600-1616.

Mattick JS, Taft RJ and Faulkner GJ (2010). A global view of genomic information--moving beyond the gene and the master regulator. *Trends Genet* 26(1): 21-28.

Maurer K, Volk S and Gerbaldo H (1997). Auguste D and Alzheimer's disease. *Lancet* 349(9064): 1546-1549.

Mawuenyega KG, Sigurdson W, Ovod V, Munsell L, Kasten T, Morris JC, Yarasheski KE and Bateman RJ (2010). Decreased clearance of CNS beta-amyloid in Alzheimer's disease. *Science* 330(6012): 1774.

McKhann G, Drachman D, Folstein M, Katzman R, Price D and Stadlan EM (1984). Clinical diagnosis of Alzheimer's disease: report of the NINCDS-ADRDA Work Group under the auspices of Department of Health and Human Services Task Force on Alzheimer's Disease. *Neurology* 34(7): 939-944.

McKhann GM, Knopman DS, Chertkow H, Hyman BT, Jack CR, Jr., Kawas CH, Klunk WE, Koroshetz WJ, Manly JJ, Mayeux R, Mohs RC, Morris JC, Rossor MN, Scheltens P, Carrillo MC, Thies B, Weintraub S and Phelps CH (2011). The diagnosis of dementia due to Alzheimer's disease: recommendations from the National Institute on Aging-Alzheimer's Association workgroups on diagnostic guidelines for Alzheimer's disease. *Alzheimers Dement* 7(3): 263-269.

McShane R, Areosa Sastre A and Minakaran N (2006). Memantine for dementia. *Cochrane Database Syst Rev(2)*: CD003154.

Miguel-Hidalgo JJ, Alvarez XA, Cacabelos R and Quack G (2002). Neuroprotection by memantine against neurodegeneration induced by beta-amyloid(1-40). *Brain Res* 958(1): 210-221.

Morgan K (2011). The three new pathways leading to Alzheimer's disease. *Neuropathol Appl Neurobiol* 37(4): 353-357.

Mullis KB and Faloona FA (1987). Specific synthesis of DNA in vitro via a polymerase-catalyzed chain reaction. *Methods Enzymol* 155: 335-350.

Naj AC, Jun G, Beecham GW, Wang LS, Vardarajan BN, Buros J, Gallins PJ, Buxbaum JD, Jarvik GP, Crane PK, Larson EB, Bird TD, Boeve BF, Graff-Radford NR, De Jager PL, Evans D, Schneider JA, Carrasquillo MM, Ertekin-Taner N, Younkin SG, Cruchaga C, Kauwe JS, Nowotny P, Kramer P, Hardy J, Huentelman MJ, Myers AJ, Barmada MM, Demirci FY, Baldwin CT, Green RC, Rogaeva E, George-Hyslop PS, Arnold SE, Barber R, Beach T, Bigio EH, Bowen JD, Boxer A, Burke JR, Cairns NJ, Carlson CS, Carney RM, Carroll SL, Chui HC, Clark DG, Corneveaux J, Cotman CW, Cummings JL, Decarli C, Dekosky ST, Diaz-Arrastia R, Dick M, Dickson DW, Ellis WG, Faber KM, Fallon KB, Farlow MR, Ferris S, Frosch MP, Galasko DR, Ganguli M, Gearing M, Geschwind DH, Ghetti B, Gilbert JR, Gilman S, Giordani B, Glass JD, Growdon JH, Hamilton RL, Harrell LE, Head E, Honig LS, Hulette CM, Hyman BT, Jicha GA, Jin LW, Johnson N, Karlawish J, Karydas A, Kaye JA, Kim R, Koo EH, Kowall NW, Lah JJ, Levey AI, Lieberman AP, Lopez OL, Mack WJ, Marson DC, Martiniuk F, Mash DC, Masliah E, McCormick WC, McCurry SM, McDavid AN, McKee AC, Mesulam M, Miller BL, Miller CA, Miller JW, Parisi JE, Perl DP, Peskind E, Petersen RC, Poon WW, Quinn JF, Rajbhandary RA, Raskind M, Reisberg B, Ringman JM, Roberson ED, Rosenberg RN, Sano M, Schneider LS, Seeley W, Shelanski ML, Slifer MA, Smith CD, Sonnen JA, Spina S, Stern RA, Tanzi RE, Trojanowski JQ, Troncoso JC, Van Deerlin VM, Vinters HV, Vonsattel JP, Weintraub S, Welsh-Bohmer KA, Williamson J, Woltjer RL, Cantwell LB, Dombroski BA, Beekly D, Lunetta KL, Martin ER, Kamboh MI, Saykin AJ, Reiman EM, Bennett DA, Morris JC, Montine TJ, Goate AM, Blacker D, Tsuang DW, Hakonarson H, Kukull WA, Foroud TM, Haines JL, Mayeux R, Pericak-Vance MA, Farrer LA and Schellenberg GD (2011). Common variants at MS4A4/MS4A6E, CD2AP, CD33 and EPHA1 are associated with late-onset Alzheimer's disease. *Nat Genet* 43(5): 436-441.

Nathans D and Smith HO (1975). Restriction endonucleases in the analysis and restructuring of dna molecules. *Annu Rev Biochem* 44: 273-293.

Nee LE, Polinsky RJ, Eldridge R, Weingartner H, Smallberg S and Ebert M (1983). A family with histologically confirmed Alzheimer's disease. *Arch Neurol* 40(4): 203-208.

Newell KL, Hyman BT, Growdon JH and Hedley-Whyte ET (1999). Application of the National Institute on Aging (NIA)-Reagan Institute criteria for the neuropathological diagnosis of Alzheimer disease. *J Neuropathol Exp Neurol* 58(11): 1147-1155.

Nuutinen T, Suuronen T, Kauppinen A and Salminen A (2009). Clusterin: a forgotten player in Alzheimer's disease. *Brain Res Rev* 61(2): 89-104.

Oddo S, Caccamo A, Shepherd JD, Murphy MP, Golde TE, Kayed R, Metherate R, Mattson MP, Akbari Y and LaFerla FM (2003). Triple-transgenic model of Alzheimer's disease with plaques and tangles: intracellular Abeta and synaptic dysfunction. *Neuron* 39(3): 409-421.

Orgogozo JM, Gilman S, Dartigues JF, Laurent B, Puel M, Kirby LC, Jouanny P, Dubois B, Eisner L, Flitman S, Michel BF, Boada M, Frank A and Hock C (2003). Subacute meningoencephalitis in a subset of patients with AD after Abeta42 immunization. *Neurology* 61(1): 46-54.

Pan Q, Shai O, Lee LJ, Frey BJ and Blencowe BJ (2008). Deep surveying of alternative splicing complexity in the human transcriptome by high-throughput sequencing. *Nat Genet* 40(12): 1413-1415.

Pareek CS, Smoczynski R and Tretyn A (2011). Sequencing technologies and genome sequencing. *J Appl Genet.*

Perlmutter LS, Barron E and Chui HC (1990). Morphologic association between microglia and senile plaque amyloid in Alzheimer's disease. Neurosci Lett 119(1): 32-36.

Perusini G (1909). Über klinisch und histologisch eigenartige psychische Erkrankungen des späteren Lebensalters. Histologische und Histopathologische Arbeiten. *Nissl F and Alzheimer* A: 297-351.

Peskind ER, Li G, Shofer J, Quinn JF, Kaye JA, Clark CM, Farlow MR, DeCarli C, Raskind MA, Schellenberg GD, Lee VM and Galasko DR (2006). Age and apolipoprotein E*4 allele effects on cerebrospinal fluid beta-amyloid 42 in adults with normal cognition. *Arch Neurol* 63(7): 936-939.

Postina R (2008). A closer look at alpha-secretase. *Curr Alzheimer Res* 5(2): 179-186.

Preece P and Cairns NJ (2003). Quantifying mRNA in postmortem human brain: influence of gender, age at death, postmortem interval, brain pH, agonal state and inter-lobe mRNA variance. *Brain Res Mol Brain Res* 118(1-2): 60-71.

Price JL, McKeel DW, Jr., Buckles VD, Roe CM, Xiong C, Grundman M, Hansen LA, Petersen RC, Parisi JE, Dickson DW, Smith CD, Davis DG, Schmitt FA, Markesbery WR, Kaye J, Kurlan R, Hulette C, Kurland BF, Higdon R, Kukull W and Morris JC (2009). Neuropathology of nondemented aging: presumptive evidence for preclinical Alzheimer disease. *Neurobiol Aging* 30(7): 1026-1036.

Pritchard JK (2001). Are rare variants responsible for susceptibility to complex diseases? *Am J Hum Genet* 69(1): 124-137.

Raina P, Santaguida P, Ismaila A, Patterson C, Cowan D, Levine M, Booker L and Oremus M (2008). Effectiveness of cholinesterase inhibitors and memantine for treating dementia: evidence review for a clinical practice guideline. *Ann Intern Med* 148(5): 379-397.

Ramskold D, Wang ET, Burge CB and Sandberg R (2009). An abundance of ubiquitously expressed genes revealed by tissue transcriptome sequence data. *PLoS Comput Biol* 5(12): e1000598.

Rapoport M, Dawson HN, Binder LI, Vitek MP and Ferreira A (2002). Tau is essential to beta -amyloid-induced neurotoxicity. *Proc Natl Acad Sci U S A* 99(9): 6364-6369.

Reiman EM, Webster JA, Myers AJ, Hardy J, Dunckley T, Zismann VL, Joshipura KD, Pearson JV, Hu-Lince D, Huentelman MJ, Craig DW, Coon KD, Liang WS, Herbert RH, Beach T, Rohrer KC, Zhao AS, Leung D, Bryden L, Marlowe L, Kaleem M, Mastroeni D, Grover A, Heward CB, Ravid R, Rogers J, Hutton ML, Melquist S, Petersen RC, Alexander GE, Caselli RJ, Kukull W, Papassotiropoulos A and Stephan DA (2007). GAB2 alleles modify Alzheimer's risk in APOE epsilon4 carriers. *Neuron* 54(5): 713-720.

Riddell DR, Zhou H, Atchison K, Warwick HK, Atkinson PJ, Jefferson J, Xu L, Aschmies S, Kirksey Y, Hu Y, Wagner E, Parratt A, Xu J, Li Z, Zaleska MM, Jacobsen JS, Pangalos MN and Reinhart PH (2008). Impact of apolipoprotein E (ApoE) polymorphism on brain ApoE levels. *J Neurosci* 28(45): 11445-11453.

Rinne JO, Brooks DJ, Rossor MN, Fox NC, Bullock R, Klunk WE, Mathis CA, Blennow K, Barakos J, Okello AA, Rodriguez Martinez de Liano S, Liu E, Koller M, Gregg KM, Schenk D, Black R and Grundman M (2010). 11C-PiB PET assessment of change in fibrillar amyloid-beta load in patients with Alzheimer's disease treated with bapineuzumab: a phase 2, double-blind, placebo-controlled, ascending-dose study. *Lancet Neurol* 9(4): 363-372.

Roberson ED, Scearce-Levie K, Palop JJ, Yan F, Cheng IH, Wu T, Gerstein H, Yu GQ and Mucke L (2007). Reducing endogenous tau ameliorates amyloid beta-induced deficits in an Alzheimer's disease mouse model. *Science* 316(5825): 750-754.

Rovelet-Lecrux A, Hannequin D, Raux G, Le Meur N, Laquerriere A, Vital A, Dumanchin C, Feuillette S, Brice A, Vercelletto M, Dubas F, Frebourg T and Campion D (2006). APP locus duplication causes autosomal dominant early-onset Alzheimer disease with cerebral amyloid angiopathy. *Nat Genet* 38(1): 24-26.

Rowe CC, Ellis KA, Rimajova M, Bourgeat P, Pike KE, Jones G, Fripp J, Tochon-Danguy H, Morandeau L, O'Keefe G, Price R, Raniga P, Robins P, Acosta O, Lenzo N, Szoeke C, Salvado O, Head R, Martins R, Masters CL, Ames D and Villemagne VL (2010). Amyloid imaging results from the Australian Imaging, Biomarkers and Lifestyle (AIBL) study of aging. *Neurobiol Aging* 31(8): 1275-1283.

Saiki RK, Scharf S, Faloona F, Mullis KB, Horn GT, Erlich HA and Arnheim N (1985). Enzymatic amplification of beta-globin genomic sequences and restriction site analysis for diagnosis of sickle cell anemia. *Science* 230(4732): 1350-1354.

Sanger F, Nicklen S and Coulson AR (1977). DNA sequencing with chain-terminating inhibitors. *Proc Natl Acad Sci U S A* 74(12): 5463-5467.

Schenk D, Barbour R, Dunn W, Gordon G, Grajeda H, Guido T, Hu K, Huang J, Johnson-Wood K, Khan K, Kholodenko D, Lee M, Liao Z, Lieberburg I, Motter R, Mutter L, Soriano F, Shopp G, Vasquez N, Vandevert C, Walker S, Wogulis M, Yednock T, Games D and Seubert P (1999). Immunization with amyloid-beta attenuates Alzheimer-disease-like pathology in the PDAPP mouse. *Nature* 400(6740): 173-177.

Schneider LS, Dagerman KS, Higgins JP and McShane R (2011). Lack of evidence for the efficacy of memantine in mild Alzheimer disease. *Arch Neurol* 68(8): 991-998.

Schottky J (1932). Ueber praesenile Verbloedungen. Z. Ges. Neurol. Psychiat. 140: 333-397.

Selkoe DJ (2002). Alzheimer's disease is a synaptic failure. *Science* 298(5594): 789-791.

Shepherd C, McCann H and Halliday GM (2009). Variations in the neuropathology of familial Alzheimer's disease. *Acta Neuropathol* 118(1): 37-52.

Simpson JE, Ince PG, Lace G, Forster G, Shaw PJ, Matthews F, Savva G, Brayne C and Wharton SB (2010). Astrocyte phenotype in relation to Alzheimer-type pathology in the ageing brain. *Neurobiol Aging* 31(4): 578-590.

Snyder EM, Nong Y, Almeida CG, Paul S, Moran T, Choi EY, Nairn AC, Salter MW, Lombroso PJ, Gouras GK and Greengard P (2005). Regulation of NMDA receptor trafficking by amyloid-beta. *Nat Neurosci* 8(8): 1051-1058.

Soldner F, Hockemeyer D, Beard C, Gao Q, Bell GW, Cook EG, Hargus G, Blak A, Cooper O, Mitalipova M, Isacson O and Jaenisch R (2009). Parkinson's disease patient-derived induced pluripotent stem cells free of viral reprogramming factors. *Cell* 136(5): 964-977.

Somorjai RL, Dolenko B and Baumgartner R (2003). Class prediction and discovery using gene microarray and proteomics mass spectroscopy data: curses, caveats, cautions. *Bioinformatics* 19(12): 1484-1491.

Southern EM (1975). Detection of specific sequences among DNA fragments separated by gel electrophoresis. *J Mol Biol* 98(3): 503-517.

Sperling RA, Aisen PS, Beckett LA, Bennett DA, Craft S, Fagan AM, Iwatsubo T, Jack CR, Jr., Kaye J, Montine TJ, Park DC, Reiman EM, Rowe CC, Siemers E, Stern Y, Yaffe K, Carrillo MC, Thies B, Morrison-Bogorad M, Wagster MV and Phelps CH (2011). Toward defining the preclinical stages of Alzheimer's disease: recommendations from the National Institute on Aging-Alzheimer's Association workgroups on diagnostic guidelines for Alzheimer's disease. *Alzheimers Dement* 7(3): 280-292.

Stern Y, Gurland B, Tatemichi TK, Tang MX, Wilder D and Mayeux R (1994). Influence of education and occupation on the incidence of Alzheimer's disease. *Jama* 271(13): 1004-1010.

Strittmatter WJ, Weisgraber KH, Huang DY, Dong LM, Salvesen GS, Pericak-Vance M, Schmechel D, Saunders AM, Goldgaber D and Roses AD (1993). Binding of human apolipoprotein E to synthetic amyloid beta peptide: isoform-specific effects and implications for late-onset Alzheimer disease. *Proc Natl Acad Sci U S A* 90(17): 8098-8102.

Sutherland GT, Janitz M and Kril JJ (2011a). Understanding the pathogenesis of Alzheimer's disease: will RNA-Seq realize the promise of transcriptomics? *J Neurochem* 116(6): 937-946.

Sutherland GT and Sidhu KS (2011). Pluripotent Stem Cells for (Neurodegenerative) Disease Modelling. *Frontiers in Pluripotent Stem Cells Research and Therapeutic Potentials; Bench-To-Bedside*. Sidhu KS, Bentham Press. (under publication).

Sutherland GT, Siebert GA, Kril JJ and Mellick GD (2011b). Knowing Me, Knowing You: Can Knowledge of Risk Factors for Alzheimer's Disease Prove Useful in Understanding the Pathogenesis of Parkinson's Disease? *J Alzheimers Dis.* 25(3): 395-415

Takahashi K, Tanabe K, Ohnuki M, Narita M, Ichisaka T, Tomoda K and Yamanaka S (2007). Induction of pluripotent stem cells from adult human fibroblasts by defined factors. *Cell* 131(5): 861-872.

Tanzi RE (1989). Molecular genetics of Alzheimer's disease and the amyloid beta peptide precursor gene. *Ann Med* 21(2): 91-94.

Tanzi RE, Bird ED, Latt SA and Neve RL (1987a). The amyloid beta protein gene is not duplicated in brains from patients with Alzheimer's disease. *Science* 238(4827): 666-669.

Tanzi RE, St George-Hyslop PH, Haines JL, Polinsky RJ, Nee L, Foncin JF, Neve RL, McClatchey AI, Conneally PM and Gusella JF (1987b). The genetic defect in familial Alzheimer's disease is not tightly linked to the amyloid beta-protein gene. *Nature* 329(6135): 156-157.

Terry RD and Katzman R (1983). Senile dementia of the Alzheimer type. *Ann Neurol* 14(5): 497-506.

The 1000 Genomes Project Consortium (2010). A map of human genome variation from population-scale sequencing. *Nature* 467(7319): 1061-1073.

The Huntington's Disease Collaborative Research Group (1993). A novel gene containing a trinucleotide repeat that is expanded and unstable on Huntington's disease chromosomes. The Huntington's Disease Collaborative Research Group. *Cell* 72(6): 971-983.

Troncoso JC, Martin LJ, Dal Forno G and Kawas CH (1996). Neuropathology in controls and demented subjects from the Baltimore Longitudinal Study of Aging. *Neurobiol Aging* 17(3): 365-371.

Twine NA, Janitz K, Wilkins MR and Janitz M (2011). Whole transcriptome sequencing reveals gene expression and splicing differences in brain regions affected by Alzheimer's disease. *PLoS One* 6(1): e16266.

Vassar R, Kovacs DM, Yan R and Wong PC (2009). The beta-secretase enzyme BACE in health and Alzheimer's disease: regulation, cell biology, function, and therapeutic potential. *J Neurosci* 29(41): 12787-12794.

Venter JC, Adams MD, Myers EW, Li PW, Mural RJ, Sutton GG, Smith HO, Yandell M, Evans CA, Holt RA, Gocayne JD, Amanatides P, Ballew RM, Huson DH, Wortman JR, Zhang Q, Kodira CD, Zheng XH, Chen L, Skupski M, Subramanian G, Thomas PD, Zhang J, Gabor Miklos GL, Nelson C, Broder S, Clark AG, Nadeau J, McKusick VA, Zinder N, Levine AJ, Roberts RJ, Simon M, Slayman C, Hunkapiller M, Bolanos R, Delcher A, Dew I, Fasulo D, Flanigan M, Florea L, Halpern A, Hannenhalli S, Kravitz S, Levy S, Mobarry C, Reinert K, Remington K, Abu-Threideh J, Beasley E, Biddick K, Bonazzi V, Brandon R, Cargill M, Chandramouliswaran I, Charlab R, Chaturvedi K, Deng Z, Di Francesco V, Dunn P, Eilbeck K, Evangelista C, Gabrielian AE, Gan W, Ge W, Gong F, Gu Z, Guan P, Heiman TJ, Higgins ME, Ji RR, Ke Z, Ketchum KA, Lai Z, Lei Y, Li Z, Li J, Liang Y, Lin X, Lu F, Merkulov GV, Milshina N, Moore HM, Naik AK, Narayan VA, Neelam B, Nusskern D, Rusch DB, Salzberg S, Shao W, Shue B, Sun J, Wang Z, Wang A, Wang X, Wang J, Wei M, Wides R, Xiao C, Yan C, Yao A, Ye J, Zhan M, Zhang W, Zhang H, Zhao Q, Zheng L, Zhong F, Zhong W, Zhu S, Zhao S, Gilbert D, Baumhueter S, Spier G, Carter C, Cravchik A, Woodage T, Ali F, An H, Awe A, Baldwin D, Baden H, Barnstead M, Barrow I, Beeson K, Busam D, Carver A, Center A, Cheng ML, Curry L, Danaher S, Davenport L, Desilets R, Dietz S, Dodson K, Doup L, Ferriera S, Garg N, Gluecksmann A, Hart B, Haynes J, Haynes C, Heiner C, Hladun S, Hostin D, Houck J, Howland T, Ibegwam C, Johnson J, Kalush F, Kline L, Koduru S, Love A, Mann F, May D, McCawley S, McIntosh T, McMullen I, Moy M, Moy L, Murphy B, Nelson K, Pfannkoch C, Pratts E, Puri V, Qureshi H, Reardon M, Rodriguez R, Rogers YH, Romblad D, Ruhfel B, Scott R, Sitter C, Smallwood M, Stewart E, Strong R, Suh E, Thomas R, Tint NN, Tse S, Vech C, Wang G, Wetter J, Williams S, Williams M, Windsor S, Winn-Deen E, Wolfe K, Zaveri J, Zaveri K, Abril JF, Guigo R, Campbell MJ, Sjolander KV, Karlak B, Kejariwal A, Mi H, Lazareva B, Hatton T, Narechania A, Diemer K, Muruganujan A, Guo N, Sato S, Bafna V, Istrail S, Lippert R, Schwartz R, Walenz B, Yooseph S, Allen D, Basu A, Baxendale J, Blick L, Caminha M, Carnes-Stine J, Caulk P, Chiang YH, Coyne M, Dahlke C, Mays A, Dombroski M, Donnelly M, Ely D, Esparham S, Fosler C, Gire H, Glanowski S, Glasser K, Glodek A, Gorokhov M, Graham K, Gropman B, Harris M, Heil J, Henderson S, Hoover J, Jennings D, Jordan C, Jordan J, Kasha J, Kagan L, Kraft C, Levitsky A, Lewis M, Liu X, Lopez J, Ma D, Majoros W, McDaniel J, Murphy S, Newman M, Nguyen T, Nguyen N, Nodell M, Pan S, Peck J, Peterson M, Rowe W, Sanders R, Scott J, Simpson M, Smith T, Sprague A, Stockwell T, Turner R, Venter E, Wang M, Wen M, Wu D, Wu M, Xia A, Zandieh A and Zhu X (2001). The sequence of the human genome. *Science* 291(5507): 1304-1351.

Vlad SC, Miller DR, Kowall NW and Felson DT (2008). Protective effects of NSAIDs on the development of Alzheimer disease. *Neurology* 70(19): 1672-1677.

Walsh DM, Klyubin I, Fadeeva JV, Rowan MJ and Selkoe DJ (2002). Amyloid-beta oligomers: their production, toxicity and therapeutic inhibition. *Biochem Soc Trans* 30(4): 552-557.

Wan Y, Kertesz M, Spitale RC, Segal E and Chang HY (2011). Understanding the transcriptome through RNA structure. *Nat Rev Genet* 12(9): 641-655.

Wang ET, Sandberg R, Luo S, Khrebtukova I, Zhang L, Mayr C, Kingsmore SF, Schroth GP and Burge CB (2008). Alternative isoform regulation in human tissue transcriptomes. *Nature* 456(7221): 470-476.

Weiner MW, Aisen PS, Jack CR, Jr., Jagust WJ, Trojanowski JQ, Shaw L, Saykin AJ, Morris JC, Cairns N, Beckett LA, Toga A, Green R, Walter S, Soares H, Snyder P, Siemers E, Potter W, Cole PE and Schmidt M (2010). The Alzheimer's disease neuroimaging initiative: progress report and future plans. Alzheimers Dement 6(3): 202-211 e207.

Weisgraber KH, Innerarity TL and Mahley RW (1982). Abnormal lipoprotein receptor-binding activity of the human E apoprotein due to cysteine-arginine interchange at a single site. *J Biol Chem* 257(5): 2518-2521.

Weller RO, Subash M, Preston SD, Mazanti I and Carare RO (2008). Perivascular drainage of amyloid-beta peptides from the brain and its failure in cerebral amyloid angiopathy and Alzheimer's disease. *Brain Pathol* 18(2): 253-266.

Wilkins MR, Sanchez JC, Gooley AA, Appel RD, Humphery-Smith I, Hochstrasser DF and Williams KL (1996). Progress with proteome projects: why all proteins expressed by a genome should be identified and how to do it. *Biotechnol Genet Eng Rev* 13: 19-50.

Wimo A, Winblad B and Jonsson L (2007). An estimate of the total worldwide societal costs of dementia in 2005. *Alzheimers Dement* 3(2): 81-91.

Wolozin B, Kellman W, Ruosseau P, Celesia GG and Siegel G (2000). Decreased prevalence of Alzheimer disease associated with 3-hydroxy-3-methyglutaryl coenzyme A reductase inhibitors. *Arch Neurol* 57(10): 1439-1443.

Yoshikai S, Sasaki H, Doh-ura K, Furuya H and Sakaki Y (1990). Genomic organization of the human amyloid beta-protein precursor gene. *Gene* 87(2): 257-263.

Yu YJ, Zhang Y, Kenrick M, Hoyte K, Luk W, Lu Y, Atwal J, Elliott JM, Prabhu S, Watts RJ and Dennis MS (2011). Boosting brain uptake of a therapeutic antibody by reducing its affinity for a transcytosis target. *Sci Transl Med* 3(84): 84ra44.

Zellner M, Veitinger M and Umlauf E (2009). The role of proteomics in dementia and Alzheimer's disease. *Acta Neuropathol* 118(1): 181-195.